# THE MAKING OF A DOCTOR PART 2
## The Sequel
VOLUME J

DR. JULIUS ADEBIYI AKANNI ṢODIPỌ

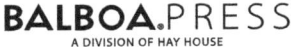

Copyright © 2022 Dr. Julius Adebiyi Akanni Ṣodipọ.

All rights reserved. No part of this book may be used or reproduced by any means, graphic, electronic, or mechanical, including photocopying, recording, taping or by any information storage retrieval system without the written permission of the author except in the case of brief quotations embodied in critical articles and reviews.

Balboa Press books may be ordered through booksellers or by contacting:

Balboa Press
A Division of Hay House
1663 Liberty Drive
Bloomington, IN 47403
www.balboapress.co.uk
UK TFN: 0800 0148647 (Toll Free inside the UK)
UK Local: (02) 0369 56325 (+44 20 3695 6325 from outside the UK)

Because of the dynamic nature of the Internet, any web addresses or links contained in this book may have changed since publication and may no longer be valid. The views expressed in this work are solely those of the author and do not necessarily reflect the views of the publisher, and the publisher hereby disclaims any responsibility for them.

The author of this book does not dispense medical advice or prescribe the use of any technique as a form of treatment for physical, emotional, or medical problems without the advice of a physician, either directly or indirectly. The intent of the author is only to offer information of a general nature to help you in your quest for emotional and spiritual well-being. In the event you use any of the information in this book for yourself, which is your constitutional right, the author and the publisher assume no responsibility for your actions.

Any people depicted in stock imagery provided by Getty Images are models, and such images are being used for illustrative purposes only.
Certain stock imagery © Getty Images.

Print information available on the last page.

ISBN: 978-1-9822-8587-6 (sc)
ISBN: 978-1-9822-8589-0 (hc)
ISBN: 978-1-9822-8588-3 (e)

Balboa Press rev. date: 05/27/2022

# CONTENTS

Dedication .................................................................................. vii
Appreciation............................................................................... ix
Aim ........................................................................................... xi
Introduction ............................................................................ xiii

Results of queries that list all consultations from the 22$^{nd}$ to
the end of April 2000 to April 2015 ........................................... 1

Results of queries that list all consultations from the 22$^{nd}$ to
the end of May 1997 to May 2015 ......................................... 159

Results of queries that list all consultations from the 22$^{nd}$ to
the end of June 1997 to June 2015 ........................................ 331

Results of queries that list all consultations from the 22$^{nd}$ to
the end of July 1997 to July 2015 .......................................... 533

Results of queries that list all consultations from the 22$^{nd}$ to
the end of August 1997 to August 2014 ................................ 745

# DEDICATION

I dedicate this book to my four sons:
Julius Adedeji Arẹmu (with his immense football knowledge and fan of Chelsea);
John Adeṣọla (fan of Arsenal);
Isaac Adetokunbọ (fan of Manchester United) and
Johnson Adeyinka Adeolu (fan of Manchester United).

Their mother Gloria Adanma Abẹkẹ Nee Okoroafor (who is a fan of the football teams that her sons and her husband support).

To the memory of my:
father's father Papa (Chief) Isaac Ademoye Ọmọlaja Ṣodipọ;
father's mother Madam Bilewunmi-ọmọ Ṣodipọ (alias Iya Ita-ọlọti);
mother's mother Nee Alice Aina Ero-Phillips (alias Iya Alakara);
mother Madam (Chief) Harriet Olufunkẹ Ibidunni Ṣodipọ (alias Mama 'Biyi);
father Dr (Chief) John Adewunmi Akanbi Ṣodipọ.

# APPRECIATION

I will like to thank my wife, Gloria Adanma Abękę (Nee Okoroafor), for showing cursory interests during the production of the whole project.

# AIM

Any proceeds from the sale(s) or distribution of this book (the whole project) should be used in setting up a Fund, which should be invested in a safe investment. This fund should be called Dr Julius Adebiyi Akanni Ṣodipọ's Fund. This should be added to fund set up from income earned from the sale (royalty) of the earlier edition of The Making of the Doctor by the same author.

All the proceeds being generated from the sale of the book (or project) as well as all the proceeds from his estate should be deposited as Capital into the fund. The managers of the Estate Fund should not get more than 10% of the income generated by the Fund each year. The proceeds in the Fund should be invested in a relatively safe investment and what is generated should be called the Fund Income.

So, should any of the remaining of my estate, after deduction of any debts and taxes should be added to the Dr Julius Adebiyi Akanni Ṣodipọ's Fund. The monies in the fund should be distributed from time to time occasionally but regularly to my biological grandchildren, biological great grandchildren, biological great great grandchildren, and biological generations yet to be born with no conditions attached other than being my proven biological descendant. For example, for those who are eligible i.e., my biological descendants, 30 percent of the yearly income should be distributed equally yearly rather than 5 percent monthly. Those who are managing the Fund and its distribution should receive 5 to 10 percent of the yearly income, as appropriate to use in maintaining the fund and as their fees.

The remaining 90% (or 95%) of the yearly income generated by the Estate Fund, reiterated here, should be equally divided between the biological posterity of Dr Julius Adebiyi Akanni Ṣodipọ for generations to come including those yet unborn for as long as possible as far as the Estate exists.

The division of the Estate Fund's income should be as follows:

Each member of his (my) biological posterity should get their own share from the age of 30 years old until the age of 55 years old, or they are no longer alive if this should happen earlier. As reiterated earlier their own share should be given to them yearly or more frequently if the managers feel it is in the best interest of the recipient to do so.

An independent legal firm (team) mutually agreeable to most of the stakeholders must be employed. The legal firm is to ensure the smooth running by the Fund Managers, to ensure that the managers keep to the protocol set out above or not to significantly deviate from it. The legal team should receive not more than 5% of the yearly income of the fund as their renumeration.

# INTRODUCTION

This book is the sequel to the Making of a doctor. It goes from Volume A to Volume S. Quite a lot of the work done in this book was done before embarking on the work in the famous previous volumes. So the work was done on the raw data. The reader may encounter some mistakes in this book which are few and subtle, and Ṣẹgun apologises for this. A challenge for the reader is to locate these mistakes and correct them. The contents of this book are query results to Ṣẹgun's consultation database over the years from January 1997 to December 2015. The databases for October, November and December 2002 are shown. The data for the remaining of 2002 are unfortunately missing. Out of hours finished in June 1998 after which the local GP co-operative and later the government took over the care of the patients out of hours. The reader can access the database from results shown below or better still access them in the previous edition of the famous Ṣẹgun's books (volumes), The Making of a Doctor, by the same author. Any other period not accounted for is when Segun was away from the Surgery on holidays. Ṣẹgun had to arrange for locum doctors to cover the period. Even though the locum doctors (GPs) were responsible for the care of the patients, Ṣẹgun was ultimately responsible for their care during his absence. Legally the patients were under Ṣẹgun's care.

Some of the data result are broken down in tables whilst majority are not. These are hundreds of query results. This could be done individually but it will take forever. To overcome this problem Ṣẹgun used the opportunity of computer programming which Ṣẹgun formulated, using Visual Basic for Application (VBA) for Access. The VBA for Access codings used are included in volume S. One of the examples below: **Result of a query to list all those referred in January 1997 (AllPatientsReferredInJan1997).**

The part in the brackets is a phrase allowed as a table or query heading in terms of number of characters and what characters are allowed in Microsoft Access. The part outside, the bracket, is a more understandable form of the enclosed phrase or statement in the bracket. To get the tabular results of query results not shown, the reader will need to have access to the databases as described above. All the results are produced using the VBA for Access codings referred to above, as enclosed in volume.

Towards the end of volume S is a football clubs/teams and internet acronyms tree view project, using codings in VBA for Excel. When the program is run, the reader will be able to view fun details of football clubs or national football teams of many countries and internet acronyms (and what they mean). Please note that the list is not exhaustive but includes what Ṣẹgun remembered or what he was able to gather from his research.

# RESULTS OF QUERIES THAT LIST ALL CONSULTATIONS FROM THE 22ND TO THE END OF APRIL 2000 TO APRIL 2015

Result of a query that lists all consultations from the 22nd to the end of April 2000 (ConsultationsSeenFrom22ndTillEndOfApr2000)

| SurgeryDate | DateOfBirth | Sex | Diagnosis | TimeIn | TimeOut | Complaints | Treatments | NumbersID | Notes |
|---|---|---|---|---|---|---|---|---|---|
| 26.04.2000 | 31.12.1953 | F | Revisit | 1640 | 1645 | Still coughing | Ciprofloxacin & Codeine Linctus | 1075 | |
| 25.04.2000 | 13.03.1954 | F | | 942 | 951 | She would like to be referred to Gynaecologist regarding HRT | Referred to Gynaecologist (Benenden) | 1172 | |
| 27.04.2000 | 18.04.1930 | F | Revisit | 1742 | 1752 | Phlebitis improving | Hirudoid cream | 118 | For serum Cholesterol. Penicillin & Neomycin allergy. |
| 25.04.2000 | 27.08.1970 | M | S/Leave | 1657 | 1701 | Injury (R) knee | | 1262 | |
| 27.04.2000 | 05.02.1946 | F | | 944 | 950 | Pain (L) hand & arm | Advised to use own analgesia | 1268 | |
| 28.04.2000 | 26.11.1935 | M | | 1823 | 1834 | ?Collapse | For FBC, U/Es & Glucose | 1276 | |
| 27.04.2000 | 01.12.1934 | F | | 900 | 915 | Script for QVar autohaler 50 mcg given | | 1371 | |
| 26.04.2000 | 04.09.1967 | M | Pain | 1746 | 1753 | Low abdominal pain & (R) testicle | For MSU, USScan of the lower abdomen & testicles | 1429 | |
| 27.04.2000 | 08.08.1924 | F | | 1806 | 1816 | Back pain again | For MSU | 1559 | |
| 25.04.2000 | 22.12.1959 | M | S/Leave | 1746 | 1754 | Crush injury (R) ring finger tip - Med. 5 | | 1595 | |
| 28.04.2000 | 17.07.1970 | F | | 1816 | 1823 | Allergic rash | Referred to Dermatologist | 1658 | |
| 27.04.2000 | 30.05.1916 | M | | 940 | 944 | Blood shot (R) eye | Chloramphenicol eye drops | 1712 | Poor hearing (L) side, referred to ENT Surgeon. |

## Result of a query that lists all consultations from the 22nd to the end of April 2000 (ConsultationsSeenFrom22ndTillEndOfApr2000)

| SurgeryDate | DateOfBirth | Sex | Diagnosis | TimeIn | TimeOut | Complaints | Treatments | NumbersID | Notes |
|---|---|---|---|---|---|---|---|---|---|
| 25.04.2000 | 09.10.1921 | M | | 1708 | 1717 | T.A.T.T. | For FBC & TFTs | 1998 | |
| 28.04.2000 | 16.07.1957 | F | | 1723 | 1728 | Advised to increase Pizotifen dose from 1.5 mg to 3 mg nocte | | 2164 | Septrin allergy. |
| 28.04.2000 | 15.01.1986 | F | Revisit | 1720 | 1723 | Itchy rash on face is back again | Referred to Dermatologist | 2168 | |
| 28.04.2000 | 10.08.1931 | M | URTI | 1728 | 1731 | Sore throat | Amoxycillin | 2182 | Aspirin allergy. |
| 26.04.2000 | 19.12.1957 | M | RTI | 1753 | 1758 | Cough | Ciprofloxacin | 2267 | He also has a mole on the (L) lower abdomen which has recently changed colour, referred to Dermatologist. |
| 25.04.2000 | 19.07.1925 | F | | 1701 | 1704 | Her cold (L) hand is better now | | 2290 | |
| 28.04.2000 | 05.11.1941 | M | | 1753 | 1803 | Uric Acid elevated | Allopurinol | 251 | |
| 26.04.2000 | 06.05.1958 | F | | 928 | 935 | Script for Amitriptyline given | | 2576 | |
| 27.04.2000 | 21.09.1950 | F | Pain | 1646 | 1654 | Pain (R) hip | Kapake | 2796 | Script for Kapake. For FSH & LH. |
| 26.04.2000 | 27.11.1950 | M | S/Leave | 923 | 928 | Pain (L) knee - Med. 5 | | 287 | |
| 26.04.2000 | 28.03.1990 | M | Revisit | 1705 | 1709 | Sore throat again | Augmentin-Duo | 2934 | |
| 28.04.2000 | 01.08.1948 | F | | 1731 | 1739 | Light-headedness | For fasting Glucose | 3009 | |
| 25.04.2000 | 22.02.1944 | M | UTI | 1717 | 1728 | Frequency | For MSU | 3203 | |
| 26.04.2000 | 20.08.1931 | F | Pain | 1043 | 1050 | Pain (L) fingers from knitting | Co-dydramol & Movelat gel | 3266 | Penicillin & Ibuprofen allergy. |

## Result of a query that lists all consultations from the 22nd to the end of April 2000 (ConsultationsSeenFrom22ndTillEndOfApr2000)

| SurgeryDate | DateOfBirth | Sex | Diagnosis | TimeIn | TimeOut | Complaints | Treatments | NumbersID | Notes |
|---|---|---|---|---|---|---|---|---|---|
| 28.04.2000 | 04.01.1983 | F | RTI | 1635 | 1640 | Cough | Co-Amoxiclav & Codeine Linctus | 3318 | |
| 26.04.2000 | 14.08.1935 | M | | 1033 | 1037 | Fore-skin & penis bleeds | Trimethoprim | 3353 | |
| 27.04.2000 | 25.09.1970 | F | URTI | 1049 | 1059 | Sore throat & fever | Amoxycillin & Ibuprofen | 3533 | |
| 25.04.2000 | 19.05.1992 | F | Rash | 1817 | 1829 | ?Allergic rash to Amoxycillin | Cetirizine & Calamine lotion | 3581 | |
| 25.04.2000 | 28.10.1930 | F | | 937 | 942 | Pain & tenderness over (L) meta-tarsal bones | For X-Ray (L) foot | 359 | |
| 25.04.2000 | 08.04.1971 | F | Pain | 1806 | 1817 | Pain & lump (L) breast | Referred to Breast Surgeon | 3633 | |
| 27.04.2000 | 12.08.1944 | M | S/Leave | 1707 | 1719 | Diverticular disease | | 364 | |
| 26.04.2000 | 19.06.1933 | M | Anaemia | 904 | 912 | Hb 11.2 g/dl | Ferrous Sulphate | 3648 | |
| 25.04.2000 | 05.06.1924 | M | RTI | 1229 | 1245 | Cough & vomiting | Ciprofloxacin, Metoclopramide & Co-dydramol | 381 | Home visit. |
| 27.04.2000 | 17.03.1957 | F | | 1733 | 1742 | Deafness in (R) ear | Referred to ENT Surgeon | 3873 | |
| 28.04.2000 | 13.03.1992 | F | | 928 | 932 | Script for Eumovate cream given | | 3919 | Penicillin allergy. |
| 27.04.2000 | 29.01.1917 | F | | 1816 | 1826 | Advised to come back for repeat prescription of Enalapril in one week | | 4079 | |
| 27.04.2000 | 19.01.1943 | F | S/Leave | 1033 | 1043 | Pain (R) knee - Private | | 4226 | For X-Ray (R) knee. |

## Result of a query that lists all consultations from the 22nd to the end of April 2000 (ConsultationsSeenFrom22ndTillEndOfApr2000)

| SurgeryDate | DateOfBirth | Sex | Diagnosis | TimeIn | TimeOut | Complaints | Treatments | NumbersID | Notes |
|---|---|---|---|---|---|---|---|---|---|
| 25.04.2000 | 08.04.1943 | M | S/Leave | 1754 | 1802 | Chest infection - Private | | 4435 | |
| 25.04.2000 | 17.09.1938 | M | S/Leave | 1741 | 1746 | Pain (L) hip - Private | | 4448 | |
| 26.04.2000 | 31.12.1922 | M | | 1240 | 1306 | Panicky | Diazepam | 4470 | Script for Atrovent & Salbutamol nebules given. Home visit. |
| 25.04.2000 | 19.07.1994 | F | RTI | 1738 | 1741 | Cough | Amoxycillin | 4535 | |
| 28.04.2000 | 25.03.1925 | F | | 1652 | 1658 | Script for Omeprazole given | | 4625 | |
| 25.04.2000 | 02.07.1943 | M | | 1027 | 1044 | Inj. Depo-Medrone with Lidocaine given to the (R) elbow | | 4667 | |
| 28.04.2000 | 11.08.1935 | F | Pain | 952 | 958 | Pain (R) arm & (R) hand | Ibuprofen & Co-dydramol | 4670 | |
| 25.04.2000 | 19.03.1967 | M | RTI | 1728 | 1738 | Cough & wheezy | Amoxycillin, Prednisolone & nebulizer | 4730 | |
| 26.04.2000 | 10.12.1944 | M | Revisit | 912 | 923 | He still has lower abdominal pain & bloated | Colpermin | 4780 | For FBC, ESR & USScan of the lower abdomen. |
| 28.04.2000 | 11.03.1961 | M | Pain | 900 | 905 | Pain (L) thigh | Referred to Physiotherapist (BUPA) | 4954 | |
| 26.04.2000 | 03.04.1949 | F | | 1037 | 1043 | Letter to whom it may concern detailing drugs | | 4975 | Penicillin allergy. Her husband came to Surgery. |

## Result of a query that lists all consultations from the 22nd to the end of April 2000 (ConsultationsSeenFrom22ndTillEndOfApr2000)

| SurgeryDate | DateOfBirth | Sex | Diagnosis | TimeIn | TimeOut | Complaints | Treatments | NumbersID | Notes |
|---|---|---|---|---|---|---|---|---|---|
| 28.04.2000 | 15.06.1973 | F | | 958 | 1006 | Script for Microgynon-30 given | | 5038 | |
| 26.04.2000 | 02.05.1985 | F | | 1709 | 1712 | Septic (R) In growing toe nail | Flucloxacillin | 5114 | |
| 27.04.2000 | 31.10.1920 | F | RTI | 1725 | 1733 | Cough | Amoxycillin & Codeine Linctus | 5160 | Wonky knees, Rx. Co-dydramol & Ibuprofen. |
| 25.04.2000 | 09.05.1927 | M | | 1155 | 1225 | Worsening dyspnoea & cachexia | Referred to Medical Dr. on call, SGH | 5162 | Home visit. |
| 28.04.2000 | 17.05.1943 | M | | 1739 | 1742 | Indigestion | Referred to Gastro-enterologist | 5208 | Penicillin allergy. |
| 27.04.2000 | 05.01.1981 | F | | 921 | 928 | Script for Cilest given | | 5226 | |
| 27.04.2000 | 07.02.1953 | M | Pain | 915 | 921 | Pain (L) calf, ?DVT | Referred to Medical Dr. on call, SGH | 5425 | |
| 27.04.2000 | 07.02.1953 | M | Revisit | 1834 | 1844 | Pain in (L) leg persists | Amitriptyline | 5425 | Insomnia, Rx. Zopiclone. |
| 26.04.2000 | 18.11.1996 | M | | 1740 | 1746 | Script for Promethazine given | | 5442 | Penicillin allergy. |
| 28.04.2000 | 31.08.1919 | F | Hypertension | 932 | 952 | BP 170/80 | Enalapril | 5489 | |
| 26.04.2000 | 08.02.1945 | M | RTI | 1635 | 1640 | Cough | Amoxycillin | 5516 | |
| 26.04.2000 | 28.04.1918 | M | | 1712 | 1722 | Tender cyst (L) temple | Flucloxacillin | 5526 | Script for Frusemide & Aqueous cream given. |

Result of a query that lists all consultations from the 22nd to the end of April 2000 (ConsultationsSeenFrom22ndTillEndOfApr2000)

| SurgeryDate | DateOfBirth | Sex | Diagnosis | TimeIn | TimeOut | Complaints | Treatments | NumbersID | Notes |
|---|---|---|---|---|---|---|---|---|---|
| 26.04.2000 | 07.04.1919 | F | | 935 | 940 | Bruising (L) breast | Advised to observe | 5558 | Penicillin allergy. |
| 27.04.2000 | 31.05.1967 | F | UTI | 1059 | 1107 | Dysuria | Trimethoprim | 5565 | For MSU. |
| 25.04.2000 | 17.01.1965 | F | Pain | 1829 | 1843 | (L) chest pain | Co-Proxamol | 5571 | She refuses to go to hospital. |
| 26.04.2000 | 24.11.1954 | F | | 1733 | 1740 | Pain (R) foot | She will come back in four weeks | 558 | |
| 27.04.2000 | 28.09.1921 | F | | 1654 | 1707 | Tearful & very depressed | Referred to CPN | 5597 | |
| 28.04.2000 | 17.04.1923 | M | Pain | 1006 | 1017 | Indigestion & Epigastric discomfort | Omeprazole | 560 | Referred to Gastro-enterologist. (R) testicle is painful & tender, referred to Urologist. Penicillin allergy. |
| 25.04.2000 | 30.03.1984 | F | Revisit | 951 | 1000 | Back pain has persisted | Ibuprofen & Co-dydramol | 5608 | T.A.T.T., for FBC & TFTs. |
| 28.04.2000 | 19.12.1978 | F | URTI | 1022 | 1028 | Sore throat | Co-Amoxiclav | 5626 | FP1001 (GMS4) form signed. |
| 27.04.2000 | 20.12.1941 | F | | 1025 | 1033 | Script for Atorvastatin given | | 5721 | For LFTs. |
| 28.04.2000 | 24.04.1935 | F | | 910 | 928 | Carbamazepine is not helping her restless legs | Referred to Neurologist | 5770 | Script for Atrovent & Salbutamol nebules given. |
| 28.04.2000 | 16.03.1998 | F | | 1017 | 1022 | Bad cold & diarrhoea yesterday | Ibuprofen | 6038 | |

Result of a query that lists all consultations from the 22nd to the end of April 2000 (ConsultationsSeenFrom22ndTillEndOfApr2000)

| SurgeryDate | DateOfBirth | Sex | Diagnosis | TimeIn | TimeOut | Complaints | Treatments | NumbersID | Notes |
|---|---|---|---|---|---|---|---|---|---|
| 25.04.2000 | 18.07.1965 | F | | 906 | 910 | Histology of mole on leg; Superficial capillary haemangioma. No malignancy | | 6042 | FP1001 (GMS4) form signed. |
| 25.04.2000 | 02.04.1958 | M | URTI | 1802 | 1806 | (R) ear ache | Otosporin ear drops | 6053 | |
| 27.04.2000 | 03.11.1960 | F | | 1021 | 1025 | Flixonase is not helping her nasal congestion any more | Referred to ENT Surgeon | 6062 | |
| 28.04.2000 | 06.03.1997 | F | | 1642 | 1650 | For CXR | | 6090 | Script for Simple Linctus given. |
| 26.04.2000 | 11.07.1967 | M | RTI | 1722 | 1733 | Cough & vomiting | Amoxycillin & Metoclopramide | 6133 | |
| 28.04.2000 | 21.07.1998 | F | | 1714 | 1720 | Advised to see P/ Nurse on advise on the use of inhaler | | 6160 | |
| 28.04.2000 | 22.07.1917 | F | | 1742 | 1753 | Feeling of a lump in her throat | Referred to ENT Surgeon | 6182 | Penicillin & Vallergan allergy. |
| 27.04.2000 | 22.07.1938 | F | URTI | 1719 | 1725 | (R) ear sore | Otomize ear spray | 6235 | |
| 26.04.2000 | 09.09.1998 | F | | 1803 | 1810 | Her mum thinks she has sore throat | Amoxycillin & Ibuprofen | 6238 | |
| 25.04.2000 | 24.02.1925 | M | | 910 | 929 | Awaiting Blood test results | | 6239 | |
| 28.04.2000 | 24.02.1925 | M | | 1028 | 1048 | Enlarged, craggy Prostate | Referred to Urologist (Urgent) | 6239 | Grossly elevated PSA. |

Result of a query that lists all consultations from the 22nd to the end of April 2000 (ConsultationsSeenFrom22ndTillEndOfApr2000)

| SurgeryDate | DateOfBirth | Sex | Diagnosis | TimeIn | TimeOut | Complaints | Treatments | NumbersID | Notes |
|---|---|---|---|---|---|---|---|---|---|
| 26.04.2000 | 25.02.1980 | F | Rash | 1758 | 1803 | Painful & itching on (L) fore-head & sore (L) ear lobe | Fucidin-H ointment | 6255 | |
| 27.04.2000 | 04.02.1972 | F | Depression | 1003 | 1021 | Unable to cope | Citalopram | 6311 | FP1001 (GMS4) form signed. |
| 25.04.2000 | 04.08.1973 | F | UTI | 1636 | 1654 | Dysuria | Trimethoprim | 6331 | HVS: Bacterial vaginosis, Rx. Metronidazole. Ears itchy, Rx. Otomize ear spray. Recurrent cystitis, for FBC, U/Es & fasting & serum Glucose. FP1001 (GMS4) form signed. |
| 25.04.2000 | 13.01.1999 | M | RTI | 1704 | 1708 | Cough | Amoxycillin | 6332 | |
| 28.04.2000 | 23.05.1948 | F | | 1658 | 1714 | For CXR & TFTs | | 6361 | |
| 27.04.2000 | 20.06.1930 | M | | 1640 | 1646 | Prostatic symptoms | Referred to Urologist (Manor House) | 6363 | |
| 26.04.2000 | 06.07.1958 | M | | 1002 | 1016 | Infected nasal wound following a fall | Erythromycin | 6366 | Penicillin allergy. For CXR. |
| 28.04.2000 | 26.06.1963 | F | Pain | 1055 | 1103 | Neck pain following RTA | Ibuprofen & Co-dydramol | 6393 | FP1001 (GMS4) form signed. |
| 27.04.2000 | 03.12.1970 | F | | 1752 | 1801 | Wart on (R) thumb | Referred to Dermatologist | 6457 | Script for Microgynon-30 ED given. |

Result of a query that lists all consultations from the 22nd to the end of April 2000 (ConsultationsSeenFrom22ndTillEndOfApr2000)

| SurgeryDate | DateOfBirth | Sex | Diagnosis | TimeIn | TimeOut | Complaints | Treatments | NumbersID | Notes |
|---|---|---|---|---|---|---|---|---|---|
| 27.04.2000 | 14.04.1978 | F |  | 928 | 935 | Advised to see P/Nurse for Inj. Depo-Provera |  | 6464 |  |
| 25.04.2000 | 26.05.1971 | M |  | 1654 | 1657 | Lump under penis | Advised to go to GUM clinic | 6503 |  |
| 26.04.2000 | 24.03.1940 | F |  | 1016 | 1032 | Script for Verapramil & Buccastem given |  | 6567 | Distalgesic allergy. |
| 26.04.2000 | 26.01.1953 | M | S/Leave | 940 | 946 | General disability |  | 6590 | He also has cough & choking, Rx. Amoxycillin. |
| 28.04.2000 | 06.06.1924 | M | Revisit | 1048 | 1055 | Persistent indigestion | Lansoprazole | 6596 | Referred to Gastro-enterologist. |
| 27.04.2000 | 20.11.1945 | M |  | 935 | 940 | Dizziness | Betahistine | 6617 | S/Leave given for CVA. Penicillin allergy. |
| 26.04.2000 | 28.11.1978 | F |  | 1830 | 1842 | Abdominal pain | Referred to Gynaecological Dr. on call, Basildon hospital | 6630 | Penicillin allergy. She is 14 weeks gestation. |
| 28.04.2000 | 22.02.1956 | M | Pain | 1803 | 1816 | Pain (R) shoulder | Ibuprofen & Co-dydramol | 6630 |  |
| 27.04.2000 | 11.07.1921 | F |  | 1826 | 1834 | Persistent WBC in urine | Trimethoprim | 6678 | She also has Glaucoma in (L) eye, referred to Ophthalmologist. |
| 25.04.2000 | 24.02.1969 | F | Revisit | 1013 | 1018 | Throat still feels uncomfortable | Co-Amoxiclav | 6700 |  |

## Result of a query that lists all consultations from the 22nd to the end of April 2000 (ConsultationsSeenFrom22ndTillEndOfApr2000)

| SurgeryDate | DateOfBirth | Sex | Diagnosis | TimeIn | TimeOut | Complaints | Treatments | NumbersID | Notes |
|---|---|---|---|---|---|---|---|---|---|
| 25.04.2000 | 25.02.1988 | F | Pain | 1018 | 1023 | Headaches | Referred to Paediatrician | 6701 | The headache is not improving with Paracetamol. |
| 25.04.2000 | 09.08.1972 | F |  | 932 | 937 | Hay fever | Beclomethasone Aqueous nasal spray & Cetirizine | 6736 |  |
| 25.04.2000 | 07.12.1966 | M |  | 929 | 932 | Hay fever | Loratadine | 6737 |  |
| 26.04.2000 | 21.07.1963 | F |  | 1645 | 1702 | Script for Loestrin 30 & Citalopram given |  | 835 |  |
| 25.04.2000 | 20.11.1923 | M |  | 1000 | 1013 | Uric Acid 477 umol/L, elevated | Allopurinol | 916 |  |
| 27.04.2000 | 09.06.1954 | F |  | 1801 | 1806 | Breast tenderness | Frusemide | 927 |  |

## Result of a query that lists all consultations from the 22nd to the end of April 2001 (ConsultationsSeenFrom22ndTillEndOfApr2001)

| SurgeryDate | DateOfBirth | Sex | Diagnosis | TimeIn | TimeOut | Complaints | Treatments | NumbersID | Notes |
|---|---|---|---|---|---|---|---|---|---|
| 25.04.2001 | 26.10.1957 | F | Depression | 1654 | 1703 | Stress & anxiety | Citalopram | NP | Pain lower back, Rx. Diclofenac enteric coated & Co-dydramol. |
| 27.04.2001 | 23.09.1954 | M | S/Leave | 1804 | 1808 | Back Pain |  | 1017 |  |
| 25.04.2001 | 21.12.1973 | M | Lump | 931 | 937 | Small subcutaneous cyst on the scrotum | Referred to Surgeon (Basildon hospital) | 1085 |  |

## Result of a query that lists all consultations from the 22nd to the end of April 2001 (ConsultationsSeenFrom22ndTillEndOfApr2001)

| SurgeryDate | DateOfBirth | Sex | Diagnosis | TimeIn | TimeOut | Complaints | Treatments | NumbersID | Notes |
|---|---|---|---|---|---|---|---|---|---|
| 25.04.2001 | 08.02.1939 | F | | 1029 | 1037 | Giddiness & sneezing | Galpseud, Prochlorperazine, Chloramphenicol eye drops & Loratadine | 113 | For CXR. |
| 23.04.2001 | 03.10.1969 | F | Pain | 1030 | 1034 | Indigestion pain | Lansoprazole | 1206 | Trimethoprim allergy. |
| 26.04.2001 | 25.03.1944 | M | | 1728 | 1733 | Palpitations | For CXR, FBC & TFTs | 125 | |
| 25.04.2001 | 27.06.1986 | M | Rash | 1801 | 1805 | Acne spots on face | Tetracycline | 1267 | |
| 27.04.2001 | 07.11.1980 | M | RTI | 1729 | 1740 | Cough | Erythromycin | 132 | |
| 25.04.2001 | 28.07.1939 | F | | 1720 | 1731 | Advised to stop Bendrofluazide because of side-effects | | 1398 | |
| 24.04.2001 | 21.09.1924 | F | URTI | 941 | 947 | Sore throat | Amoxycillin | 1419 | Script for Simvastatin given. |
| 26.04.2001 | 03.03.1925 | M | Pain | 925 | 939 | (R) hip & neck pain | Diclofenac, Rabeprazole & Paracetamol | 1558 | For X-Ray (R) hip & Cervical X-Ray. |
| 23.04.2001 | 15.11.1940 | F | Conjunctivitis | 1751 | 1754 | Sticky & painful (R) eye | Chloramphenicol eye drops | 1619 | |
| 24.04.2001 | 24.12.1955 | F | | 1755 | 1801 | Wound is infected & sore | Flucloxacillin & Fucidin cream | 1638 | |
| 24.04.2001 | 17.10.1967 | F | S/Leave | 1037 | 1041 | Pain in (R) shoulder, lower back, (R) hip & neck | | 1646 | |
| 26.04.2001 | 27.06.1944 | M | | 1749 | 1757 | He will contact the Surgeon directly about his neck lump | | 1673 | |

Result of a query that lists all consultations from the 22nd to the end of April 2001 (ConsultationsSeenFrom22ndTillEndOfApr2001)

| SurgeryDate | DateOfBirth | Sex | Diagnosis | TimeIn | TimeOut | Complaints | Treatments | NumbersID | Notes |
|---|---|---|---|---|---|---|---|---|---|
| 24.04.2001 | 26.06.1953 | M | Rash | 953 | 1000 | Rash both groins | Terbinafine cream | 1681 | |
| 24.04.2001 | 02.09.1941 | F | | 1000 | 1005 | Advised to get her Co-Proxamol as a repeat prescription | | 1797 | |
| 27.04.2001 | 14.12.1912 | F | ?DVT | 1345 | 1410 | (R) leg is swollen & painful | Referred to DVT clinic, SGH | 1805 | Home visit. |
| 23.04.2001 | 05.06.1944 | M | Hypertension | 920 | 932 | BP 170/100 | Bendrofluozide | 1874 | |
| 23.04.2001 | 04.01.1962 | F | UTI | 1648 | 1702 | Dysuria | Cefalexin | 1884 | For MSU. Trimethoprim allergy. |
| 26.04.2001 | 31.08.1982 | F | | 1022 | 1036 | Chlamydial swabs positive | GUM referral suggested | 1924 | |
| 27.04.2001 | 29.11.1929 | F | | 1649 | 1657 | CXR: Heart is not enlarged | | 193 | |
| 26.04.2001 | 20.09.1946 | F | Rash | 939 | 944 | Rash on neck & fingers | 1% Hydrocortisone cream | 1973 | |
| 24.04.2001 | 11.03.1968 | F | Revisit | 1730 | 1739 | Her migraine headaches are still bad | Referred to Neurologist | 2 | |
| 27.04.2001 | 30.05.1985 | M | Pain | 1657 | 1702 | Pain in the knees | Paracetamol & Ibuprofen | 2096 | |
| 27.04.2001 | 06.07.1936 | F | | 1743 | 1755 | Script for Bisoprolol & Sotalol given | | 2150 | |
| 23.04.2001 | 16.07.1957 | F | S/Leave | 1702 | 1712 | Diarrhoea & unwell - Private | | 2164 | Script for Electrolade, Loperamide, Buscopan & Co-dydramol given. Stool for C&S. |

13

Result of a query that lists all consultations from the 22nd to the end of April 2001 (ConsultationsSeenFrom22ndTillEndOfApr2001)

| SurgeryDate | DateOfBirth | Sex | Diagnosis | TimeIn | TimeOut | Complaints | Treatments | NumbersID | Notes |
|---|---|---|---|---|---|---|---|---|---|
| 27.04.2001 | 16.07.1957 | F | | 950 | 959 | Campylobacter culture in the stool | Erythromycin | 2164 | Septrin allergy. |
| 25.04.2001 | 22.03.1933 | F | Pain | 957 | 1001 | Pain (R) knee | For X-Ray (R) knee | 2179 | |
| 27.04.2001 | 21.10.1982 | M | Rash | 925 | 930 | Brown patches on chest | Oilatum Plus emollient & Unguentum Merck | 2196 | |
| 23.04.2001 | 14.08.1927 | M | Pain | 944 | 953 | Pain (L) side of neck | Co-dydramol & Diclofenac enteric coated | 2289 | For Cervical X-Ray. |
| 23.04.2001 | 01.04.1988 | F | | 1754 | 1758 | She gets wheezy | Advised to see P/ Nurse for asthma check | 2318 | |
| 25.04.2001 | 24.09.1937 | M | | 1805 | 1808 | Cholesterol 6 mmols/L | Simvastatin | 2329 | |
| 26.04.2001 | 01.03.1984 | F | Pain | 1116 | 1123 | Injury (R) foot & ankle | For X-Ray | 2349 | |
| 26.04.2001 | 08.05.1986 | F | Revisit | 1105 | 1113 | Warts on fingers are still present | Referred to Dermatologist (Basildon hospital) | 2350 | |
| 26.04.2001 | 11.05.1959 | F | | 1113 | 1116 | Outbreak of Scabies at her work place | Lyclear Dermal cream | 2351 | Penicillin, Septrin & Tetracycline allergy. |
| 25.04.2001 | 28.03.1970 | F | S/Leave | 1001 | 1015 | Pain & numbness of (R) hand | | 2375 | Migraine headaches, Rx. Pizotifen & Sumatriptan. |

Result of a query that lists all consultations from the 22nd to the end of April 2001 (ConsultationsSeenFrom22ndTillEndOfApr2001)

| SurgeryDate | DateOfBirth | Sex | Diagnosis | TimeIn | TimeOut | Complaints | Treatments | NumbersID | Notes |
|---|---|---|---|---|---|---|---|---|---|
| 23.04.2001 | 02.11.1977 | F | | 905 | 914 | For FBC & Fasting Glucose | | 2487 | |
| 27.04.2001 | 22.09.1939 | F | | 917 | 925 | U/Es - all normal | | 2510 | |
| 27.04.2001 | 07.03.1935 | F | RTI | 1740 | 1743 | Cough | Amoxycillin | 2522 | |
| 24.04.2001 | 06.01.1943 | F | | 1801 | 1814 | Inj. Depo-Medrone with Lidocaine given to (L) shoulder | | 2642 | |
| 25.04.2001 | 08.04.1990 | M | | 1641 | 1649 | Nose is blocked | Beclomethasone nasal spray | 2789 | Cefaclor allergy. |
| 23.04.2001 | 07.07.1983 | F | URTI | 1038 | 1041 | Sore throat | Amoxycillin | 3085 | FP1001 (GMS4) form signed. |
| 23.04.2001 | 30.04.1985 | M | Revisit | 1718 | 1726 | Osteochondritis of the (R) third metatarsal | Referred to Orthopaedic Surgeon (Basildon hospital) | 318 | Script for Co-dydramol & Diclofenac enteric coated given. |
| 27.04.2001 | 17.07.1942 | M | | 1643 | 1649 | Smelly discharge from the penis | Erythromycin | 3244 | Penicillin allergy. |
| 26.04.2001 | 20.11.1965 | M | Pain | 900 | 910 | Chest pain | Co-dydramol & Diclofenac enteric coated | 3254 | |
| 26.04.2001 | 25.06.1938 | F | | 1055 | 1105 | Bilateral pedal oedema | Furosemide | 3415 | |
| 25.04.2001 | 03.12.1949 | F | Rash | 1649 | 1654 | Rash on shoulder | Fucidin-H cream | 3509 | Script for Frusemide given. |
| 24.04.2001 | 25.11.1946 | M | UTI | 947 | 953 | Dysuria | Trimethoprim | 3558 | For MSU. |
| 23.04.2001 | 19.05.1956 | F | S/Leave | 1712 | 1718 | Bilateral Chevron Osteotomy | | 3568 | |

15

Result of a query that lists all consultations from the 22nd to the end of April 2001 (ConsultationsSeenFrom22ndTillEndOfApr2001)

| SurgeryDate | DateOfBirth | Sex | Diagnosis | TimeIn | TimeOut | Complaints | Treatments | NumbersID | Notes |
|---|---|---|---|---|---|---|---|---|---|
| 23.04.2001 | 28.10.1930 | F | Pain | 1034 | 1038 | Pain in the back & hips | For X-Ray of the hips & Lumbo-Sacral spine | 359 | |
| 27.04.2001 | 08.04.1971 | F | UTI | 1051 | 1101 | Dysuria | Trimethoprim | 3633 | |
| 25.04.2001 | 05.12.1937 | M | RTI | 937 | 952 | Chesty cough | Erythromycin | 3646 | |
| 23.04.2001 | 10.03.1946 | F | Pain | 1809 | 1817 | Pain (L) side of neck | Dihydrocodeine, Diclofenac enteric coated tablets & injection | 3710 | |
| 25.04.2001 | 23.07.1953 | M | S/Leave | 904 | 922 | | | 3725 | Script for Phenytoin given. |
| 25.04.2001 | 16.11.1987 | F | | 1808 | 1813 | PER VAGINA discharge | Erythromycin | 3770 | |
| 24.04.2001 | 19.03.1919 | M | Pain | 933 | 941 | Pain (L) hip | Co-dydramol | 3892 | For X-Ray. |
| 23.04.2001 | 04.09.1985 | M | RTI | 1758 | 1803 | Cough | Amoxycillin | 3959 | Nuts allergy. |
| 27.04.2001 | 19.05.1964 | M | Pain | 1021 | 1026 | Injury (L) wrist | For X-Ray | 3995 | |
| 23.04.2001 | 06.05.1993 | F | URTI | 1041 | 1045 | (R) ear ache | Amoxycillin & Paracetamol | 4040 | |
| 26.04.2001 | 08.04.1961 | F | S/Leave | 950 | 953 | Headaches | | 407 | |
| 27.04.2001 | 29.01.1917 | F | | 1015 | 1021 | Advised to see P/Nurse regarding appropriate inhaler for her breathlessness | | 4079 | |
| 23.04.2001 | 14.07.1906 | F | URTI | 1205 | 1212 | Infected rhinorrhoea | Amoxycillin & Soluble Paracetamol | 413 | Home visit. |
| 27.04.2001 | 26.07.1924 | M | | 959 | 1006 | Script for Cefalexin given | | 4270 | |

Result of a query that lists all consultations from the 22nd to the end of April 2001 (ConsultationsSeenFrom22ndTillEndOfApr2001)

| SurgeryDate | DateOfBirth | Sex | Diagnosis | TimeIn | TimeOut | Complaints | Treatments | NumbersID | Notes |
|---|---|---|---|---|---|---|---|---|---|
| 26.04.2001 | 30.10.1969 | F | | 1805 | 1819 | Irregular heavy bleeding | Norethisterone | 4275 | |
| 23.04.2001 | 11.12.1968 | M | RTI | 1731 | 1735 | Cough | Amoxycillin | 4315 | |
| 25.04.2001 | 12.08.1967 | F | | 1015 | 1025 | Bacterial vaginosis | Metronidazole | 4402 | Script for Citalopram given. |
| 27.04.2001 | 13.10.1944 | M | | 947 | 950 | (L) Gum abscess | Amoxycillin | 441 | |
| 26.04.2001 | 31.12.1922 | M | RTI | 1759 | 1805 | Cough | Amoxycillin & Erythromycin | 4470 | Script for Salmeterol & Difflam spray given. |
| 27.04.2001 | 29.09.1932 | F | | 1006 | 1010 | To come in for a weight check in one month for Xenical | | 4487 | |
| 27.04.2001 | 01.02.1959 | M | | 1708 | 1716 | For Uric Acid | | 4523 | |
| 26.04.2001 | 19.06.1927 | F | RTI | 1757 | 1759 | Cough | Amoxycillin | 4527 | |
| 23.04.2001 | 28.08.1994 | F | Rash | 1726 | 1731 | Itchy rash on the back | Loratadine & Calamine lotion | 4545 | |
| 26.04.2001 | 25.02.1947 | F | | 1835 | 1844 | Inj. Depo-Medrone with Lidocaine given to (L) shoulder | | 4576 | |
| 23.04.2001 | 22.11.1983 | F | Revisit | 1741 | 1751 | Itchy rash is still present | Referred to Dermatologist (Basildon hospital) | 464 | Script for Co-dydramol & Balneum Plus Bath oil given. |
| 25.04.2001 | 23.05.1987 | F | URTI | 1707 | 1719 | Pain on (R) ear | Erythromycin | 4653 | |
| 25.04.2001 | 16.11.1962 | F | | 1714 | 1720 | Cyst on (R) side of face | Flucloxacillin & Penicillin V | 4655 | Penicillin allergy. |

Result of a query that lists all consultations from the 22nd to the end of April 2001 (ConsultationsSeenFrom22ndTillEndOfApr2001)

| SurgeryDate | DateOfBirth | Sex | Diagnosis | TimeIn | TimeOut | Complaints | Treatments | NumbersID | Notes |
|---|---|---|---|---|---|---|---|---|---|
| 24.04.2001 | 11.08.1935 | F | | 1649 | 1653 | Advised to continue with the Bendrofluazide | | 4670 | |
| 24.04.2001 | 30.05.1938 | F | | 1657 | 1709 | Script for Felodipine given | | 4706 | Penicillin allergy. |
| 23.04.2001 | 11.07.1933 | M | | 914 | 920 | Night cramps | Quinine Sulphate | 4968 | |
| 26.04.2001 | 21.08.1986 | F | | 1819 | 1835 | PR bleeding | Referred to Surgical Dr. on call, SGH | 4997 | |
| 26.04.2001 | 11.11.1932 | F | | 1733 | 1744 | Script for Clotrimazole & Lansoprazole given | | 5290 | |
| 24.04.2001 | 14.10.1928 | M | | 1005 | 1018 | Constipation | Senna & Glycerine suppositories | 537 | Pain in the knees, Rx. Inj. Depo-Medrone with Lidocaine. |
| 24.04.2001 | 25.02.1929 | F | | 1018 | 1030 | Bleeding & painful haemorrhoids | Referred to Bowel Surgeon | 538 | Script for Waxsol & EarCalm spray given. |
| 24.04.2001 | 10.11.1957 | F | | 1748 | 1755 | Palpitations | Propranolol | 5385 | |
| 24.04.2001 | 04.07.1986 | F | URTI | 1744 | 1748 | Sore throat | Amoxycillin | 5386 | |
| 27.04.2001 | 18.02.1926 | F | | 1010 | 1015 | Bilateral cataracts | Referred to Ophthalmologist | 5543 | |
| 25.04.2001 | 23.07.1976 | M | Pain | 1703 | 1707 | Fell & landed on his (R) knee | For X-Ray | 5555 | |
| 26.04.2001 | 02.12.1993 | M | | 1650 | 1657 | Verrucae on the (R) heel | Occlusal | 5569 | Penicillin allergy. |
| 26.04.2001 | 17.01.1965 | F | | 1006 | 1012 | Offensive per vagina discharge | Advised to see the P/Nurse for HVS | 5571 | 3 months pregnant. |

Result of a query that lists all consultations from the 22nd to the end of April 2001 (ConsultationsSeenFrom22ndTillEndOfApr2001)

| SurgeryDate | DateOfBirth | Sex | Diagnosis | TimeIn | TimeOut | Complaints | Treatments | NumbersID | Notes |
|---|---|---|---|---|---|---|---|---|---|
| 24.04.2001 | 23.10.1996 | F | Rash | 1713 | 1718 | Dry skin, red & inflamed | Erythromycin, Oilatum Plus emollient & Fucidin-H cream | 5593 | |
| 23.04.2001 | 05.12.1924 | F | | 935 | 944 | For repeat TFTs in 6 months | | 5649 | For MSU. |
| 26.04.2001 | 26.10.1962 | M | | 1012 | 1022 | Hot, sweaty & pain (R) loin | Amoxycillin & Co-dydramol | 5691 | |
| 27.04.2001 | 12.01.1929 | M | | 1034 | 1051 | Uric Acid 486 mcmol/L, elevated | Allopurinol | 5703 | |
| 27.04.2001 | 27.12.1941 | F | | 1716 | 1729 | Smarting anus | Scheriproct suppositories & Xyloproct ointment | 5790 | |
| 25.04.2001 | 20.02.1937 | F | URTI | 1025 | 1029 | Sinusitis | Amoxycillin | 5798 | |
| 25.04.2001 | 30.03.1946 | M | | 1037 | 1056 | Advised to contact the Orthopaedic Surgeon to write letter required from Halifax | | 5845 | |
| 24.04.2001 | 25.12.1963 | F | URTI | 1644 | 1649 | Blocked nose | Amoxycillin | 5934 | |
| 24.04.2001 | 20.04.1984 | M | URTI | 1653 | 1657 | Sore throat | Penicillin V | 5937 | |
| 27.04.2001 | 08.01.1998 | F | RTI | 1639 | 1643 | Cough | Erythromycin | 5948 | Penicillin allergy. |
| 23.04.2001 | 23.03.1926 | M | | 1638 | 1648 | Script for Esomeprazole given | | 5954 | |
| 23.04.2001 | 29.09.1975 | F | | 1008 | 1013 | Late period | For Pregnancy test | 5970 | Penicillin allergy. |
| 26.04.2001 | 29.09.1975 | F | | 1701 | 1718 | Pregnancy test is positive | | 5970 | Penicillin allergy. |

Result of a query that lists all consultations from the 22nd to the end of April 2001 (ConsultationsSeenFrom22ndTillEndOfApr2001)

| SurgeryDate | DateOfBirth | Sex | Diagnosis | TimeIn | TimeOut | Complaints | Treatments | NumbersID | Notes |
|---|---|---|---|---|---|---|---|---|---|
| 23.04.2001 | 12.02.1938 | M | Revisit | 1803 | 1809 | He still has claudication pain in (L) leg | Referred to Vascular Surgeon (Basildon hospital) | 5997 | |
| 26.04.2001 | 05.12.1920 | M | | 1036 | 1055 | Giddy & neck pain | Betahistine & Cervical X-Ray | 6015 | Script for Bendrofluazide given. |
| 24.04.2001 | 13.12.1948 | F | | 1721 | 1730 | Dizzy spells | Prochlorperazine | 6033 | Sore & red ears, Rx. Otomize ear spray. For FBC & Fasting Glucose. |
| 25.04.2001 | 22.02.1924 | M | | 1739 | 1755 | Abscess on chest is still quite big | Referred to Surgical Dr. on call, (Basildon hospital) | 6094 | |
| 23.04.2001 | 23.05.1998 | M | | 1023 | 1030 | Tip of the penis balloons out | Referred to Urologist (BUPA) | 6098 | |
| 25.04.2001 | 22.01.1944 | M | RTI | 1731 | 1739 | Cough | Erythromycin | 6183 | Penicillin allergy. Script for Simvastin given. |
| 24.04.2001 | 19.12.1974 | M | | 911 | 919 | Both groin pull | Reassured | 6319 | |
| 27.04.2001 | 04.05.1961 | M | S/Leave | 930 | 947 | Blurred vision & weakness - Private | | 6340 | Penicillin allergy. |
| 23.04.2001 | 11.03.1999 | F | | 953 | 1008 | Constipation & Vomiting | Metoclopramide, Lactulose & Glycerine suppositories | 6382 | |
| 26.04.2001 | 08.05.1974 | M | RTI | 1718 | 1728 | Cough | Amoxycillin & Codeine Linctus | 6532 | Depression, Rx. Citalopram. |

Result of a query that lists all consultations from the 22nd to the end of April 2001 (ConsultationsSeenFrom22ndTillEndOfApr2001)

| SurgeryDate | DateOfBirth | Sex | Diagnosis | TimeIn | TimeOut | Complaints | Treatments | NumbersID | Notes |
|---|---|---|---|---|---|---|---|---|---|
| 24.04.2001 | 15.08.1961 | M | | 919 | 933 | Pain (L) big toe, ?Gout | For Uric Acid | 6569 | |
| 26.04.2001 | 16.07.1915 | F | | 1345 | 1415 | Unwell, pedal oedema | Referred to MAU, SGH | 6585 | Home visit. |
| 25.04.2001 | 09.11.1978 | F | | 1755 | 1801 | She wants her period delayed | Advised to take her Cilest without leaving the one week gap in between the two packets | 6622 | |
| 25.04.2001 | 08.05.1939 | F | Lump | 952 | 957 | Cyst on the fore-head | Referred to Surgeon | 6643 | |
| 24.04.2001 | 02.05.1929 | F | RTI | 1638 | 1644 | Cough | Ciprofloxacin & Codeine Linctus | 6693 | |
| 24.04.2001 | 26.06.1955 | F | Pain | 900 | 911 | Back pain | Co-dydramol & Diclofenac enteric coated | 6753 | For X-Ray of the Lumbo-Sacral spine. |
| 26.04.2001 | 10.03.1987 | M | Pain | 1657 | 1701 | Pain knees & heel | Ibuprofen | 6778 | |
| 26.04.2001 | 16.05.1967 | M | | 1744 | 1749 | Letter to expedite Orthopaedic appointment | | 6815 | |
| 27.04.2001 | 28.11.1969 | M | | 1702 | 1708 | Recurrent mouth ulcers | Amoxycillin & Metronidazole | 6827 | |
| 27.04.2001 | 11.07.1963 | M | | 1755 | 1804 | Script for Lansoprazole given | | 6832 | Penicillin allergy. |
| 27.04.2001 | 23.09.1998 | M | | 1817 | 1823 | Vomiting & sore throat | Metoclopramide, Paracetamol, Amoxycillin | 6864 | Script for Calamine lotion given. |

21

Result of a query that lists all consultations from the 22nd to the end of April 2001 (ConsultationsSeenFrom22ndTillEndOfApr2001)

| SurgeryDate | DateOfBirth | Sex | Diagnosis | TimeIn | TimeOut | Complaints | Treatments | NumbersID | Notes |
|---|---|---|---|---|---|---|---|---|---|
| 25.04.2001 | 16.05.1976 | M | | 922 | 931 | Sore (R) loin | For U/Es, MSU & USScan of the kidneys | 6874 | |
| 26.04.2001 | 20.10.1998 | F | Revisit | 910 | 925 | Still unwell & abdominal pain | Referred to Paediatric Dr. on call, Basildon hospital | 6919 | |
| 26.04.2001 | 20.02.1971 | F | | 944 | 950 | Late period | For Pregnancy test | 6954 | Penicillin allergy. |
| 27.04.2001 | 20.02.1971 | F | | 1808 | 1817 | Pregnancy test positive | | 6954 | Penicillin allergy. |
| 24.04.2001 | 11.01.1964 | F | | 1030 | 1037 | Script for Dihydrocodeine given | | 6976 | |
| 26.04.2001 | 01.02.1988 | M | | 1646 | 1650 | Wart on (L) palm | Occlusal | 6977 | |
| 24.04.2001 | 01.04.1937 | M | S/Leave | 1041 | 1045 | (R) knee joint replacement | | 6987 | |
| 27.04.2001 | 28.10.1931 | M | | 906 | 917 | Night cramps | Quinine Sulphate | 7031 | Script for Ramipril given. |
| 27.04.2001 | 26.02.1940 | F | URTI | 1026 | 1034 | (L) ear is itchy & sore | Otomize ear spray | 7047 | |
| 23.04.2001 | 12.10.1985 | M | | 1013 | 1023 | Recurrent epistaxes | Naseptin cream & Amoxycillin | 7074 | |
| 25.04.2001 | 16.07.1972 | M | Revisit | 1813 | 1822 | Repeat script given for a lost one | | 782 | |
| 26.04.2001 | 10.09.1919 | F | | 1123 | 1126 | Script for Prednisolone enteric coated given | | 823 | |

Result of a query that lists all consultations from the 22nd to the end of April 2001 (ConsultationsSeenFrom22ndTillEndOfApr2001)

| SurgeryDate | DateOfBirth | Sex | Diagnosis | TimeIn | TimeOut | Complaints | Treatments | NumbersID | Notes |
|---|---|---|---|---|---|---|---|---|---|
| 26.04.2001 | 04.07.1959 | F | Revisit | 953 | 1006 | Still has neck pain | Referred to Orthopaedic Surgeon (BUPA) | 96 | |
| 24.04.2001 | 31.12.1930 | F | URTI | 1709 | 1713 | Bilateral ear ache | Amoxycillin & Sofradex ear drops | 989 | |

Result of a query that lists all consultations from the 22nd to the end of April 2003 (ConsultationsSeenFrom22ndTillEndOfApr2003)

| SurgeryDate | DateOfBirth | Sex | Diagnosis | TimeIn | TimeOut | Complaints | Treatments | NumbersID | Notes |
|---|---|---|---|---|---|---|---|---|---|
| 23.04.2003 | 05.01.1971 | F | | 1750 | 1808 | Late Period | For Pregnancy test | 1003 | |
| 22.04.2003 | 20.04.1947 | F | URTI | 1112 | 1124 | Sore throat | Erythromycin | 11 | Penicillin allergy. S/Leave for Depression & Flu symptoms given. |
| 28.04.2003 | 26.11.1935 | M | Pain | 1701 | 1705 | Pain under (L) 1st & 2nd toes | Co-codamol | 1276 | |
| 22.04.2003 | 03.02.1977 | M | Rash | 1712 | 1717 | Dry itchy skin | Fusidic Acid 2% + 1% Hydrocortisone cream & Oilatum Plus shower gel | 1306 | |
| 22.04.2003 | 06.07.1948 | M | | 1712 | 1720 | To take OTC migraine medication | | 1356 | |

Result of a query that lists all consultations from the 22nd to the end of April 2003 (ConsultationsSeenFrom22ndTillEndOfApr2003)

| SurgeryDate | DateOfBirth | Sex | Diagnosis | TimeIn | TimeOut | Complaints | Treatments | NumbersID | Notes |
|---|---|---|---|---|---|---|---|---|---|
| 22.04.2003 | 26.10.1943 | F | | 1014 | 1021 | To contact the Liver Unit in Cambridge regarding her painful leg | | 1365 | |
| 28.04.2003 | 15.06.1987 | M | Lump | 1753 | 1801 | (R) Inguinal hernia | Referred to Surgeon | 1447 | |
| 24.04.2003 | 05.01.1984 | M | | 1036 | 1045 | Painful piles & boils on thighs | Scheriproct ointment, Scheriproct suppositories, Flucloxacillin & Fusidic Acid cream | 1504 | |
| 24.04.2003 | 25.12.1948 | M | | 930 | 946 | To see P/Nurse in 6 months | For repeat HBA1c | 165 | |
| 29.04.2003 | 25.02.1988 | F | | 1720 | 1724 | Hay fever | Fexofenadine | 1701 | Itchy eczema rash on the thighs, Rx. 1% Hydrocortisone cream. |
| 22.04.2003 | 30.04.1917 | M | UTI | 1245 | 1305 | Abdominal pain & dysuria | Trimethoprim | 1733 | Home visit. Depressed, Rx. Fluoxetine. Script for Ensure Plus & Enlive given. |
| 25.04.2003 | 30.04.1917 | M | Pain | 1345 | 1400 | Abdominal pain | Sevredol | 1733 | Home visit. |
| 23.04.2003 | 23.07.1923 | M | | 959 | 1011 | Frequency of micturition & nocturia | For MSU | 175 | Script for Injection Methlprednisolone 40mg, Lidocaine 10mg/ml. |

24

Result of a query that lists all consultations from the 22nd to the end of April 2003 (ConsultationsSeenFrom22ndTillEndOfApr2003)

| SurgeryDate | DateOfBirth | Sex | Diagnosis | TimeIn | TimeOut | Complaints | Treatments | NumbersID | Notes |
|---|---|---|---|---|---|---|---|---|---|
| 25.04.2003 | 29.12.1983 | M | Rash | 1009 | 1026 | Itchy reddish rash on the back | Fusidic Acid 2% + 1% Hydrocortisone cream | 1903 | |
| 29.04.2003 | 06.07.1957 | F | | 1039 | 1043 | Referred to Gastro-enterologist regarding her abdominal & back pain | | 1954 | |
| 25.04.2003 | 22.09.1928 | F | | 1728 | 1736 | Script for Frusemide given | | 2137 | |
| 25.04.2003 | 26.08.1960 | M | Rash | 1736 | 1745 | Lesion on chin | Referred to Dermatologist | 2187 | |
| 25.04.2003 | 25.11.1985 | F | Rash | 1721 | 1728 | Itchy red rash on hands | Miconazole 2% + 1% Hydrocortisone cream | 2201 | FP1001 (GMS4) form completed. |
| 28.04.2003 | 22.03.1936 | F | | 1009 | 1027 | Diabetic Clinic | | 2345 | Script for Enalapril given. |
| 24.04.2003 | 28.03.1970 | F | | 1009 | 1018 | Script for Co-codamol given | | 2375 | Referred to Endocrinologist. |
| 28.04.2003 | 28.05.1985 | F | S/Leave | 1737 | 1745 | Diarrhoea & Vomiting - Private | | 2387 | |
| 25.04.2003 | 07.11.1984 | F | URTI | 1745 | 1752 | Sore throat | Amoxycillin | 2438 | FP1001 (GMS4) form completed. |
| 25.04.2003 | 21.11.1988 | F | Pain | 1649 | 1656 | Pain & tenderness (L) 4th metatarsal | Advised to go to A/E for X-Ray | 2507 | |
| 29.04.2003 | 21.11.1988 | F | Revisit | 907 | 918 | Area of the (L) foot is swollen & tender | Erythromycin & Ibuprofen | 2507 | Penicillin allergy. |

Result of a query that lists all consultations from the 22nd to the end of April 2003 (ConsultationsSeenFrom22ndTillEndOfApr2003)

| SurgeryDate | DateOfBirth | Sex | Diagnosis | TimeIn | TimeOut | Complaints | Treatments | NumbersID | Notes |
|---|---|---|---|---|---|---|---|---|---|
| 24.04.2003 | 28.06.1934 | M | Hypertension | 903 | 910 | BP 186/103 | Atenolol | 2512 | |
| 22.04.2003 | 16.02.1984 | F | | 1720 | 1730 | Itchy rash on legs & face | Fusidic Acid 2% + 1% Hydrocortisone cream | 2524 | |
| 29.04.2003 | 07.09.1980 | F | | 1049 | 1115 | HGV Medical Examination done | | 2577 | |
| 29.04.2003 | 08.06.1984 | M | | 1802 | 1806 | X-Ray (R) shoulder: Possible injury to the epiphyses of the acromion, probably insignificant | | 2670 | |
| 23.04.2003 | 24.03.1973 | M | S/Leave | 1647 | 1652 | Injury to (L) ankle - Private | | 2784 | |
| 28.04.2003 | 05.09.1956 | F | URTI | 1647 | 1651 | Sore throat | Amoxycillin | 2844 | |
| 28.04.2003 | 09.02.1956 | M | Revisit | 1651 | 1701 | Sore throat again | Erythromycin | 2846 | |
| 22.04.2003 | 15.02.1932 | F | RTI | 1029 | 1036 | Cough | Erythromycin | 3043 | Penicillin allergy. |
| 22.04.2003 | 18.03.1978 | M | | 1039 | 1043 | Hay fever | Loratadine | 3115 | |
| 24.04.2003 | 26.03.1980 | F | Lump | 1032 | 1036 | Cyst on (L) side of face | Referred to Plastic Surgeon | 3116 | |
| 28.04.2003 | 31.05.1947 | F | | 918 | 923 | USScan of abdomen results are not yet available | | 3316 | Penicillin allergy. |
| 25.04.2003 | 28.08.1986 | M | Revisit | 1003 | 1009 | Both ears are blocked | To try warm Olive oil | 3428 | |
| 25.04.2003 | 02.12.1923 | M | Pain | 1330 | 1345 | Pain both legs | Co-codamol & Nafiidrofuryl | 3429 | Home visit. |

26

Result of a query that lists all consultations from the 22nd to the end of April 2003 (ConsultationsSeenFrom22ndTillEndOfApr2003)

| SurgeryDate | DateOfBirth | Sex | Diagnosis | TimeIn | TimeOut | Complaints | Treatments | NumbersID | Notes |
|---|---|---|---|---|---|---|---|---|---|
| 28.04.2003 | 09.06.1953 | M | S/Leave | 923 | 929 | Fractured (R) Humerus - Med. 5 | | 3695 | Penicillin allergy. Duplicate copy. |
| 24.04.2003 | 02.08.1963 | F | | 1119 | 1124 | Viral rash | | 3796 | |
| 23.04.2003 | 21.05.1971 | F | Pain | 951 | 959 | Ache inside vagina | For MSU & USScan of the Pelvis/lower abdomen | 39 | Penicillin allergy. |
| 23.04.2003 | 03.02.1971 | F | | 1746 | 1750 | Drugs reauthorised | | 4003 | |
| 22.04.2003 | 05.07.1931 | F | | 1136 | 1144 | Script for Atenolol given | | 4008 | |
| 28.04.2003 | 07.10.1933 | M | | 942 | 944 | Script for Olanzapine given | | 4055 | |
| 23.04.2003 | 28.04.1934 | F | | 918 | 923 | Serum Cholesterol 5.9 mmols/L | | 4056 | |
| 23.04.2003 | 08.04.1961 | F | | 902 | 909 | Inflamed & itchy abrasion on the (L) upper arm | Flucloxacillin & Fusidic Acid 2% + 1% Hydrocortisone cream | 407 | |
| 24.04.2003 | 26.07.1924 | M | RTI | 946 | 957 | Chesty cough & wheezy | Amoxycillin, Erythromycin & Tiotropium | 4270 | |
| 28.04.2003 | 15.02.1927 | F | URTI | 929 | 934 | Sore throat | Erythromycin | 4495 | Script for Adcal D3 given. |
| 22.04.2003 | 28.06.1994 | F | Pain | 1124 | 1127 | Sore (R) arm for 2 weeks | Ibuprofen | 4502 | |

Result of a query that lists all consultations from the 22nd to the end of April 2003 (ConsultationsSeenFrom22ndTillEndOfApr2003)

| SurgeryDate | DateOfBirth | Sex | Diagnosis | TimeIn | TimeOut | Complaints | Treatments | NumbersID | Notes |
|---|---|---|---|---|---|---|---|---|---|
| 25.04.2003 | 03.04.1969 | F |  | 1026 | 1045 | Script for Salbutamol easi breathe inhaler & Lansoprazole given |  | 4508 | Referred to One Stop Endoscopy Unit, SGH. Penicillin allergy. |
| 29.04.2003 | 23.05.1987 | F |  | 1726 | 1731 | Recurrent sore throats | Erythromycin | 4563 | Penicillin allergy. |
| 28.04.2003 | 24.11.1973 | M | Revisit | 1745 | 1749 | Gets bad headaches in Sunlight from his (R) dilated pupil | Referred to Ophthalmologist | 4565 |  |
| 25.04.2003 | 19.02.1974 | M | Rash | 1718 | 1721 | Small lesion on scalp, ?BCC | Referred to Dermatologist | 4566 |  |
| 23.04.2003 | 17.10.1928 | M |  | 1017 | 1024 | To take the Fleet enema for Barium enema preparation of his bowels |  | 4611 |  |
| 22.04.2003 | 22.04.1959 | F | S/Leave | 1657 | 1706 | Depression - Private |  | 463 |  |
| 28.04.2003 | 22.04.1959 | F | S/Leave | 1722 | 1724 | Depression |  | 463 |  |
| 23.04.2003 | 22.11.1983 | F | RTI | 1808 | 1815 | Cough & fever | Amoxycillin & Ibuprofen | 464 |  |
| 25.04.2003 | 21.09.1923 | M | Rash | 944 | 949 | Shingles rash on S1 distribution on the (L) side | Famciclovir | 4692 |  |
| 25.04.2003 | 13.03.1932 | M |  | 1752 | 1804 | Injection Zoladex given |  | 4699 |  |
| 29.04.2003 | 28.11.1991 | M |  | 1638 | 1648 | Possible balanitis | Trimethoprim | 5079 |  |

Result of a query that lists all consultations from the 22nd to the end of April 2003 (ConsultationsSeenFrom22ndTillEndOfApr2003)

| SurgeryDate | DateOfBirth | Sex | Diagnosis | TimeIn | TimeOut | Complaints | Treatments | NumbersID | Notes |
|---|---|---|---|---|---|---|---|---|---|
| 25.04.2003 | 11.01.1957 | F |  | 1632 | 1641 | PER VAGINA bleeding for the past 4 weeks after stopping Depo-Provera injection | Norethisterone | 5113 |  |
| 23.04.2003 | 31.10.1920 | F | Pain | 1024 | 1031 | Pain & swelling (R) knee following fall | For X-Ray | 5160 | For TSH. |
| 28.04.2003 | 06.01.1978 | M | Pain | 1749 | 1753 | Pain (L) Achilles tendon area | For Physiotherapy | 555 |  |
| 25.04.2003 | 09.02.1963 | F |  | 935 | 9440 | Ears are blocked with wax | Ear syringing to be done by P/Nurse | 5567 |  |
| 25.04.2003 | 29.10.1949 | F |  | 949 | 1003 | Heavy irregular periods with clots over the past 3 cycles | Referred to Gynaecologist (Basildon Hospital) | 5567 | For USScan of the uterus (urgent), B12, Folate & serum Ferritin. |
| 29.04.2003 | 12.09.1964 | M | Rash | 1703 | 1714 | Mole on the back | Referred to Dermatologist | 5568 | Low back pain, Rx. Dihydrocodeine. For Lumbar Spine X-Ray. |
| 29.04.2003 | 27.07.1983 | F |  | 1731 | 1745 | Septic abrasion on (L) thigh | Flucloxacillin & Fusidic Acid cream | 5588 | FP1001 (GMS4) form completed. |
| 25.04.2003 | 13.06.1997 | F |  | 1703 | 1705 | Hay fever | Loratadine suspension | 5632 |  |
| 29.04.2003 | 09.07.1964 | F |  | 1240 | 1250 | Diarrhoea, dizziness & cough | Erythromycin & Prochlorperazine | 5729 | FP1001 (GMS4) form completed. Home visit. |

Result of a query that lists all consultations from the 22nd to the end of April 2003 (ConsultationsSeenFrom22ndTillEndOfApr2003)

| SurgeryDate | DateOfBirth | Sex | Diagnosis | TimeIn | TimeOut | Complaints | Treatments | NumbersID | Notes |
|---|---|---|---|---|---|---|---|---|---|
| 28.04.2003 | 05.07.1970 | F | | 1636 | 1641 | Deafness in (R) ear following cold | Amoxycillin & Otomize ear spray | 5774 | |
| 23.04.2003 | 16.08.1950 | F | Revisit | 923 | 933 | Still has neck ache | For Physiotherapy | 583 | Penicillin allergy. |
| 22.04.2003 | 08.09.1964 | F | RTI | 1741 | 1751 | Cough | Amoxycillin | 5895 | |
| 22.04.2003 | 19.01.1983 | F | | 1751 | 1806 | Script for Dianette given | | 5907 | Penicillin allergy. FP1001 (GMS4) form signed. |
| 23.04.2003 | 12.02.1938 | M | | 1630 | 1647 | X-Ray (R) knee: some degenerative OA changes seen. A small joint effusion is seen. No bony injury | | 5997 | |
| 25.04.2003 | 20.04.1933 | F | Pain | 920 | 929 | Pain in the muscles of the neck | Intralgin | 6110 | Script for Bumetanide given. |
| 24.04.2003 | 01.07.1998 | M | RTI | 910 | 914 | Chesty cough | Amoxycillin | 6120 | |
| 29.04.2003 | 19.01.1964 | F | | 1714 | 1720 | Run down & depressed | Referred to Practice Counsellor | 6196 | |
| 22.04.2003 | 20.12.1922 | F | | 1650 | 1657 | Paronychia (R) thumb | Flucloxacillin, Fusidic Acid cream & Co-codamol | 6237 | |
| 29.04.2003 | 20.12.1922 | F | UTI | 1657 | 1703 | Dysuria | For MSU | 6237 | |
| 23.04.2003 | 01.11.1998 | M | URTI | 1742 | 1746 | Bilateral ear ache | Amoxycillin & Paracetamol | 6266 | |

Result of a query that lists all consultations from the 22nd to the end of April 2003 (ConsultationsSeenFrom22ndTillEndOfApr2003)

| SurgeryDate | DateOfBirth | Sex | Diagnosis | TimeIn | TimeOut | Complaints | Treatments | NumbersID | Notes |
|---|---|---|---|---|---|---|---|---|---|
| 25.04.2003 | 24.04.1948 | F | | 929 | 935 | To continue on own medication for her arthritis | | 6321 | |
| 25.04.2003 | 22.07.1968 | F | RTI | 904 | 911 | Cough | Amoxycillin | 6339 | FP1001 (GMS4) form completed. |
| 22.04.2003 | 04.05.1961 | M | S/Leave | 1127 | 1136 | Chest infection - Private | | 6340 | Script for Erythromycin given. Penicillin allergy. |
| 28.04.2003 | 04.05.1961 | M | | 1027 | 1036 | Diabetic Clinic | | 6340 | Penicillin allergy. |
| 23.04.2003 | 21.05.1936 | M | Rash | 933 | 938 | Warry lesion on the (L) upper arm | Referred to Dermatologist | 6396 | |
| 23.04.2003 | 29.03.1974 | F | | 1725 | 1742 | Contact with Chicken Pox | For serum Varicella Zoster antibodies | 6489 | Trimethoprim allergy. 16/40 gestation. |
| 25.04.2003 | 01.09.1999 | M | | 1641 | 1649 | D&V | Electrolade | 6564 | |
| 24.04.2003 | 28.11.1978 | F | S/Leave | 1055 | 1101 | Gall stones & Pregnant | Paracetamol | 6636 | |
| 22.04.2003 | 08.05.1939 | F | | 1021 | 1029 | For repeat FBC in 6 months | | 6643 | |
| 22.04.2003 | 02.05.1929 | F | | 1043 | 1102 | Painful & tender (R) calf | Referred to DVT Clinic, SGH | 6693 | |
| 29.04.2003 | 24.02.1969 | F | | 1724 | 1726 | (L) eye goes itchy & blood shot | To see own Optician | 6700 | |
| 24.04.2003 | 04.05.1937 | F | | 1018 | 1032 | USScan Abdomen/ Pelvis: Huge parapelvic cyst possibly on (L) kidney | Referred to Urologist | 6723 | |

31

Result of a query that lists all consultations from the 22nd to the end of April 2003 (ConsultationsSeenFrom22ndTillEndOfApr2003)

| SurgeryDate | DateOfBirth | Sex | Diagnosis | TimeIn | TimeOut | Complaints | Treatments | NumbersID | Notes |
|---|---|---|---|---|---|---|---|---|---|
| 29.04.2003 | 18.07.1955 | M | UTI | 1020 | 1024 | Fever, joint ache & dysuria | Trimethoprim | 6841 | For MSU. |
| 29.04.2003 | 25.07.2000 | F | URTI | 1024 | 1031 | Infected rhinorrhoea | Amoxycillin & Ibuprofen | 6849 | |
| 29.04.2003 | 15.07.1955 | F | S/Leave | 918 | 921 | Stress | | 6857 | |
| 29.04.2003 | 29.04.1955 | F | Rash | 931 | 937 | Eczema on face, very itchy | 1% Hydrocortisone ointment | 6862 | |
| 23.04.2003 | 01.01.1962 | M | S/Leave | 938 | 943 | Anxiety - Med. 5 | | 6879 | |
| 24.04.2003 | 19.10.1971 | M | | 957 | 1009 | He will go & think about the options of getting the vasectomy done | | 6891 | |
| 25.04.2003 | 16.05.1964 | M | | 1710 | 1718 | Slightly itchy lump near the anus | Scheriproct ointment | 6940 | For Physiotherapy. |
| 22.04.2003 | 27.03.1935 | M | | 1730 | 1741 | The Parking Badge Scheme for Disabled People Medical Practitioner Report completed | | 6942 | |
| 29.04.2003 | 03.03.1934 | M | | 1748 | 1802 | I explained to him that I cannot give injection to his scapula region for his pain | | 6984 | |
| 24.04.2003 | 31.10.2000 | M | URTI | 1051 | 1055 | Infected rhinorrhoea & vomiting | Amoxycillin, Metoclopramide & Paracetamol | 6986 | |

Result of a query that lists all consultations from the 22nd to the end of April 2003 (ConsultationsSeenFrom22ndTillEndOfApr2003)

| SurgeryDate | DateOfBirth | Sex | Diagnosis | TimeIn | TimeOut | Complaints | Treatments | NumbersID | Notes |
|---|---|---|---|---|---|---|---|---|---|
| 23.04.2003 | 09.02.1980 | F | | 1034 | 1041 | Eyes are very itchy | Sodium Cromoglycate eye drops | 7148 | Penicillin allergy. 21/40 gestation. |
| 28.04.2003 | 05.11.1980 | M | Pain | 955 | 1002 | (L) shoulder pain & back pain | Diclofenac enteric coated | 7169 | Dizziness & polyuria. For FBC & Fasting Glucose. |
| 25.04.2003 | 15.03.1922 | F | Pain | 911 | 920 | Pain & swelling (L) knee | Co-codamol | 7229 | For X-Ray. Script for Salbutamol easi-breathe inhaler given. |
| 29.04.2003 | 14.11.1949 | F | Revisit | 925 | 931 | Still has neck & (R) shoulder pain | Referred to Physiotherapy | 7283 | |
| 25.04.2003 | 17.08.1952 | F | S/Leave | 900 | 904 | Back Pain | | 7291 | |
| 29.04.2003 | 03.07.1938 | M | | 957 | 1020 | (L) sided weakness, ?(L) CVA | Referred to Medical Dr. on call, SGH | 7305 | |
| 25.04.2003 | 23.11.1975 | M | URTI | 1705 | 1710 | Sore throat | Amoxycillin | 7318 | |
| 22.04.2003 | 12.11.1999 | M | RTI | 1642 | 1650 | Cough | Amoxycillin & Paracetamol | 7335 | |
| 23.04.2003 | 01.10.1990 | F | | 1103 | 1113 | Social Services annual Medical examination done | | 7365 | |
| 23.04.2003 | 20.05.1988 | F | | 1050 | 1103 | Social Services annual Medical examination done | | 7367 | |
| 25.04.2003 | 06.01.1946 | M | RTI | 1320 | 1330 | Cough, diarrhoea & dizziness | Erythromycin & Prochlorperazine | 7383 | Home visit. |

33

## Result of a query that lists all consultations from the 22nd to the end of April 2003 (ConsultationsSeenFrom22ndTillEndOfApr2003)

| SurgeryDate | DateOfBirth | Sex | Diagnosis | TimeIn | TimeOut | Complaints | Treatments | NumbersID | Notes |
|---|---|---|---|---|---|---|---|---|---|
| 24.04.2003 | 13.02.2002 | F | URTI | 1045 | 1051 | Infected rhinorrhoea & vomiting | Amoxycillin, Metoclopramide & Paracetamol | 7392 | |
| 29.04.2003 | 11.05.1941 | F | | 921 | 925 | For repeat Cholesterol with P/Nurse in 6 months | | 7396 | |
| 22.04.2003 | 23.04.1947 | M | S/Leave | 1706 | 1712 | MUA & Injection bilateral shoulders | | 7440 | Penicillin allergy. |
| 23.04.2003 | 30.09.1923 | M | RTI | 1722 | 1725 | Chesty cough | Amoxycillin | 7457 | Ciprofloxacin allergy. |
| 29.04.2003 | 27.08.1997 | F | | 1046 | 1049 | Vomiting | Electrolade & Metoclopramide | 7459 | |
| 29.04.2003 | 30.01.2001 | F | | 1043 | 1046 | D&V | Electrolade | 7461 | |
| 29.04.2003 | 03.05.1944 | F | | 1031 | 1039 | Script for Bendrofluazide given | | 7499 | Script for Lamotrigine given. |
| 29.04.2003 | 25.08.1937 | M | Pain | 937 | 945 | Pain (R) elbow | Injection MethylPrednisolone 40mg, Lidocaine 10mg/ml | 7510 | |
| 23.04.2003 | 31.08.1971 | M | | 909 | 918 | Male fertility test normal | | 7523 | |
| 29.04.2003 | 20.12.1943 | F | | 1634 | 1638 | For TFTs | | 7524 | Penicillin allergy. |
| 25.04.2003 | 21.11.1948 | M | Revisit | 1045 | 1053 | Ear ache again after swimming | Amoxycillin & Otomize ear spray | 7542 | |
| 22.04.2003 | 11.08.1952 | F | S/Leave | 1036 | 1039 | Injury to (R) foot - Med. 5 | | 7544 | |

Result of a query that lists all consultations from the 22nd to the end of April 2003 (ConsultationsSeenFrom22ndTillEndOfApr2003)

| SurgeryDate | DateOfBirth | Sex | Diagnosis | TimeIn | TimeOut | Complaints | Treatments | NumbersID | Notes |
|---|---|---|---|---|---|---|---|---|---|
| 29.04.2003 | 31.07.1918 | F | | 907 | 907 | X-Ray (L) toe: Prominent hallux valgus deformity of the 1st MTPJ | Referred to Podiatrist | 7568 | For Urates. |
| 28.04.2003 | 12.01.1982 | M | Pain | 934 | 942 | Chest Pain | Co-codamol & Diclofenac enteric coated | 7581 | |
| 28.04.2003 | 09.02.1940 | M | | 1641 | 1647 | For MSU | | 7596 | |
| 22.04.2003 | 22.05.1920 | F | URTI | 1102 | 1112 | Sore throat | Erythromycin | 7601 | Penicillin allergy. |
| 29.04.2003 | 09.10.1974 | F | | 1648 | 1651 | Recurrent UTIs | Referred to ENT Surgeon | 7618 | |
| 25.04.2003 | 18.10.1966 | F | | 1053 | 1110 | Routine A/Natal check | | 7634 | |
| 24.04.2003 | 09.12.1962 | F | | 914 | 921 | (R) Cervical lymphadenopathy | For FBC | 764 | FP1001 (GMS4) form completed. |
| 24.04.2003 | 25.06.1919 | F | | 1101 | 1112 | Referred to Gynaecologist (Basildon Hospital) regarding her Ring Pessary | | 7654 | |
| 28.04.2003 | 27.08.1952 | F | | 910 | 918 | USScan of the abdomen - large solitary gallbladder calculus | Referred to Surgeon (BUPA) | 7676 | For TFTs. |
| 23.04.2003 | 03.11.1993 | F | Rash | 1011 | 1017 | Sore & itchy spots on (L) arm & (L) nipple area | Flucloxacillin & Fusidic Acid 2% + 1% Hydrocortisone cream | 7711 | |

35

Result of a query that lists all consultations from the 22nd to the end of April 2003 (ConsultationsSeenFrom22ndTillEndOfApr2003)

| SurgeryDate | DateOfBirth | Sex | Diagnosis | TimeIn | TimeOut | Complaints | Treatments | NumbersID | Notes |
|---|---|---|---|---|---|---|---|---|---|
| 29.04.2003 | 27.12.2000 | F | RTI | 1745 | 1748 | Cough | Erythromycin | 7733 | Penicillin allergy. |
| 28.04.2003 | 20.02.1990 | M | Rash | 1719 | 1722 | Itchy rash on the (L) sole of the foot | Miconazole 2% + 1% Hydrocortisone cream | 7737 | |
| 23.04.2003 | 17.02.1949 | M | | 1652 | 1708 | To get drugs as repeat prescription | | 7758 | |
| 28.04.2003 | 15.05.1989 | F | | 1705 | 1715 | Awaiting a list of her repeat medication | | 7780 | |
| 23.04.2003 | 01.09.1961 | M | Pain | 1815 | 1819 | Pain (R) knee after skiing | For X-Ray | 832 | |
| 25.04.2003 | 04.03.1947 | M | Revisit | 1656 | 1703 | Sinus problems is still as bad | Budesonide aqua nasal spray | 88 | Referred to ENT Surgeon. |
| 23.04.2003 | 16.07.1983 | F | | 1708 | 1722 | Inflamed area over the head of the (L) 5th metacarpal | Fusidic Acid cream | 967 | |
| 22.04.2003 | 08.05.1962 | M | Depression | 1631 | 1639 | Anxiety & Panic attacks | Fluoxetine | Temp | |
| 25.04.2003 | 25.09.1984 | M | Rash | 1804 | 1810 | Psoriatic plaque lesions | Clobetasol 0.05% cream | Temp | |
| 28.04.2003 | 30.09.1934 | F | Pain | 1002 | 1009 | Pain (R) arm & tingling in fingers | Ibuprofen, Ranitidine & Co-codamol | Temp | |
| 28.04.2003 | 31.01.1985 | F | Pain | 1715 | 1719 | Post LSCS pain | Co-codamol | Temp | |

## Result of a query that lists all consultations from the 22nd to the end of April 2004 (ConsultationsSeenFrom22ndTillEndOfApr2004)

| SurgeryDate | DateOfBirth | Sex | Diagnosis | TimeIn | TimeOut | Complaints | Treatments | NumbersID | Notes |
|---|---|---|---|---|---|---|---|---|---|
| 26.04.2004 | 08.02.1939 | F | | 1032 | 1044 | Script for Amoxycillin, Chloramphenicol eye drops & Co-codamol given | | 113 | Trimethoprim allergy. |
| 22.04.2004 | 26.08.1966 | M | | 1007 | 1014 | Septic wound on fore-head | Flucloxacillin | 115 | |
| 26.04.2004 | 09.05.1969 | M | Conjunctivitis | 1752 | 1757 | Sticky, red & sore eyes | Chloramphenicol eye drops | 1152 | |
| 27.04.2004 | 22.08.1963 | M | Pain | 900 | 907 | (L) knee is painful & clicks | For X-Ray (L) knee | 1370 | |
| 26.04.2004 | 21.09.1924 | F | | 910 | 933 | Subconjunctival hemorrhage (L) eye | Chloramphenicol eye drops | 1419 | Script for Flucloxacillin given. |
| 28.04.2004 | 06.08.1941 | M | | 941 | 948 | To try own Paracetamol for the pain at the back of the eyes | | 1425 | |
| 27.04.2004 | 28.07.1936 | M | | 956 | 1009 | Script for Flucloxacillin, Zopiclone & Fusidic Acid 2% + 1% Hydrocortisone cream given | | 1508 | |
| 29.04.2004 | 11.11.1940 | M | Revisit | 932 | 941 | Still feels he has chest infection | Amoxycillin | 1611 | |
| 23.04.2004 | 02.09.1941 | F | Pain | 1648 | 1707 | Migraine | Ergotamine with cyclizine & caffeine | 1797 | Script for Propranolol given. |

37

Result of a query that lists all consultations from the 22nd to the end of April 2004 (ConsultationsSeenFrom22ndTillEndOfApr2004)

| SurgeryDate | DateOfBirth | Sex | Diagnosis | TimeIn | TimeOut | Complaints | Treatments | NumbersID | Notes |
|---|---|---|---|---|---|---|---|---|---|
| 23.04.2004 | 11.03.1968 | F | | 917 | 924 | For Fasting Glucose | | 2 | |
| 29.04.2004 | 12.02.1917 | M | RTI | 1318 | 1340 | Chesty cough | Amoxycillin & Erythromycin | 2006 | Home visit. |
| 28.04.2004 | 03.11.1957 | F | | 1644 | 1651 | LH & FSH results suggest that she is menopausal | | 2210 | |
| 26.04.2004 | 16.01.1982 | F | | 1745 | 1752 | For FBC & Rheumatoid Factor | | 2220 | Penicillin allergy. |
| 26.04.2004 | 16.06.1915 | M | | 1632 | 1644 | Unwell, jaundiced & no appetite | Referred to MAU, SGH | 245 | |
| 23.04.2004 | 09.01.1938 | F | S/Leave | 1753 | 1801 | (L) knee replacement - Med. 5 | | 2508 | |
| 23.04.2004 | 19.03.1925 | F | | 1021 | 1040 | Polyuria & polydipsia | For U/Es, Fasting Glucose & FBC | 2634 | |
| 23.04.2004 | 30.11.1936 | M | RTI | 924 | 929 | Tickly cough | Amoxycillin | 2793 | |
| 26.04.2004 | 06.04.1924 | F | RTI | 1010 | 1016 | Difficulty breathing | Erythromycin | 2909 | Penicillin allergy. |
| 26.04.2004 | 11.09.1914 | F | Rash | 945 | 950 | Multiple wounds on the limbs | Referred to Dermatologist (Basildon Hospital) | 3004 | |
| 23.04.2004 | 06.12.1952 | F | | 900 | 907 | Persistent cough for 5 years | Referred to Chest Physician | 3082 | Palpitations, referred to Cardiologist. |
| 28.04.2004 | 20.02.1920 | F | Pain | 932 | 936 | Pain at the back of the neck | Etodolac | 323 | |
| 27.04.2004 | 31.10.1915 | F | | 135 | 1050 | USScan of Thyroid showed multiple nodules | Referred to Physician | 336 | |

## Result of a query that lists all consultations from the 22nd to the end of April 2004 (ConsultationsSeenFrom22ndTillEndOfApr2004)

| SurgeryDate | DateOfBirth | Sex | Diagnosis | TimeIn | TimeOut | Complaints | Treatments | NumbersID | Notes |
|---|---|---|---|---|---|---|---|---|---|
| 28.04.2004 | 20.01.1969 | M | Revisit | 1015 | 1021 | Lump on lower back is getting bigger | Referred to Surgeon (BUPA) | 3471 | |
| 23.04.2004 | 19.06.1944 | F | | 942 | 950 | 2nd EDOS study visit | | 3475 | |
| 27.04.2004 | 28.10.1960 | M | | 1029 | 1035 | Fever & diarrhoea | FBC, Malarial parasites & Stool for C&S | 3501 | |
| 28.04.2004 | 12.08.1944 | M | S/Leave | 1745 | 1800 | Pain in (R) heel - Med. 5 | | 364 | Script for Co-codamol, Ibuprofen & Rabeprazole given. |
| 26.04.2004 | 05.12.1937 | M | | 958 | 1005 | Infected stye (L) lower eye lid | Chloramphenicol eye drops | 3646 | |
| 26.04.2004 | 16.11.1987 | F | | 1651 | 1703 | To try OTC Canesten cream for her vulvar-vaginal itching | | 3770 | |
| 23.04.2004 | 31.03.1986 | F | | 907 | 917 | Hay fever | Levocetirizine | 4001 | Hyperhidrosis, Rx. Aluminium chloride hexahydrate solution 20%. |
| 29.04.2004 | 09.03.1993 | F | | 926 | 932 | Hay fever | Cetirizine | 4048 | |
| 29.04.2004 | 04.09.1952 | M | Rash | 1020 | 1028 | His psoriasis has flared up | Referred to Dermatologist (Basildon Hospital) | 4128 | |
| 23.04.2004 | 03.03.1994 | M | | 1723 | 1728 | Abscess (L) upper gum | Amoxycillin | 4386 | |

Result of a query that lists all consultations from the 22nd to the end of April 2004 (ConsultationsSeenFrom22ndTillEndOfApr2004)

| SurgeryDate | DateOfBirth | Sex | Diagnosis | TimeIn | TimeOut | Complaints | Treatments | NumbersID | Notes |
|---|---|---|---|---|---|---|---|---|---|
| 29.04.2004 | 04.10.1928 | F | Pain | 950 | 1005 | Multiple joints pains | Referred to Rheumatologist | 4403 | |
| 27.04.2004 | 09.04.1938 | M | | 907 | 914 | To Persevere for now with Coracten | | 4519 | Tetracycline allergy. |
| 26.04.2004 | 28.08.1994 | F | Rash | 1703 | 1713 | Mole on face | Referred to Dermatologist (BUPA) | 4545 | |
| 26.04.2004 | 24.11.1973 | M | S/Leave | 1016 | 1026 | Throat infection - Private & Med. 3 | | 4565 | |
| 22.04.2004 | 21.02.1976 | F | Depression | 922 | 932 | Weepy & separated from partner | Referred to P/ Counsellor | 4586 | |
| 23.04.2004 | 13.03.1932 | M | | 1050 | 1055 | Injection Zoladex given | | 4699 | |
| 28.04.2004 | 30.05.1938 | F | Lump | 904 | 912 | Sebaceous cyst behind (L) ear lobe | Referred to Surgeon | 4760 | Penicillin allergy. |
| 22.04.2004 | 28.01.1953 | F | | 932 | 950 | To try Oil of evening Primrose for her bilateral breast tenderness | | 4781 | |
| 28.04.2004 | 09.12.1939 | M | | 920 | 932 | Script for Salicylates with Nicotinate cream given | | 4902 | |
| 29.04.2004 | 14.10.1969 | F | S/Leave | 1050 | 1059 | (R) Carpal tunnel decompression - Med. 5 | | 5122 | |
| 29.04.2004 | 07.10.1944 | M | S/Leave | 1028 | 1032 | Depression - Med. 5 | | 5141 | |
| 28.04.2004 | 12.02.1996 | M | | 1010 | 1015 | Blocked tear ducts | Referred to Ophthalmologist | 5165 | Plaster allergy. |

Result of a query that lists all consultations from the 22nd to the end of April 2004 (ConsultationsSeenFrom22ndTillEndOfApr2004)

| SurgeryDate | DateOfBirth | Sex | Diagnosis | TimeIn | TimeOut | Complaints | Treatments | NumbersID | Notes |
|---|---|---|---|---|---|---|---|---|---|
| 28.04.2004 | 23.10.1956 | F | S/Leave | 948 | 951 | Depression - Med. 5 | | 5177 | |
| 26.04.2004 | 18.02.1943 | M | | 1713 | 1720 | Getting more deaf | Referred to ENT Surgeon | 519 | |
| 26.04.2004 | 17.05.1943 | M | | 1725 | 1735 | Script for Fexofenadine given | | 5208 | |
| 22.04.2004 | 29.08.1976 | M | Rash | 901 | 908 | Itchy & sore rash all over | Referred to Dermatologist (Basildon Hospital) | 522 | Script for Erythromycin given. Penicillin allergy. |
| 23.04.2004 | 27.10.1988 | F | | 1728 | 1732 | Warts on the (R) hand | Salicylic acid topical solution 26% | 5235 | |
| 26.04.2004 | 04.04.1996 | M | | 940 | 945 | Script for Salbutamol inhaler given | | 5282 | |
| 28.04.2004 | 01.02.1996 | M | | 1707 | 1716 | For MSU, FBC, LFTs, Clotting screen & Fasting Glucose | | 5336 | |
| 26.04.2004 | 14.10.1928 | M | RTI | 1335 | 1345 | Chesty cough | Amoxycillin | 537 | Home visit. |
| 26.04.2004 | 02.06.1994 | F | Rash | 1644 | 1647 | Impetigo rash on face | Mupirocin cream | 5375 | |
| 22.04.2004 | 04.07.1986 | F | | 1014 | 1018 | To try OTC Co-codamol & Ibuprofen for her whiplash injury | | 5386 | |
| 22.04.2004 | 25.06.1921 | M | | 1036 | 1050 | Script for Atenolol, Quinine Sulphate & Chloramphenicol eye drops given | | 5474 | |

Result of a query that lists all consultations from the 22nd to the end of April 2004 (ConsultationsSeenFrom22ndTillEndOfApr2004)

| SurgeryDate | DateOfBirth | Sex | Diagnosis | TimeIn | TimeOut | Complaints | Treatments | NumbersID | Notes |
|---|---|---|---|---|---|---|---|---|---|
| 29.04.2004 | 25.06.1921 | M | RTI | 1032 | 1038 | Chesty cough | Amoxycillin | 5474 | |
| 28.04.2004 | 09.12.1964 | F | | 1702 | 1707 | For FBC & Fasting Glucose | | 5534 | |
| 27.04.2004 | 04.05.1989 | M | | 1009 | 1014 | To go to A/E regarding injury (R) ankle | | 5585 | Penicillin allergy. |
| 26.04.2004 | 09.07.1969 | M | | 1647 | 1651 | Hay fever | Cetirizine | 563 | |
| 28.04.2004 | 25.08.1949 | F | Pain | 951 | 958 | Epigastric pain | Rabeprazole | 5846 | Septrin & Penicillin allergy. |
| 23.04.2004 | 02.06.1977 | M | | 1746 | 1753 | Septic wound on the (R) Index finger | Erythromycin | 585 | |
| 26.04.2004 | 13.12.1982 | M | S/Leave | 950 | 958 | Injury (L) thumb - Med. 5 | | 586 | Penicillin allergy. |
| 27.04.2004 | 03.12.1955 | F | S/Leave | 1014 | 1020 | Depression - Med. 5 | | 614 | |
| 28.04.2004 | 11.09.1978 | M | Pain | 1632 | 1640 | Pain (R) knee | For X-Ray | 6244 | Penicillin allergy. |
| 29.04.2004 | 05.11.1993 | M | URTI | 921 | 926 | Sore throat | Amoxycillin | 6309 | Script for Loratadine given. |
| 28.04.2004 | 05.03.1973 | F | | 1805 | 1810 | Weepy | Referred to P/ Counsellor | 6320 | Penicillin allergy. |
| 26.04.2004 | 14.09.1972 | F | | 1757 | 1805 | T.A.T.T | For FBC, TFTs & Fasting Glucose | 6337 | Penicillin allergy. |
| 29.04.2004 | 06.12.1962 | M | Pain | 941 | 950 | Persistent dull ache in the chest | Referred to Cardiologist | 6415 | |
| 26.04.2004 | 15.12.1965 | F | | 1044 | 1050 | Burst condom | Levonorgestrel | 6422 | |
| 28.04.2004 | 29.07.1938 | M | | 1716 | 1720 | Script for Co-codamol given | | 6445 | For X-Ray of the (L) hip. |
| 26.04.2004 | 27.07.1999 | M | | 1050 | 1059 | Hay fever | Loratadine syrup | 6534 | |
| 29.04.2004 | 25.01.1988 | F | RTI | 1015 | 1020 | Cough | Amoxycillin | 6586 | |

Result of a query that lists all consultations from the 22nd to the end of April 2004 (ConsultationsSeenFrom22ndTillEndOfApr2004)

| SurgeryDate | DateOfBirth | Sex | Diagnosis | TimeIn | TimeOut | Complaints | Treatments | NumbersID | Notes |
|---|---|---|---|---|---|---|---|---|---|
| 28.04.2004 | 19.09.1925 | F | | 1810 | 1817 | Script for Etodolac given | | 665 | Penicillin allergy. |
| 28.04.2004 | 04.05.1937 | F | | 936 | 941 | Small wounds on the (R) leg | Flucloxacillin | 6723 | |
| 22.04.2004 | 22.02.1963 | M | S/Leave | 1000 | 1007 | Back Pain | Dihydrocodeine & Diclofenac e/c | 6739 | |
| 28.04.2004 | 23.11.1946 | M | S/Leave | 912 | 920 | Back Pain | | 6822 | |
| 22.04.2004 | 28.04.1936 | F | | 1018 | 1023 | For Physiotherapy | | 6953 | Aspirin allergy. |
| 23.04.2004 | 26.05.1941 | F | | 957 | 1017 | To lose 2.5kg in 4 weeks before she can go on Xenical | | 701 | |
| 26.04.2004 | 01.01.1968 | F | | 1740 | 1745 | Script for Tranexamic Acid given | | 7021 | |
| 26.04.2004 | 06.12.1940 | M | | 933 | 940 | Mucus at the back of the throat | Amoxycillin | 7145 | Script for Betahistine given. |
| 23.04.2004 | 24.06.2001 | M | Revisit | 1017 | 1021 | Still has chesty cough despite antibiotics | For CXR | 7155 | |
| 26.04.2004 | 17.08.1952 | F | | 1720 | 1725 | Script for Dihydrocodeine & Rabeprazole given | | 7291 | |
| 22.04.2004 | 09.09.1944 | M | Hypertension | 908 | 922 | BP 174/86 | Nifedipine m/r capsule | 7324 | |
| 23.04.2004 | 25.08.1933 | F | | 1638 | 1648 | Script for Prochlorperazine & Atenolol given | | 7428 | |
| 29.04.2004 | 03.07.1950 | F | | 912 | 921 | Prickly heat rash | Chlorpheniramine | 7468 | |

Result of a query that lists all consultations from the 22nd to the end of April 2004 (ConsultationsSeenFrom22ndTillEndOfApr2004)

| SurgeryDate | DateOfBirth | Sex | Diagnosis | TimeIn | TimeOut | Complaints | Treatments | NumbersID | Notes |
|---|---|---|---|---|---|---|---|---|---|
| 23.04.2004 | 21.04.1990 | M | Revisit | 1716 | 1723 | Tender lump on (R) face is still present | Referred to Maxillo-facial Surgeon (Basildon Hospital) | 7560 | |
| 22.04.2004 | 27.10.1966 | M | Pain | 950 | 1000 | Pain (L) groin & haematuria | Referred to Surgical Dr. on call, Basildon (Hospital) | 7571 | |
| 27.04.2004 | 22.06.1974 | F | S/Leave | 948 | 956 | Diarrhoea & vomiting | | 7596 | Stool for C&S. |
| 22.04.2004 | 17.07.1940 | F | | 1030 | 1036 | To take Atenolol 50mg daily | | 7627 | |
| 23.04.2004 | 03.10.1937 | F | RTI | 1740 | 1746 | Cough | Erythromycin | 7633 | Script for Clotrimazole 1% + 1% Hydrocortisone cream. Penicillin allergy. |
| 26.04.2004 | 05.12.2002 | M | | 1026 | 1032 | To apply own Calamine lotion to viral rash | | 7637 | |
| 27.04.2004 | 29.10.1989 | M | | 927 | 942 | Mum to contact hospital regarding writing to us for USScan of his kidneys for him | | 7660 | Penicillin allergy. |
| 27.04.2004 | 28.03.1970 | F | Pain | 942 | 948 | Low back pain | For X-Ray | 7661 | |
| 28.04.2004 | 01.06.1932 | M | Revisit | 958 | 1005 | (L) thumb is still swollen | Etodolac | 7685 | For X-Ray. |

## Result of a query that lists all consultations from the 22nd to the end of April 2004 (ConsultationsSeenFrom22ndTillEndOfApr2004)

| SurgeryDate | DateOfBirth | Sex | Diagnosis | TimeIn | TimeOut | Complaints | Treatments | NumbersID | Notes |
|---|---|---|---|---|---|---|---|---|---|
| 28.04.2004 | 04.01.1950 | F | Revisit | 1005 | 1010 | She still has boils on her leg | Erythromycin | 7685 | Penicillin allergy. |
| 28.04.2004 | 26.04.1943 | M | URTI | 1730 | 1735 | Sore throat | Amoxycillin | 7697 | |
| 23.04.2004 | 15.02.1943 | F | Lump | 1105 | 1110 | Lump in (L) breast | Referred to Breast Surgeon | 7708 | |
| 23.04.2004 | 13.04.1944 | M | Lump | 1632 | 1638 | (R) Inguinal hernia | Referred to Surgeon | 7753 | |
| 29.04.2004 | 15.01.1938 | F | Revisit | 1005 | 1015 | Rash on (R) leg has got worse & spread | Referred to Dermatologist (Basildon Hospital) | 7798 | Erythromycin allergy. |
| 28.04.2004 | 11.11.1961 | M | | 1720 | 1730 | Dizzy spells | For FBC & Fasting Glucose | 7902 | |
| 29.04.2004 | 18.08.1963 | M | | 900 | 912 | Awaiting his Medical records regarding referral for his Lyme disease | | 7920 | |
| 27.04.2004 | 05.10.1976 | M | | 1020 | 1029 | Furuncles in (L) axilla | Flucloxacillin | 913 | For FBC & Fasting Glucose. |
| 26.04.2004 | 30.10.1984 | F | | 1805 | 1810 | To continue antibiotics far cat bites on her finger | | 980 | |
| 23.04.2004 | 10.10.1969 | M | URTI | 937 | 942 | Sore throat | Amoxycillin | NP (DS) | |
| 23.04.2004 | 27.08.1965 | M | S/Leave | 1707 | 1716 | Pain in both heels | | NP (DT) | |
| 26.04.2004 | 19.11.1977 | F | | 901 | 906 | Bleeds from back passage when she wipes herself | Prednisolone with Cinchocaine ointment | NP (KM) | |

45

### Result of a query that lists all consultations from the 22nd to the end of April 2004 (ConsultationsSeenFrom22ndTillEndOfApr2004)

| SurgeryDate | DateOfBirth | Sex | Diagnosis | TimeIn | TimeOut | Complaints | Treatments | NumbersID | Notes |
|---|---|---|---|---|---|---|---|---|---|
| 26.04.2004 | 15.05.1980 | F | Pain | 906 | 910 | (R) knee swelling & pain | For X-Ray | NP (SP) | Erythromycin allergy. |
| 28.04.2004 | 15.05.1980 | F | Pain | 1800 | 1805 | Pain in the (R) upper gum | Amoxycillin | NP (SP) | Erythromycin allergy. |
| 22.04.2004 | 15.11.1969 | M | Pain | 1023 | 1030 | Pain in (R) groin | Dihydrocodeine | Temp | |
| 28.04.2004 | 03.03.1973 | F | URTI | 1640 | 1644 | Running nose | Amoxycillin | Temp | |

### Result of a query that lists all consultations from the 22nd to the end of April 2005 (ConsultationsSeenFrom22ndTillEndOfApr2005)

| SurgeryDate | DateOfBirth | Sex | Diagnosis | TimeIn | TimeOut | Complaints | Treatments | NumbersID | Notes |
|---|---|---|---|---|---|---|---|---|---|
| 25.04.2005 | 07.01.1954 | F | Rash | 1746 | 1759 | Rosacea rash | Tetracycline | 1094 | |
| 29.04.2005 | 21.04.1959 | M | | 1716 | 1721 | To see Nurse regarding dietary advice about her high Cholesterol | | 1184 | |
| 29.04.2005 | 14.11.1963 | F | | 1712 | 1716 | Script for Tamoxifen given | | 1185 | |
| 28.04.2005 | 15.07.1936 | F | | 928 | 937 | Script for Simvastatin given | | 1309 | |
| 28.04.2005 | 15.02.1929 | F | Conjunctivitis | 1001 | 1012 | Weepy painful eyes | Chloramphenicol eye drops | 16 | Penicillin allergy. |
| 27.04.2005 | 23.01.1968 | F | URTI | 1004 | 1015 | Itchy ears | Dexamethasone with neomycin ear spray | 1679 | For FBC. |
| 25.04.2005 | 15.10.1923 | F | Pain | 927 | 946 | Sciatica pain | For Physiotherapy | 1711 | |

Result of a query that lists all consultations from the 22nd to the end of April 2005 (ConsultationsSeenFrom22ndTillEndOfApr2005)

| SurgeryDate | DateOfBirth | Sex | Diagnosis | TimeIn | TimeOut | Complaints | Treatments | NumbersID | Notes |
|---|---|---|---|---|---|---|---|---|---|
| 25.04.2005 | 19.01.1940 | F | | 1640 | 1651 | Script for Atenolol given | | 1850 | |
| 27.04.2005 | 19.08.1926 | F | | 1015 | 1024 | Script for Metformin given | | 1907 | |
| 29.04.2005 | 29.11.1929 | F | | 1035 | 1050 | Script for Prednisolone e/c, Frusemide & Simvastatin given | | 193 | |
| 26.04.2005 | 06.07.1936 | F | | 1650 | 1702 | Waiting to see the Cardiologist | | 2150 | |
| 26.04.2005 | 19.12.1949 | M | Revisit | 1748 | 1755 | Still has chesty cough | For CXR | 216 | |
| 29.04.2005 | 06.11.1915 | M | Pain | 923 | 931 | Pain in (R) groin | Co-codamol | 229 | |
| 25.04.2005 | 19.07.1925 | F | | 1657 | 1704 | To continue with soluble Aspirin | | 2290 | |
| 28.04.2005 | 07.11.1984 | F | | 1021 | 1031 | Routine P/Natal with baby in the Surgery | | 2438 | |
| 26.04.2005 | 05.11.1941 | M | | 1806 | 1813 | Private script for Viagra given | | 251 | Script for Diclofenac e/c given. |
| 25.04.2005 | 24.03.1959 | M | | 1014 | 1024 | To come back if alternating bowel habit continues or re-occurs | | 2580 | |
| 28.04.2005 | 17.12.1924 | M | | 1031 | 1041 | Insomnia | Temazepam | 2635 | |
| 27.04.2005 | 17.02.1958 | M | | 918 | 926 | Tender gland (R) chin | Amoxycillin | 3 | For FBC. For X-Ray (R) hip. |
| 26.04.2005 | 19.02.1942 | F | | 955 | 1006 | Script for Nicotine patch '20' given | | 3481 | |

47

## Result of a query that lists all consultations from the 22nd to the end of April 2005 (ConsultationsSeenFrom22ndTillEndOfApr2005)

| SurgeryDate | DateOfBirth | Sex | Diagnosis | TimeIn | TimeOut | Complaints | Treatments | NumbersID | Notes |
|---|---|---|---|---|---|---|---|---|---|
| 27.04.2005 | 18.02.1926 | F | | 1024 | 1032 | Script for Sodium bicarbonate ear drops given | | 3502 | Trimethoprim & Aspirin allergy. |
| 29.04.2005 | 15.07.1956 | M | Revisit | 920 | 923 | Recurrent (R) ear infection with discharge | Referred to ENT Surgeon (BUPA) | 352 | |
| 26.04.2005 | 21.11.1923 | M | URTI | 1713 | 1717 | Sore throat | Amoxycillin | 3730 | |
| 25.04.2005 | 24.09.1941 | F | | 1759 | 1808 | Rectal bleeding | Referred to Rectal Surgeon (urgent) | 3760 | |
| 28.04.2005 | 20.04.1936 | M | | 1741 | 1755 | For KUB USScan | | 3840 | |
| 25.04.2005 | 20.12.1931 | M | | 946 | 951 | (R) ear infection | Amoxycillin | 4020 | |
| 27.04.2005 | 22.02.1923 | F | | 1722 | 1736 | For FBC & CXR | | 4119 | |
| 29.04.2005 | 14.10.1958 | M | | 1819 | 1823 | Mouth ulcers | Amoxycillin | 4250 | |
| 28.04.2005 | 25.05.1931 | F | | 1644 | 1651 | Her son came in to enquire regarding holiday Sickness cancellation form | | 4339 | |
| 25.04.2005 | 25.03.1925 | F | | 1024 | 1029 | To observer her BP for now | | 4625 | |
| 28.04.2005 | 10.12.1944 | M | | 1755 | 1801 | T.A.T.T. | For FBC & TFTs | 4780 | For Lumbar Spine X-Ray. |
| 25.04.2005 | 28.02.1927 | M | | 1140 | 1153 | Inj. Zoladex given | | 4838 | |
| 26.04.2005 | 03.01.1904 | F | RTI | 910 | 928 | Cough | Amoxycillin | 4877 | For CXR. Script for Candesartan given. Lederfen allergy. |
| 25.04.2005 | 09.02.1965 | F | | 1721 | 1726 | For LH & FSH | | 5077 | |
| 27.04.2005 | 14.10.1969 | F | | 1651 | 1704 | For CXR | | 5122 | |

Result of a query that lists all consultations from the 22nd to the end of April 2005 (ConsultationsSeenFrom22ndTillEndOfApr2005)

| SurgeryDate | DateOfBirth | Sex | Diagnosis | TimeIn | TimeOut | Complaints | Treatments | NumbersID | Notes |
|---|---|---|---|---|---|---|---|---|---|
| 27.04.2005 | 04.12.1957 | F | | 938 | 950 | Script for Salmeterol with fluticasone cfc free inhaler (MDI) 25mcg + 250mcg & Prednisolone given | | 5228 | |
| 26.04.2005 | 17.10.1965 | F | URTI | 1025 | 1030 | Sore throat | Amoxycillin | 5571 | |
| 29.04.2005 | 24.11.1954 | F | | 1739 | 1743 | T.A.T.T. | For FBC & TFTs | 558 | |
| 28.04.2005 | 17.08.1947 | F | RTI | 1651 | 1656 | Chesty cough | Cefpodoxime | 56 | Script for Fluconazole given. |
| 27.04.2005 | 17.04.1923 | M | RTI | 1736 | 1742 | Cough | Ampicillin | 560 | |
| 29.04.2005 | 12.06.1946 | M | S/Leave | 1633 | 1646 | Acute Coronary Syndrome | | 584 | |
| 27.04.2005 | 13.04.1942 | M | | 1051 | 1058 | Script for Injection Methylprednisolone with lidocaine given | | 5876 | |
| 27.04.2005 | 13.04.1942 | M | | 1803 | 1820 | Injection Depo-Medrone with Lidocaine given to (L) shoulder | | 5876 | |
| 25.04.2005 | 01.01.1953 | M | | 901 | 908 | Private script for Cialis given | | 5975 | |
| 29.04.2005 | 17.12.1931 | M | | 912 | 920 | For Fasting Cholesterol, U/Es & FBC | | 5978 | |
| 28.04.2005 | 08.03.1961 | M | Revisit | 946 | 951 | Pain (R) elbow is worse | Referred to Orthopaedic Surgeon (BUPA) | 6198 | |

Result of a query that lists all consultations from the 22nd to the end of April 2005 (ConsultationsSeenFrom22ndTillEndOfApr2005)

| SurgeryDate | DateOfBirth | Sex | Diagnosis | TimeIn | TimeOut | Complaints | Treatments | NumbersID | Notes |
|---|---|---|---|---|---|---|---|---|---|
| 28.04.2005 | 10.01.1973 | F | | 957 | 1001 | Script for Metronidazole given | | 6305 | |
| 26.04.2005 | 13.10.1969 | F | | 1637 | 1650 | Script for NiQuitin CQ patch given | | 6327 | |
| 29.04.2005 | 29.07.1938 | M | RTI | 942 | 949 | Chesty cough | Amoxycillin | 6445 | |
| 26.04.2005 | 14.11.1916 | F | | 1710 | 1713 | Cough | Amoxycillin | 6591 | Daughter came to Surgery. |
| 26.04.2005 | 09.04.1944 | F | | 1702 | 1710 | Patient is to contact the Orthopaedic Surgeon's secretary directly | | 6592 | |
| 28.04.2005 | 07.07.1992 | M | | 925 | 928 | To see own Dentist regarding (L) upper jaw lump | | 6658 | |
| 26.04.2005 | 19.12.1974 | F | | 1755 | 1806 | Script for NiQuitin CQ patch given | | 6729 | |
| 27.04.2005 | 16.09.1936 | M | | 1000 | 1004 | Private script for Viagra given | | 693 | |
| 25.04.2005 | 25.02.1949 | M | | 1736 | 1746 | Lloyds TSB Insurance Medical Claim form completed | | 6956 | |
| 28.04.2005 | 11.01.1964 | F | S/Leave | 1635 | 1644 | EAU & Hysteroscopy - Med. 5 | | 6976 | |
| 25.04.2005 | 05.02.1943 | F | | 1726 | 1733 | Dizziness & nausea | Prochlorperazine | 7066 | |
| 26.04.2005 | 26.10.1959 | F | Pain | 1736 | 1741 | Painful (R) knee | For X-Ray | 7223 | |

Result of a query that lists all consultations from the 22nd to the end of April 2005 (ConsultationsSeenFrom22ndTillEndOfApr2005)

| SurgeryDate | DateOfBirth | Sex | Diagnosis | TimeIn | TimeOut | Complaints | Treatments | NumbersID | Notes |
|---|---|---|---|---|---|---|---|---|---|
| 28.04.2005 | 19.06.1944 | F | | 920 | 925 | To try OTC Nurofen & Gaviscon for her arthritis | | 7267 | |
| 29.04.2005 | 08.10.1963 | M | | 1743 | 1757 | Script for Gliclazide & Simvastatin given | | 7400 | |
| 29.04.2005 | 06.12.1964 | M | | 1757 | 1807 | Migraine headache | Frovatriptan | 7405 | |
| 29.04.2005 | 04.08.1936 | M | | 1002 | 1016 | Script for Co-codamol given | | 7443 | |
| 26.04.2005 | 04.04.1953 | M | Revisit | 1717 | 1720 | Lump on the penis is still sore | Referred to Urologist | 7467 | |
| 27.04.2005 | 03.05.1944 | F | | 1751 | 1754 | On Atorvastatin | | 7499 | Lamotrigine allergy. |
| 28.04.2005 | 19.09.1938 | F | | 937 | 946 | Script for Erythromycin given | | 7513 | |
| 25.04.2005 | 28.03.1960 | F | URTI | 1651 | 1657 | Sore throat | Amoxycillin | 7518 | Script for Dihydrocodeine given. |
| 27.04.2005 | 11.06.1972 | M | | 926 | 938 | For Physiotherapy | | 7552 | |
| 29.04.2005 | 25.07.1934 | M | | 931 | 942 | Script for Gliclazide given | | 7609 | |
| 27.04.2005 | 06.04.1938 | M | | 1712 | 1722 | Script for Allopurinol given | | 7626 | |
| 29.04.2005 | 05.12.2002 | M | | 955 | 1002 | Diarrhoea & vomiting | Oral rehydration salts oral powder | 7637 | Stool for C&S. |
| 27.04.2005 | 04.07.1938 | F | UTI | 1032 | 1047 | Pyrexial & low back pain | Amoxycillin | 7647 | Script for Bendrofluazide given. For MSU. |

Result of a query that lists all consultations from the 22nd to the end of April 2005 (ConsultationsSeenFrom22ndTillEndOfApr2005)

| SurgeryDate | DateOfBirth | Sex | Diagnosis | TimeIn | TimeOut | Complaints | Treatments | NumbersID | Notes |
|---|---|---|---|---|---|---|---|---|---|
| 27.04.2005 | 29.10.1989 | M | Rash | 902 | 918 | Acne rash on back | Tetracycline topical solution | 7660 | |
| 26.04.2005 | 27.02.19.8 | F | | 928 | 946 | Script for Simvastatin & Lisinopril given | | 7706 | Pain (L) knee, referred to Orthopaedic Surgeon (BUPA). |
| 29.04.2005 | 29.06.1934 | M | URTI | 949 | 955 | Smelly discharge from (R) ear | Dexamethasone with neomycin ear spray | 7727 | Penicillin allergy. |
| 29.04.2005 | 20.11.1950 | F | | 1721 | 1730 | Script for Dihydrocodeine & Nicotine patch given | | 7764 | Referred to Pain Management Specialist. |
| 27.04.2005 | 01.12.1970 | M | Rash | 1047 | 1051 | Scabies rash | Permethrin cream 5% w/w | 7773 | |
| 26.04.2005 | 11.08.1948 | M | | 900 | 910 | For FBC & USScan of the abdomen | | 7784 | |
| 25.04.2005 | 23.08.1944 | F | | 911 | 920 | Patient came in regarding Disability Benefit form/report | | 7841 | |
| 27.04.2005 | 05.03.1938 | F | Pain | 1105 | 1111 | Low back pain | Co-codamol | 7846 | |
| 25.04.2005 | 19.10.1938 | M | | 920 | 927 | To continue with the Meloxicam | | 7847 | |
| 25.04.2005 | 26.06.1945 | F | S/Leave | 1715 | 1721 | Ovarian Cancer – Med. 5 | | 939 | |

## Result of a query that lists all consultations from the 22nd to the end of April 2005 (ConsultationsSeenFrom22ndTillEndOfApr2005)

| SurgeryDate | DateOfBirth | Sex | Diagnosis | TimeIn | TimeOut | Complaints | Treatments | NumbersID | Notes |
|---|---|---|---|---|---|---|---|---|---|
| 28.04.2005 | 07.12.1986 | F | | 1041 | 1048 | She doesn't want any letter to whom it may concern regarding the damaged tendon in her (R) Index finger | | 95 | |
| 25.04.2005 | 03.03.1929 | F | | 951 | 1004 | Script for Dihydrocodeine given | | 979 | |
| 28.04.2005 | 30.10.1984 | F | | 1703 | 1711 | To stop the Amitriptyline | | 980 | |
| 28.04.2005 | 13.08.1996 | M | Rash | 1012 | 1021 | Butterfly rash across the face & abdominal pain | Referred to Paediatrician | NP (AA) | |
| 26.04.2005 | 14.12.1973 | M | | 1720 | 1725 | To try OTC analgesia | | NP (AP) | |
| 29.04.2005 | 20.12.2004 | F | | 1811 | 1819 | To take own Calpol | | NP (AP) | |
| 27.04.2005 | 22.01.1991 | M | | 1747 | 151 | Verruca (R) foot | Salicylic acid topical solution | NP (BH) | |
| 25.04.2005 | 06.11.1961 | F | S/Leave | 1808 | 1816 | Dizziness | | NP (BP) | Penicillin allergy. |
| 29.04.2005 | 10.10.1969 | M | RTI | 1807 | 1811 | Cough | Amoxycillin | NP (DS) | Referred to Dermatologist (Basildon Hospital). |
| 26.04.2005 | 09.12.2003 | F | URTI | 1019 | 1025 | Infected rhinorrhoea | Amoxycillin | NP (EAMO) | |
| 26.04.2005 | 29.05.1937 | M | RTI | 1040 | 1052 | Chesty cough | Amoxycillin | NP (FAS) | |
| 29.04.2005 | 07.06.1924 | F | | 1730 | 1739 | Script for Dihydrocodeine given | | NP (ILV) | Referred to Care of the Elderly Physician. |
| 29.04.2005 | 22.04.1942 | F | | 1016 | 1023 | Script for Simvastatin given | | NP (JAS) | |

53

Result of a query that lists all consultations from the 22nd to the end of April 2005 (ConsultationsSeenFrom22ndTillEndOfApr2005)

| SurgeryDate | DateOfBirth | Sex | Diagnosis | TimeIn | TimeOut | Complaints | Treatments | NumbersID | Notes |
|---|---|---|---|---|---|---|---|---|---|
| 28.04.2005 | 29.10.1985 | M | | 1656 | 1700 | T.A.T.T. | For FBC, TFTs & Fasting Glucose | NP (JB) | |
| 27.04.2005 | 04.06.1958 | F | Hypertension | 1704 | 1712 | BP 155/103 | Bendrofluazide | NP (JC) | |
| 27.04.2005 | 12.07.1948 | F | S/Leave | 950 | 1000 | Removal of brain tumour - Med. 5 | | NP (JE) | For FBC. |
| 25.04.2005 | 10.08.1973 | M | URTI | 1704 | 1715 | Sore throat | Amoxycillin | NP (JK) | |
| 26.04.2005 | 27.11.2004 | F | URTI | 1006 | 1013 | Pulling her ears | Amoxycillin | NP (JLR) | |
| 26.04.2005 | 01.12.1973 | F | | 1725 | 1730 | Abscess (R) upper gum | Erythromycin | NP (JM) | Penicillin allergy. |
| 26.04.2005 | 31.01.1938 | F | | 1030 | 1040 | Script for Temazepam given | | NP (JMS) | |
| 28.04.2005 | 21.12.2004 | F | URTI | 951 | 957 | Infected rhinorrhoea | Amoxycillin & Paracetamol | NP (JO) | Script for Oilatum cream given. |
| 28.04.2005 | 12.04.2004 | M | | 1801 | 1807 | Off his feeds & pyrexial | Amoxycillin | NP (JO) | |
| 29.04.2005 | 03.01.1995 | F | | 1823 | 1830 | Itchy rash | Desloratadine | NP (JT) | |
| 28.04.2005 | 20.10.1925 | F | | 905 | 920 | She stopped Thyroxine long time ago | | NP (MH) | Penicillin allergy. |
| 26.04.2005 | 26.01.1966 | F | | 1741 | 1748 | Pre-menstrual tension | Dydrogesterone | NP (MI) | |
| 27.04.2005 | 19.06.1983 | F | S/Leave | 1754 | 1803 | Depression - Med. 5 | | NP (NS) | Duplicate. |
| 26.04.2005 | 25.01.1939 | F | RTI | 1013 | 1019 | Chesty cough | Erythromycin | NP (PC) | |
| 29.04.2005 | 06.10.1933 | M | | 902 | 912 | Script for Atenolol given | | NP (RK) | |
| 26.04.2005 | 19.02.1942 | F | | 946 | 955 | Script for Gliclazide given | | NP (SW) | Septrin allergy. |

54

Result of a query that lists all consultations from the 22nd to the end of April 2005 (ConsultationsSeenFrom22ndTillEndOfApr2005)

| SurgeryDate | DateOfBirth | Sex | Diagnosis | TimeIn | TimeOut | Complaints | Treatments | NumbersID | Notes |
|---|---|---|---|---|---|---|---|---|---|
| 27.04.2005 | 26.05.1936 | M | Pain | 1742 | 1747 | Painful & swollen (L) wrist | Diclofenac, Omeprazole & Flucloxacillin | NP (TC) | |
| 29.04.2005 | 15.09.1939 | M | | 1023 | 1035 | Script for Simvastatin given | | NP (WJS) | |

Result of a query that lists all consultations from the 22nd to the end of April 2006 (ConsultationsSeenFrom22ndTillEndOfApr2006)

| SurgeryDate | DateOfBirth | Sex | Diagnosis | TimeIn | TimeOut | Complaints | Treatments | Initials | Notes |
|---|---|---|---|---|---|---|---|---|---|
| 24.04.2006 | 27.03.1940 | F | | 936 | 950 | For X-Ray of (R) Clavicle & (L) hand | | MAD | Script for Cinchocaine with hydrocortisone suppositories given. |
| 24.04.2006 | 25.02.1934 | M | RTI | 950 | 957 | Cough & wheezy | Ciprofloxacin, Loratadine & Prednisolone e/c given | BAC | |
| 24.04.2006 | 22.08.1980 | F | | 957 | 1004 | To see me in 4 to 6 weeks for repeat FBC & ESR | | CJW | |
| 24.04.2006 | 07.03.1968 | F | | 1004 | 1015 | Menorrhagia & Dysmenorrhoea | Referred to Gynaecologist | JES | |
| 24.04.2006 | 25.08.1963 | M | S/Leave | 1015 | 1020 | (L) thigh injury | | PW | |
| 24.04.2006 | 26.07.1960 | F | | 1020 | 1028 | Script for Amitriptyline given | | DP | |

55

Result of a query that lists all consultations from the 22nd to the end of April 2006 (ConsultationsSeenFrom22ndTillEndOfApr2006)

| SurgeryDate | DateOfBirth | Sex | Diagnosis | TimeIn | TimeOut | Complaints | Treatments | Initials | Notes |
|---|---|---|---|---|---|---|---|---|---|
| 24.04.2006 | 23.07.1984 | F | Depression | 1033 | 1043 | Script for Citalopram, Amoxycillin & Fusidic acid with hydrocortisone cream 2% + 1% given | | MNW | |
| 24.04.2006 | 16.04.1949 | M | | 1043 | 1049 | Script for Sildenafil - "SLS" given | | DRT | |
| 24.04.2006 | 20.10.1935 | F | | 1049 | 1057 | Referred to Neurologist regarding her tremor | | MM | |
| 24.04.2006 | 03.08.1968 | F | S/Leave | 1057 | 1102 | Depression | | JM | |
| 24.04.2006 | 03.07.1939 | M | | 1102 | 1114 | Yearly Diabetic Monitoring Done | | RFL | |
| 24.04.2006 | 29.10.1949 | F | Pain | 1114 | 1127 | Back Pain | Diclofenac e/c & Dihydrocodeine | DT | For MSU. |
| 24.04.2006 | 08.11.1931 | F | | 1127 | 1142 | Script for Amitriptyline & Soya with lauromacrogols bath oil given | | JC | |
| 24.04.2006 | 16.03.1927 | F | | 1142 | 1154 | Yearly Diabetic Monitoring Done | | JPW | |
| 24.04.2006 | 23.02.1941 | M | | 1154 | 1209 | Script for Co-codamol given | | RWM | |
| 24.04.2006 | 31.12.1953 | F | RTI | 1246 | 1250 | Cough | Amoxycillin | JH | |
| 24.04.2006 | 08.07.1952 | F | | 1644 | 1656 | Referred to Physiotherapist regarding her back pain | | PMA | |

Result of a query that lists all consultations from the 22nd to the end of April 2006 (ConsultationsSeenFrom22ndTillEndOfApr2006)

| SurgeryDate | DateOfBirth | Sex | Diagnosis | TimeIn | TimeOut | Complaints | Treatments | Initials | Notes |
|---|---|---|---|---|---|---|---|---|---|
| 24.04.2006 | 10.05.1968 | F | | 1656 | 1700 | Phlebitis on (L) leg | Flucloxacillin | AB | |
| 24.04.2006 | 28.03.1960 | F | | 1700 | 1708 | Script for Temazepam given | | DK | |
| 24.04.2006 | 29.05.1960 | M | | 1708 | 1713 | Script for Dihydrocodeine & Diclofenac given | | RCK | |
| 24.04.2006 | 20.10.1983 | F | RTI | 1713 | 1717 | Chesty cough | Amoxycillin | ARS | |
| 24.04.2006 | 05.12.1956 | M | | 1717 | 1725 | He came to inform me that his back pain got worse since a bus ran into the back of his car | | DTB | |
| 24.04.2006 | 25.07.1939 | F | | 1737 | 1754 | For CXR | | PMC | |
| 24.04.2006 | 22.02.1960 | M | S/Leave | 1754 | 1806 | (L) radical Orchidectomy | | MDG | |
| 24.04.2006 | 08.01.1972 | M | | 1806 | 1815 | Wound next to (L) eye, septic | Flucloxacillin & Fusidic acid cream | EM | |
| 24.04.2006 | 20.03.1952 | F | S/Leave | 1818 | 1825 | Laparoscopic Cholecystectomy - Med. 5 | | LJF | Weepy around & sickness feeling, Rx. Flucloxacillin & Metoclopramide. |
| 24.04.2006 | 05.08.1980 | M | | 1825 | 1832 | Referred to Paediatrician regarding his persistent chesty cough | | JMMO | |

57

Result of a query that lists all consultations from the 22nd to the end of April 2006 (ConsultationsSeenFrom22ndTillEndOfApr2006)

| SurgeryDate | DateOfBirth | Sex | Diagnosis | TimeIn | TimeOut | Complaints | Treatments | Initials | Notes |
|---|---|---|---|---|---|---|---|---|---|
| 24.04.2006 | 21.11.1994 | F | Rash | 1832 | 1840 | Itchy rash on arms & face | Loratadine | HJA | |
| 25.04.2006 | 15.05.1945 | M | | 945 | 958 | Referred to Eye Dr. on call, SGH regarding wart/lump in the medial angle of the (L) eye | | VCC | |
| 25.04.2006 | 02.04.1962 | F | S/Leave | 958 | 1005 | Painful lower ribs | | PJL | |
| 25.04.2006 | 02.05.1990 | F | Conjunctivitis | 1005 | 1009 | Sticky eyes & discharge | Chloramphenicol eye drops | CSA | |
| 25.04.2006 | 25.12.1942 | M | URTI | 1009 | 1014 | Sore throat | Amoxycillin | RFL | Script for Beclomethasone aqueous nasal spray given. |
| 25.04.2006 | 06.03.1926 | F | | 1014 | 1026 | Script for Co-codamol & MethylPrednisolone with Lidocaine given | | MHT | |
| 25.04.2006 | 20.05.2003 | M | RTI | 1026 | 1030 | Chesty cough | Amoxycillin | CJM | |
| 25.04.2006 | 05.07.1931 | F | | 1036 | 1050 | Script for Rosiglitazone with Metformin given | | AVD | |
| 25.04.2006 | 11.04.1982 | F | S/Leave | 1054 | 1107 | Injury to (L) ankle & (R) knee - Private | | JLS | |
| 25.04.2006 | 15.03.1940 | F | UTI | 1107 | 1118 | Dysuria | Amoxycillin | BRS | For MSU. |
| 25.04.2006 | 10.03.1936 | F | | 1134 | 1150 | Yearly Diabetic Monitoring Done | | JBS | Script for Coracten XL given. |
| 25.04.2006 | 19.04.1984 | F | | 1150 | 1158 | Post-natal with Baby check done | | AJD | |

58

Result of a query that lists all consultations from the 22nd to the end of April 2006 (ConsultationsSeenFrom22ndTillEndOfApr2006)

| SurgeryDate | DateOfBirth | Sex | Diagnosis | TimeIn | TimeOut | Complaints | Treatments | Initials | Notes |
|---|---|---|---|---|---|---|---|---|---|
| 25.04.2006 | 23.03.1926 | M | | 1649 | 1706 | For USScan of the kidneys | | JWH | |
| 25.04.2006 | 06.10.1981 | F | | 1706 | 1716 | Constipation | Lactulose & Glycerol suppositories | WK | |
| 25.04.2006 | 26.04.1984 | M | Rash | 1716 | 1723 | (L) T10 Shingles | Acyclovir tablets | PAB | |
| 25.04.2006 | 05.06.1924 | M | | 1723 | 1735 | Script for Ciprofloxacin given | | DAC | Referred to Care of the Elderly Doctor regarding his restless legs. Penicillin allergy. |
| 25.04.2006 | 10.03.1968 | M | Lump | 1735 | 1742 | (R) Inguinal hernia | Referred to General Surgeon | MAC | |
| 25.04.2006 | 11.03.1968 | F | | 1742 | 1753 | Referred to Gynaecologist (BUPA) regarding her menorrhagia | | EJA | |
| 25.04.2006 | 25.08.1989 | F | Conjunctivitis | 1753 | 1758 | Her baby daughter has bilateral sticky eyes | Chloramphenicol eye drops | LMD | |
| 25.04.2006 | 25.11.1968 | M | Pain | 1758 | 1805 | (L) wrist pain | Diclofenac e/c & Co-codamol | CAR | Penicillin allergy. |
| 25.04.2006 | 27.11.1952 | F | | 1805 | 1811 | Script for Atenolol & Bendrofluazide given | | JD | |
| 25.04.2006 | 23.12.1974 | M | Lump | 1811 | 1818 | Possible lump (R) testicle | For USScan of the testicles (urgent) | BS | |
| 25.04.2006 | 08.01.1972 | M | | 1818 | 1826 | Script for Co-codamol given | | EM | |

Result of a query that lists all consultations from the 22nd to the end of April 2006 (ConsultationsSeenFrom22ndTillEndOfApr2006)

| SurgeryDate | DateOfBirth | Sex | Diagnosis | TimeIn | TimeOut | Complaints | Treatments | Initials | Notes |
|---|---|---|---|---|---|---|---|---|---|
| 26.04.2006 | 05.06.1935 | F | | 938 | 954 | For repeat FBC & U/Es in 3 to 6 months | | PCB | |
| 26.04.2006 | 11.12.1944 | F | | 954 | 1004 | Script for Sodium Valproate e/c & Diclofenac e/c given | | GNW | |
| 26.04.2006 | 07.10.1933 | M | | 1004 | 1009 | Script for Olanzapine given | | FDF | |
| 26.04.2006 | 18.02.1943 | M | | 1009 | 1026 | Ezetrol stopped as it was giving him nightmares | | JC | |
| 26.04.2006 | 28.03.1926 | F | | 1026 | 1040 | Referred to Dermatologist regarding warts on face & leg | | JD | |
| 26.04.2006 | 21.02.1976 | F | | 1040 | 1050 | Script for Nizoral shampoo given | | FPT | |
| 26.04.2006 | 03.12.1924 | F | | 1054 | 1102 | To take all her BP medications | | AH | |
| 26.04.2006 | 29.10.1949 | F | S/Leave | 1102 | 1110 | Back Pain | | DT | |
| 26.04.2006 | 26.03.1951 | F | | 1125 | 1133 | For HBA1c & other blood tests | | LEP | |
| 26.04.2006 | 24.02.1990 | F | | 1133 | 1147 | To attend FP clinic for her pill | | LC | |
| 26.04.2006 | 09.10.1924 | F | RTI | 1147 | 1159 | Chesty cough | Ciprofloxacin | VOM | |
| 26.04.2006 | 20.03.1987 | M | | 1159 | 1228 | Awaiting what specialist says about his going back to work | | CRS | |
| 26.04.2006 | 04.12.2003 | F | | 1228 | 1234 | Script for Timodine cream given | | EAMEO | |

60

Result of a query that lists all consultations from the 22nd to the end of April 2006 (ConsultationsSeenFrom22ndTillEndOfApr2006)

| SurgeryDate | DateOfBirth | Sex | Diagnosis | TimeIn | TimeOut | Complaints | Treatments | Initials | Notes |
|---|---|---|---|---|---|---|---|---|---|
| 26.04.2006 | 10.01.1973 | F | | | 1234 | 1238 | Script for Citalopram given | | NEO | |
| 27.04.2006 | 19.01.1924 | F | | 945 | 1000 | Script for Coracten XL & Atorvastatin given | | MRD | |
| 27.04.2006 | 28.03.1961 | M | S/Leave | 1000 | 1018 | Pain in Private x 2 | | RAB | |
| 27.04.2006 | 13.08.1996 | M | Depressed | 1018 | 1030 | Weepy & insomnia | Referred to Child Psychiatrist | ADA | Mum came to Surgery. |
| 27.04.2006 | 20.01.1935 | F | Pain | 1030 | 1036 | Neck Pain | Co-codamol | JW | |
| 27.04.2006 | 25.05.1973 | F | S/Leave | 1036 | 1050 | Back Pain Med. 5 | | TJ | |
| 27.04.2006 | 29.11.1969 | M | | 1050 | 1057 | Septic (R) in growing toe nail | Flucloxacillin | CW | |
| 27.04.2006 | 19.05.1969 | F | URTI | 1057 | 1104 | Sore throat | Amoxycillin | LH | Script for Co-codamol given. |
| 27.04.2006 | 11.03.1939 | F | Pain | 1104 | 1110 | Pain in fingers | Co-codamol & Diclofenac e/c | JPD | |
| 27.04.2006 | 04.11.1969 | M | | 1110 | 1119 | Script for Chlorpromazine given | | PJD | Mum came to Surgery. |
| 27.04.2006 | 25.02.1934 | M | | 1119 | 1123 | To ask for more Loratadine if he gets more hay fever symptoms | | BAC | |
| 27.04.2006 | 25.12.1948 | M | RTI | 1123 | 1145 | Chesty cough | Amoxycillin | CGB | Yearly Diabetic Monitoring Done. Script for Coracten XL given. For CXR. |

Result of a query that lists all consultations from the 22nd to the end of April 2006 (ConsultationsSeenFrom22ndTillEndOfApr2006)

| SurgeryDate | DateOfBirth | Sex | Diagnosis | TimeIn | TimeOut | Complaints | Treatments | Initials | Notes |
|---|---|---|---|---|---|---|---|---|---|
| 27.04.2006 | 17.07.1981 | F | | 1145 | 1153 | If she notices any breast lump to come back | | XL | |
| 27.04.2006 | 27.04.1925 | M | | 1153 | 1204 | Yearly Diabetic Monitoring Done | | SAB | |
| 27.04.2006 | 25.06.1996 | F | | 1648 | 1653 | To see nurse to keep an eye on the lump behind her (R) nipple | | ERY | |
| 27.04.2006 | 08.05.1993 | M | | 1653 | 1658 | Hay fever | Desloratadine | ATB | |
| 27.04.2006 | 13.09.1942 | F | | 1709 | 1719 | Referred to General Surgeon (BUPA) regarding her abdominal pain | | JOH | |
| 27.04.2006 | 03.12.1960 | M | Conjunctivitis | 1719 | 1725 | Sticky (R) eye | Chloramphenicol eye drops | GTR | |
| 27.04.2006 | 25.07.1955 | F | | 1725 | 1736 | Script for Kliovance given | | LR | |
| 27.04.2006 | 15.10.1923 | F | | 1736 | 1743 | Septic cryotherapy wounds on the hands | Flucloxacillin | DWR | |
| 27.04.2006 | 13.09.1944 | M | | 1743 | 1749 | Script for Dexamethasone ear spray given | | AW | |
| 27.04.2006 | 01.02.1931 | M | | 1751 | 1804 | Copy of CXR result given to patient | | MDS | |
| 27.04.2006 | 01.08.1947 | F | | 1804 | 1811 | Script for Co-codamol given | | JLC | |
| 27.04.2006 | 06.11.1948 | M | | 1811 | 1820 | Diarrhoea | Co-phenotrope & Oral rehydration salts oral powder | LAL | |

Result of a query that lists all consultations from the 22nd to the end of April 2006 (ConsultationsSeenFrom22ndTillEndOfApr2006)

| SurgeryDate | DateOfBirth | Sex | Diagnosis | TimeIn | TimeOut | Complaints | Treatments | Initials | Notes |
|---|---|---|---|---|---|---|---|---|---|
| 27.04.2006 | 20.02.2003 | M | | 1820 | 1824 | Script for Salbutamol inhaler given | | CJM | |
| 28.04.2006 | 27.08.1933 | M | | 944 | 954 | Referred to General Surgeon regarding (R) lower abdominal pain | | HGH | |
| 28.04.2006 | 14.01.1965 | M | | 958 | 1005 | Hay fever | Fexofenadine | DCB | |
| 28.04.2006 | 23.05.1927 | M | | 1005 | 1022 | Yearly Diabetic Monitoring Done | | JHM | |
| 28.04.2006 | 01.11.1936 | M | | 1022 | 1035 | Script for Lisinopril & Simvastatin given | | JJS | |
| 28.04.2006 | 23.10.1929 | F | | 1035 | 1047 | Yearly Diabetic Monitoring Done | | MOL | |
| 28.04.2006 | 24.04.1935 | F | Pain | 1055 | 1112 | Back Pain | Tramadol | DAS | For Lumbar Spine X-Ray. Mouth ulcers, Rx. Metronidazole. |
| 28.04.2006 | 24.03.1973 | M | S/Leave | 1118 | 1128 | Eczema flare-up - Private | | JCM | |
| 28.04.2006 | 26.06.1954 | M | S/Leave | 1128 | 1137 | (L) knee pain | | CDP | |
| 28.04.2006 | 18.10.1920 | F | | 1137 | 1145 | Script for Co-codamol given | | QK | |
| 28.04.2006 | 15.03.1922 | F | | 1145 | 1156 | For serum BNP | | WBB | |
| 28.04.2006 | 06.03.1926 | F | | 1156 | 1216 | Injection Depo-Medrone with Lidocaine given to the (L) shoulder | | MHT | |
| 28.04.2006 | 26.10.1943 | F | | 1216 | 1230 | Dog bite on the (R) hand | Co-Amoxiclav | APM | |

Result of a query that lists all consultations from the 22nd to the end of April 2006 (ConsultationsSeenFrom22ndTillEndOfApr2006)

| SurgeryDate | DateOfBirth | Sex | Diagnosis | TimeIn | TimeOut | Complaints | Treatments | Initials | Notes |
|---|---|---|---|---|---|---|---|---|---|
| 28.04.2006 | 14.12.2001 | F | URTI | 1230 | 1239 | Sore throat | Erythromycin | ABLAK | Referred to Paediatrician regarding her recurrent sore throats. |
| 28.04.2006 | 03.01.1914 | F | RTI | 1350 | 1405 | Chesty cough | Erythromycin & Amoxycillin | LG | Home visit. Lederfen allergy. |
| 28.04.2006 | 09.01.1949 | M | Lump | 1645 | 1709 | Inguinal hernia | Referred to General Surgeon | DFH | |
| 28.04.2006 | 24.12.1972 | F | | 1709 | 1722 | For FBC, U/Es, Fasting Lipids & Fasting Glucose | | CM | |
| 28.04.2006 | 06.12.1945 | M | S/Leave | 1722 | 1728 | Weakness in the (L) hand | | BS | |
| 28.04.2006 | 25.12.1946 | F | | 1728 | 1733 | Script for Kliovance given | | AS | |
| 28.04.2006 | 22.07.1961 | M | S/Leave | 1733 | 1739 | Shingles | | PWL | |
| 28.04.2006 | 10.11.2001 | F | Revisit | 1739 | 1744 | Still has chesty cough despite taking Amoxycillin | Cefalexin | GLB | For CXR. |
| 28.04.2006 | 20.03.1952 | F | | 1744 | 1752 | Script for Penicillin V & Flucloxacillin given | | LJF | |
| 28.04.2006 | 01.12.1967 | M | | 1752 | 1758 | Referred to ENT Surgeon regarding his recurrent sore crusty nostrils | | RAJ | |
| 28.04.2006 | 04.05.1947 | F | | 1758 | 1807 | MSU - normal | | MPW | |

### Result of a query that lists all consultations from the 22nd to the end of April 2006 (ConsultationsSeenFrom22ndTillEndOfApr2006)

| SurgeryDate | DateOfBirth | Sex | Diagnosis | TimeIn | TimeOut | Complaints | Treatments | Initials | Notes |
|---|---|---|---|---|---|---|---|---|---|
| 28.04.2006 | 07.02.1972 | F | | 1807 | 1814 | Letter to whom it may concern regarding her hospitalizations for Asthma exacerbation daughter being on frequent antibiotics | | SVR | |
| 28.04.2006 | 06.06.1947 | F | Conjunctivitis | 1814 | 1820 | Sticky (R) eye with swelling of surrounding cheek | Chloramphenicol eye drops & Amoxycillin | MM | |
| 28.04.2006 | 08.01.1972 | M | | 1820 | 1828 | Advised to put in a self-certificate for first week | | EM | |

### Result of a query that lists all consultations from the 22nd to the end of April 2007 (ConsultationsSeenFrom22ndTillEndOfApr2007)

| SurgeryDate | DateOfBirth | Sex | Diagnosis | TimeIn | TimeOut | Complaints | Treatments | Initials | Notes |
|---|---|---|---|---|---|---|---|---|---|
| 23.04.2007 | 05.08.1988 | F | | 945 | 952 | Script for Ethinyloestradiol with Levonorgestrel given | | ESC | |
| 23.04.2007 | 08.12.1938 | F | | 959 | 1011 | USScan of neck showed large goitrous thyroid mass | | EVB | |
| 23.04.2007 | 08.03.1961 | M | S/Leave | 1011 | 1016 | Pain in the (R) elbow - Private | | RAB | |
| 23.04.2007 | 24.12.1950 | F | RTI | 1016 | 1022 | Chesty cough | Amoxycillin | GB | |
| 23.04.2007 | 26.06.1991 | F | | 1022 | 1027 | Sore lip | Amoxycillin | JMJG | |
| 23.04.2007 | 19.01.1924 | F | | 1027 | 1041 | Lisinopril | | MRD | |

Result of a query that lists all consultations from the 22$^{nd}$ to the end of April 2007 (ConsultationsSeenFrom22ndTillEndOfApr2007)

| SurgeryDate | DateOfBirth | Sex | Diagnosis | TimeIn | TimeOut | Complaints | Treatments | Initials | Notes |
|---|---|---|---|---|---|---|---|---|---|
| 23.04.2007 | 08.04.1943 | F | S/Leave | 1046 | 1104 | Pain in the (L) heel - Private & Med. 3 | | JMM | Script for Diclofenac e/c & Omeprazole given. |
| 23.04.2007 | 09.05.1936 | F | | 1104 | 1109 | Script for Flucloxacillin given | | DLS | |
| 23.04.2007 | 06.04.1938 | M | | 1109 | 1117 | I explained to him that it will be inappropriate to discuss his wife's Medical problems in her absence | | RA | |
| 23.04.2007 | 16.04.1966 | M | | 1117 | 1126 | Referred to the One Stop Haematuria clinic regarding his persistent haematuria | | AJDP | |
| 23.04.2007 | 17.09.1965 | F | S/Leave | 1126 | 1140 | Back Pain - Med. 5 | | PAE | |
| 23.04.2007 | 25.05.1936 | M | | 1140 | 1200 | Script for Salbutamol inhaler & Prednisolone e/c given | | TC | |
| 23.04.2007 | 02.12.1923 | M | | 1405 | 1415 | Referred to General Surgeon regarding (R) Inguinal hernia | | RA | Home visit. |
| 23.04.2007 | 21.03.1973 | M | | 1641 | 1650 | To see nurse in 6 months for repeat FBC & U/Es | | DRK | |
| 23.04.2007 | 13.12.1957 | F | | 1700 | 1716 | Referred to Colorectal Surgeon regarding rectal bleeding & alternating bowel habits | | LM | |

Result of a query that lists all consultations from the 22nd to the end of April 2007 (ConsultationsSeenFrom22ndTillEndOfApr2007)

| SurgeryDate | DateOfBirth | Sex | Diagnosis | TimeIn | TimeOut | Complaints | Treatments | Initials | Notes |
|---|---|---|---|---|---|---|---|---|---|
| 23.04.2007 | 09.07.1969 | M | | 1716 | 1723 | Script for Cetirizine given | | DBJD | |
| 23.04.2007 | 02.06.1936 | M | | 1723 | 1727 | Medication review done | | AJG | |
| 23.04.2007 | 04.09.1928 | M | | 1727 | 1744 | Referred to General Surgeon regarding (R) groin pain & discomfort | | RJJ | Script for Tolterodine m/r given. |
| 23.04.2007 | 16.05.1975 | F | S/Leave | 1744 | 1749 | DVT - Med. 5 | | ELG | |
| 23.04.2007 | 06.10.1952 | M | RTI | 1749 | 1755 | Cough | Amoxycillin | CJG | |
| 23.04.2007 | 22.03.1967 | F | | 1755 | 1805 | Script for Gaviscon Advance given | | BAB | SSMG (cert) form completed. |
| 23.04.2007 | 29.12.1956 | M | | 1805 | 1813 | Referred to Dermatologist regarding lesions on his (R) upper arm & fore-head | | FJF | For X-Ray (R) shoulder. |
| 23.04.2007 | 06.03.1973 | F | S/Leave | 1813 | 1820 | Work related stress | | KLSL | |
| 24.04.2007 | 19.06.1944 | F | | 942 | 954 | Script for Lisinopril given | | PJL | |
| 24.04.2007 | 27.04.1928 | M | | 954 | 1011 | BP 127/63 | | RFV | |
| 24.04.2007 | 25.07.1939 | F | | 1020 | 1030 | Script for Rosiglitazone given | | JLB | |
| 24.04.2007 | 18.11.1937 | F | | 1030 | 1042 | For X-Ray of the (L) wrist | | RM | |

Result of a query that lists all consultations from the 22nd to the end of April 2007 (ConsultationsSeenFrom22ndTillEndOfApr2007)

| SurgeryDate | DateOfBirth | Sex | Diagnosis | TimeIn | TimeOut | Complaints | Treatments | Initials | Notes |
|---|---|---|---|---|---|---|---|---|---|
| 24.04.2007 | 20.04.1938 | M | | 1042 | 1047 | Script for Chloramphenicol eye ointment & Flucloxacillin given | | DAD | |
| 24.04.2007 | 28.12.1962 | M | S/Leave | 1047 | 1058 | Pain in the (L) hip | | KF | For X-Ray of the Cervical Spine & of the (L) hip. Script for Dihydrocodeine given. |
| 24.04.2007 | 16.01.1952 | F | | 1058 | 1105 | Referred to Rheumatologist regarding pain in the (R) shoulder & down the (R) arm | | SJW | |
| 24.04.2007 | 05.07.1942 | M | | 1119 | 1127 | Script for Varenicline (starter pack) given | | LTW | |
| 24.04.2007 | 07.09.1927 | F | | 1140 | 1148 | Script for Fexofenadine given | | PLW | |
| 24.04.2007 | 08.06.1974 | M | URTI | 1637 | 1652 | Sore throat | Amoxycillin | SWM | |
| 24.04.2007 | 19.02.1975 | F | | 1652 | 1701 | For Chest X-Ray | | JIM | |
| 24.04.2007 | 29.09.1932 | F | | 1709 | 1715 | Injection MethyPrednisolone with Lidocaine given | | SMD | |
| 24.04.2007 | 28.06.1991 | F | URTI | 1717 | 1723 | Sore throat | Amoxycillin | LC | |

Result of a query that lists all consultations from the 22nd to the end of April 2007 (ConsultationsSeenFrom22ndTillEndOfApr2007)

| SurgeryDate | DateOfBirth | Sex | Diagnosis | TimeIn | TimeOut | Complaints | Treatments | Initials | Notes |
|---|---|---|---|---|---|---|---|---|---|
| 24.04.2007 | 13.09.1948 | F | | 1728 | 1738 | Referred to General Surgeon regarding the lump on the medial aspect of the top of the (L) thigh | | LP | |
| 24.04.2007 | 11.02.1938 | M | | 1738 | 1747 | His diarrhoea & crampy abdominal pain are much better with the prescribed medications | | RJH | |
| 24.04.2007 | 23.07.1953 | M | S/Leave | 1805 | 1820 | Throat infection - Private | | THM | Script for Erythromycin given. Stool for C&S. |
| 24.04.2007 | 26.08.1997 | M | | 1820 | 1825 | To use own Calamine lotion for his viral rash | | JEB | |
| 25.04.2007 | 04.10.1968 | F | | 941 | 952 | For Urine Pregnancy test | | AW | |
| 25.04.2007 | 30.06.1973 | M | | 952 | 1000 | Script for Omeprazole & Ferrous Sulphate given | | LAS | |
| 25.04.2007 | 09.06.1934 | M | | 1000 | 1007 | Script for Omeprazole given | | MKC | |
| 25.04.2007 | 20.10.1983 | F | S/Leave | 1026 | 1031 | Asthma attack | | ARS | |
| 25.04.2007 | 09.01.1987 | M | | 1031 | 1040 | Script for Flucloxacillin given | | MPS | |
| 25.04.2007 | 11.05.1959 | F | | 1040 | 1047 | Script for Lisinopril given | | LJE | |

Result of a query that lists all consultations from the 22nd to the end of April 2007 (ConsultationsSeenFrom22ndTillEndOfApr2007)

| SurgeryDate | DateOfBirth | Sex | Diagnosis | TimeIn | TimeOut | Complaints | Treatments | Initials | Notes |
|---|---|---|---|---|---|---|---|---|---|
| 25.04.2007 | 14.06.1957 | F | S/Leave | 1047 | 1055 | Operation on the (R) ankle - Med. 5 | | AB | |
| 25.04.2007 | 14.08.1946 | M | | 1055 | 1110 | Private script for Tadalafil given | | RBG | |
| 25.04.2007 | 29.11.1946 | F | | 1110 | 1125 | Script for Lisinopril & Conjugated oestrogens equine with medroxyprogesterone (continuous) given | | CMT | |
| 25.04.2007 | 26.03.1991 | F | | 1125 | 1130 | Urine pregnancy test was negative | | KLR | |
| 25.04.2007 | 20.12.1960 | M | RTI | 1130 | 1136 | Chesty cough | Amoxycillin | RP | |
| 25.04.2007 | 05.02.1946 | F | | 1136 | 1150 | Barclays Sickness claim form completed | | ML | |
| 25.04.2007 | 12.02.1943 | F | | 1646 | 1655 | Script for Atorvastatin given | | SAW | |
| 25.04.2007 | 20.08.1939 | F | | 1655 | 1706 | Script for Levothyroxine given | | SLT | For Thyroid antibodies. |
| 25.04.2007 | 23.09.1948 | M | | 1706 | 1712 | Script for Ferrous Sulphate given | | KWK | |
| 25.04.2007 | 19.05.1944 | F | | 1712 | 1724 | Script for Quinine Sulphate & Zoton Fastab given | | AWB | |
| 25.04.2007 | 28.02.1981 | M | S/Leave | 1726 | 1734 | Operation on the (R) little finger - Med. 5 | | DJC | |
| 25.04.2007 | 27.08.1933 | M | RTI | 1734 | 1739 | Chesty cough | Amoxycillin | HGH | |
| 25.04.2007 | 10.10.1992 | F | | 1739 | 1744 | For X-Ray (L) elbow | | AEH | |

70

Result of a query that lists all consultations from the 22nd to the end of April 2007 (ConsultationsSeenFrom22ndTillEndOfApr2007)

| SurgeryDate | DateOfBirth | Sex | Diagnosis | TimeIn | TimeOut | Complaints | Treatments | Initials | Notes |
|---|---|---|---|---|---|---|---|---|---|
| 25.04.2007 | 23.04.1950 | F | | 1744 | 1751 | Referred to Rheumatologist regarding high Rheumatoid factor & multiple joints pain | | PEH | |
| 25.04.2007 | 17.03.1968 | F | | 1751 | 1800 | Referred to Gynaecologist regarding persistent intermenstrual bleeding & menorrhagia | | NJB | For USScan of the pelvis. |
| 25.04.2007 | 23.05.1927 | M | RTI | 1800 | 1813 | Chesty cough | Amoxycillin | JHM | |
| 25.04.2007 | 07.09.2001 | F | URTI | 1813 | 1818 | Sore throat | Amoxycillin | TEK | |
| 25.04.2007 | 23.03.2000 | M | Conjunctivitis | 1820 | 1829 | Sticky & red (L) eye with cellulitis (L) lower eye lid | Flucloxacillin & Chloramphenicol eye drops | LAB | Script for Loratadine given. |
| 26.04.2007 | 19.04.1991 | F | | 941 | 954 | Referred to Neurologist regarding her fainting episodes | | LMB | Referred to General Surgeon regarding lump on the back of her head. |
| 26.04.2007 | 03.12.1924 | F | | 954 | 1000 | Medication review done | | AH | |
| 26.04.2007 | 07.10.1933 | M | | 1000 | 1010 | Script for Olanzapine & Erythromycin given | | FDF | Penicillin allergy. |
| 26.04.2007 | 05.11.1941 | M | | 1010 | 1024 | Private script for Viagra given | | WB | Script for Tramadol m/r given. |

71

Result of a query that lists all consultations from the 22nd to the end of April 2007 (ConsultationsSeenFrom22ndTillEndOfApr2007)

| SurgeryDate | DateOfBirth | Sex | Diagnosis | TimeIn | TimeOut | Complaints | Treatments | Initials | Notes |
|---|---|---|---|---|---|---|---|---|---|
| 26.04.2007 | 24.04.1931 | F | RTI | 1026 | 1032 | Chesty cough | Amoxycillin & Prednisolone e/c | JWB | |
| 26.04.2007 | 01.06.1907 | F | RTI | 1032 | 1037 | Chesty cough | Erythromycin | WEKT | Daughter came to Surgery. |
| 26.04.2007 | 15.03.1922 | F | | 1043 | 1058 | Referred to Colorectal Surgeon regarding piles | | WBB | For X-Ray of both feet. |
| 26.04.2007 | 12.05.1936 | M | | 1058 | 1112 | Script for Co-codamol given | | AM | |
| 26.04.2007 | 13.10.1969 | F | | 1112 | 1124 | Referred to General Surgeon regarding lump in the (R) groin area | | PG | Script for Microgynon 30 given. |
| 26.04.2007 | 01.04.1962 | F | S/Leave | 1124 | 1132 | Laparoscopic Cholecystectomy - Med. 5 | | TKC | |
| 26.04.2007 | 27.05.2000 | M | URTI | 1132 | 1137 | Sore throat | Amoxycillin | NCB | |
| 26.04.2007 | 24.02.1932 | F | | 1137 | 1147 | Script for Clotrimazole cream & Pramipexole given | | EM | |
| 26.04.2007 | 16.03.1956 | F | | 1147 | 1157 | Referred to Gastroenterologist regarding passing jelly like material rectally | | SPD | Script for Hyoscine butylbromide given. |
| 26.04.2007 | 30.03.1923 | M | | 1157 | 1222 | Script for Salbutamol inhaler given | | PGH | |
| 26.04.2007 | 09.12.2003 | F | URTI | 1222 | 1227 | Sore throat | Amoxycillin | EAMEO | |

Result of a query that lists all consultations from the 22nd to the end of April 2007 (ConsultationsSeenFrom22ndTillEndOfApr2007)

| SurgeryDate | DateOfBirth | Sex | Diagnosis | TimeIn | TimeOut | Complaints | Treatments | Initials | Notes |
|---|---|---|---|---|---|---|---|---|---|
| 26.04.2007 | 02.07.1926 | M | RTI | 1425 | 1435 | Chesty cough | Amoxycillin & Prednisolone e/c | BLB | Home visit. |
| 26.04.2007 | 06.03.2000 | M | | 1654 | 1700 | Mum given letter to whom it may concern that he is healthy | | MA | |
| 26.04.2007 | 12.10.1946 | F | | 1700 | 1714 | Script for Allopurinol given | | CPS | |
| 26.04.2007 | 02.12.1994 | F | | 1714 | 1728 | Referred to Orthopaedic Surgeon regarding Freiberg's disease of the 2nd (L) metatarsal head | | AAP | |
| 26.04.2007 | 27.08.1922 | M | | 1728 | 1736 | Script for Co-codamol given | | AC | |
| 26.04.2007 | 27.05.1951 | F | | 1736 | 1743 | Script for Flucloxacillin & Diclofenac e/c given | | BH | |
| 26.04.2007 | 06.01.1955 | M | | 1743 | 1747 | Private script for Viagra given | | MAS | |
| 26.04.2007 | 23.07.1923 | M | | 1747 | 1800 | Pyrexial | Amoxycillin | KWB | |
| 26.04.2007 | 30.08.1977 | M | S/Leave | 1800 | 1806 | Painful (L) lower chest - Med. 5 | | RBC | |
| 26.04.2007 | 03.08.1957 | F | S/Leave | 1806 | 1819 | Chest infection - Private & Med. 5 | | CK | Script for Co-Amoxiclav given. |
| 26.04.2007 | 10.05.1968 | F | | 1819 | 1827 | Script for Erythromycin & Otomize ear spray given | | AB | Referred to Practice Counsellor regarding feeling low. |
| 26.04.2007 | 13.05.1982 | F | URTI | 1827 | 1832 | sinusitis | Amoxycillin | DMB | |

73

Result of a query that lists all consultations from the 22nd to the end of April 2007 (ConsultationsSeenFrom22ndTillEndOfApr2007)

| SurgeryDate | DateOfBirth | Sex | Diagnosis | TimeIn | TimeOut | Complaints | Treatments | Initials | Notes |
|---|---|---|---|---|---|---|---|---|---|
| 26.04.2007 | 12.02.1996 | M | URTI | 1832 | 1840 | Breath smells & pyrexial | Erythromycin | JW | |
| 26.04.2007 | 29.12.1930 | F | | 1925 | 1955 | Script for Enlive given | | AK | Home visit. Penicillin allergy. |
| 27.04.2007 | 29.12.1930 | F | | 925 | 935 | Patient certified dead | | AK | Home visit. Penicillin allergy. |
| 27.04.2007 | 28.03.1945 | M | | 947 | 954 | To enquire about the stockings size etc. from the chemist | | APD | |
| 27.04.2007 | 28.08.1946 | F | | 954 | 1001 | She will discuss about any concerns about going on statin as she is on Methotrexate with the specialist | | APD | |
| 27.04.2007 | 03.06.1967 | F | | 1001 | 1011 | Referred to Dermatologist under the NHS regarding atopic eczema | | NLB | |
| 27.04.2007 | 09.04.1926 | M | | 1011 | 1024 | Referred to Chest Physician for high resolution CT Scan of her chest as suggested on the result of his Chest X-Ray result | | TS | |
| 27.04.2007 | 11.04.1982 | F | | 1024 | 1030 | To come back once the spots on her chin re-appears | | JLS | |

74

Result of a query that lists all consultations from the 22nd to the end of April 2007 (ConsultationsSeenFrom22ndTillEndOfApr2007)

| SurgeryDate | DateOfBirth | Sex | Diagnosis | TimeIn | TimeOut | Complaints | Treatments | Initials | Notes |
|---|---|---|---|---|---|---|---|---|---|
| 27.04.2007 | 17.05.1935 | F |  | 1030 | 1036 | She is not keen to be referred for further evaluation of her inconclusive Chest X-Ray result |  | CSS |  |
| 27.04.2007 | 13.07.1946 | F |  | 1042 | 1052 | Referred to Orthopaedic Surgeon regarding pain in the (R) knee & in her (L) hand/wrist region |  | JFRH |  |
| 27.04.2007 | 28.02.1934 | F | RTI | 1052 | 1057 | Chesty cough | Amoxycillin | DIM |  |
| 27.04.2007 | 14.05.1927 | F |  | 1057 | 1114 | For monthly urinalysis for proteinuria with the nurse |  | 43070 |  |
| 27.04.2007 | 23.04.1936 | F |  | 1114 | 1131 | The Parking Badge Scheme for Disabled People Medical Practitioner Report completed with the patient |  | PEB |  |
| 27.04.2007 | 25.10.1966 | M |  | 1131 | 1139 | Script for Amoxycillin, Flucloxacillin, Sibutramine & Fusidic acid cream given |  | WBG |  |
| 27.04.2007 | 16.02.1975 | F |  | 1139 | 1149 | Referred to Chest Physician regarding persistent chest pain |  | JIM |  |

Result of a query that lists all consultations from the 22nd to the end of April 2007 (ConsultationsSeenFrom22ndTillEndOfApr2007)

| SurgeryDate | DateOfBirth | Sex | Diagnosis | Complaints | TimeIn | TimeOut | Treatments | Initials | Notes |
|---|---|---|---|---|---|---|---|---|---|
| 27.04.2007 | 31.10.1943 | M | RTI | Chesty cough | 1149 | 1154 | Amoxycillin | NFH | |
| 27.04.2007 | 25.02.1986 | F | | For Pregnancy test | 1648 | 1656 | | SJH | |
| 27.04.2007 | 24.03.1959 | M | | For Chest X-Ray | 1656 | 1702 | | KMH | |
| 27.04.2007 | 06.07.1957 | F | | For TFTs | 1702 | 1714 | | WS | Script for Amoxycillin given. |
| 27.04.2007 | 11.03.1944 | M | | Advised to go to A/E as advised by Minor Injuries for neck X-Ray having had a fall | 1714 | 1721 | | KRW | |
| 27.04.2007 | 05.12.1956 | M | | Referred to Gastroenterologist regarding recurrent abdominal pain | 1721 | 1732 | | DTB | Script for Rabeprazole given. |
| 27.04.2007 | 06.12.1964 | M | | Septic insect bites on legs & arm | 1732 | 1737 | Flucloxacillin | PJC | |
| 27.04.2007 | 12.05.2000 | M | | Script for Amoxycillin, Fusidic acid with hydrocortisone cream & neomycin sulphate with chlorhexidine nasal cream given | 1731 | 1743 | | CTD | |
| 27.04.2007 | 29.01.1993 | M | | Hay fever | 1743 | 1747 | Loratadine | JM | |
| 27.04.2007 | 22.02.1971 | M | | Script for Co-codamol & Diclofenac e/c given | 1747 | 1754 | | SB | For KUB USScan & USScan of the testicles. |
| 27.04.2007 | 03.08.1957 | F | | Script for Erythromycin given | 1803 | 1812 | | CK | Penicillin allergy. |

Result of a query that lists all consultations from the 22nd to the end of April 2007 (ConsultationsSeenFrom22ndTillEndOfApr2007)

| SurgeryDate | DateOfBirth | Sex | Diagnosis | TimeIn | TimeOut | Complaints | Treatments | Initials | Notes |
|---|---|---|---|---|---|---|---|---|---|
| 27.04.2007 | 08.03.1982 | F | | 1812 | 1817 | For TFTs | | TMW | |
| 27.04.2007 | 29.09.1932 | F | | 1817 | 1829 | Injection Depo-Medrone with Lidocaine 2mls given to the (L) knee | | SMD | |

Result of a query that lists all consultations from the 22nd to the end of April 2008 (ConsultationsSeenFrom22ndTillEndOfApr2008)

| SurgeryDate | DateOfBirth | Sex | Diagnosis | TimeIn | TimeOut | Complaints | Treatments | Initials | Notes |
|---|---|---|---|---|---|---|---|---|---|
| 22.04.2008 | 16.09.1980 | F | S/Leave | 941 | 947 | Back Pain | | LCP | |
| 22.04.2008 | 18.04.1965 | M | S/Leave | 951 | 956 | Stress | | MGF | |
| 22.04.2008 | 27.08.1969 | F | | 1003 | 1011 | For B12, Folate & Ferritin | | MLS | |
| 22.04.2008 | 28.10.1960 | M | | 1011 | 1025 | Script for Amoxycillin & Prednisolone with Cinchocaine ointment given | | JJK | |
| 22.04.2008 | 31.10.1950 | F | | 1025 | 1036 | Referred to Orthopaedic Surgeon (BUPA) regarding injured (R) middle finger | | WG | Script for Co-dydramol & Diclofenac e/c given. |
| 22.04.2008 | 06.04.1924 | F | | 1036 | 1044 | Medication Review Done | | EJB | |
| 22.04.2008 | 23.08.1925 | F | | 1044 | 1056 | Script for Doxazosin given | | REP | |

77

Result of a query that lists all consultations from the 22nd to the end of April 2008 (ConsultationsSeenFrom22ndTillEndOfApr2008)

| SurgeryDate | DateOfBirth | Sex | Diagnosis | TimeIn | TimeOut | Complaints | Treatments | Initials | Notes |
|---|---|---|---|---|---|---|---|---|---|
| 22.04.2008 | 23.01.1991 | F | RTI | 1102 | 1108 | Chesty cough | Amoxycillin | DSLB | |
| 22.04.2008 | 03.02.2008 | F | | 1108 | 1113 | To get OTC Normal Saline nasal drops | | AAL | |
| 22.04.2008 | 16.06.1915 | M | | 1113 | 1122 | Referred to Surgical Dr. on call, SGH regarding (R) upper abdominal pain | | LB | |
| 22.04.2008 | 12.04.1938 | M | | 1122 | 1135 | Injection Depo-Medrone with Lidocaine given to the (R) shoulder | | MAF | |
| 22.04.2008 | 22.01.1932 | M | | 1355 | 1405 | Fairly well in himself, no need for 2 weekly visits for now | | RM | Home visit. |
| 22.04.2008 | 03.10.1958 | F | | 1642 | 1650 | Medication Review Done | | DJP | |
| 22.04.2008 | 03.07.1995 | F | | 1705 | 1720 | Referred to Child Psychiatrist regarding getting very angry & naughty at school | | KLPW | |
| 22.04.2008 | 18.06.1993 | F | | 1720 | 1729 | Script for Clindamycin with benzoyl peroxide gel & Salicylic acid topical solution 26% given | | LT | |
| 22.04.2008 | 06.02.1944 | M | | 1729 | 1734 | Medication Review Done | | AMC | |

Result of a query that lists all consultations from the 22nd to the end of April 2008 (ConsultationsSeenFrom22ndTillEndOfApr2008)

| SurgeryDate | DateOfBirth | Sex | Diagnosis | TimeIn | TimeOut | Complaints | Treatments | Initials | Notes |
|---|---|---|---|---|---|---|---|---|---|
| 22.04.2008 | 03.04.1987 | M | | 1734 | 1738 | For Fasting Blood Glucose | | CJBH | |
| 22.04.2008 | 24.03.1969 | M | | 1738 | 1746 | Referred to Dermatologist regarding discolouration of his (L) arm | | PO | Script for Dihydrocodeine given. |
| 22.04.2008 | 25.11.1949 | M | | 1749 | 1800 | Referred to ENT Surgeon regarding his hoarse voice | | GJD | |
| 22.04.2008 | 15.03.1967 | F | | 1807 | 1815 | Script for Varenicline given | | MP | |
| 22.04.2008 | 17.05.1939 | M | | 1815 | 1822 | Private script for Viagra given | | JTN | |
| 23.04.2008 | 23.03.1926 | M | | 946 | 1008 | Script for Oxybutynin given | | JWH | |
| 23.04.2008 | 28.10.1930 | F | | 1008 | 1012 | Reassured regarding her marginally elevated serum Creatinine level | | KBC | |
| 23.04.2008 | 20.01.1987 | F | | 1012 | 1018 | Re-referred to Psychiatrist as she missed earlier appointment | | DLG | |
| 23.04.2008 | 03.12.1948 | M | RTI | 1018 | 1026 | Chesty cough | Amoxycillin | HF | |
| 23.04.2008 | 20.09.1934 | M | RTI | 1026 | 1041 | Chesty cough | Amoxycillin | EWM | |
| 23.04.2008 | 11.06.1987 | M | S/Leave | 1041 | 1052 | (R) ankle Injury - Private | | DP | |

Result of a query that lists all consultations from the 22nd to the end of April 2008 (ConsultationsSeenFrom22ndTillEndOfApr2008)

| SurgeryDate | DateOfBirth | Sex | Diagnosis | TimeIn | TimeOut | Complaints | Treatments | Initials | Notes |
|---|---|---|---|---|---|---|---|---|---|
| 23.04.2008 | 17.02.1957 | F | | 1052 | 1057 | For Chest X-Rays | | VMF | |
| 23.04.2008 | 02.01.1983 | F | S/Leave | 1111 | 1130 | Strress - Private | | FMN | |
| 23.04.2008 | 18.05.1975 | F | | 1130 | 1146 | Routine mum & baby post-natal check | | EGHG | |
| 23.04.2008 | 24.05.1909 | F | RTI | 1340 | 135 | Chesty cough | Amoxycillin | HMP | Home visit. |
| 23.04.2008 | 06.07.1957 | F | | 1642 | 1648 | For MSU | | WS | |
| 23.04.2008 | 27.11.1955 | F | S/Leave | 1656 | 1701 | Depression | | JVH | |
| 23.04.2008 | 19.07.1968 | M | | 1704 | 1720 | Referred to Urologist regarding his (L) varicocele | | LJB | |
| 23.04.2008 | 01.09.1961 | M | | 1720 | 1727 | Referred to Orthopaedic Surgeon regarding tingling in his (L) fingers | | CJG | |
| 23.04.2008 | 20.07.1956 | M | | 1727 | 1733 | Script for Omeprazole given | | MDJ | |
| 23.04.2008 | 17.02.1958 | M | RTI | 1733 | 1740 | Chesty cough | Amoxycillin | RFA | |
| 23.04.2008 | 27.08.1948 | F | | 1744 | 1755 | Referred to Ophthalmologist regarding watery eyes | | BJH | |
| 23.04.2008 | 24.12.1989 | F | RTI | 1755 | 1801 | Chesty cough | Amoxycillin | AJR | |
| 23.04.2008 | 12.06.1948 | F | Rash | 1810 | 1817 | Itchy rash on the sole of the (L) foot | Miconazole with Hydrocortisone cream | GEP | |
| 23.04.2008 | 19.05.1988 | F | | 1821 | 1828 | Referred for TOP | | DRC | |
| 23.04.2008 | 29.01.1956 | M | | 1843 | 1853 | Feels giddy & has nausea | Prochlorperazine | AJH | Home visit. |

Result of a query that lists all consultations from the 22nd to the end of April 2008 (ConsultationsSeenFrom22ndTillEndOfApr2008)

| SurgeryDate | DateOfBirth | Sex | Diagnosis | TimeIn | TimeOut | Complaints | Treatments | Initials | Notes |
|---|---|---|---|---|---|---|---|---|---|
| 24.04.2008 | 11.06.1962 | F | | 951 | 1005 | Medication Review Done | | KLB | |
| 24.04.2008 | 23.05.1927 | M | | 1005 | 1030 | Medication Review Done | | JHM | |
| 24.04.2008 | 13.07.1946 | F | | 1030 | 1036 | Script for Simvastatin given | | JFRH | |
| 24.04.2008 | 05.10.1969 | F | | 1036 | 1041 | Referred to Dermatologist regarding spots all over | | NJS | |
| 24.04.2008 | 27.03.1935 | M | | 1041 | 1050 | To discuss with Darrent Valley hospital, Kent regarding his abnormal U/Es & single kidney | | RH | |
| 24.04.2008 | 28.08.1946 | F | RTI | 1050 | 1102 | Chesty cough | Amoxycillin | VAG | Referred to Neurologist regarding tingling in the (L) hand & (L) foot. |
| 24.04.2008 | 31.10.1920 | F | | 1102 | 1112 | For repeat MSU | | NMB | |
| 24.04.2008 | 17.07.1940 | F | | 1112 | 1120 | Referred to Orthopaedic Surgeon regarding painful (R) knee | | MPA | |
| 24.04.2008 | 19.02.1947 | M | | 1120 | 1132 | Script for Dihydrocodeine given | | SMB | |

Result of a query that lists all consultations from the 22nd to the end of April 2008 (ConsultationsSeenFrom22ndTillEndOfApr2008)

| SurgeryDate | DateOfBirth | Sex | Diagnosis | TimeIn | TimeOut | Complaints | Treatments | Initials | Notes |
|---|---|---|---|---|---|---|---|---|---|
| 24.04.2008 | 17.10.1928 | M | | 1132 | 1140 | Script for Doxepin given | | CDW | |
| 24.04.2008 | 31.05.1930 | F | | 1403 | 1413 | Script for Loperamide, Electrolade & Buscopan given | | SAW | Penicillin & Paracetamol allergy. Home visit. |
| 24.04.2008 | 16.10.1921 | F | | 1420 | 1440 | For FBC, U/Es, TFTs, Fasting Glucose, MSU & CRP | | EPF | Home visit. |
| 24.04.2008 | 07.02.1940 | F | | 1645 | 1701 | Medication Review Done | | MEC | |
| 24.04.2008 | 12.10.1946 | F | | 1701 | 1708 | Script for Ferrous Sulphate given | | CPS | |
| 24.04.2008 | 06.04.1930 | M | | 1708 | 1714 | Script for Ferrous Sulphate given | | JHS | |
| 24.04.2008 | 05.04.1952 | M | | 1714 | 1720 | Medication Review Done | | LFC | |
| 24.04.2008 | 11.02.1955 | M | RTI | 1720 | 1725 | Chesty cough | Amoxycillin | MC | |
| 24.04.2008 | 09.04.1997 | F | URTI | 1725 | 1730 | Sore throat & Vomiting | Metoclopramide & Amoxycillin | HBS | |
| 24.04.2008 | 15.06.1988 | M | | 1742 | 1749 | Script for Omeprazole given | | SK | |
| 24.04.2008 | 03.10.1951 | M | | 1749 | 1759 | Script for Otomize ear spray & Peppermint oil e/c m/r capsules | | JWS | |
| 24.04.2008 | 15.05.1945 | M | | 1759 | 1806 | Script for Amoxycillin given | | VCC | |
| 24.04.2008 | 02.11.2006 | F | RTI | 1806 | 1812 | Chesty cough | Amoxycillin | KLA | |

Result of a query that lists all consultations from the 22$^{nd}$ to the end of April 2008 (ConsultationsSeenFrom22ndTillEndOfApr2008)

| SurgeryDate | DateOfBirth | Sex | Diagnosis | TimeIn | TimeOut | Complaints | Treatments | Initials | Notes |
|---|---|---|---|---|---|---|---|---|---|
| 24.04.2008 | 16.04.1971 | M | | 1812 | 1822 | Script for Co-codamol & Diclofenac e/c given | | DO | For MSU. |
| 25.04.2008 | 16.07.1952 | F | S/Leave | 924 | 931 | Fibromyalgia | | KAM | |
| 25.04.2008 | 08.03.1946 | F | | 931 | 937 | Medication Review Done | | GRC | |
| 25.04.2008 | 06.06.1947 | M | RTI | 942 | 951 | Chesty cough | Erythromycin | TLS | |
| 25.04.2008 | 01.12.1967 | M | RTI | 951 | 955 | Chesty cough | Erythromycin | RAJ | Penicillin allergy. |
| 25.04.2008 | 21.05.1930 | F | RTI | 958 | 1009 | Chesty cough | Erythromycin | DMD | Penicillin allergy. |
| 25.04.2008 | 17.04.1923 | M | | 1012 | 1018 | Medication Review Done | | JWD | |
| 25.04.2008 | 26.09.1983 | F | | 1026 | 1035 | For Lumbar spine X-Rays (Oblique views) | | JADF | |
| 25.04.2008 | 03.02.1968 | M | | 1035 | 1041 | To attend stop smoking clinic | | MP | |
| 25.04.2008 | 11.12.1943 | F | | 1041 | 1054 | Script for Trimethoprim given | | PAH | For MSU. |
| 25.04.2008 | 03.08.1933 | F | RTI | 1054 | 1102 | Chesty cough | Cefalexin | BB | Penicillin allergy. |
| 25.04.2008 | 24.10.1989 | F | S/Leave | 1102 | 1118 | Back Pain | | HSI | |
| 25.04.2008 | 21.02.1959 | F | | 1108 | 1119 | Referred to Gynaecologist regarding post coital bleeding | | GT | For MSU for fastidious organisms. |
| 25.04.2008 | 24.11.1954 | F | RTI | 1126 | 1132 | Chesty cough | Amoxycillin | HD | |
| 25.04.2008 | 16.06.1915 | M | | 1330 | 1340 | To continue with own analgesia | | LB | Home visit. |

83

Result of a query that lists all consultations from the 22nd to the end of April 2008 (ConsultationsSeenFrom22ndTillEndOfApr2008)

| SurgeryDate | DateOfBirth | Sex | Diagnosis | TimeIn | TimeOut | Complaints | Treatments | Initials | Notes |
|---|---|---|---|---|---|---|---|---|---|
| 28.04.2008 | 13.03.1932 | M | | 946 | 954 | Referred to Physiotherapist regarding upper abdominal muscular pain | | RJW | |
| 28.04.2008 | 06.04.1937 | M | | 954 | 1002 | Script for Diazepam given | | GWH | |
| 28.04.2008 | 12.07.1967 | M | | 1002 | 1011 | Script for Lysine acetylsalicylate with Metoclopramide given | | KRG | |
| 28.04.2008 | 06.01.1943 | F | | 1011 | 1023 | Referred to Dermatologist regarding small crusty lesion on the (R) side of the bridge of the nose | | PC | |
| 28.04.2008 | 12.08.1936 | M | | 1023 | 1030 | For MSU | | RHP | |
| 28.04.2008 | 15.06.1942 | M | | 1030 | 1038 | Private script for Cialis given | | SJF | For B12, Folate & serum Ferritin. |
| 28.04.2008 | 22.12.1945 | F | | 1038 | 1046 | Referred to ENT Surgeon regarding fuzzy head & feeling of being drunk when she lies down | | CYW | |
| 28.04.2008 | 19.05.1935 | F | | 1055 | 1100 | Script for Erythromycin given | | SMK | |

84

## Result of a query that lists all consultations from the 22nd to the end of April 2008 (ConsultationsSeenFrom22ndTillEndOfApr2008)

| SurgeryDate | DateOfBirth | Sex | Diagnosis | TimeIn | TimeOut | Complaints | Treatments | Initials | Notes |
|---|---|---|---|---|---|---|---|---|---|
| 28.04.2008 | 27.08.1922 | M | | 1100 | 1112 | Referred to Dermatologist regarding punched out ulcer on the lateral malleolus | | AC | |
| 28.04.2008 | 11.11.1934 | M | | 1112 | 1122 | Pruritus | Fexofenadine | VRB | |
| 28.04.2008 | 23.09.1936 | M | | 1122 | 1129 | Lower (R) chest pain following RTA | Co-codamol | TH | |
| 28.04.2008 | 15.09.1939 | F | | 1129 | 1136 | Happy with own analgesia following RTA | | EH | |
| 28.04.2008 | 15.01.1927 | M | | 1411 | 1420 | Script for Trimethoprim given | | HD | Home visit. For MSU. |
| 28.04.2008 | 03.08.1995 | F | | 1652 | 1702 | Re-referred to Paediatrician as she missed earlier appointment | | JT | |
| 28.04.2008 | 16.05.1964 | M | | 1702 | 1710 | To take own Co-codamol for his neck pain | | GDC | |
| 28.04.2008 | 31.01.1964 | F | | 1710 | 1715 | To mention to the Physiotherapist regarding pain in her (R) ankle | | DH | |
| 28.04.2008 | 19.01.1964 | F | | 1715 | 1720 | Script for Amoxycillin given | | NAB | |
| 28.04.2008 | 15.06.1974 | F | S/Leave | 1720 | 1726 | Arthroscopy (L) shoulder - Med. 5 | | SAH | |

85

Result of a query that lists all consultations from the 22nd to the end of April 2008 (ConsultationsSeenFrom22ndTillEndOfApr2008)

| SurgeryDate | DateOfBirth | Sex | Diagnosis | TimeIn | TimeOut | Complaints | Treatments | Initials | Notes |
|---|---|---|---|---|---|---|---|---|---|
| 28.04.2008 | 19.06.1933 | M | | 1729 | 1738 | Awaiting histology of polyp taken during colonoscopy | | BAT | |
| 28.04.2008 | 17.09.1986 | F | S/Leave | 1738 | 1805 | Sexual Assault - Private | | AK | Referred to Practice Counsellor. Script for Erythromycin & Temazepam given. |
| 28.04.2008 | 08.11.1921 | F | | 1805 | 1815 | To take half tablet of Frusemide 20mg on alternate days | | JW | |
| 28.04.2008 | 21.11.1923 | M | | 1815 | 1829 | To stop the Cardicor & Diclofenac as they upset him until he is reviewed in hospital | | RU | |
| 28.04.2008 | 15.10.1974 | M | | 1829 | 1835 | Script for Amoxycillin given | | CSP | For Chest X-Rays. |
| 29.04.2008 | 24.08.1946 | M | | 944 | 953 | Script for Fusidic acid with Hydrocortisone cream given | | RL | |
| 29.04.2008 | 06.12.1947 | M | | 953 | 1007 | Script for Ferrous Sulphate given | | BSK | |
| 29.04.2008 | 21.05.1958 | F | | 1007 | 1012 | Script for Paracetamol with Metoclopramide | | SB | |
| 29.04.2008 | 24.10.1929 | F | | 1012 | 1034 | Referred to General Surgeon regarding lump/thickening on the (L) side of the neck | | LL | |

## Result of a query that lists all consultations from the 22nd to the end of April 2008 (ConsultationsSeenFrom22ndTillEndOfApr2008)

| SurgeryDate | DateOfBirth | Sex | Diagnosis | TimeIn | TimeOut | Complaints | Treatments | Initials | Notes |
|---|---|---|---|---|---|---|---|---|---|
| 29.04.2008 | 24.08.1969 | F | RTI | 1034 | 1044 | Chesty cough | Amoxycillin | MLS | |
| 29.04.2008 | 20.12.1931 | M | | 1044 | 1100 | Script for Amoxycillin & Bendroflumethiazide given | | FWW | |
| 29.04.2008 | 25.08.1939 | F | | 1100 | 1106 | Script for Amoxycillin & Chloramphenicol eye drops given | | DET | |
| 29.04.2008 | 10.09.1945 | F | RTI | 1108 | 1116 | Chesty cough | Amoxycillin | JP | |
| 29.04.2008 | 23.12.1942 | F | | 1116 | 1130 | Script for Doxazosin given | | JASP | |
| 29.04.2008 | 21.04.1990 | M | | 1130 | 1136 | To get OTC Canesten cream for the red pimply rash on his glans penis | | BFC | |
| 29.04.2008 | 25.01.1939 | F | | 1645 | 1653 | Medication Review Done | | PMC | |
| 29.04.2008 | 08.04.2008 | F | | 1653 | 1706 | Child is feeding well & has no evidence of chicken pox at present | | CR | |
| 29.04.2008 | 16.01.1998 | F | | 1706 | 1711 | Letter to Dermatologist to expedite hospital appointment | | MJZ | |
| 29.04.2008 | 29.04.1925 | M | | 1711 | 1718 | Medication Review Done | | ADR | |
| 29.04.2008 | 04.11.1924 | F | | 1718 | 1730 | Medication Review Done | | OJR | |

87

Result of a query that lists all consultations from the 22nd to the end of April 2008 (ConsultationsSeenFrom22ndTillEndOfApr2008)

| SurgeryDate | DateOfBirth | Sex | Diagnosis | TimeIn | TimeOut | Complaints | Treatments | Initials | Notes |
|---|---|---|---|---|---|---|---|---|---|
| 29.04.2008 | 11.08.1962 | F | | 1730 | 1736 | For FBC | | KRD | |
| 29.04.2008 | 03.07.1974 | F | RTI | 1736 | 1742 | Chesty cough | Amoxycillin | SAK | Referred to Orthopaedic Surgeon regarding pains with pins & needles in both hands along the median nerves distribution. |
| 29.04.2008 | 24.02.2007 | M | RTI | 1742 | 1750 | Chesty cough | Amoxycillin | ASMP | Script for Chloramphenicol eye drops given. |
| 29.04.2008 | 17.03.1940 | F | | 1802 | 1812 | Script for Trimethoprim given | | MER | For MSU. |
| 29.04.2008 | 06.09.1964 | F | | 1812 | 1821 | Script for Gaviscon Advance given | | ELB | For FBC & Glandular fever screen. |

Result of a query that lists all consultations from the 22nd to the end of April 2009 (ConsultationsSeenFrom22ndTillEndOfApr2009)

| SurgeryDate | DateOfBirth | Sex | Diagnosis | TimeIn | TimeOut | Complaints | Treatments | Initials | Notes |
|---|---|---|---|---|---|---|---|---|---|
| 22.04.2009 | 20.09.1965 | M | | 942 | 955 | Referred to Breast Surgeon regarding tenderness in (L) Breast nipple | | VJC | For FBC, U/Es, TFTs, LFTs, Fasting cholesterol & fasting Glucose. |
| 22.04.2009 | 27.08.1933 | M | | 955 | 1001 | Script for Amoxycillin given | | HGH | |

Result of a query that lists all consultations from the 22nd to the end of April 2009 (ConsultationsSeenFrom22ndTillEndOfApr2009)

| SurgeryDate | DateOfBirth | Sex | Diagnosis | TimeIn | TimeOut | Complaints | Treatments | Initials | Notes |
|---|---|---|---|---|---|---|---|---|---|
| 22.04.2009 | 28.08.1946 | F |  | 1001 | 1010 | To see me in one month for review of the (L) arm swelling |  | MPB |  |
| 22.04.2009 | 21.11.1923 | M |  | 1010 | 1023 | Referred to Urologist (urgent) regarding elevated PSA level |  | RU |  |
| 22.04.2009 | 17.02.1957 | F | RTI | 1023 | 1028 | Chesty cough | Amoxycillin | VMC |  |
| 22.04.2009 | 16.08.1927 | F |  | 1037 | 1047 | Script for Buprenorphine 35mcg/hr given |  | EFM |  |
| 22.04.2009 | 24.02.1952 | F |  | 1047 | 1054 | Referred to Oral Surgeon regarding her bad oral odour |  | JMB |  |
| 22.04.2009 | 23.03.1926 | M |  | 1054 | 1104 | Bilateral pedal oedema | Furosemide | JWH |  |
| 22.04.2009 | 25.07.1939 | F | RTI | 1104 | 1110 | Chesty cough | Amoxycillin | JLB | Script for Chloramphenicol eye drops given. |
| 22.04.2009 | 26.08.1913 | F |  | 1240 | 1250 | Script for Amoxycillin & Salbutamol inhaler given |  | AEC | Home visit. |
| 22.04.2009 | 14.02.1976 | M | URTI | 1637 | 1646 | (L) ear ache | Amoxycillin | JG | Script for Prochlorperazine given. |
| 22.04.2009 | 04.11.1924 | F |  | 1646 | 1652 | Rash on the loser legs | 1% Hydrocortisone cream | OJR |  |
| 22.04.2009 | 03.10.1937 | F |  | 1701 | 1710 | Script for Trimethoprim given |  | DG |  |

Result of a query that lists all consultations from the 22nd to the end of April 2009 (ConsultationsSeenFrom22ndTillEndOfApr2009)

| SurgeryDate | DateOfBirth | Sex | Diagnosis | TimeIn | TimeOut | Complaints | Treatments | Initials | Notes |
|---|---|---|---|---|---|---|---|---|---|
| 22.04.2009 | 18.02.1968 | F |  | 1717 | 1728 | To contact Queens hospital, Romford to check if they can see her again regarding her dystonia |  | PAC |  |
| 22.04.2009 | 30.07.1983 | F |  | 1728 | 1732 | To have cryotherapy for the fibro-adenomas on her (L) fore-arm & anterior chest |  | YP |  |
| 22.04.2009 | 18.05.1975 | F | RTI | 1732 | 1742 | Chesty cough | Amoxycillin | EGHG | For Fasting Glucose. |
| 22.04.2009 | 06.05.1971 | M | RTI | 1742 | 1749 | Chesty cough | Amoxycillin | RHG | Referred to Orthopaedic Surgeon regarding his (L) knee that gives way & swells up. |
| 22.04.2009 | 31.07.2006 | F |  | 1749 | 1758 | Script for Amoxycillin & Fusidic acid 1% eye drops given |  | MC | For MSU. |
| 22.04.2009 | 24.01.1957 | M |  | 1758 | 1803 | Script for Bendroflumethiazide given |  | PGI |  |
| 23.04.2009 | 17.01.1956 | F |  | 948 | 956 | Script for Co-Amoxiclav given |  | SR |  |
| 23.04.2009 | 16.08.1927 | F |  | 956 | 1004 | For Chest X-Rays |  | GC |  |
| 23.04.2009 | 05.12.1934 | F |  | 1004 | 1010 | BP 144/64 |  | JS |  |

Result of a query that lists all consultations from the 22nd to the end of April 2009 (ConsultationsSeenFrom22ndTillEndOfApr2009)

| SurgeryDate | DateOfBirth | Sex | Diagnosis | TimeIn | TimeOut | Complaints | Treatments | Initials | Notes |
|---|---|---|---|---|---|---|---|---|---|
| 23.04.2009 | 20.04.1938 | M | | 1010 | 1014 | Script for Omeprazole given | | DAD | |
| 23.04.2009 | 13.08.1970 | F | | 1014 | 1026 | Script for Clenil Modulite inhaler, Conjugated Estrogens & Salbutamol inhaler given | | MCG | |
| 23.04.2009 | 19.02.1942 | F | | 1026 | 1031 | Medication Review Done | | EF | |
| 23.04.2009 | 16.03.1956 | F | | 1031 | 1051 | Script for Dihydrocodeine & Metformin given | | SPD | |
| 23.04.2009 | 02.07.1937 | M | RTI | 1051 | 1056 | Chesty cough | Erythromycin | GG | Penicillin allergy. |
| 23.04.2009 | 01.02.1997 | M | | 1056 | 1102 | Worms in stool | Mebendazole | MSG | |
| 23.04.2009 | 15.04.1973 | F | URTI | 1642 | 1649 | Nasal congestion | Amoxycillin | LJB | |
| 23.04.2009 | 13.09.1948 | F | | 1649 | 1658 | Referred to Endocrinologist regarding her persistently abnormal TFTs despite increasing the Levothyroxine dose | | LP | |
| 23.04.2009 | 18.10.1974 | F | | 1658 | 1706 | Script for Diclofenac e/c & Dihydrocodeine given | | HAW | |
| 23.04.2009 | 09.08.1971 | M | | 1706 | 1713 | He may need cervical collar for his whiplash injury | | JCW | |
| 23.04.2009 | 13.05.1982 | F | | 1727 | 1735 | For Pregnancy test | | DMB | |

91

**Result of a query that lists all consultations from the 22nd to the end of April 2009 (ConsultationsSeenFrom22ndTillEndOfApr2009)**

| SurgeryDate | DateOfBirth | Sex | Diagnosis | TimeIn | TimeOut | Complaints | Treatments | Initials | Notes |
|---|---|---|---|---|---|---|---|---|---|
| 23.04.2009 | 21.10.2008 | F | Conjunctivitis | 1733 | 1739 | Sticky eyes | Chloramphenicol eye drops | EC | |
| 23.04.2009 | 31.03.1967 | F | | 1744 | 1750 | Patient informed that her laparoscopy was normal & she can contact the hospital if she wants a follow-up | | LJS | |
| 23.04.2009 | 14.10.1993 | M | | 1750 | 1756 | Script for Benzoyl Peroxide 4% cream given | | JJS | |
| 23.04.2009 | 26.09.1994 | M | | 1804 | 1817 | Referred to Orthopaedic Surgeon regarding pain in the (L) hip region after having the slipped epiphyses screwed bilaterally 2 years ago | | RJR | |
| 24.04.2009 | 03.09.1951 | M | S/Leave | 935 | 945 | Back Pain - Med. 5 | | GLH | Script for Dihydrocodeine given. |
| 24.04.2009 | 27.03.1931 | F | | 945 | 950 | Script for Amoxycillin given | | MMA | |
| 24.04.2009 | 24.03.1972 | M | S/Leave | 950 | 955 | Back Pain | | EAS | |
| 24.04.2009 | 28.03.1945 | M | | 955 | 1000 | Script for Co-codamol given | | APD | |

Result of a query that lists all consultations from the 22nd to the end of April 2009 (ConsultationsSeenFrom22ndTillEndOfApr2009)

| SurgeryDate | DateOfBirth | Sex | Diagnosis | TimeIn | TimeOut | Complaints | Treatments | Initials | Notes |
|---|---|---|---|---|---|---|---|---|---|
| 24.04.2009 | 22.12.1953 | F | | 1016 | 1031 | Script for Erythromycin given | | IR | For TFTs. Referred to Orthopaedic Surgeon regarding tightness & discomfort behind the (R) knee. |
| 24.04.2009 | 13.08.1985 | M | URTI | 1031 | 1044 | Sore throat | Erythromycin | KJH | Penicillin allergy. For FBC in 4 months with the nurse. |
| 24.04.2009 | 18.02.1978 | F | RTI | 1044 | 1056 | Chesty cough | Amoxycillin | KJW | Referred to Podiatrist regarding her increasing more prominent & more painful bunion on the (L) foot. Script for Qvar inhaler given. |
| 24.04.2009 | 15.04.1943 | F | | 1056 | 1104 | Script for Simvastatin given | | SEN | |
| 24.04.2009 | 28.06.2007 | M | | 1104 | 1114 | Referred to Paediatrician regarding overriding 2nd (R) toe on the 3rd toe | | SS | Letter to ENT Surgeon to expedite appointment regarding his discharge from the (R) ear. |
| 24.04.2009 | 28.09.1924 | F | | 1416 | 1455 | Script for Trimethoprim given | | VMG | Home visit. For FBC, U/Es & MSU. Macrodantin allergy. |

93

Result of a query that lists all consultations from the 22nd to the end of April 2009 (ConsultationsSeenFrom22ndTillEndOfApr2009)

| SurgeryDate | DateOfBirth | Sex | Diagnosis | TimeIn | TimeOut | Complaints | Treatments | Initials | Notes |
|---|---|---|---|---|---|---|---|---|---|
| 27.04.2009 | 14.08.1947 | F | | 945 | 951 | Script for Lamotrigine given | | PJH | |
| 27.04.2009 | 17.11.1919 | M | | 1003 | 1012 | The Parking Badge Scheme for Disabled People Medical Practitioner Report form ESS208B completed with his daughter in Surgery | | HHP | His daughter came to the Surgery. |
| 27.04.2009 | 10.05.1968 | F | | 1022 | 1031 | Referred to Gynaecologist regarding her heavy irregular painful periods | | AB | |
| 27.04.2009 | 28.09.1939 | F | | 1031 | 1036 | Advised to see the Practice nurse regarding dieting for her elevated serum cholesterol | | LR | |
| 27.04.2009 | 27.03.1940 | F | | 1036 | 1044 | Advised to see the Practice nurse for cryotherapy for her fibroma | | MAD | |
| 27.04.2009 | 16.09.1936 | M | | 1106 | 1112 | Private script for Viagra given | | LPCE | |
| 27.04.2009 | 29.08.1924 | M | | 1425 | 1455 | Referred to Medical, Dr. on call, SGH, regarding being very pale | | VRH | Home visit. |

94

Result of a query that lists all consultations from the 22nd to the end of April 2009 (ConsultationsSeenFrom22ndTillEndOfApr2009)

| SurgeryDate | DateOfBirth | Sex | Diagnosis | TimeIn | TimeOut | Complaints | Treatments | Initials | Notes |
|---|---|---|---|---|---|---|---|---|---|
| 27.04.2009 | 31.05.1997 | F | Rash | 1644 | 1650 | Impetigo-like rash on face | Erythromycin & Fusidic acid cream | SC | Penicillin allergy. |
| 27.04.2009 | 01.09.1997 | F | RTI | 1654 | 1659 | Chesty cough | Amoxycillin | SAG | |
| 27.04.2009 | 01.02.1996 | M | | 1659 | 1715 | Referred to Paediatrician to be assessed regarding having ADHD | | CTH | |
| 27.04.2009 | 23.11.1975 | F | | 1715 | 1722 | Sore swelling (L) axilla | Flucloxacillin | TRHS | |
| 27.04.2009 | 24.07.1956 | M | | 1723 | 1736 | Script for Ezetimibe & Bendroflumethiazide given | | SS | |
| 27.04.2009 | 19.04.1996 | M | | 1736 | 1747 | Re-referred to Child Psychiatrist regarding his behaviour problem | | SAM | |
| 27.04.2009 | 04.07.1986 | F | | 1747 | 1800 | She will look into being referred for gastric banding under the NHS & come back to us | | CA | |
| 27.04.2009 | 18.02.1968 | F | | 1800 | 1808 | Referred to Neurologist regarding her Dystonia disorder | | PAC | |
| 27.04.2009 | 27.09.1931 | M | RTI | 1808 | 1814 | Chesty cough | Amoxycillin | JJ | Script for Prednisolone e/c given. |

Result of a query that lists all consultations from the 22nd to the end of April 2009 (ConsultationsSeenFrom22ndTillEndOfApr2009)

| SurgeryDate | DateOfBirth | Sex | Diagnosis | TimeIn | TimeOut | Complaints | Treatments | Initials | Notes |
|---|---|---|---|---|---|---|---|---|---|
| 28.04.2009 | 02.09.1941 | F | | 942 | 953 | Script for Dihydrocodeine given | | MS | For Lumbar Spine X-Rays. |
| 28.04.2009 | 11.08.1935 | F | | 953 | 959 | Script for Co-codamol given | | CH | |
| 28.04.2009 | 20.06.1984 | M | URTI | 959 | 1004 | Sinusitis | Amoxycillin | PD | |
| 28.04.2009 | 23.11.1946 | M | | 1009 | 1021 | Private script for Tadalafil given | | TSM | |
| 28.04.2009 | 05.03.1954 | F | | 1021 | 1030 | Script for Trimethoprim given | | PSC | For MSU & Fasting Glucose. |
| 28.04.2009 | 16.05.1944 | F | | 1030 | 1037 | Referred to Rheumatologist regarding arthritis in her fingers with multiple nodes at the ip joints | | JRL | |
| 28.04.2009 | 13.07.2008 | M | | 1049 | 1058 | Script for Amoxycillin given | | MJD | |
| 28.04.2009 | 12.12.1959 | M | | 1058 | 1103 | Script for Dihydrocodeine & Amitriptyline given | | RJW | |
| 28.04.2009 | 15.01.2001 | F | URTI | 1103 | 1109 | (R) ear ache | Amoxycillin | HLA | Script for Malathion 0.5% aqueous liquid. |

Result of a query that lists all consultations from the 22nd to the end of April 2009 (ConsultationsSeenFrom22ndTillEndOfApr2009)

| SurgeryDate | DateOfBirth | Sex | Diagnosis | TimeIn | TimeOut | Complaints | Treatments | Initials | Notes |
|---|---|---|---|---|---|---|---|---|---|
| 28.04.2009 | 21.01.1962 | F | | 1109 | 1149 | For FBC, U/Es, TFTs & serum cholesterol | | JCC | Form AH, Adult Health Report, Medical report on prospective application for a short-term fostering / adoption / inter-country adoption / respite care form completed. |
| 28.04.2009 | 05.03.1972 | M | | 1644 | 1700 | Dizziness - Med. 5 | | WDJGW | Script for Amoxycillin given. |
| 28.04.2009 | 23.01.1994 | F | | 1700 | 1709 | Script for Clotrimazole 1% cream & Loratadine given | | WMS | |
| 28.04.2009 | 18.10.1964 | F | | 1709 | 1714 | She will like her period postponed for holidays | Norethisterone | LVG | |
| 28.04.2009 | 22.07.1939 | F | RTI | 1714 | 1719 | Chesty cough | Amoxycillin | AP | For Chest X-Rays. |
| 28.04.2009 | 25.04.1951 | F | Conjunctivitis | 1719 | 1725 | Discharge from both eyes | Chloramphenicol eye drops | SM | Penicillin & Trimethoprim allergy. |
| 28.04.2009 | 05.01.1994 | M | | 1728 | 1732 | Script for Loratadine given | | JDPC | For FBC. |
| 28.04.2009 | 27.10.1996 | F | | 1741 | 1749 | Script for Amoxycillin given | | KLA | |

Result of a query that lists all consultations from the 22nd to the end of April 2009 (ConsultationsSeenFrom22ndTillEndOfApr2009)

| SurgeryDate | DateOfBirth | Sex | Diagnosis | TimeIn | TimeOut | Complaints | Treatments | Initials | Notes |
|---|---|---|---|---|---|---|---|---|---|
| 28.04.2009 | 19.05.1969 | F | | 1749 | 1801 | Referred to ENT Surgeon regarding getting frequent recurrent tonsilitis | | KLA | |
| 28.04.2009 | 25.01.1957 | M | | 1801 | 1835 | Form AH. Adult Health Report Medical report on prospective application for short-term fostering / long-term fostering / adoption / intercountry adoption / respite care form completed with the patient | | GWC | |
| 29.04.2009 | 30.09.1969 | M | S/Leave | 945 | 956 | Back Pain | Co-codamol 30mg/500mg | SGM | |
| 29.04.2009 | 28.02.1975 | M | | 956 | 1003 | Script for Fusidic acid 2% / Hydrocortisone 1% cream given | | SN | |
| 29.04.2009 | 05.10.1969 | F | | 1003 | 1012 | She says she does not want to see the Dermatologist again for now | | NJS | |
| 29.04.2009 | 28.06.1968 | F | S/Leave | 1012 | 1025 | Chest Infection & Back Pain | | RA | Script for Amoxycillin & Co-codamol given. |

Result of a query that lists all consultations from the 22nd to the end of April 2009 (ConsultationsSeenFrom22ndTillEndOfApr2009)

| SurgeryDate | DateOfBirth | Sex | Diagnosis | TimeIn | TimeOut | Complaints | Treatments | Initials | Notes |
|---|---|---|---|---|---|---|---|---|---|
| 29.04.2009 | 05.03.1934 | M | | 1025 | 1039 | For Lumbar Spine X-Rays, MSU & PSA | | CHD | |
| 29.04.2009 | 16.04.1971 | M | | 1039 | 1049 | Referred to Cardiologist regarding chest pain & being breathless on exertion | | DO | |
| 29.04.2009 | 14.03.1930 | F | | 1049 | 1058 | Script for Lisinopril given | | LMHS | |
| 29.04.2009 | 17.08.1947 | F | | 1058 | 1112 | Referred to Endocrinologist regarding possible hypothyroidism | | SAA | Referred to Podiatrist regarding her (R) bunion. |
| 29.04.2009 | 29.01.1956 | M | | 1112 | 1120 | Referred to Dermatologist regarding blood blisters on the dorsal surface of his (R) fore-arm | | AJH | |
| 29.04.2009 | 05.01.1922 | F | | 1120 | 1138 | Referred to Chest Physician (urgent) regarding collapse, consolidation & effusion on the (R) side on the Chest X-Rays | | MEMP | |
| 29.04.2009 | 28.09.1924 | F | | 1412 | 1455 | Discussed with Social services regarding arranging for a respite or interim care away from home for her | | VMG | Home visit. |

Result of a query that lists all consultations from the 22nd to the end of April 2009 (ConsultationsSeenFrom22ndTillEndOfApr2009)

| SurgeryDate | DateOfBirth | Sex | Diagnosis | TimeIn | TimeOut | Complaints | Treatments | Initials | Notes |
|---|---|---|---|---|---|---|---|---|---|
| 29.04.2009 | 28.02.1981 | M | | 1645 | 1659 | Script for Fluoxetine given | | DJC | Referred to Dermatologist regarding lesions on his face. |
| 29.04.2009 | 15.04.1956 | M | | 1659 | 1713 | Script for Ferrous Sulphate & Metoclopramide given | | MAO | |
| 29.04.2009 | 02.07.1924 | M | | 1713 | 1721 | Script for Furosemide given | | TCC | For X-Rays of the proximal end of the (L) femur to exclude foreign body or bony damage. |
| 29.04.2009 | 29.08.1939 | M | | 1721 | 1730 | Referred to Dermatologist regarding skin tags on his upper thighs & lesion on his back | | JFP | |
| 29.04.2009 | 26.01.2003 | F | | 1730 | 1742 | Script for Chlorphenamine, Clenil Modulite inhaler & Fusidic acid with Hydrocortisone cream given | | CSIB | |

Result of a query that lists all consultations from the 22nd to the end of April 2010 (ConsultationsSeenFrom22ndTillEndOfApr2010)

| SurgeryDate | DateOfBirth | Sex | Diagnosis | TimeIn | TimeOut | Complaints | Treatments | Initials | Notes |
|---|---|---|---|---|---|---|---|---|---|
| 22.04.2010 | 10.04.1937 | F | | 943 | 956 | Medication Review Done | | MC | |
| 22.04.2010 | 13.11.1976 | F | | 956 | 1002 | Script for Tramadol capsules given | | LEM | |
| 22.04.2010 | 27.08.1935 | M | | 1002 | 1019 | Script for Amoxycillin given | | AAS | |
| 22.04.2010 | 29.03.1930 | M | | 1019 | 1032 | For X-Rays of the hips | | EDT | |
| 22.04.2010 | 27.01.1934 | F | | 1032 | 1050 | Script for Levothyroxine given | | JWC | For B12, Folate, Thyroid antibodies & Ferritin. |
| 22.04.2010 | 19.01.1964 | F | RTI | 1050 | 1055 | Cough | Erythromycin | NAB | |
| 22.04.2010 | 04.05.2009 | F | | 1055 | 1059 | Referred to Paediatrician regarding her persistent cough | | ELW | |
| 22.04.2010 | 11.03.2010 | M | | 1116 | 1130 | Routine 6 weeks post-natal check done | | RTS | Script for Infant Gaviscon given. |
| 22.04.2010 | 11.03.2010 | M | | 1130 | 1155 | Routine 6 weeks post-natal check done | | BCS | Script for Infant Gaviscon given. Mum prescribed Ferrous Sulphate & Erythromycin. |
| 22.04.2010 | 12.04.1998 | M | | 1653 | 1700 | Script for Loratadine given | | ADT | |
| 22.04.2010 | 25.06.1938 | F | | 1705 | 1725 | Medication Review Done | | JEL | |

Result of a query that lists all consultations from the 22nd to the end of April 2010 (ConsultationsSeenFrom22ndTillEndOfApr2010)

| SurgeryDate | DateOfBirth | Sex | Diagnosis | TimeIn | TimeOut | Complaints | Treatments | Initials | Notes |
|---|---|---|---|---|---|---|---|---|---|
| 22.04.2010 | 21.06.1942 | M | | 1725 | 1734 | Script for Lisinopril given | | WJB | |
| 22.04.2010 | 01.08.1951 | F | | 1734 | 1752 | Script for Allopurinol & Diclofenac e/c given | | JM | Referred to Counsellor regarding stress of housing her son & his family of 3 children. |
| 22.04.2010 | 01.09.1961 | M | | 1752 | 1756 | Script for Flucloxacillin given | | CJG | |
| 22.04.2010 | 29.09.1992 | M | | 1756 | 1801 | For FBC & U/Es | | EGC | |
| 22.04.2010 | 28.01.1969 | M | | 1801 | 1808 | Referred to ENT Surgeon regarding lump in his throat | | NW | |
| 22.04.2010 | 05.04.1964 | F | | 1808 | 1818 | Script for Furosemide given | | JL | |
| 22.04.2010 | 21.12.2000 | F | | 1818 | 1824 | Script for Amoxycillin & Fusidic acid with Hydrocortisone cream given | | DH | |
| 22.04.2010 | 07.03.2008 | F | | 1824 | 1830 | Script for Maxolon Paediatric & Trimethoprim given | | KCHG | |
| 22.04.2010 | 20.09.2006 | F | | 1830 | 1835 | Referred to ENT Surgeon for tonsillectomy regarding her enlarged tonsils | | IEHG | |
| 23.04.2010 | 14.05.1971 | M | RTI | 929 | 941 | Chesty cough | Amoxycillin | NJF | |

102

Result of a query that lists all consultations from the 22nd to the end of April 2010 (ConsultationsSeenFrom22ndTillEndOfApr2010)

| SurgeryDate | DateOfBirth | Sex | Diagnosis | TimeIn | TimeOut | Complaints | Treatments | Initials | Notes |
|---|---|---|---|---|---|---|---|---|---|
| 23.04.2010 | 23.08.1963 | F | | 941 | 953 | Script for Trimethoprim given | | GPB | Referred to One Stop Haematuria clinic. |
| 23.04.2010 | 22.05.1988 | M | | 953 | 1001 | Referred to Ophthalmologist regarding his recurrent styes | | MCC | |
| 23.04.2010 | 23.08.1963 | F | | 941 | 953 | Referred to Pain Management specialist regarding his back & (R) hip pain | | EJG | For X-Rays of Lumbar spine & hips. |
| 23.04.2010 | 18.07.1929 | F | | 1018 | 1024 | Script for Otomize ear spray & Prochlorperazine given | | JMMG | |
| 23.04.2010 | 12.06.1968 | M | | 1024 | 1043 | To have the Amitriptyline reduced gradually, ways of reducing it explained to him | | ATR | |
| 23.04.2010 | 29.08.1924 | M | | 1043 | 1100 | Referred to Cardiologist regarding his chest pains | | JFL | For Chest X-Rays, FBC, B12, folate, Ferritin & Bence Jones Protein. |
| 23.04.2010 | 30.08.1977 | M | | 1100 | 1112 | (L) lower gum abscess | Amoxycillin | RBC | |

Result of a query that lists all consultations from the 22nd to the end of April 2010 (ConsultationsSeenFrom22ndTillEndOfApr2010)

| SurgeryDate | DateOfBirth | Sex | Diagnosis | TimeIn | TimeOut | Complaints | Treatments | Initials | Notes |
|---|---|---|---|---|---|---|---|---|---|
| 23.04.2010 | 05.11.1924 | F | | 1112 | 1126 | The Blue Badge Parking Scheme of Parking Concessions for Disabled and Blind form completed with the patient in the Surgery | | BM | |
| 23.04.2010 | 29.04.1935 | F | | 1126 | 1134 | Script for Ciprofloxacin & Pavacol D given | | CM | For Chest X-Rays. |
| 23.04.2010 | 24.06.2001 | M | URTI | 1134 | 1140 | Sore throat | Amoxycillin | JSB | |
| 23.04.2010 | 03.10.2003 | M | | 1140 | 1151 | Script for Amoxycillin, Flucloxacillin & Metoclopramide given | | BTA | Referred to Paediatrician regarding recurrent heart pain. |
| 23.04.2010 | 26.10.1925 | M | | 1448 | 1500 | (L) toes are rather red & inflamed | Flucloxacillin | EGS | Home visit. |
| 26.04.2010 | 25.07.1963 | M | | 944 | 954 | Enalapril dose increased from 10mg to 20mg daily | | CPC | |
| 26.04.2010 | 19.07.1925 | F | | 954 | 1003 | Script for Betamethasone Valerate scalp application, Gaviscon Advance suspension & Temazepam given | | RMW | |
| 26.04.2010 | 06.10.1952 | M | | 1003 | 1021 | Medication Review Done | | CJG | |

Result of a query that lists all consultations from the 22nd to the end of April 2010 (ConsultationsSeenFrom22ndTillEndOfApr2010)

| SurgeryDate | DateOfBirth | Sex | Diagnosis | TimeIn | TimeOut | Complaints | Treatments | Initials | Notes |
|---|---|---|---|---|---|---|---|---|---|
| 26.04.2010 | 29.08.1939 | M | | 1021 | 1036 | Referred to Dermatologist regarding the feeling of stinging nettles all over his body on & off | | JFP | |
| 26.04.2010 | 03.03.1946 | M | | 1036 | 1045 | Script for Co-codamol given | | SP | |
| 26.04.2010 | 31.07.1956 | M | RTI | 1045 | 1052 | Chesty cough | Amoxycillin | RVGH | |
| 26.04.2010 | 03.12.1924 | F | | 1052 | 1058 | Script for Amoxycillin given | | AH | |
| 26.04.2010 | 08.04.2008 | F | RTI | 1058 | 1104 | Chesty cough | Amoxycillin | CER | |
| 26.04.2010 | 22.03.1931 | F | | 1104 | 1111 | For FBC, serum Ferritin & U/Es | | HH | |
| 26.04.2010 | 27.08.1922 | M | | 1447 | 1510 | He is finding it hard to come to terms with the fact that he may have cancer | | AC | Home visit. |
| 26.04.2010 | 12.12.1935 | M | | 1645 | 1650 | Medication Review Done | | KAR | |
| 26.04.2010 | 05.06.1960 | M | | 1650 | 1701 | Referred to ENT Surgeon regarding loss of sense of taste & smell | | GWP | Referred to Urologist regarding his frequency & nocturia. For PSA. |
| 26.04.2010 | 18.05.1975 | F | URTI | 1701 | 1705 | Sore throat | Erythromycin | EGEG | |
| 26.04.2010 | 28.10.2004 | F | URTI | 1705 | 1711 | Sore throat | Amoxycillin | FAP | |
| 26.04.2010 | 01.01.1936 | F | | 1724 | 1741 | Script for Omeprazole given | | ALC | For FBC, U/Es, LFTs, MSU & serum cholesterol. |

**Result of a query that lists all consultations from the 22nd to the end of April 2010 (ConsultationsSeenFrom22ndTillEndOfApr2010)**

| SurgeryDate | DateOfBirth | Sex | Diagnosis | TimeIn | TimeOut | Complaints | Treatments | Initials | Notes |
|---|---|---|---|---|---|---|---|---|---|
| 26.04.2010 | 27.10.1997 | M | | 1741 | 1745 | Referred to ENT Surgeon regarding his recurrent nose bleeds | | LRS | |
| 26.04.2010 | 25.07.1984 | F | | 1745 | 1752 | Script for Chloramphenicol eye drops given | | DDW | |
| 26.04.2010 | 02.10.1945 | F | | 1752 | 1757 | Dizziness | Prochlorperazine | BT | |
| 27.04.2010 | 15.04.1951 | F | | 944 | 954 | Script for Folic acid given | | MM | Referred for Sigmoidoscopy. |
| 27.04.2010 | 18.05.1946 | F | | 954 | 1003 | Medication Review Done | | JMS | |
| 27.04.2010 | 10.08.1931 | M | | 1003 | 1015 | Script for Macrogol compound half-strength powder sachets NPF given | | REW | |
| 27.04.2010 | 04.01.1967 | F | | 1015 | 1021 | Script for Ferrous Sulphate given | | MC | |
| 27.04.2010 | 02.04.1962 | F | | 1021 | 1031 | Script for Acyclovir tablets given | | PJL | |
| 27.04.2010 | 17.04.1945 | F | | 1031 | 1037 | Script for Erythromycin given | | MC | |
| 27.04.2010 | 06.12.1940 | F | | 1037 | 1041 | Referred to Cardiologist regarding her frequent & more severe chest pains | | MC | |
| 27.04.2010 | 08.04.1945 | M | Pain | 1041 | 1050 | (L) shoulder pain | Co-codamol, Diclofenac e/c & Omeprazole | GTW | |

Result of a query that lists all consultations from the 22nd to the end of April 2010 (ConsultationsSeenFrom22ndTillEndOfApr2010)

| SurgeryDate | DateOfBirth | Sex | Diagnosis | TimeIn | TimeOut | Complaints | Treatments | Initials | Notes |
|---|---|---|---|---|---|---|---|---|---|
| 27.04.2010 | 07.02.1997 | M | | 1103 | 1113 | Referred to Ophthalmologist regarding his recurrent (L) upper eye lid styes | | JAW | |
| 27.04.2010 | 27.08.1935 | M | | 1115 | 1130 | Referred for Colonoscopy (urgent) regarding the persistent discharge from the back passage | | AAS | |
| 27.04.2010 | 26.09.1919 | F | | 1645 | 1655 | The Blue Badge Parking scheme of the Parking Concessions for Disabled and Blind form ECC1190 (ESS208B) completed with the patient in the Surgery | | EMW | |
| 27.04.2010 | 04.12.1989 | F | | 1659 | 1705 | (L) plantar warts | Salicylic acid 26% solution | AJR | |
| 27.04.2010 | 25.08.1949 | F | | 1705 | 1711 | For X-Rays of the hands | | JP | |
| 27.04.2010 | 20.06.1950 | M | | 1722 | 1731 | Referred to One Stop Haematuria clinic regarding his persistent haematuria | | PH | |
| 27.04.2010 | 25.12.1959 | M | | 1755 | 1838 | Fostering Medical Examination done | | MH | For MSU, U/Es, LFTs, Fasting Lipids & FBC. |

107

Result of a query that lists all consultations from the 22nd to the end of April 2010 (ConsultationsSeenFrom22ndTillEndOfApr2010)

| SurgeryDate | DateOfBirth | Sex | Diagnosis | TimeIn | TimeOut | Complaints | Treatments | Initials | Notes |
|---|---|---|---|---|---|---|---|---|---|
| 27.04.2010 | 31.07.1961 | F | | 1838 | 1855 | Script for Norethisterone given | | CMW | Referred to Gynaecologist (urgent) regarding her frequent irregular per vagina bleeding. |
| 27.04.2010 | 21.06.1959 | M | | 1855 | 1904 | Referred to Dermatologist regarding widespread rash, possibly chicken pox | | SJW | |
| 27.04.2010 | 21.04.1959 | M | | 1904 | 1910 | Script for Fucithalmic eye drops given | | MK | |
| 27.04.2010 | 17.03.1968 | F | | 1910 | 1933 | Script for Levothyroxine & Lisinopril given | | NJB | Referred to Endocrinologist regarding her newly diagnosed hypothyroidism. |
| 28.04.2010 | 19.05.1992 | F | | 946 | 1000 | Script for Microgynon 30 given | | FLM | |
| 28.04.2010 | 27.08.1933 | M | | 1000 | 1009 | Script for Omeprazole given | | HGH | Referred for Gastroscopy regarding his indigestion. |
| 28.04.2010 | 27.05.1941 | F | | 1008 | 1021 | Referred to Dermatologist regarding red itchy rash on her arms & legs | | MDR | Referred to Rheumatologist regarding her multiple joints pains. |

Result of a query that lists all consultations from the 22nd to the end of April 2010 (ConsultationsSeenFrom22ndTillEndOfApr2010)

| SurgeryDate | DateOfBirth | Sex | Diagnosis | TimeIn | TimeOut | Complaints | Treatments | Initials | Notes |
|---|---|---|---|---|---|---|---|---|---|
| 28.04.2010 | 07.09.1928 | M | | 1021 | 1026 | Medication Review Done | | LW | |
| 28.04.2010 | 14.11.1963 | F | | 1026 | 1043 | Script for Letrozole & Acetazolamide given | | SJK | |
| 28.04.2010 | 21.02.1916 | F | | 1043 | 1057 | Script for Macrogol compound half-strength oral powder sachets NPF, Mebendazole chewable tablets & Trimethoprim given | | EFH | |
| 28.04.2010 | 09.08.1927 | F | | 1057 | 1109 | Script for Co-codamol & Lisinopril given | | SW | |
| 28.04.2010 | 23.07.1943 | F | | 1109 | 1116 | Medication Review Done | | JFA | |
| 28.04.2010 | 23.04.1923 | F | URTI | 1646 | 1653 | (L) ear ache | Amoxycillin & Otomize ear spray | JD | |
| 28.04.2010 | 26.09.1937 | M | | 1653 | 1700 | Cramps in the (L) leg | Quinine Sulphate | DJD | |
| 28.04.2010 | 27.02.1992 | M | | 1700 | 1710 | Script for Erythromycin given | | CPH | For FBC, U/Es & Fasting Glucose. |
| 28.04.2010 | 12.01.1992 | F | | 1724 | 130 | Script for Gaviscon Advance & Sudocrem given | | SAL | |
| 28.04.2010 | 21.09.1983 | M | | 1735 | 1741 | Referred to Breast Surgeon regarding the lumps behind his nipples | | JH | |

Result of a query that lists all consultations from the 22nd to the end of April 2010 (ConsultationsSeenFrom22ndTillEndOfApr2010)

| SurgeryDate | DateOfBirth | Sex | Diagnosis | TimeIn | TimeOut | Complaints | Treatments | Initials | Notes |
|---|---|---|---|---|---|---|---|---|---|
| 28.04.2010 | 23.01.1961 | F | | 1741 | 1828 | Fostering Medical examination done | | JJH | For MSU. |
| 28.04.2010 | 06.02.1944 | M | | 1828 | 1833 | Script for Dihydrocodeine & Tramadol given | | AMC | |
| 29.04.2010 | 30.08.1977 | M | S/Leave | 945 | 951 | Med. 3 04/10 given for Fractured (R) knee | | RBC | |
| 29.04.2010 | 13.04.1942 | M | | 955 | 1019 | For U/Es, FBC, BNP, serum cholesterol & Chest X-Rays | | HJM | |
| 29.04.2010 | 06.05.1929 | F | | 1019 | 1025 | Referred to Dermatologist regarding punched out ulcer on the (L) lower shin | | JAE | |
| 29.04.2010 | 03.12.1924 | F | | 1026 | 1033 | To stop the Amoxycillin having developed red rash on the lower legs while taking them | | AH | |
| 29.04.2010 | 01.01.1926 | M | | 1034 | 1045 | For FBC & U/Es | | HAJB | |
| 29.04.2010 | 21.03.2010 | F | | 1045 | 1055 | Routine 6 weeks baby's postnatal check done, no abnormalities found | | LMRS | |
| 29.04.2010 | 17.12.1990 | F | | 1055 | 1104 | Routine 6 weeks mum's post-natal check done | | CS | |

Result of a query that lists all consultations from the 22nd to the end of April 2010 (ConsultationsSeenFrom22ndTillEndOfApr2010)

| SurgeryDate | DateOfBirth | Sex | Diagnosis | TimeIn | TimeOut | Complaints | Treatments | Initials | Notes |
|---|---|---|---|---|---|---|---|---|---|
| 29.04.2010 | 02.07.1924 | M | | 1108 | 1115 | Medication Review Done | | TCC | |
| 29.04.2010 | 28.06.1956 | M | | 1115 | 1130 | Script for Co-codamol, Diclofenac e/c, Flucloxacillin & Fusidic acid cream given | | BGM | |
| 29.04.2010 | 02.10.1992 | M | Conjunctivitis | 1130 | 1136 | Sore red (R) eye | Chloramphenicol eye drop | LF | |
| 29.04.2010 | 06.06.1958 | M | | 1648 | 1653 | Private script for Viagra given | | PRP | |
| 29.04.2010 | 07.03.1999 | F | URTI | 1653 | 1658 | Sore throat | Amoxycillin | SAW | Script for Chloramphenicol eye drops given. |
| 29.04.2010 | 12.02.1996 | M | | 1658 | 1702 | For Chest X-Rays | | JW | |
| 29.04.2010 | 21.08.1934 | F | | 1724 | 1730 | Medication Review Done | | IEW | |
| 29.04.2010 | 01.11.1939 | M | | 1732 | 1740 | Script for Co-codamol, Diclofenac e/c & Omeprazole given | | JN | |
| 29.04.2010 | 01.01.1976 | M | | 1740 | 1744 | For FBC, U/Es, Fasting Lipids, Fasting Glucose & LFTs | | JJH | |
| 29.04.2010 | 23.05.1971 | F | | 1744 | 1755 | Pregnancy test positive | | BCR | |

### Result of a query that lists all consultations from the 22nd to the end of April 2010 (ConsultationsSeenFrom22ndTillEndOfApr2010)

| SurgeryDate | DateOfBirth | Sex | Diagnosis | TimeIn | TimeOut | Complaints | Treatments | Initials | Notes |
|---|---|---|---|---|---|---|---|---|---|
| 29.04.2010 | 19.05.1969 | F | | 1755 | 1800 | She will like her period postponed | Norethisterone | LH | |
| 29.04.2010 | 27.05.1959 | F | | 1800 | 1805 | Script for Co-codamol & Hyoscine butylbromide given | | SM | For USScan of the upper abdomen (urgent). |
| 29.04.2010 | 24.02.1992 | F | | 1805 | 1813 | Referred to Dermatologist regarding persistent rash on both feet | | ELP | For FBC & U/Es. |

### Result of a query that lists all consultations from the 22nd to the end of April 2011 (ConsultationsSeenFrom22ndTillEndOfApr2011)

| SurgeryDate | DateOfBirth | Sex | Diagnosis | TimeIn | TimeOut | Complaints | Treatments | Initials | Notes |
|---|---|---|---|---|---|---|---|---|---|
| 26.04.2011 | 03.02.1949 | F | | 949 | 1001 | Medication Review Done | | DPH | |
| 26.04.2011 | 27.07.1948 | M | | 1004 | 1017 | Script for Bendroflumethiazide & Lisinopril given | | BAG | |
| 26.04.2011 | 06.07.1936 | F | RTI | 1017 | 1027 | Chesty cough | Erythromycin | MLW | Penicillin allergy. |
| 26.04.2011 | 23.10.1947 | F | URTI | 1027 | 1035 | Sore throat | Amoxycillin | EEV | |
| 26.04.2011 | 03.03.1937 | M | | 1035 | 1058 | Medication Review Done | | EJC | |
| 26.04.2011 | 20.12.1928 | M | | 1058 | 1116 | For serum Ferritin, Folate & B12 | | RM | |

Result of a query that lists all consultations from the 22nd to the end of April 2011 (ConsultationsSeenFrom22ndTillEndOfApr2011)

| SurgeryDate | DateOfBirth | Sex | Diagnosis | TimeIn | TimeOut | Complaints | Treatments | Initials | Notes |
|---|---|---|---|---|---|---|---|---|---|
| 26.04.2011 | 03.07.1940 | F | | 1116 | 1125 | Medication Review Done | | JMM | |
| 26.04.2011 | 04.03.1947 | M | RTI | 1125 | 1131 | Chesty cough | Amoxycillin | GSB | |
| 26.04.2011 | 22.11.1966 | M | | 1649 | 1707 | Script for Omeprazole & Peppermint oil e/c m/r capsules given | | SFR | |
| 26.04.2011 | 25.11.1946 | M | | 1707 | 1711 | Script for Amitriptyline given | | DBY | |
| 26.04.2011 | 13.01.1957 | F | | 1711 | 1724 | Medication Review Done | | PAW | |
| 26.04.2011 | 16.03.1978 | M | | 1724 | 1734 | Medication Review Done | | JWPS | His mum came to the Surgery. |
| 26.04.2011 | 25.11.1943 | M | | 1734 | 1740 | Referred to Dermatologist regarding the rash on the lateral aspect of his (L) lower leg | | AES | |
| 26.04.2011 | 11.09.1933 | M | | 1740 | 1750 | Referred to Dermatologist regarding the darkish mole on his (L) elbow | | FM | |
| 26.04.2011 | 03.07.1939 | M | | 1750 | 1758 | Medication Review Done | | RFL | |
| 26.04.2011 | 18.04.1957 | F | | 1758 | 1813 | Script for Pioglitazone/ Metformin given | | SK | |
| 27.04.2011 | 15.04.1927 | M | | 946 | 1002 | Medication Review Done | | JB | |

Result of a query that lists all consultations from the 22nd to the end of April 2011 (ConsultationsSeenFrom22ndTillEndOfApr2011)

| SurgeryDate | DateOfBirth | Sex | Diagnosis | TimeIn | TimeOut | Complaints | Treatments | Initials | Notes |
|---|---|---|---|---|---|---|---|---|---|
| 27.04.2011 | 10.04.1937 | F | | 1002 | 1019 | Script for Methylprednisolone with Lidocaine injection given | | MC | The Blue Badge Parking Scheme of Parking Concessions for Disabled and Medical Practitioner Report form ECC 1190 (ESS208B) completed with the patient in the Surgery. |
| 27.04.2011 | 06.01.1943 | F | | 1019 | 1031 | Script for Levothyroxine & Slow-K tablets given | | PC | |
| 27.04.2011 | 14.04.1946 | F | RTI | 1031 | 1037 | Chesty cough | Amoxycillin | VBB | |
| 27.04.2011 | 29.11.1937 | F | | 1037 | 1052 | Referred to Orthopaedic Surgeon for toe nail avulsion as requested by the Podiatrist | | MRS | |
| 27.04.2011 | 19.05.1944 | F | URTI | 1052 | 1059 | (L) ear ache | Amoxycillin & Otomize ear spray | AWB | |
| 27.04.2011 | 20.11.1936 | M | | 1059 | 1109 | Script for Ferrous Sulphate & Levothyroxine given | | NN | |
| 27.04.2011 | 10.12.1951 | F | | 1109 | 1117 | Script for Metformin given | | FMM | |

## Result of a query that lists all consultations from the 22nd to the end of April 2011 (ConsultationsSeenFrom22ndTillEndOfApr2011)

| SurgeryDate | DateOfBirth | Sex | Diagnosis | TimeIn | TimeOut | Complaints | Treatments | Initials | Notes |
|---|---|---|---|---|---|---|---|---|---|
| 27.04.2011 | 04.02.1918 | F | | 1320 | 1330 | Script for Flucloxacillin & Metoclopramide given | | JM | Home visit. |
| 27.04.2011 | 02.01.1933 | F | | 1335 | 1355 | Script for Diazepam, Erythromycin & Prednisolone given | | DLW | Home visit. |
| 27.04.2011 | 09.10.1976 | F | RTI | 1650 | 1707 | Chesty cough | Amoxycillin | SM | |
| 27.04.2011 | 24.09.1999 | F | Rash | 1707 | 1712 | Itchy red rash | Calamine lotion & Loratadine | KJG | |
| 27.04.2011 | 10.07.1962 | F | | 1712 | 1718 | Script for Mometasone nasal spray given | | PL | |
| 27.04.2011 | 30.03.1960 | F | Pain | 1718 | 1724 | Back Pain | Diclofenac e/c & Dihydrocodeine | MTP | |
| 27.04.2011 | 06.01.1969 | F | | 1728 | 1736 | Referred to Orthopaedic Surgeon regarding her (R) knee pain & it giving way | | KEL | |
| 27.04.2011 | 10.10.1992 | F | | 1746 | 1755 | She wants her period postponed whilst on holidays | Norethisterone | AGH | |
| 27.04.2011 | 09.09.1949 | M | | 1755 | 1800 | Script for Amoxycillin given | | CSM | |
| 28.04.2011 | 10.11.1984 | F | Pain | 945 | 957 | Sprained (L) foot | Co-codamol & Diclofenac e/c | AH | |
| 28.04.2011 | 06.12.1947 | M | | 957 | 1007 | Script for Ciprofloxacin & Loperamide given | | BSK | |

Result of a query that lists all consultations from the 22nd to the end of April 2011 (ConsultationsSeenFrom22ndTillEndOfApr2011)

| SurgeryDate | DateOfBirth | Sex | Diagnosis | TimeIn | TimeOut | Complaints | Treatments | Initials | Notes |
|---|---|---|---|---|---|---|---|---|---|
| 28.04.2011 | 06.11.1990 | M | URTI | 1007 | 1012 | (R) ear ache | Amoxycillin | MEGL | |
| 28.04.2011 | 05.09.1956 | F | | 1012 | 1022 | Throbbing (R) facial swelling | Erythromycin & Metronidazole | LPH | |
| 28.04.2011 | 07.06.1972 | M | | 1022 | 1037 | Script for Dihydrocodeine & Diclofenac e/c given | | MJL | Referred to Physiotherapist regarding injury to (R) shoulder whilst playing rugby. |
| 28.04.2011 | 20.05.1987 | F | | 1104 | 1122 | Routine immediate post-natal mum & baby check | | DAD | Script for Cilest & Infacol given. |
| 28.04.2011 | 13.12.1968 | M | | 1641 | 1647 | Referred to ENT Surgeon regarding his bilateral deafness as requested from the Audiology clinic | | GAC | |
| 28.04.2011 | 18.02.1968 | F | | 1647 | 1708 | Script for Uniphyllin continus given | | PAC | |
| 28.04.2011 | 31.08.1964 | M | | 1708 | 1717 | Referred to Physiotherapist regarding being unable to fully supinate his (R) fore-arm | | CJW | |

116

Result of a query that lists all consultations from the 22nd to the end of April 2011 (ConsultationsSeenFrom22ndTillEndOfApr2011)

| SurgeryDate | DateOfBirth | Sex | Diagnosis | TimeIn | TimeOut | Complaints | Treatments | Initials | Notes |
|---|---|---|---|---|---|---|---|---|---|
| 28.04.2011 | 02.12.1980 | M | | 1729 | 1750 | Advised to speak to the Gynaecologist looking after his wife's infertility problems regarding him having male fertility test done | | SW | |
| 28.04.2011 | 10.11.1976 | F | RTI | 1750 | 1755 | Chesty cough | Amoxycillin | DPS | |
| 28.04.2011 | 01.01.1976 | M | | 1755 | 1802 | Referred for Vasectomy | | JJH | |

Result of a query that lists all consultations from the 22nd to the end of April 2012 (ConsultationsSeenFrom22ndTillEndOfApr2012)

| SurgeryDate | DateOfBirth | Sex | Diagnosis | TimeIn | TimeOut | Complaints | Treatments | Initials | Notes |
|---|---|---|---|---|---|---|---|---|---|
| 23.04.2012 | 04.11.1924 | F | | 942 | 959 | Script for Indapamide given | | OJR | |
| 23.04.2012 | 28.03.1970 | F | S/Leave | 959 | 1008 | Med.3 04/10 given for Excision of a melanocytic lesion on her back from 14.04.12 for 1 month | | LJ | |
| 23.04.2012 | 20.04.1938 | M | | 1008 | 1018 | Script for Chloramphenicol eye ointment given | | DAD | |

Result of a query that lists all consultations from the 22nd to the end of April 2012 (ConsultationsSeenFrom22ndTillEndOfApr2012)

| SurgeryDate | DateOfBirth | Sex | Diagnosis | TimeIn | TimeOut | Complaints | Treatments | Initials | Notes |
|---|---|---|---|---|---|---|---|---|---|
| 23.04.2012 | 11.09.1958 | M | S/Leave | 1018 | 1026 | Med.3 04/10 given for Septoplasty and trimming of the inferior turbinates from 23.04.12 until 24.04.12 | | DJS | |
| 23.04.2012 | 17.07.1983 | M | | 1027 | 1037 | Script for Flucloxacillin given | | JCR | Referred to Orthopaedic Surgeon regarding possible (L) carpal tunnel syndrome. |
| 23.04.2012 | 20.01.1941 | F | | 1037 | 1048 | For X-Rays of her (R) knee & her (R) hip | | BDD | |
| 23.04.2012 | 26.10.1961 | M | | 1048 | 1056 | Medication Review Done | | CB | |
| 23.04.2012 | 23.03.1950 | F | | 1056 | 1104 | For X-Rays of her (L) knee & (L) hip | | YC | |
| 23.04.2012 | 13.12.1934 | F | | 1643 | 1649 | To take the Metformin tds | | SDH | |
| 23.04.2012 | 26.04.1944 | F | | 1656 | 1703 | For Lumbar spine X-Rays & MSU | | AW | |
| 23.04.2012 | 29.12.1975 | F | | 1703 | 1710 | Script for Ferrous Fumarate given | | JC | |
| 23.04.2012 | 16.03.1963 | F | S/Leave | 1710 | 1728 | Med.3 04/10 given for Depression from 23.04.12 for 3 months | | TJC | Referred to Counsellor regarding her depression. |
| 23.04.2012 | 11.08.1935 | F | | 1728 | 1736 | Script for Furosemide given | | CH | |

118

Result of a query that lists all consultations from the 22nd to the end of April 2012 (ConsultationsSeenFrom22ndTillEndOfApr2012)

| SurgeryDate | DateOfBirth | Sex | Diagnosis | TimeIn | TimeOut | Complaints | Treatments | Initials | Notes |
|---|---|---|---|---|---|---|---|---|---|
| 23.04.2012 | 13.03.1973 | F | | 1738 | 1744 | BP 112/72 | | LNS | |
| 23.04.2012 | 19.09.1984 | M | | 1744 | 1804 | Script for Amoxycillin & Metronidazole given | | RLWL | Referred to Urologist regarding his epididymal cysts. |
| 23.04.2012 | 05.03.1994 | M | | 1804 | 1812 | Script for Occlusal given | | JMW | |
| 23.04.2012 | 26.06.1997 | F | | 1822 | 1829 | Script for Flucloxacillin given | | EBF | |
| 24.04.2012 | 02.07.1943 | M | | 943 | 950 | For Cervical spine X-Rays | | WRW | |
| 24.04.2012 | 08.10.1940 | M | | 950 | 1003 | Script for Amoxycillin given | | GAFM | For Fasting Glucose. |
| 24.04.2012 | 27.04.1939 | F | | 1003 | 1013 | For U/Es, LFTs, FBC & serum cholesterol | | DBS | |
| 24.04.2012 | 13.03.1932 | M | | 1013 | 1032 | He came in with the new Easyhalers which I showed him how to use | | BJC | |
| 24.04.2012 | 22.05.1988 | M | S/Leave | 1032 | 1042 | Med.3 04/10 given for Depression from 23.04.12 for 3 months | | MCC | |
| 24.04.2012 | 10.04.1969 | F | S/Leave | 1045 | 1053 | Med.3 04/10 given for Depression and Heavy bleeding from 24.04.12 for 3 months | | LAJ | |

Result of a query that lists all consultations from the 22nd to the end of April 2012 (ConsultationsSeenFrom22ndTillEndOfApr2012)

| SurgeryDate | DateOfBirth | Sex | Diagnosis | TimeIn | TimeOut | Complaints | Treatments | Initials | Notes |
|---|---|---|---|---|---|---|---|---|---|
| 24.04.2012 | 27.07.1940 | M | | 1053 | 1104 | Script for Lansoprazole & Transvasin Heat Rub cream given | | BAG | For Cervical spine X-Rays. |
| 24.04.2012 | 01.12.1942 | M | | 1104 | 1118 | Referred to Cardiologist following his sudden loss of consciousness whilst driving on A13 | | | |
| 24.04.2012 | 01.09.1946 | M | | 1108 | 1134 | Script for Amoxycillin given | | PAH | |
| 24.04.2012 | 29.08.1915 | F | | 1310 | 1320 | To increase the Fortisip drinks from bd to tds | | FJ | Home visit. |
| 24.04.2012 | 02.11.1949 | M | RTI | 1324 | 1334 | Chesty cough | Amoxycillin | SJW | Home visit. |
| 24.04.2012 | 31.07.1923 | M | | 1646 | 1656 | Cryotherapy blasts applied to scalp lesion | | HO | |
| 24.04.2012 | 08.04.1945 | M | | 1656 | 1702 | Cryotherapy blasts applied to warts on the (R) fingers | | GTW | |
| 24.04.2012 | 05.03.1950 | M | S/Leave | 1702 | 1712 | Med.3 04/10 given for (L) toe amputation from 24.04.12 until 08.05.12 | | LAJ | |
| 24.04.2012 | 09.08.1961 | M | | 1712 | 1720 | Script for Symbicort given | | SRC | |
| 24.04.2012 | 04.10.1968 | F | | 1720 | 1728 | Script for Omeprazole given | | AW | Script for Janumet given. |

Result of a query that lists all consultations from the 22nd to the end of April 2012 (ConsultationsSeenFrom22ndTillEndOfApr2012)

| SurgeryDate | DateOfBirth | Sex | Diagnosis | TimeIn | TimeOut | Complaints | Treatments | Initials | Notes |
|---|---|---|---|---|---|---|---|---|---|
| 24.04.2012 | 10.01.1958 | M | | 1728 | 1735 | Script for Otosporin ear drops given | | ARH | |
| 24.04.2012 | 05.10.1974 | M | | 1744 | 1754 | Script for Tramadol capsules given | | SMG | For MSU. |
| 24.04.2012 | 31.10.1969 | F | | 1754 | 1800 | Script for Amoxycillin & Co-codamol given | | SJY | Referred to Physiotherapist regarding her neck pain. |
| 24.04.2012 | 25.09.1996 | F | | 1800 | 1809 | Script for Cetraben emollient cream & Trimovate cream given | | ERY | |
| 25.04.2012 | 16.03.1956 | F | | 942 | 1001 | Script for Janumet given | | SPD | |
| 25.04.2012 | 04.11.1966 | F | | 1001 | 1010 | For FBC, B12, Folate & serum Ferritin | | SJOB | |
| 25.04.2012 | 04.11.1934 | M | | 1010 | 1024 | Script for Movicol-Half oral powder sachets given | | TEE | |
| 25.04.2012 | 31.01.1969 | F | | 1024 | 1029 | Script for Mebeverine given | | JP | |
| 25.04.2012 | 03.01.1987 | F | | 1029 | 1042 | Routine 6 weeks post-natal check done | | KSP | |
| 25.04.2012 | 26.04.1943 | M | | 1042 | 1058 | Script for Trimethoprim given | | WWH | For MSU, PSA & USScan of the testicles. Penicillin allergy. |

Result of a query that lists all consultations from the 22nd to the end of April 2012 (ConsultationsSeenFrom22ndTillEndOfApr2012)

| SurgeryDate | DateOfBirth | Sex | Diagnosis | TimeIn | TimeOut | Complaints | Treatments | Initials | Notes |
|---|---|---|---|---|---|---|---|---|---|
| 25.04.2012 | 24.12.1929 | F | | 1100 | 1110 | Script for Cetraben cream & Transvasin Heat Rub cream given | | ECH | Penicillin allergy. |
| 25.04.2012 | 30.01.1987 | M | S/Leave | 1110 | 1116 | Med.3 04/10 given for Fracture (R) clavicle from 23.04.12 for 1 month | | NJW | |
| 25.04.2012 | 31.05.1930 | F | | 1116 | 1123 | For X-Rays of the pelvis & (R) hip | | SAW | |
| 25.04.2012 | 22.06.1979 | F | | 1123 | 1132 | Script for Amoxycillin, Codeine, Noriday & Prednisolone tablets given | | JLW | |
| 25.04.2012 | 24.12.1932 | F | | 1320 | 1330 | Script for Furosemide & Co-Amoxiclav given | | EM | Home visit. |
| 25.04.2012 | 02.05.1990 | F | | 1646 | 1655 | Script for 1% Hydrocortisone cream given | | MIG | |
| 25.04.2012 | 28.11.1925 | F | | 1657 | 1708 | Script for Amoxycillin & Otosporin ear drops given | | JIF | |
| 25.04.2012 | 12.05.1953 | M | | 1708 | 1717 | For GTT | | AG | |
| 25.04.2012 | 13.04.1942 | M | | 1717 | 1734 | Script for Furosemide given | | HJM | |

Result of a query that lists all consultations from the 22nd to the end of April 2012 (ConsultationsSeenFrom22ndTillEndOfApr2012)

| SurgeryDate | DateOfBirth | Sex | Diagnosis | TimeIn | TimeOut | Complaints | Treatments | Initials | Notes |
|---|---|---|---|---|---|---|---|---|---|
| 25.04.2012 | 13.04.1971 | M | | 1734 | 1744 | Script for Co-codamol, Ibuprofen, Orlistat & Balneum Plus bath oil given | | NJF | |
| 25.04.2012 | 25.03.1925 | F | | 1754 | 1814 | Script for Trimethoprim given | | JC | |
| 26.04.2012 | 19.06.1944 | F | | 944 | 956 | BP 143/83 | | PJL | |
| 26.04.2012 | 22.02.1936 | M | | 956 | 1001 | Script for Omeprazole given | | HPA | |
| 26.04.2012 | 18.10.1958 | F | | 1001 | 1009 | She came to inform me about the lump on the (R) side of her Thyroid gland already being investigated at Basildon hospital | | GGM | |
| 26.04.2012 | 05.03.1934 | M | | 1013 | 1020 | Script for Co-codamol & Vardenafil given | | CHD | |
| 26.04.2012 | 11.11.1934 | M | | 1020 | 1026 | Script for Salbutamol given | | VRB | |
| 26.04.2012 | 19.02.1942 | F | | 1026 | 1036 | Script for Lisinopril given | | EF | |
| 26.04.2012 | 26.05.1936 | M | | 1042 | 1055 | Script for Gliclazide & 1% Hydrocortisone cream given | | TC | |

123

Result of a query that lists all consultations from the 22nd to the end of April 2012 (ConsultationsSeenFrom22ndTillEndOfApr2012)

| SurgeryDate | DateOfBirth | Sex | Diagnosis | TimeIn | TimeOut | Complaints | Treatments | Initials | Notes |
|---|---|---|---|---|---|---|---|---|---|
| 26.04.2012 | 18.07.1956 | F | S/Leave | 1055 | 1109 | Med.3 04/10 given for Multiple joints pains & injury to (R) foot from 24.04.12 for 3 months | | MTC | Referred for Colonoscopy regarding rectal bleeding. For FBC, Fasting Glucose, fasting lipids & U/Es. |
| 26.04.2012 | 07.02.1948 | M | | 1645 | 1704 | Script for Flucloxacillin given | | GRC | Referred to Oral Surgeon regarding the very bad taste in his mouth. |
| 26.04.2012 | 13.11.1976 | F | | 1704 | 1710 | Script for Erythromycin given | | LEM | Penicillin allergy. |
| 26.04.2012 | 02.05.1949 | M | | 1710 | 1717 | Referred to Podiatrist regarding pain in both feet worse on the (R) side | | RB | |
| 26.04.2012 | 08.08.1956 | M | S/Leave | 1717 | 1725 | Med.3 04/10 given for Stress from 23.04.12 for 2 weeks | | JR | |
| 26.04.2012 | 09.04.2000 | M | | 1725 | 1744 | For FBC, U/Es, TFTs & Fasting Glucose given | | OO | Script for Buscopan given. |
| 26.04.2012 | 11.02.1972 | M | | 1744 | 1750 | Script for Lansoprazole & Tramadol given | | DJB | |
| 26.04.2012 | 13.03.1973 | F | S/Leave | 1750 | 1756 | Med.3 04/10 given for Stress from 26.04.12 for 1 month | | LNS | |

Result of a query that lists all consultations from the 22nd to the end of April 2012 (ConsultationsSeenFrom22ndTillEndOfApr2012)

| SurgeryDate | DateOfBirth | Sex | Diagnosis | TimeIn | TimeOut | Complaints | Treatments | Initials | Notes |
|---|---|---|---|---|---|---|---|---|---|
| 26.04.2012 | 29.06.1947 | F | | 1756 | 1804 | Script for Furosemide & Ibuprofen given | | SLS | |
| 26.04.2012 | 06.07.1948 | M | | 1804 | 1810 | He will take own Paracetamol for his arthritic (L) knee | | DRS | |
| 27.04.2012 | 18.03.1967 | F | | 943 | 956 | Script for Co-codamol, Ibuprofen & Omeprazole given | | SO | |
| 27.04.2012 | 18.02.1968 | F | | 956 | 1014 | Script for Oseltamivir given | | PAC | |
| 27.04.2012 | 13.08.1978 | M | | 1014 | 1021 | Referred to Physiotherapist regarding his (R) knee injury & pain | | RED | |
| 27.04.2012 | 05.04.1952 | M | | 1021 | 1030 | Script for Amitriptyline given | | LFC | |
| 27.04.2012 | 25.05.1970 | F | | 1035 | 1045 | Script for Codeine given | | SA | For X-Rays of the Lumbar Spine & (R) shoulder. |
| 27.04.2012 | 25.11.1975 | M | | 1045 | 1054 | Script for Canesten HC cream given | | TAM | For FBC, U/Es & serum cholesterol. |
| 27.04.2012 | 19.09.1964 | M | | 1054 | 1106 | Script for Co-codamol & Ibuprofen given | | DJM | Aware of the BMA fee. |
| 27.04.2012 | 01.09.1983 | F | | 1106 | 1113 | Script for Trimethoprim given | | KLH | Penicillin allergy. |

Result of a query that lists all consultations from the 22nd to the end of April 2013 (ConsultationsSeenFrom22ndTillEndOfApr2013)

| SurgeryDate | DateOfBirth | Sex | Diagnosis | TimeIn | TimeOut | Complaints | Treatments | Initials | Notes |
|---|---|---|---|---|---|---|---|---|---|
| 22.04.2013 | 07.08.1971 | F | S/Leave | 944 | 956 | Med. 3 04/10 given for Depression for 3 months from 21.04.13 | | LPH | Script for Serrtraline, Penicillin V & Flucloxacillin given. |
| 22.04.2013 | 10.09.1945 | F | | 956 | 1010 | Script for Fucidin H cream given | | JP | |
| 22.04.2013 | 17.09.1965 | F | | 1010 | 1015 | To stop the Amitriptyline to see if the redness in her legs improve | | PAE | |
| 22.04.2013 | 02.07.1943 | M | | 1015 | 1020 | Script for Beclomethasone nasal spray & Sodium cromoglicate eye drops given | | WRW | |
| 22.04.2013 | 16.08.1943 | M | | 1022 | 1033 | Script for Codeine tablets, Naproxen & Transvasin Heat Rub cream given | | MJG | |
| 22.04.2013 | 31.01.1959 | M | | 1033 | 1039 | Script for Forxiga given | | DH | |
| 22.04.2013 | 23.05.1927 | M | | 1039 | 1100 | Script for Erythromycin given | | JM | |
| 22.04.2013 | 16.06.1965 | F | | 1100 | 1108 | Script for Naproxen given | | JLP | |
| 22.04.2013 | 16.11.1944 | F | | 1108 | 1116 | For TFTs, Fasting Glucose, B12, Folate, Ferritin & HbA1c | | JH | |

Result of a query that lists all consultations from the 22nd to the end of April 2013 (ConsultationsSeenFrom22ndTillEndOfApr2013)

| SurgeryDate | DateOfBirth | Sex | Diagnosis | TimeIn | TimeOut | Complaints | Treatments | Initials | Notes |
|---|---|---|---|---|---|---|---|---|---|
| 22.04.2013 | 09.04.1997 | F | | 1116 | 1121 | Script for Co-Amoxiclav given | | HBS | |
| 22.04.2013 | 03.05.1977 | M | | 1646 | 1656 | Script for Lisinopril given | | CC | |
| 22.04.2013 | 05.09.1998 | F | | 1656 | 1703 | Script for Rigevidon tablets given | | EVW | |
| 22.04.2013 | 02.12.1954 | M | | 1703 | 1712 | For U/Es | | OAK | |
| 22.04.2013 | 10.12.1971 | M | | 1712 | 1721 | Script for Amitriptyline given | | PT | |
| 22.04.2013 | 26.03.1951 | F | | 1721 | 1728 | Script for Codeine tablets & Naproxen given | | LEP | |
| 22.04.2013 | 27.07.1995 | F | | 1750 | 1802 | Script for Cetirizine, Fostair inhaler, Salbutamol inhaler & Tramadol capsules given | | BM | |
| 22.04.2013 | 01.07.1976 | M | | 1802 | 1807 | Script for Amoxycillin given | | LJM | |
| 22.04.2013 | 18.03.1987 | F | | 1807 | 1814 | Script for Norethisterone tablets given | | LP | |
| 22.04.2013 | 03.12.1989 | F | | 1814 | 1820 | Script for Lansoprazole capsules given | | EDB | |

Result of a query that lists all consultations from the 22nd to the end of April 2013 (ConsultationsSeenFrom22ndTillEndOfApr2013)

| SurgeryDate | DateOfBirth | Sex | Diagnosis | TimeIn | TimeOut | Complaints | Treatments | Initials | Notes |
|---|---|---|---|---|---|---|---|---|---|
| 23.04.2013 | 15.12.1939 | M | | 940 | 950 | Referred to Ophthalmologist (Dr. Idre) regarding his droopy (R) lower eye lid | | ERC | |
| 23.04.2013 | 07.11.1946 | M | | 951 | 1001 | BP 145/90 | | GJW | |
| 23.04.2013 | 02.12.1994 | F | | 1006 | 1015 | Counsellor has arranged for her to attend anxiety course, anger management & one to one therapy | | AAP | |
| 23.04.2013 | 16.09.1936 | M | | 1015 | 1037 | Private script for Viagra given | | LPCE | |
| 23.04.2013 | 31.01.1933 | M | | 1043 | 1057 | Script for Levothyroxine given | | MPB | |
| 23.04.2013 | 31.07.1923 | M | | 1057 | 1105 | He will bring the name of the cream he will like prescribed next time | | HO | |
| 23.04.2013 | 15.09.1925 | F | | 1105 | 1124 | Script for Buprenorphine 70mcg patch & Transvasin Heat Rub cream prescribed | | DFS | |
| 23.04.2013 | 18.07.1956 | F | S/Leave | 1642 | 1653 | Med. 3 04/10 given for Multiple joint pains and injury to (R) foot for 3 months from 23.04.13 | | MTC | |

Result of a query that lists all consultations from the 22nd to the end of April 2013 (ConsultationsSeenFrom22ndTillEndOfApr2013)

| SurgeryDate | DateOfBirth | Sex | Diagnosis | TimeIn | TimeOut | Complaints | Treatments | Initials | Notes |
|---|---|---|---|---|---|---|---|---|---|
| 23.04.2013 | 11.05.1972 | M | | 1653 | 1702 | Script for Hyoscine butylbromide & Omeprazole given | | JRG | For USScan of the upper abdomen. |
| 23.04.2013 | 02.06.1970 | M | S/Leave | 1702 | 1717 | Med. 3 04/10 given for Depression for 3 months from 09.03.13 | | DLM | |
| 23.04.2013 | 03.03.1951 | M | | 1732 | 1740 | Medications Review Done | | SWP | |
| 23.04.2013 | 19.12.1949 | M | | 1740 | 1748 | For X-Rays of the (L) foot | | DJB | |
| 23.04.2013 | 11.03.1986 | M | | 1753 | 1803 | Script for Trimethoprim given | | LTB | |
| 24.04.2013 | 11.07.1960 | M | | 946 | 951 | To see the nurse in 9 to 12 months for repeat U/Es | | KBT | |
| 24.04.2013 | 20.12.1928 | M | | 951 | 1010 | Dementia annual review done with his wife | | RM | |
| 24.04.2013 | 26.03.1958 | F | | 1010 | 1021 | Script for Codeine tablets & Naproxen given | | JLS | For X-Rays of the (L) wrist. |
| 24.04.2013 | 29.11.1967 | M | RTI | 1021 | 1030 | Chesty cough | Amoxycillin | MAW | |
| 24.04.2013 | 06.10.2009 | F | | 1030 | 1039 | Constipation | Laculose | LP | |
| 24.04.2013 | 01.08.1947 | F | | 1039 | 1044 | Script for Prochlorperazine given | | JLC | |

Result of a query that lists all consultations from the 22nd to the end of April 2013 (ConsultationsSeenFrom22ndTillEndOfApr2013)

| SurgeryDate | DateOfBirth | Sex | Diagnosis | TimeIn | TimeOut | Complaints | Treatments | Initials | Notes |
|---|---|---|---|---|---|---|---|---|---|
| 24.04.2013 | 01.01.1924 | M | | 1044 | 1052 | Referred to Incontinence clinic regarding his anus getting wet | | HAJB | |
| 24.04.2013 | 17.11.1992 | F | | 1052 | 1059 | Script for Amoxycillin given | | SJH | For MSU |
| 24.04.2013 | 23.01.1009 | M | | 1059 | 1104 | Script for Erythromycin given | | SKF | |
| 24.04.2013 | 03.07.1992 | M | | 1104 | 1116 | Script for Propranolol given | | RFC | Referred to Counsellor regarding his anxiety attacks. |
| 24.04.2013 | 08.03.1946 | F | | 1644 | 1651 | She is due to start physiotherapy in early May 2013 | | GRC | |
| 24.04.2013 | 23.06.1962 | M | | 1651 | 1702 | Medications Review Done | | MD | |
| 24.04.2013 | 07.03.1999 | F | | 1702 | 1711 | Referred to ENT Surgeon regarding deafness in the (L) ear | | SAW | |
| 24.04.2013 | 06.05.1971 | M | | 1711 | 1719 | Advised to get a letter from his specialist to attach with his jobcentreplus application form if necessary | | RHG | |

Result of a query that lists all consultations from the 22nd to the end of April 2013 (ConsultationsSeenFrom22ndTillEndOfApr2013)

| SurgeryDate | DateOfBirth | Sex | Diagnosis | TimeIn | TimeOut | Complaints | Treatments | Initials | Notes |
|---|---|---|---|---|---|---|---|---|---|
| 24.04.2013 | 06.02.1944 | M | | 1719 | 1730 | Script for Benzydamine cream given | | AMC | Referred to Oral Surgeon regarding the persistent ulcer on the edge of his tongue. |
| 24.04.2013 | 13.11.1996 | F | | 1730 | 1739 | Script for Microgynon 30 given | | GAH | |
| 24.04.2013 | 23.01.1961 | F | | 1739 | 1746 | Script for Transvasin Heat Rub cream given | | JJH | |
| 24.04.2013 | 24.09.1976 | M | | 1746 | 1752 | Script for Omeprazole given | | DIB | |
| 24.04.2013 | 17.02.1987 | F | | 1752 | 1800 | Script for Sertraline given | | KMT | |
| 25.04.2013 | 24.04.1966 | M | | 945 | 1000 | Script for Canesten HC cream given | | BSE | |
| 25.04.2013 | 22.11.1981 | M | S/Leave | 1000 | 1007 | Med. 3 04/10 given for Back Pain for 3 months from 21.04.13 | | DPP | |
| 25.04.2013 | 08.05.1956 | F | | 1007 | 1017 | Script for Amoxycillin & Zolmitriptan given | | SH | |
| 25.04.2013 | 01.12.1942 | M | | 1017 | 1027 | Script for Codeine tablets given | | MP | For ESR & CRP. |
| 25.04.2013 | 10.04.1937 | F | | 1027 | 1032 | Script for Chloramphenicol eye drops given | | MC | |
| 25.04.2013 | 26.01.1953 | M | | 1037 | 1047 | Script for Metformin/ Sitagliptin given | | BGN | |

Result of a query that lists all consultations from the 22nd to the end of April 2013 (ConsultationsSeenFrom22ndTillEndOfApr2013)

| SurgeryDate | DateOfBirth | Sex | Diagnosis | TimeIn | TimeOut | Complaints | Treatments | Initials | Notes |
|---|---|---|---|---|---|---|---|---|---|
| 25.04.2013 | 09.04.1944 | F | | 1047 | 1057 | For Ferritin, B12 & Folate | | JN | |
| 25.04.2013 | 12.10.1973 | F | | 1057 | 1105 | Script for Flucloxacillin given | | DMB | |
| 25.04.2013 | 02.06.1936 | M | | 1105 | 1123 | Family advised to contact Social Services as they feel he should bot be discharged from rehabilitation which is due to happen in about 2 weeks | | AJG | |
| 25.04.2013 | 08.11.1929 | M | | 1647 | 1657 | For repeat PSA in 6 to 8 weeks, form given to the patient | | FAD | |
| 25.04.2013 | 20.01.1941 | F | RTI | 1657 | 1702 | Chesty cough | Erythromycin | BDD | Penicillin allergy. |
| 25.04.2013 | 16.06.1967 | M | | 1702 | 1712 | Script for Flucloxacillin given | | PBK | |
| 25.04.2013 | 28.09.1959 | F | | 1712 | 1718 | Script for Amoxycillin given | | CAW | |
| 25.04.2013 | 18.04.1965 | M | | 1736 | 1742 | Script for Citalopram given | | MGF | |
| 25.04.2013 | 03.02.1957 | M | S/Leave | 1746 | 1803 | Med. 3 04/10 given for Diabetes Mellitus with (R) foot complications for 3 months from 25.04.13 | | ER | |

Result of a query that lists all consultations from the 22nd to the end of April 2013 (ConsultationsSeenFrom22ndTillEndOfApr2013)

| SurgeryDate | DateOfBirth | Sex | Diagnosis | TimeIn | TimeOut | Complaints | Treatments | Initials | Notes |
|---|---|---|---|---|---|---|---|---|---|
| 26.04.2013 | 05.03.1950 | M | | 943 | 953 | Script for Amitriptyline, Naproxen, Omeprazole & Tramadol capsules given | | TMJC | |
| 26.04.2013 | 08.08.1940 | F | | 953 | 1003 | For X-Rays of both knees | | WAW | |
| 26.04.2013 | 12.10.1948 | F | | 1003 | 1011 | Script for Atorvastatin & Transvasin Heat Rub cream given | | SFC | |
| 26.04.2013 | 08.04.1945 | M | | 1011 | 1025 | For Fasting Glucose | | GTW | |
| 26.04.2013 | 22.05.1931 | F | | 1025 | 1031 | Script for Solaraze 3% gel given | | DK | |
| 26.04.2013 | 20.02.1930 | M | | 1031 | 1049 | Medications Review Done | | AL | |
| 26.04.2013 | 01.02.2010 | M | | 1049 | 1054 | Script for Chloramphenicol eye drops given | | SJL | |
| 26.04.2013 | 25.03.1944 | M | | 1219 | 1233 | Script for Oxybutynin & Transvasin Heat Rub cream given | | CJH | For PSA. |
| 29.04.2013 | 13.11.1952 | F | | 945 | 955 | To see her optician to review her cataract | | LH | |
| 29.04.2013 | 07.03.1955 | F | | 955 | 1003 | Medications Review Done | | DN | |
| 29.04.2013 | 24.03.1935 | F | | 1003 | 1009 | Script for Codeine tablets & Lansoprazole given | | PW | |

Result of a query that lists all consultations from the 22nd to the end of April 2013 (ConsultationsSeenFrom22ndTillEndOfApr2013)

| SurgeryDate | DateOfBirth | Sex | Diagnosis | TimeIn | TimeOut | Complaints | Treatments | Initials | Notes |
|---|---|---|---|---|---|---|---|---|---|
| 29.04.2013 | 17.09.1965 | F | | 1009 | 1018 | Medications Review Done | | PAE | |
| 29.04.2013 | 02.12.1973 | F | | 1018 | 1028 | For Pregnancy test, FBC, Ferritin, Folate & B12 | | MC | |
| 29.04.2013 | 13.05.1977 | F | | 1028 | 1034 | Script for Ovranette tablets given | | RBW | |
| 29.04.2013 | 08.10.1950 | F | | 1050 | 1104 | Script for Ferrous Fumarate given | | CAH | |
| 29.04.2013 | 26.08.1947 | F | | 1110 | 1116 | To see the nurse in 6 months for repeat FBC | | CYB | |
| 29.04.2013 | 31.10.2009 | M | | 1116 | 1122 | Script for Dioralyte given | | TJJM | |
| 29.04.2013 | 28.04.1936 | F | | 1645 | 1652 | BP 128/79 | | ORB | |
| 29.04.2013 | 21.06.1975 | F | | 1652 | 1702 | Script for Amoxycillin & Otosporin ear drops given | | AKE | Referred to Dermatologist regarding mole on the (L) side of her neck. |
| 29.04.2013 | 01.11.1936 | M | | 1711 | 1717 | Medications Review Done | | JJS | |
| 29.04.2013 | 17.05.1935 | F | | 1717 | 1725 | For FBC, U/Es, TFTs, Fasting Glucose, LFTs, Bone Profile & Fasting lipids | | CSS | |

## Result of a query that lists all consultations from the 22nd to the end of April 2013 (ConsultationsSeenFrom22ndTillEndOfApr2013)

| SurgeryDate | DateOfBirth | Sex | Diagnosis | TimeIn | TimeOut | Complaints | Treatments | Initials | Notes |
|---|---|---|---|---|---|---|---|---|---|
| 29.04.2013 | 04.06.2007 | F | | 1744 | 1754 | Script for Clenil Modulite inhaler & Volumatic with paediatric mask given | | RLT | For Chest X-Rays. |
| 29.04.2013 | 13.10.1955 | F | | 1754 | 1803 | To contact Orthopaedic Surgeon regarding operation on her (L) knee | | TK | |
| 29.04.2013 | 05.06.1924 | M | | 1803 | 1814 | Script for Trimethoprim given | | DAC | |
| 29.04.2013 | 08.04.1995 | F | | 1814 | 1818 | Script for Naseptin nasal cream given | | SB | |
| 29.04.2013 | 12.11.1993 | F | | 1818 | 1822 | Script for Elidel 1% cream given | | MB | |

## Result of a query that lists all consultations from the 22nd to the end of April 2014 (ConsultationsSeenFrom22ndTillEndOfApr2014)

| SurgeryDate | DateOfBirth | Sex | Diagnosis | TimeIn | TimeOut | Complaints | Treatments | Initials | Notes |
|---|---|---|---|---|---|---|---|---|---|
| 22.04.2014 | 20.02.1930 | M | | 945 | 959 | Script for Lansoprazole given | | AL | |
| 22.04.2014 | 21.06.1975 | F | | 959 | 1007 | She will come back later for sick leave | | AKE | |
| 22.04.2014 | 09.09.1962 | F | S/Leave | 1007 | 1014 | Med. 3 04/10 given for Bariatric Surgery from 21.04.14 to 23.04.14 | | MLF | |

Result of a query that lists all consultations from the 22nd to the end of April 2014 (ConsultationsSeenFrom22ndTillEndOfApr2014)

| SurgeryDate | DateOfBirth | Sex | Diagnosis | TimeIn | TimeOut | Complaints | Treatments | Initials | Notes |
|---|---|---|---|---|---|---|---|---|---|
| 22.04.2014 | 08.03.1961 | M | S/Leave | 1014 | 1024 | Med. 3 04/10 given for Pain in the (R) knee for 6 months from 18.04.14 | | RAB | Script for Citalopram & Co-codamol given. |
| 22.04.2014 | 13.11.1953 | M | | 1024 | 1033 | For X-Rays of both knees | | GJK | |
| 22.04.2014 | 04.11.1924 | F | | 1033 | 1054 | Script for Co-codamol & Metoclopramide given | | OJR | |
| 22.04.2014 | 27.05.1954 | F | | 1054 | 1103 | Medications Review done | | CAA | |
| 22.04.2014 | 11.07.1962 | M | | 1103 | 1118 | Script for Amlodipine given | | JEG | |
| 22.04.2014 | 30.12.1994 | F | | 1130 | 1144 | Referred for Termination of Pregnancy | | CVJ | |
| 22.04.2014 | 16.04.1930 | F | | 1346 | 1416 | Referred to Gastroenterologist (?Dr. Bray) regarding her alternating diarrhoea/constipation | | IDB | Home visit. |
| 22.04.2014 | 16.09.1997 | F | | 1648 | 1655 | Referred to Ophthalmologist (Dr. Idre) regarding her (R) squint & poor vision in the (R) eye | | GJJ | |
| 22.04.2014 | 11.04.1990 | F | | 1655 | 1712 | For Urine Pregnancy test | | TJT | |

Result of a query that lists all consultations from the 22nd to the end of April 2014 (ConsultationsSeenFrom22ndTillEndOfApr2014)

| SurgeryDate | DateOfBirth | Sex | Diagnosis | TimeIn | TimeOut | Complaints | Treatments | Initials | Notes |
|---|---|---|---|---|---|---|---|---|---|
| 22.04.2014 | 23.01.2009 | M | URTI | 1712 | 1719 | Sore throat | Co-Amoxiclav | SKF | |
| 22.04.2014 | 16.09.1997 | M | URTI | 1719 | 1725 | Bilateral ear ache | Amoxycillin | DCMF | |
| 22.04.2014 | 27.01.1940 | F | Rash | 1725 | 1733 | Shingles rash (R) S1 region | Acyclovir tablets, Amitripyline & Co-codamol | JD | |
| 22.04.2014 | 13.02.1971 | M | | 1733 | 1740 | Script for Co-Amoxiclav given | | PME | |
| 22.04.2014 | 29.03.1978 | M | | 1744 | 1804 | Script for Codeine tablets given | | NFH | |
| 22.04.2014 | 25.12.1948 | M | | 1804 | 1825 | Script for Amitripyline & Transvasin Heat Rub spray given | | CGB | |
| 22.04.2014 | 06.03.1998 | F | RTI | 1825 | 1831 | Chesty cough | Doxycycline | PB | |
| 22.04.2014 | 21.09.1983 | M | | 1831 | 1837 | Script for Flucloxacillin given | | JH | |
| 23.04.2014 | 22.02.1944 | M | | 942 | 1009 | Script for Gabapentin given | | AS | |
| 23.04.2014 | 03.02.1957 | M | | 1009 | 1035 | He may come in to have a Taxi Medical examination done | | ER | |
| 23.04.2014 | 27.03.1935 | M | | 1035 | 1052 | Script for Co-codamol & Transvasin Heat Rub cream given | | RH | For USScan of the (R) shoulder given. |
| 23.04.2014 | 27.05.1979 | F | | 1052 | 1102 | Script for Sertraline given | | DLP | Referred to Counsellor regarding her depression. |

137

Result of a query that lists all consultations from the 22nd to the end of April 2014 (ConsultationsSeenFrom22ndTillEndOfApr2014)

| SurgeryDate | DateOfBirth | Sex | Diagnosis | TimeIn | TimeOut | Complaints | Treatments | Initials | Notes |
|---|---|---|---|---|---|---|---|---|---|
| 23.04.2014 | 08.03.1946 | F | | 1102 | 1107 | To see the nurse in 6 months for repeat serum cholesterol | | GRC | |
| 23.04.2014 | 19.01.1964 | F | | 1107 | 1113 | Script for Lisinopril given | | NAB | |
| 23.04.2014 | 06.02.1944 | M | | 1113 | 1120 | For FBC, U/Es, Fasting Glucose & Bone profile | | AMC | |
| 23.04.2014 | 09.10.1974 | F | | 1120 | 1129 | Script for Ferrous Fumarate given | | MJF | |
| 23.04.2014 | 10.11.1969 | F | | 1129 | 1142 | Script for Nitrofurantoin given | | PS | For MSU. Penicillin allergy. |
| 23.04.2014 | 23.03.1967 | F | | 1647 | 1657 | Script for Doxycycline, Otomize ear spray & Prochlorperazine given | | TPW | |
| 23.04.2014 | 12.02.1996 | M | | 1657 | 1705 | Script for Doxycycline given | | JW | |
| 23.04.2014 | 11.03.1968 | F | | 1705 | 1718 | Script for Doxycycline, Betahistine & Hyoscine butylbromide given | | EJA | For USScan of the upper abdomen. |
| 23.04.2014 | 30.12.1962 | F | | 1718 | 1736 | For FBC, U/Es, LFTs, TFTs, Fasting Lipids, Fasting Glucose & FSH | | KLS | |

Result of a query that lists all consultations from the 22nd to the end of April 2014 (ConsultationsSeenFrom22ndTillEndOfApr2014)

| SurgeryDate | DateOfBirth | Sex | Diagnosis | TimeIn | TimeOut | Complaints | Treatments | Initials | Notes |
|---|---|---|---|---|---|---|---|---|---|
| 23.04.2014 | 07.12.1968 | M | | 1736 | 1743 | Referred to ENT Surgeon regarding the feeling of congealed milk being stuck in his throat on & off over the past 2 months | | SKF | |
| 23.04.2014 | 07.08.1971 | F | | 1743 | 1751 | Script for Doxycycline given | | LPH | Managing neck and Back pain booklet & The STarT Back Musculoskeletal Screening Tool leaflet given. |
| 23.04.2014 | 11.03.1986 | M | | 1751 | 1801 | For MSU | | LTB | |
| 23.04.2014 | 20.02.1990 | M | S/Leave | 1806 | 1813 | Med. 3 04/10 given for Back Pain for 1 week from 21.04.14 | | JLG | |
| 24.04.2014 | 02.09.1951 | F | | 944 | 955 | BP 120/83 | | CMS | |
| 24.04.2014 | 27.01.2013 | F | | 955 | 1002 | Referred to Paediatrician regarding sudden development of squint over the past 2 weeks | | AIH | |
| 24.04.2014 | 31.08.1964 | M | S/Leave | 1002 | 1008 | Med. 3 04/10 given for Pain in the (R) arm for 2 weeks from 23.04.14 | | CJW | |

Result of a query that lists all consultations from the 22nd to the end of April 2014 (ConsultationsSeenFrom22ndTillEndOfApr2014)

| SurgeryDate | DateOfBirth | Sex | Diagnosis | TimeIn | TimeOut | Complaints | Treatments | Initials | Notes |
|---|---|---|---|---|---|---|---|---|---|
| 24.04.2014 | 09.03.1947 | F | | 1008 | 1019 | For Fasting Glucose, FBC, U/Es, Cholesterol & Bone profile | | PAN | |
| 24.04.2014 | 26.02.1934 | F | | 1019 | 1027 | Script for Doxycycline & Indapamide given | | DIM | |
| 24.04.2014 | 28.03.1945 | M | | 1032 | 1044 | Referred to Colorectal Surgeon (urgent) regarding soiling himself with faeces | | APD | |
| 24.04.2014 | 14.06.1945 | M | | 1044 | 1052 | Script for Doxycycline given | | BL | For Chest X-Rays. |
| 24.04.2014 | 03.12.1924 | F | | 1052 | 1103 | For serum BNP | | AH | |
| 24.04.2014 | 04.11.1924 | F | | 1103 | 1127 | Inj. Depo-Medrone with Lidocaine 2mls given to the (L) knee | | OJR | |
| 24.04.2014 | 01.02.1931 | M | | 1307 | 1324 | Referred to Gastroenterologist (urgent) regarding his jaundice & pale stools | | MDS | For FBC, U/Es, LFTs, Clotting screen & USScan of the abdomen (urgent). Home visit. |
| 24.04.2014 | 28.02.1941 | F | | 1644 | 1657 | Script for Diazepam given | | SJW | |
| 24.04.2014 | 17.07.1983 | F | | 1657 | 1705 | Script for Citalopram given | | DLR | |
| 24.04.2014 | 19.08.1939 | F | | 1705 | 1712 | Script for Doxycycline given | | JEN | |

Result of a query that lists all consultations from the 22nd to the end of April 2014 (ConsultationsSeenFrom22ndTillEndOfApr2014)

| SurgeryDate | DateOfBirth | Sex | Diagnosis | TimeIn | TimeOut | Complaints | Treatments | Initials | Notes |
|---|---|---|---|---|---|---|---|---|---|
| 24.04.2014 | 21.11.1954 | M | | 1712 | 1724 | For U/Es in 5 weeks, form given to the patient | | GLS | |
| 24.04.2014 | 16.06.1967 | M | | 1728 | 1738 | Script for Co-Amoxiclav & Chloramphenicol eye drops given | | PBK | For Chest X-Rays. |
| 24.04.2014 | 03.11.2000 | F | | 1738 | 1744 | Script for Beconase Aqueous nasal spray, Clarithromycin, Piriton & Sodium Cromoglicate eye drops given | | RPK | |
| 24.04.2014 | 21.11.1997 | M | | 1744 | 1750 | Referred to ENT Surgeon regarding his recurrent epistaxes | | ACM | |
| 24.04.2014 | 04.09.1963 | F | | 1754 | 1804 | Script for Cetraben emollient cream given | | AR | |
| 25.04.2014 | 20.07.1961 | M | | 944 | 957 | Script for Doxycycline given | | DIC | For Chest X-Rays. |
| 25.04.2014 | 16.12.1970 | F | | 957 | 1004 | Script for Doxycycline given | | KMB | For Chest X-Rays. |
| 25.04.2014 | 24.06.2001 | M | | 1004 | 1014 | To see me in 3 months for repeat FBC | | JSB | |
| 25.04.2014 | 20.12.2009 | F | | 1014 | 1024 | To see the nurse for gentle introital swab | | KL | |
| 25.04.2014 | 02.02.1976 | F | | 1024 | 1031 | For Urine Pregnancy test | | NBB | |

141

Result of a query that lists all consultations from the 22nd to the end of April 2014 (ConsultationsSeenFrom22ndTillEndOfApr2014)

| SurgeryDate | DateOfBirth | Sex | Diagnosis | TimeIn | TimeOut | Complaints | Treatments | Initials | Notes |
|---|---|---|---|---|---|---|---|---|---|
| 25.04.2014 | 20.05.1991 | F | URTI | 1043 | 1054 | Sore throat | Doxycycline | JS | For FBC, U/Es, Fasting Glucose & TFTs. |
| 25.04.2014 | 25.11.1949 | M | | 1054 | 1100 | He will have his PSA checked with the nurse in 6 months | | GJD | |
| 25.04.2014 | 26.06.1946 | M | | 1100 | 1121 | For X-Rays of the (L) middle finger | | PGB | |
| 25.04.2014 | 29.11.1946 | F | | 1121 | 1136 | She will come back later for injection of the hips at different times | | CMT | |
| 25.04.2014 | 06.04.1950 | M | | 1130 | 1135 | He is gradually weaning himself off the steroid tablets | | PAD | |
| 25.04.2014 | 12.11.2000 | M | | 1135 | 1144 | Script for Difflam spray & Amoxycillin given | | JLW | |
| 28.04.2014 | 06.12.1940 | F | | 943 | 959 | Referred to Orthopaedic Surgeon (Mr. White) regarding pain in the (R) hip | | MC | For X-Rays of the (R) hip. |
| 28.04.2014 | 06.05.1968 | M | | 1009 | 1024 | For X-Rays of the (L) elbow | | BGV | |
| 28.04.2014 | 14.03.1934 | M | | 1024 | 1041 | Referred to Neurologist regarding him shaking vigorously whilst asleep | | KRF | For FBC, U/Es, Bone profile, LFTs, B12, Folate & Ferritin. |

## Result of a query that lists all consultations from the 22nd to the end of April 2014 (ConsultationsSeenFrom22ndTillEndOfApr2014)

| SurgeryDate | DateOfBirth | Sex | Diagnosis | TimeIn | TimeOut | Complaints | Treatments | Initials | Notes |
|---|---|---|---|---|---|---|---|---|---|
| 28.04.2014 | 31.01.1941 | F | | 1041 | 1049 | Script for Toviaz given | | JAE | |
| 28.04.2014 | 05.03.1950 | M | S/Leave | 1049 | 1105 | Med. 3 04/10 given for (R) Shoulder dislocation for 6 months from 24.04.14 | | TMJC | Script for Tramadol capsules given. |
| 28.04.2014 | 20.02.1953 | F | | 1105 | 1114 | Script for Doxycycline & Otomize ear spray given | | SLF | |
| 28.04.2014 | 06.02.1946 | F | | 1114 | 1121 | Script for Prochlorperazine given | | KMT | |
| 28.04.2014 | 24.05.1976 | F | | 1645 | 1654 | Script for Fluoxetine given | | HCLE | |
| 28.04.2014 | 15.01.1935 | F | | 1654 | 1708 | Script for Transvasin Heat Rub cream given | | JRS | For X-Rays of the (L) hip. |
| 28.04.2014 | 29.02.1944 | F | | 1708 | 1714 | Referred to ENT Surgeon regarding the | | CFC | |
| 28.04.2014 | 22.04.1975 | F | | 1714 | 1721 | Script for Co-Amoxiclav given | | SAG | |
| 28.04.2014 | 27.03.1987 | F | S/Leave | 1721 | 1733 | Med. 3 04/10 given for Possible Urticarial Rash for 3 months from 25.04.14 | | MMW | For FBC, U/Es, TFTs & Fasting Glucose. |
| 28.04.2014 | 17.02.2001 | M | | 1733 | 1740 | Referred to ENT Surgeon regarding the re-emergent of a small papilloma near the tip of the nose which was excised in 2013 | | HJS | |

Result of a query that lists all consultations from the 22$^{nd}$ to the end of April 2014 (ConsultationsSeenFrom22ndTillEndOfApr2014)

| SurgeryDate | DateOfBirth | Sex | Diagnosis | TimeIn | TimeOut | Complaints | Treatments | Initials | Notes |
|---|---|---|---|---|---|---|---|---|---|
| 28.04.2014 | 05.03.1934 | M | | 1743 | 1750 | Script for Doxycycline & Omeprazole given | | CHD | |
| 28.04.2014 | 14.09.1980 | M | | 1750 | 1756 | To see the nurse monthly for BP check | | LH | |
| 28.04.2014 | 26.06.1968 | M | | 1756 | 1801 | Script for Amorolfine 5% medicated nail lacquer given | | NRC | |
| 29.04.2014 | 28.09.1973 | F | | 941 | 956 | Script for Co-codamol & Naproxen given | | DMS | Referred to Counsellor regarding feeling stressed in view of problem from her ex-partner. |
| 29.04.2014 | 13.09.1992 | F | | 956 | 1006 | Script for Sofradex ear drops & Doxycycline given | | MRW | |
| 29.04.2014 | 31.03.1956 | F | | 1006 | 1020 | Advised to see her Occupational physician or plan to retire in order to be able to address her asthma exacerbations at work | | SD | |
| 29.04.2014 | 02.02.1976 | F | | 1020 | 1028 | Urine Pregnancy test is positive | | NBB | |
| 29.04.2014 | 23.01.2009 | M | | 1028 | 1035 | To take own Calpol & apply own Calamine otion for his viral rash | | SKF | |
| 29.04.2014 | 18.09.1977 | M | | 1035 | 1041 | BP 124/84 | | KJR | |

144

Result of a query that lists all consultations from the 22nd to the end of April 2014 (ConsultationsSeenFrom22ndTillEndOfApr2014)

| SurgeryDate | DateOfBirth | Sex | Diagnosis | TimeIn | TimeOut | Complaints | Treatments | Initials | Notes |
|---|---|---|---|---|---|---|---|---|---|
| 29.04.2014 | 23.01.1950 | F | | 1041 | 1056 | Script for Propranolol given | | SM | Referred to |
| 29.04.2014 | 23.09.1954 | M | | 1056 | 1105 | Referred to Physiotherapist regarding his persistent back pain | | RRWH | |
| 29.04.2014 | 23.01.1947 | F | | 1105 | 1115 | Script for Buscopan & Co-codamol given | | BW | |
| 29.04.2014 | 15.10.1969 | F | | 1115 | 1121 | Script for Codeine tablets given | | MAC | |
| 29.04.2014 | 25.11.1985 | F | | 1642 | 1657 | Script for Fucidin H cream given | | RLW | Referred to Dermatologist (Community) regarding the contact dermatitis on her hands. |
| 29.04.2014 | 09.12.2003 | F | | 1657 | 1705 | Script for Flucloxacillin & Fusidic acid cream given | | EAMEA | For FBC, U/Es & Fasting Glucose. |
| 29.04.2014 | 18.02.1968 | F | | 1705 | 1715 | Script for Doxycycline & Fenbid 5% gel given | | PAC | |
| 29.04.2014 | 01.08.1947 | F | | 1715 | 1721 | For X-Rays of the (R) foot | | JLC | |
| 29.04.2014 | 28.12.1962 | M | | 1721 | 1729 | Script for Clarithromycin given | | KF | For serum Uric acid & U/Es. |

**Result of a query that lists all consultations from the 22nd to the end of April 2014 (ConsultationsSeenFrom22ndTillEndOfApr2014)**

| SurgeryDate | DateOfBirth | Sex | Diagnosis | TimeIn | TimeOut | Complaints | Treatments | Initials | Notes |
|---|---|---|---|---|---|---|---|---|---|
| 29.04.2014 | 02.01.1988 | M | | 1729 | 1737 | Script for Beconase Aqueous nasal spray, Codeine tablets, Fexofenadine & Montelukast given | | AHK | |
| 29.04.2014 | 03.05.1968 | F | | 1747 | 1757 | Script for Paroxetine given | | DAP | Referred to Counsellor regarding her depression. |
| 29.04.2014 | 06.03.1966 | F | | 1757 | 1805 | Referred to Vascular Surgeon (BUPA) regarding her painful varicose veins | | JLL | |

**Result of a query that lists all consultations from the 22nd to the end of April 2015 (ConsultationsSeenFrom22ndTillEndOfApr2015)**

| SurgeryDate | DateOfBirth | Sex | Diagnosis | TimeIn | TimeOut | Complaints | Treatments | Initials | Notes |
|---|---|---|---|---|---|---|---|---|---|
| 22.04.2015 | 06.11.1935 | F | | 947 | 1002 | Script for Zapain given | | SRB | |
| 22.04.2015 | 07.03.1933 | M | | 1002 | 1021 | Referred to Orthopaedic Surgeon (Knee Surgeon) regarding pain & swelling in the (R) knee post TKR | | EJM | |

Result of a query that lists all consultations from the 22nd to the end of April 2015 (ConsultationsSeenFrom22ndTillEndOfApr2015)

| SurgeryDate | DateOfBirth | Sex | Diagnosis | TimeIn | TimeOut | Complaints | Treatments | Initials | Notes |
|---|---|---|---|---|---|---|---|---|---|
| 22.04.2015 | 06.01.1969 | F | S/Leave | 1021 | 1031 | Med. 3 04/10 given for Tonsillitis for 2 weeks from 22.04.15 | | KEL | Script for Co-Amoxiclav given. For Chest X-Rays. |
| 22.04.2015 | 23.02.1951 | F | | 1036 | 1046 | She will see me around June for blood test for LFTs | | JPN | |
| 22.04.2015 | 23.07.1953 | M | | 1046 | 1100 | Script for Fucidin H cream given | | THM | For TFTs & Fasting Glucose. |
| 22.04.2015 | 23.09.1951 | F | | 1100 | 1125 | Referred to Urologist (One stop Haematuria clinic) regarding her recurrent microscopic haematuria | | DJS | |
| 22.04.2015 | 08.02.1995 | F | S/Leave | 1649 | 1713 | Med. 3 04/10 given for Depression for 3 months from 22.04.15 | | PC | Script for Citalopram given. Referred to Orthopaedic Surgeon regarding firm lump on the back of her (R) thigh with view to excision. |
| 22.04.2015 | 06.03.1966 | F | S/Leave | 1713 | 1721 | Med. 3 04/10 given for Stress for 3 months from 22.04.15 | | JLL | |
| 22.04.2015 | 18.08.1963 | M | | 1721 | 1730 | To attend GUM clinic regarding the probable warts he has on his scrotum & the groin region | | GCB | |

Result of a query that lists all consultations from the 22nd to the end of April 2015 (ConsultationsSeenFrom22ndTillEndOfApr2015)

| SurgeryDate | DateOfBirth | Sex | Diagnosis | TimeIn | TimeOut | Complaints | Treatments | Initials | Notes |
|---|---|---|---|---|---|---|---|---|---|
| 22.04.2015 | 17.03.1985 | F | | 1730 | 1739 | Script for Cetirizine & Fucidin H cream given | | KAB | |
| 22.04.2015 | 08.09.1957 | M | | 1750 | 1758 | To go to A/E if he becomes unwell | | TJG | |
| 22.04.2015 | 06.04.1960 | M | | 1758 | 1818 | Script for Citalopram, Gabapentin & Tramadol given | | AMB | |
| 23.04.2015 | 28.06.1963 | M | S/Leave | 945 | 952 | Med. 3 04/10 given for (R) Carpal tunnel decompression for 2 weeks from 23.04.15 | | PS | |
| 23.04.2015 | 08.10.1940 | F | | 952 | 1002 | Referred to Psychiatrist to see if an alternative to Trifluoperazine solution can be recommended as she is intolerant of the liquid preparation | | MRH | |
| 23.04.2015 | 09.08.1946 | F | | 1002 | 1010 | Script for Codeine tablets given | | JMW | |
| 23.04.2015 | 02.11.1938 | M | | 1010 | 1020 | Script for Fucidin H cream given | | MSH | for FBC, U/Es, Cholesterol, Fasting Glucose & TFTs. |

Result of a query that lists all consultations from the 22nd to the end of April 2015 (ConsultationsSeenFrom22ndTillEndOfApr2015)

| SurgeryDate | DateOfBirth | Sex | Diagnosis | TimeIn | TimeOut | Complaints | Treatments | Initials | Notes |
|---|---|---|---|---|---|---|---|---|---|
| 23.04.2015 | 05.06.1947 | M | | 1020 | 1032 | Script for Loratadine given | | DTR | for FBC, U/Es & Cholesterol. Referred to Physiotherapist regarding the persistent neck pain. |
| 23.04.2015 | 19.10.1965 | F | | 1032 | 1042 | Referred to Orthopaedic Surgeon (Hip Surgeon) regarding pain in the (R) hip & lower back | | DLS | |
| 23.04.2015 | 03.01.1987 | F | | 1042 | 1049 | For MSU | | KSP | |
| 23.04.2015 | 15.01.1959 | M | | 1049 | 1057 | Script for Clarithromycin given | | ROW | |
| 23.04.2015 | 21.08.1934 | F | | 1644 | 1700 | Script for Doxycycline & Gliclazide given | | IEW | Referred to Community Diabetes specialist nurses regarding her very high HbA1c. |
| 23.04.2015 | 15.11.1993 | F | | 1700 | 1705 | Her urine Pregnancy test is positive | | LKC | |
| 23.04.2015 | 20.03.1952 | F | | 1705 | 1710 | Script for Co-Amoxiclav given | | LJF | |

Result of a query that lists all consultations from the 22nd to the end of April 2015 (ConsultationsSeenFrom22ndTillEndOfApr2015)

| SurgeryDate | DateOfBirth | Sex | Diagnosis | TimeIn | TimeOut | Complaints | Treatments | Initials | Notes |
|---|---|---|---|---|---|---|---|---|---|
| 23.04.2015 | 07.12.2011 | M | | 1726 | 1736 | Script for Vermox, Ketoconazole 2% cream & Ketoconazole 2% shampoo given | | NDM | Referred to Paediatric Dermatologist regarding her scalp ringworm as he missed previous appointment. |
| 23.04.2015 | 12.05.1949 | F | | 1736 | 1743 | Script for Omeprazole given | | MK | |
| 23.04.2015 | 28.06.1959 | M | | 1743 | 1750 | Script for Doxazosin & Lisinopril given | | SCU | |
| 23.04.2015 | 27.09.1975 | F | | 1750 | 1757 | Script for Dioralyte given | | LAM | |
| 23.04.2015 | 03.11.2000 | F | | 1757 | 1710 | Script for Piriton given | | RPK | For FBC, U/Es, TFTs, Fasting Glucose, Bone profile, LFTs, Fasting lipids. The Managing Neck & Back Pain booklet with the STarT Back Musculoskeletal Screening Tool leaflet given to the patient. |
| 24.04.2015 | 02.04.1963 | M | | 945 | 954 | To see me in 6 months for repeat HbA1c blood test | | AIM | |

Result of a query that lists all consultations from the 22nd to the end of April 2015 (ConsultationsSeenFrom22ndTillEndOfApr2015)

| SurgeryDate | DateOfBirth | Sex | Diagnosis | Complaints | TimeIn | TimeOut | Treatments | Initials | Notes |
|---|---|---|---|---|---|---|---|---|---|
| 24.04.2015 | 23.12.1952 | F | | Script for Atorvastatin given | 954 | 1005 | | GCB | |
| 24.04.2015 | 05.02.1960 | F | | Script for Codeine tablets & Fenbid 5% gel given | 1005 | 1019 | | SJW | For X-Rays of the Sacro-iliac joints. The Managing Neck and Back Pain booklet & The STarT Back Musculoskeletal Screening Tool leaflet given to the patient. |
| 24.04.2015 | 22.02.1944 | M | | Referred to Orthopaedic Surgeon (Mr. Hearth - BUPA) regarding pain in the (R) knee for review of the knee & in-situ prosthesis | 1019 | 1034 | | AS | |
| 27.04.2015 | 25.12.1959 | M | | Script for Lisinopril given | 947 | 959 | | MH | For U/Es. |
| 27.04.2015 | 01.01.1953 | M | | He will come back later for the repeat prescription of the Sildenafil | 959 | 1007 | | TPH | |
| 27.04.2015 | 20.11.1944 | M | | To try OTC Senna & Gaviscon regularly | 1007 | 1016 | | JE | |

Result of a query that lists all consultations from the 22nd to the end of April 2015 (ConsultationsSeenFrom22ndTillEndOfApr2015)

| SurgeryDate | DateOfBirth | Sex | Diagnosis | TimeIn | TimeOut | Complaints | Treatments | Initials | Notes |
|---|---|---|---|---|---|---|---|---|---|
| 27.04.2015 | 22.11.1992 | F | | 1016 | 1024 | Referred to Pain Management specialist regarding pain in her lower limbs for years & getting worse | | RKC | |
| 27.04.2015 | 02.12.1973 | F | | 1024 | 1032 | Script for Metoclopramide given | | MC | |
| 27.04.2015 | 31.12.1953 | F | | 1032 | 1042 | Script for Ranitidine given | | JWH | |
| 27.04.2015 | 25.04.1931 | M | RTI | 1042 | 1050 | Chesty cough | Doxycycline | FCW | |
| 27.04.2015 | 20.11.1992 | F | | 1050 | 1059 | Script for Amoxycillin & Otomize ear spray given | | JLC | |
| 27.04.2015 | 02.04.1962 | F | | 1059 | 1106 | Script for Lansoprazole given | | PJL | Referred for Gastroscopy. |
| 27.04.2015 | 30.03.1943 | M | | 1106 | 1114 | Script for Ranolazine given | | BWF | |
| 27.04.2015 | 16.01.1986 | M | | 1644 | 1653 | Referred to Counsellor regarding his depression & being unable to cope | | ANI | |

152

Result of a query that lists all consultations from the 22nd to the end of April 2015 (ConsultationsSeenFrom22ndTillEndOfApr2015)

| SurgeryDate | DateOfBirth | Sex | Diagnosis | TimeIn | TimeOut | Complaints | Treatments | Initials | Notes |
|---|---|---|---|---|---|---|---|---|---|
| 27.04.2015 | 16.08.1983 | F | | 1653 | 1710 | Script for Dermovate scalp application given | | CEC | Referred to Dermatologist (Community) regarding bubbly rash on the front of the neck. For FBC, U/Es, Fasting Glucose, LFTs, TFTs, Fasting lipids & bone profile. |
| 27.04.2015 | 16.04.1995 | F | S/Leave | 1714 | 1724 | Med. 3 04/10 given for Prolactinoma for 3 months from 17.04.15 | | SMG | |
| 27.04.2015 | 02.02.1963 | F | | 1724 | 1732 | Medications Review Done | | JB | |
| 27.04.2015 | 08.05.1968 | M | | 1732 | 1738 | He goes to hospital yearly for review | | BGV | |
| 27.04.2015 | 26.09.2014 | M | RTI | 1738 | 1744 | Chesty cough | Amoxycillin | FJF | |
| 27.04.2015 | 23.01.1947 | F | | 1744 | 1751 | Script for Buscopan tablets given | | BW | |
| 27.04.2015 | 22.07.1961 | M | | 1751 | 1800 | Script for Sumatriptan given | | PWL | |
| 28.04.2015 | 04.10.1947 | F | | 944 | 955 | Script for Amoxycillin given | | PVD | |
| 28.04.2015 | 15.09.1957 | M | S/Leave | 955 | 1004 | Med. 3 04/10 given for Injury to the (R) injury to the (R) knee for 3 months from 27.04.15 | | PSB | |

Result of a query that lists all consultations from the 22nd to the end of April 2015 (ConsultationsSeenFrom22ndTillEndOfApr2015)

| SurgeryDate | DateOfBirth | Sex | Diagnosis | TimeIn | TimeOut | Complaints | Treatments | Initials | Notes |
|---|---|---|---|---|---|---|---|---|---|
| 28.04.2015 | 29.11.1937 | F | | 1004 | 1023 | Script for Cetirizine & Hirudoid 0.3% cream given | | MRS | |
| 28.04.2015 | 03.07.1942 | F | | 1023 | 1035 | Referred to Dermatologist (Basildon Hospital) regarding raised lesion her upper lip | | HM | |
| 28.04.2015 | 02.09.1934 | M | | 1035 | 1043 | Script for Co-codamol given | | DBM | |
| 28.04.2015 | 01.12.1934 | F | | 1043 | 1053 | Script for Doxycycline given | | LFM | |
| 28.04.2015 | 23.01.2015 | F | | 1053 | 1105 | Referred to Paediatric Dr. on call (Basildon Hospital) regarding her chest infection | | MAPL | |
| 28.04.2015 | 23.02.1991 | M | | 1105 | 1113 | Script for Lymecycline given | | MSK | |
| 28.04.2015 | 25.12.1948 | M | | 1113 | 1123 | Script for Amoxycillin given | | CGB | |
| 28.04.2015 | 18.04.1930 | F | | 1644 | 1703 | Referred to Physiotherapist (Domiciliary visit) regarding pain & swelling in the (R) ankle | | IDB | |
| 28.04.2015 | 23.09.1948 | M | | 1703 | 1712 | For repeat U/Es | | KWK | |
| 28.04.2015 | 10.04.1937 | F | | 1712 | 1725 | Script for Ferrous Sulphate given | | MC | |

Result of a query that lists all consultations from the 22nd to the end of April 2015 (ConsultationsSeenFrom22ndTillEndOfApr2015)

| SurgeryDate | DateOfBirth | Sex | Diagnosis | TimeIn | TimeOut | Complaints | Treatments | Initials | Notes |
|---|---|---|---|---|---|---|---|---|---|
| 28.04.2015 | 26.06.2004 | F | | 1725 | 1734 | Referred to Paediatrician regarding persistent lump behind her (R) ear | | FGW | For FBC & U/Es. |
| 28.04.2015 | 12.02.1959 | F | | 1734 | 1745 | She is waiting to see the dietician & the physiotherapist regarding her problems | | JEG | |
| 28.04.2015 | 18.06.1960 | F | | 1745 | 1755 | Script for Amoxycillin given | | AMF | For Chest X-Rays. |
| 28.04.2015 | 21.06.1959 | M | | 1755 | 1805 | Script for Trimethoprim given | | SJW | For MSU. |
| 29.04.2015 | 15.07.1956 | M | | 944 | 1013 | Referred to Psychiatrist for the review of his anti-depressant medications & his depression which is getting worse | | DHC | For FBC, U/Es, Fasting Glucose, LFTs, Cholesterol, Bone profile, TFTs, MSU & PSA. |
| 29.04.2015 | 16.03.1956 | F | | 1013 | 1031 | Referred to Orthopaedic Surgeon (Knee Surgeon) regarding pain in her (L) knee as advised by Pain Management Specialist | | SPD | Referred to Community Diabetic Specialist nurses regarding poor control of her Diabetes. Script for Doxycycline given. |

Result of a query that lists all consultations from the 22nd to the end of April 2015 (ConsultationsSeenFrom22ndTillEndOfApr2015)

| SurgeryDate | DateOfBirth | Sex | Diagnosis | TimeIn | TimeOut | Complaints | Treatments | Initials | Notes |
|---|---|---|---|---|---|---|---|---|---|
| 29.04.2015 | 03.10.1941 | M |  | 1031 | 1037 | Medications Review Done |  | JJD |  |
| 29.04.2015 | 12.09.1936 | F |  | 1037 | 1047 | Script for Lisinopril given |  | HDH |  |
| 29.04.2015 | 30.11.1945 | F | RTI | 1047 | 1055 | Chesty cough | Amoxycillin | PIW |  |
| 29.04.2015 | 02.02.2009 | M |  | 1055 | 1104 | Script for Amoxycillin given |  | OCM | Referred to ENT Surgeon regarding his persistent painful (L) ear & discharge. |
| 29.04.2015 | 05.10.1999 | F |  | 1104 | 1114 | Script for Amoxycillin & Chloramphenicol eye drops given |  | MMCC |  |
| 29.04.2015 | 25.01.1939 | F |  | 1114 | 1135 | Script for Fenbid 5% gel given |  | PMC | Referred to Physiotherapist regarding pain in the (R) knee. |
| 29.04.2015 | 08.10.1940 | F |  | 1135 | 1155 | Referred to Gynaecologist (Mr. Raz - 2ww) regarding probable liver metastasis found on USScan of abdomen, who is treating her for endometrial cancer |  | MRH |  |
| 29.04.2015 | 16.12.1956 | M |  | 1644 | 1658 | He will come back with evidence that he is on Diazepam to get the prescription |  | PGT |  |

Result of a query that lists all consultations from the 22nd to the end of April 2015 (ConsultationsSeenFrom22ndTillEndOfApr2015)

| SurgeryDate | DateOfBirth | Sex | Diagnosis | TimeIn | TimeOut | Complaints | Treatments | Initials | Notes |
|---|---|---|---|---|---|---|---|---|---|
| 29.04.2015 | 07.09.1928 | M | | 1658 | 1706 | Script for Amlodipine given | | LW | |
| 29.04.2015 | 23.01.1950 | F | | 1706 | 1712 | Script for Doxycycline & Co-codamol given | | SM | |
| 29.04.2015 | 24.10.1989 | F | | 1719 | 1725 | Script for Amoxycillin given | | HSI | |
| 29.04.2015 | 28.11.2012 | F | | 1725 | 1732 | Script for Amoxycillin & Simple Linctus paediatric given | | ARM | |
| 29.04.2015 | 02.06.1970 | M | | 1732 | 1740 | Script for Co-codamol & Ibuprofen given | | DLM | |
| 29.04.2015 | 10.11.1957 | F | | 1740 | 1747 | For X-Rays of the (L) foot | | CMA | |
| 29.04.2015 | 14.01.1994 | F | | 1747 | 1800 | Script for Fenbid 5% gel given | | GJG | For MSU. |

157

# RESULTS OF QUERIES THAT LIST ALL CONSULTATIONS FROM THE 22ND TO THE END OF MAY 1997 TO MAY 2015

Result of a query that lists all consultations from the 22nd to the end of May 1997 (ConsultationsSeenFrom22ndTillEndOfMay1997)

| SurgeryDate | DateOfBirth | Sex | Diagnosis | TimeIn | TimeOut | Complaints | Treatments | NumbersID | Notes |
|---|---|---|---|---|---|---|---|---|---|
| 24.05.97 | 18.10.48 | F | Conjunctivitis | 1250 | 1300 | Discharge from (L) eye | Fucithalmic eye drops | 1009 | Home visit. |
| 22.05.97 | 31.07.56 | M | S/Leave | 1655 | 1707 | Angina & migraine | | 1027 | Also has depression, referred to CPN. Prozac script also given. |
| 23.05.97 | 22.01.80 | F | URTI | 1635 | 1641 | Sore throat | Penicillin V | 1440 | |
| 23.05.97 | 19.11.68 | M | | 1819 | 1822 | Septic blister (R) foot (sole) | Flucloxacillin & Amoxycillin | 148 | |
| 23.05.97 | 15.04.28 | F | Pain | 935 | 949 | Pain (L) hip | To Physiotherapy | 1576 | |
| 23.05.97 | 17.07.70 | F | URTI | 1812 | 1818 | Sinusitis | Amoxycillin | 1658 | Her Triludan was changed to Clarityn. FP1001 (GMS4) form signed. |
| 23.05.97 | 16.10.42 | F | Rash | 1642 | 1648 | Rash in groins & lower back | Fucidin H | 1667 | She also has bad indigestion & epigastric discomfort, referred to Gastroenterologist. |
| 22.05.97 | 01.08.42 | F | Pain | 1000 | 1006 | Fell over roller skate | To A/E | 1687 | Pain (L) shoulder. |
| 22.05.97 | 02.02.20 | M | | 1707 | 1712 | FBC results not yet back | | 2135 | |
| 23.05.97 | 01.03.84 | F | URTI | 1713 | 1718 | Sore throat | Amoxycillin | 2349 | |
| 23.05.97 | 02.12.48 | M | | 1801 | 1801 | BP 140/90 | | 2380 | BP is noted to be high at work. She is on Enalapril. |

Result of a query that lists all consultations from the 22nd to the end of May 1997 (ConsultationsSeenFrom22ndTillEndOfMay1997)

| SurgeryDate | DateOfBirth | Sex | Diagnosis | TimeIn | TimeOut | Complaints | Treatments | NumbersID | Notes |
|---|---|---|---|---|---|---|---|---|---|
| 24.05.97 | 27.08.68 | F | | 1146 | 1152 | Burst condom | Schering PC4 | 2626 | Dianette script also given. |
| 22.05.97 | 10.02.24 | F | | 1642 | 1654 | Arthrotec & Gaviscon script | | 2812 | |
| 23.05.97 | 01.02.31 | M | RTI | 1707 | 1710 | Cough | Amoxycillin | 2965 | |
| 23.05.97 | 30.09.51 | M | | 902 | 911 | Low back ache | Co-dydramol & Ibuprofen | 3021 | Also constipated, Rx. Senna tablets. Scheriproct suppositories also given. |
| 24.05.97 | 06.03.91 | M | URTI | 1005 | 1008 | Sore throat | Amoxycillin | 3158 | |
| 24.05.97 | 28.07.83 | F | URTI | 1011 | 1018 | Sore throat | Amoxycillin | 317 | |
| 23.05.97 | 30.04.65 | F | | 1756 | 1800 | Per vagina bleeding | To come back if it persists | 3253 | She is at present on Cilest & she is otherwise well. |
| 24.05.97 | 30.04.65 | F | Revisit | 1158 | 1209 | Per vagina bleeding heavier | To Gynaecologist on call | 3253 | |
| 23.05.97 | 18.12.64 | F | Pain | 1649 | 1654 | Pain (L) lower abdomen | Buscopan | 3282 | |
| 23.05.97 | 05.11.88 | F | RTI | 1654 | 1657 | Cough | Amoxycillin | 3297 | |
| 23.05.97 | 31.05.47 | F | | 1004 | 1013 | Paramax script given | | 3316 | |
| 22.05.97 | 17.06.29 | F | Pain | 948 | 959 | (L) shoulder pain | Motifene & Kapake | 3476 | For Physiotherapy. |
| 23.05.97 | 19.02.42 | F | Pain | 923 | 928 | Pain at the back of the neck | Co-dydramol | 3481 | Recent smear done was normal. |
| 22.05.97 | 26.05.63 | F | | 1756 | 1801 | Infected lower lip | Amoxycillin | 3532 | FP1001 (GMS4) form signed. |

## Result of a query that lists all consultations from the 22nd to the end of May 1997 (ConsultationsSeenFrom22ndTillEndOfMay1997)

| SurgeryDate | DateOfBirth | Sex | Diagnosis | TimeIn | TimeOut | Complaints | Treatments | NumbersID | Notes |
|---|---|---|---|---|---|---|---|---|---|
| 22.05.97 | 10.08.68 | F | | 1814 | 1818 | Suprecur Nasal spray script | | 3629 | |
| 22.05.97 | 23.05.43 | M | S/Leave | 902 | 908 | Fracture (L) foot - Med 4 | | 3684 | |
| 22.05.97 | 25.08.83 | F | URTI | 1823 | 1825 | Sore throat | Penicillin V | 3765 | |
| 22.05.97 | 23.11.57 | M | Pain | 1635 | 1641 | (L) tendo Achilles sore | Referred to Orthopaedic Surgeon BUPA | 3836 | |
| 23.05.97 | 07.04.69 | M | Revisit | 1425 | 1445 | He is worse with his Chicken pox | To Medical Dr on call | 3870 | Home visit. |
| 22.05.97 | 21.05.74 | M | | 1214 | 1225 | D&V | Amoxycillin & Dioralyte | 3911 | Home visit. Also has abdominal pain, Rx. Buscopan & Buccastem. |
| 22.05.97 | 29.07.54 | F | S/Leave | 942 | 947 | Anxiety state | | 4197 | Prozac script also given. |
| 22.05.97 | 12.11.93 | F | Rash | 1025 | 1032 | Chicken pox | Paracetamol & Calamine lotion | 4256 | |
| 23.05.97 | 23.12.88 | M | | 1719 | 1725 | Itchy scalp & hair loss | Polytar shampoo | 4347 | |
| 22.05.97 | 12.08.67 | F | RTI | 912 | 924 | Cough | Amoxycillin | 4402 | Prozac script also given. |
| 22.05.97 | 16.04.94 | M | URTI | 1732 | 1736 | Infected rhinorrhoea | Augmentin-Duo | 4409 | |
| 23.05.97 | 19.03.34 | M | RTI | 1022 | 1027 | Cough | Amoxycillin & Prednisolone | 445 | |
| 22.05.97 | 01.08.59 | F | | 1036 | 1054 | 7/40 gestation | To Gynaecologist on call | 4473 | She has low abdominal pain. |
| 23.05.97 | 24.07.18 | F | RTI | 1300 | 1312 | Cough | Amoxycillin & Simple Linctus | 4511 | Home visit. |

Result of a query that lists all consultations from the 22nd to the end of May 1997 (ConsultationsSeenFrom22ndTillEndOfMay1997)

| SurgeryDate | DateOfBirth | Sex | Diagnosis | TimeIn | TimeOut | Complaints | Treatments | NumbersID | Notes |
|---|---|---|---|---|---|---|---|---|---|
| 24.05.97 | 06.03.92 | M | URTI | 1052 | 1056 | (R) ear ache | Amoxycillin | 4515 | Also has cough, Rx. Simple Linctus Paediatric. |
| 22.05.97 | 01.07.65 | M | URTI | 1826 | 1836 | Sore throat | Erythromycin | 4593 | Penicillin allergy. Pain (R) knee. To Orthopaedic Surgeon. |
| 23.05.97 | 20.09.53 | F | | 1736 | 1741 | Sun tan infection upper arms | Flucloxacillin | 4683 | Ibuprofen & Solpadol script also given. |
| 23.05.97 | 09.05.72 | F | | 1729 | 1735 | Pregnancy test positive | | 4789 | |
| 23.05.97 | 21.03.92 | F | URTI | 1726 | 1729 | Sore throat | Amoxycillin | 4794 | |
| 23.05.97 | 26.04.68 | M | S/Leave | 1746 | 1749 | Undergoing Physiotherapy in SGH | | 4925 | |
| 24.05.97 | 18.09.55 | F | | 1112 | 1115 | Fishy vaginal discharge | Tetracycline | 5071 | |
| 24.05.97 | 05.12.61 | M | | 1115 | 1118 | wife has vaginal discharge | Tetracycline | 5072 | |
| 23.05.97 | 26.10.95 | M | URTI | 1806 | 1811 | Rubbing (R) ear | Amoxycillin | 5080 | |
| 22.05.97 | 11.08.38 | M | Angina | 1713 | 1723 | For operation at London Chest hosp. | To expedite appointment | 5093 | |
| 23.05.97 | 26.07.91 | F | RTI | 1658 | 1702 | Cough | Amoxycillin | 5095 | |
| 23.05.97 | 20.06.84 | M | | 949 | 952 | Diarrhoea | Now better | 5158 | |
| 23.05.97 | 31.10.20 | F | | 953 | 1004 | Inadequately controlled TFTs | Referred to Endocrinologist | 5160 | |

163

Result of a query that lists all consultations from the 22nd to the end of May 1997 (ConsultationsSeenFrom22ndTillEndOfMay1997)

| SurgeryDate | DateOfBirth | Sex | Diagnosis | TimeIn | TimeOut | Complaints | Treatments | NumbersID | Notes |
|---|---|---|---|---|---|---|---|---|---|
| 22.05.97 | 20.04.51 | M | | 1724 | 1731 | Can't get erection | On Zantac | 5183 | Reversible impotence reported. To stop Zantac & use own Gaviscon. |
| 22.05.97 | 30.03.56 | F | | 1737 | 1746 | Stormed out of the Surgery | | 5186 | |
| 22.05.97 | 18.02.43 | M | Rash | 1802 | 1807 | ?Allergic rash on face | Clarityn | 519 | |
| 24.05.97 | 18.02.43 | M | Revisit | 1043 | 1052 | Rash oozy & worse | Fucidin H cream | 519 | Amoxycillin, Flucloxacillin & Aqueous cream also prescribed. |
| 22.05.97 | 08.12.78 | F | | 1747 | 1755 | PER VAGINA bleeding whilst on Cilest | | 5293 | If she has no proper period at the end of the packet, to come for pregnancy test. |
| 22.05.97 | 31.10.72 | F | | 1819 | 1822 | Lustral script | | 5322 | |
| 22.05.97 | 06.08.96 | F | | 1011 | 1015 | Persistent (L) watery eyes | Chloramphenicol eye drops | 5345 | Referred to Ophthalmologist. |
| 22.05.97 | 06.11.46 | M | URTI | 927 | 930 | Sore throat | Co-Amoxiclav | 5356 | |
| 22.05.97 | 30.06.73 | M | S/Leave | 1007 | 1011 | Fracture (R) tibia - Med 4 | | 5408 | |
| 23.05.97 | 18.04.63 | F | Depression | 1823 | 1830 | Under a lot of stress | Prozac | 5415 | Also has fever & unwell, R. Amoxycillin. |

## Result of a query that lists all consultations from the 22nd to the end of May 1997 (ConsultationsSeenFrom22ndTillEndOfMay1997)

| SurgeryDate | DateOfBirth | Sex | Diagnosis | TimeIn | TimeOut | Complaints | Treatments | NumbersID | Notes |
|---|---|---|---|---|---|---|---|---|---|
| 23.05.97 | 06.03.31 | M | | 912 | 922 | Migraine | Sanomigran | 5484 | He also complained of his (R) ankle giving way, referred to Orthopaedic Surgeon privately. He also has ?nasal polyp, referred to ENT Surgeon also privately. |
| 23.05.97 | 03.04.65 | M | | 1750 | 1755 | Moist navel | To use Surgical wipes | 5566 | |
| 23.05.97 | 26.08.25 | M | | 929 | 934 | Ranitidine script given | | 5581 | |
| 24.05.97 | 21.07.87 | M | URTI | 1024 | 1026 | Sore throat | Amoxycillin | 569 | |
| 22.05.97 | 26.08.49 | F | S/Leave | 931 | 941 | Cellulitis (R) leg | | 610 | |
| 22.05.97 | 29.04.84 | M | | 1859 | 1903 | Diarrhoea & fever | Loperamide & Amoxycillin | 77 | |
| 24.05.97 | 13.09.18 | M | | 1103 | 1111 | Mellolin & micropore dressing | | 841 | FBC, U/Es & Glucose normal. |
| 23.05.97 | 28.06.79 | M | Pain | 1038 | 1043 | Clash of shins | Transvasin cream | 875 | |
| 23.05.97 | 28.08.33 | M | | 1027 | 1037 | Persistent diarrhoea | Loperamide & Amoxycillin | 959 | Stool for C&S. |
| 23.05.97 | 16.02.31 | M | | 1014 | 1021 | Wheel chair to be arranged with Social Services | | 996 | |
| 23.05.97 | 21.06.78 | F | | 1703 | 1706 | Burst condom | Schering PC4 | NP | |

Result of a query that lists all consultations from the 22nd to the end of May 1997 (ConsultationsSeenFrom22ndTillEndOfMay1997)

| SurgeryDate | DateOfBirth | Sex | Diagnosis | TimeIn | TimeOut | Complaints | Treatments | NumbersID | Notes |
|---|---|---|---|---|---|---|---|---|---|
| 23.05.97 | 19.12.74 | F | | 1831 | 1836 | Unprotected sex | Schering PC4 | NP | She also requests pill, Rx. Cilest. |
| 24.05.97 | 01.06.94 | M | | 1119 | 1122 | Laceration (L) index finger | To A/E | Temp | |

Result of a query that lists all consultations from the 22nd to the end of May 1998 (ConsultationsSeenFrom22ndTillEndOfMay1998)

| SurgeryDate | DateOfBirth | Sex | Diagnosis | TimeIn | TimeOut | Complaints | Treatments | NumbersID | Notes |
|---|---|---|---|---|---|---|---|---|---|
| 23.05.98 | 03.10.69 | F | Pain | 1023 | 1035 | Pain (R) upper abdomen | Amoxycillin, Co-dydramol & Diclofenac enteric coated. For USScan of the Gall bladder. | 1206 | |
| 29.05.98 | 20.11.46 | M | | 1041 | 1051 | Gets manic | He will contact CPN | 1011 | He is to continue Prozac. |
| 26.05.98 | 31.10.69 | F | | 1000 | 1009 | Amitriptyline script | | 1022 | |
| 26.05.98 | 31.07.56 | M | | 1644 | 1653 | LFTs & MCV are abnormal in view of alcohol abuse | | 1027 | |
| 22.05.98 | 11.10.52 | M | | 957 | 1000 | Inflamed varicose veins | Flucloxacillin & Hirudoid cream | 1141 | |
| 26.05.98 | 14.10.76 | M | | 1808 | 1815 | Hay fever | Clarityn | 141 | Betnovate scalp application script also given. |

Result of a query that lists all consultations from the 22nd to the end of May 1998 (ConsultationsSeenFrom22ndTillEndOfMay1998)

| SurgeryDate | DateOfBirth | Sex | Diagnosis | TimeIn | TimeOut | Complaints | Treatments | NumbersID | Notes |
|---|---|---|---|---|---|---|---|---|---|
| 22.05.98 | 13.05.14 | M | RTI | 1430 | 1440 | Chesty cough | Ciproxin | 1466 | Home visit. He also has bruised ribs following a fall. |
| 22.05.98 | 23.01.30 | M | | 1100 | 1110 | Certified dead | | 1495 | Home visit. |
| 26.05.98 | 11.09.47 | M | | 915 | 920 | Prednisolone enteric coated script given | | 1503 | His colitis has flared up. |
| 29.05.98 | 14.05.25 | M | | 856 | 901 | Irish passport form completed | | 1523 | |
| 26.05.98 | 03.05.51 | F | RTI | 1756 | 1803 | Cough | Amoxycillin | 162 | Phenytoin script also given. |
| 26.05.98 | 30.03.16 | M | URTI | 1735 | 1737 | Sore throat | Amoxycillin | 1712 | |
| 22.05.98 | 18.02.30 | M | | 1021 | 1026 | Lansoprazole script | | 1926 | |
| 28.05.98 | 19.12.57 | M | | 1754 | 1803 | Letter to whom it may concern | | 2267 | Regarding fitness for work. |
| 26.05.98 | 17.02.22 | F | | 1022 | 1034 | To reduce Prednisolone script | | 2285 | |
| 28.05.98 | 06.11.15 | M | | 1002 | 1019 | Sore (R) groin | Fucidin cream | 229 | |
| 22.05.98 | 08.05.86 | F | Pain | 1046 | 1055 | Abdominal pain | Buscopan & Lactulose | 2350 | |
| 28.05.98 | 06.05.58 | F | | 946 | 955 | Pain at the back of the eyes & fever | Amoxycillin, Stemetil & Co-dydramol | 2576 | |
| 22.05.98 | 28.07.39 | M | S/leave | 1000 | 1005 | Schizophrenia | | 2596 | |
| 27.05.98 | 16.04.41 | M | RTI | 1011 | 1017 | Cough | Amoxycillin | 268 | |
| 28.05.98 | 08.11.21 | F | UTI | 1050 | 1056 | Dysuria | Trimethoprim | 2729 | For MSU. Has cystitis again. |
| 29.05.98 | 13.09.13 | F | | 1025 | 1033 | Verruca (L) index finger | Cuplex gel | 2838 | |

## Result of a query that lists all consultations from the 22nd to the end of May 1998 (ConsultationsSeenFrom22ndTillEndOfMay1998)

| SurgeryDate | DateOfBirth | Sex | Diagnosis | TimeIn | TimeOut | Complaints | Treatments | NumbersID | Notes |
|---|---|---|---|---|---|---|---|---|---|
| 28.05.98 | 27.09.37 | F | | 1034 | 1037 | Diclofenac enteric coated script | | 2893 | |
| 27.05.98 | 05.07.90 | F | | 925 | 937 | ESR elevate just | For rpt. ESR in 6/12 | 2912 | |
| 28.05.98 | 23.04.39 | M | RTI | 1739 | 1744 | Cough | Ciprofloxacin | 3022 | |
| 27.05.98 | 25.01.86 | F | Conjunctivitis | 1435 | 1440 | (L) red painful eye | Fucithalmic eye drops | 3031 | Home visit. |
| 27.05.98 | 23.08.63 | F | | 1420 | 1435 | Routine P/Natal check | | 3038 | Home visit. |
| 22.05.98 | 06.12.52 | F | URTI | 1018 | 1020 | Sore throat | Amoxycillin | 3082 | |
| 22.05.98 | 07.07.83 | F | URTI | 1015 | 1018 | Sore throat | Amoxycillin | 3085 | |
| 22.05.98 | 27.11.49 | M | S/leave | 944 | 956 | Pain (L) knee - Med 5 | | 3132 | |
| 23.05.98 | 07.07.62 | M | URTI | 1013 | 1021 | Sore throat | Co-Amoxiclav | 3240 | He also has gripping abdominal pain, Rx. Spasmonal & Buscopan. He also has headaches, Rx. Co-dydramol. |
| 22.05.98 | 06.09.84 | M | | 940 | 943 | To be reviewed cardiologically at St. George's hospital, Tooting at 16 year old | | 3340 | |
| 22.05.98 | 13.01.87 | F | | 932 | 940 | To be reviewed cardiologically at St. George's hospital, Tooting at 16 year old | | 3343 | |
| 27.05.98 | 23.08.91 | M | | 1003 | 1007 | Verruca (L) foot | Cuplex gel | 3358 | |

Result of a query that lists all consultations from the 22nd to the end of May 1998 (ConsultationsSeenFrom22ndTillEndOfMay1998)

| SurgeryDate | DateOfBirth | Sex | Diagnosis | TimeIn | TimeOut | Complaints | Treatments | NumbersID | Notes |
|---|---|---|---|---|---|---|---|---|---|
| 29.05.98 | 24.01.70 | F | | 908 | 920 | Flixonase & Microgynon 30 script | | 3452 | FP1001 (GMS4) form signed. |
| 28.05.98 | 16.08.27 | F | Hypertension | 1809 | 1820 | BP 180/100 | Doxazosin | 3477 | She also probably had TIA, Rx. Aspirin. |
| 26.05.98 | 19.02.42 | F | RTI | 1749 | 1755 | Cough | Amoxycillin | 3481 | |
| 29.05.98 | 10.01.92 | M | | 1033 | 1037 | Verruca (R) foot | Cuplex gel | 3492 | |
| 27.05.98 | 26.08.67 | F | | 1022 | 1027 | Rhinocort Aqua nasal spray script | | 3497 | |
| 28.05.98 | 03.12.44 | F | RTI | 929 | 932 | Cough | Ciprofloxacin | 3509 | |
| 27.05.98 | 04.04.92 | M | | 1024 | 1030 | Epistaxes | Amoxycillin, Naseptin cream & Ibuprofen | 3569 | |
| 29.05.98 | 13.07.17 | F | RTI | 1007 | 1012 | Cough | Ciprofloxacin | 3611 | She also has pedal oedema, Rx. Co-Amilofruse. |
| 28.05.98 | 05.12.39 | M | S/leave | 1703 | 1710 | Chest infection Med 3 & Med 5 | | 3646 | |
| 28.05.98 | 20.08.39 | F | | 1634 | 1640 | Letter to whom it may concern | | 3650 | Regarding injury at work. |
| 26.05.98 | 24.04.86 | M | Pain | 1744 | 1748 | Low back pain | Ibuprofen | 3659 | |
| 23.05.98 | 19.05.69 | F | | 1055 | 1104 | Anaemic | See in 3 weeks for Iron tablets | 3688 | She is at present 11 weeks gestation. |
| 29.05.98 | 07.06.40 | M | Pain | 1059 | 1110 | Pain in neck & arms | Amitriptyline | 38 | Unable to sleep. Kapake script also given. |
| 23.05.98 | 20.04.36 | M | Lump | 1038 | 1054 | Infected sebaceous cyst (L) upper eye lid | Flucloxacillin | 3840 | He also has pain in his (L) arm, Rx. GTN spray |

169

Result of a query that lists all consultations from the 22nd to the end of May 1998 (ConsultationsSeenFrom22ndTillEndOfMay1998)

| SurgeryDate | DateOfBirth | Sex | Diagnosis | TimeIn | TimeOut | Complaints | Treatments | NumbersID | Notes |
|---|---|---|---|---|---|---|---|---|---|
| 26.05.98 | 16.07.67 | F | | 1731 | 1735 | Vaginal thrush | Diflucan | 3993 | |
| 27.05.98 | 25.12.48 | M | | 1112 | 1145 | HGV medical - 58.50 pounds paid | | 4062 | |
| 22.05.98 | 10.06.70 | F | Pain | 1029 | 1033 | Aching pains both axillae | To observe | 4104 | |
| 27.05.98 | 22.03.11 | F | Pain | 1355 | 1415 | Abdominal pains | Buscopan | 4205 | Home visit. |
| 26.05.98 | 11.11.92 | F | | 1803 | 1808 | Letter to expedite Ts & As operation date | | 4304 | |
| 26.05.98 | 16.02.94 | F | RTI | 1630 | 1644 | Cough | Amoxycillin | 4339 | She gets recurrent chest infections, referred to Paediatrician (BUPA). |
| 26.05.98 | 10.03.10 | F | | 1435 | 1445 | Fainting attacks & dizziness | Stemetil | 4341 | Home visit. For FBC, Glucose & U/Es. |
| 29.05.98 | 10.03.10 | F | | 1052 | 1059 | Recurrent cystitis | Trimethoprim | 4341 | |
| 27.05.98 | 09.03.63 | F | URTI | 937 | 947 | Infected rhinorrhoea | Amoxycillin | 4368 | Ibuprofen script also given. |
| 28.05.98 | 10.12.78 | F | Pain | 1719 | 1725 | Pain both elbows | referred to Orthopaedic Surgeon | 4379 | |
| 27.05.98 | 27.04.48 | M | S/leave | 1019 | 1022 | Diabetes | | 4538 | |
| 27.05.98 | 31.03.42 | F | | 922 | 924 | Infected sutured ear lobe | Co-Amoxiclav | 4609 | |
| 26.05.98 | 01.03.30 | F | | 1240 | 1250 | Diarrhoea | Loperamide | 4652 | Home visit. She also has abdominal pain, Rx. Buscopan. |

Result of a query that lists all consultations from the 22nd to the end of May 1998 (ConsultationsSeenFrom22ndTillEndOfMay1998)

| SurgeryDate | DateOfBirth | Sex | Diagnosis | TimeIn | TimeOut | Complaints | Treatments | NumbersID | Notes |
|---|---|---|---|---|---|---|---|---|---|
| 27.05.98 | 01.02.30 | M | | 913 | 921 | Letter from hospital that he has mild Diabetes | | 4905 | |
| 28.05.98 | 20.04.92 | M | | 911 | 928 | Abnormal FBC | Referred to Paediatrician (Rapid Access clinic) | 4909 | |
| 23.05.98 | 27.11.92 | F | RTI | 1115 | 1121 | Cough | Amoxycillin | 4913 | |
| 26.05.98 | 24.05.70 | F | | 1254 | 1305 | Routine P/Natal visit | | 4921 | Home visit. |
| 26.05.98 | 18.09.92 | F | | 1715 | 1721 | (R) thumb paronychia | Flucloxacillin | 4956 | |
| 27.05.98 | 18.09.92 | F | | 1044 | 1052 | Repeat script of Flucloxacillin | | 4956 | |
| 28.05.98 | 06.03.63 | M | | 1804 | 1809 | X-Ray Nasal bones - NBI | | 4958 | |
| 28.05.98 | 10.06.20 | F | Pain | 1654 | 1703 | Arthritis pains | Ibuprofen | 4969 | |
| 28.05.98 | 29.09.95 | M | | 1041 | 1050 | Vomiting & abdominal pain | Metoclopramide & Merbentyl | 5022 | |
| 22.05.98 | 27.02.31 | F | | 1034 | 1045 | Multivitamins script | | 5036 | Her mum died recently in hospital. |
| 23.05.98 | 27.09.71 | F | URTI | 1036 | 1038 | Sore throat | Amoxycillin | 5089 | |
| 29.05.98 | 03.03.77 | M | | 1003 | 1006 | Blistery spots on the penis | Advised to go to GUM clinic, SGH | 5104 | |
| 27.05.98 | 17.05.86 | F | Pain | 956 | 1002 | Pain (L) foot | Ibuprofen & Transvasin cream | 5135 | |
| 28.05.98 | 16.10.75 | F | | 922 | 928 | Microgynon 30 script | | 5180 | FP1001 (GMS4) form signed. |

Result of a query that lists all consultations from the 22nd to the end of May 1998 (ConsultationsSeenFrom22ndTillEndOfMay1998)

| SurgeryDate | DateOfBirth | Sex | Diagnosis | TimeIn | TimeOut | Complaints | Treatments | NumbersID | Notes |
|---|---|---|---|---|---|---|---|---|---|
| 26.05.98 | 09.07.72 | M | Pain | 1048 | 1102 | Chest pain & unwell | GTN spray & Erythromycin | 520 | Penicillin allergy. Pulse 46/min, referred to Cardiologist. |
| 29.05.98 | 05.01.81 | F | RTI | 938 | 946 | Cough | Amoxycillin & Simple Linctus | 5226 | |
| 28.05.98 | 31.01.34 | F | Lump | 1038 | 1041 | Mole on lower abdomen, flaky | See back in 3 months | 5234 | |
| 29.05.98 | 04.04.96 | M | Lump | 902 | 908 | Cervical lymphadenopathy | See in 2 weeks | 5282 | |
| 26.05.98 | 26.05.96 | M | URTI | 1040 | 1047 | Sore throat | Amoxycillin | 5292 | Letter to expedite tongue-tie operation date. |
| 26.05.98 | 12.04.72 | M | S/leave | 945 | 952 | Injury (L) ankle - Med 3 & Med 5 | | 5294 | |
| 28.05.98 | 02.12.43 | F | UTI | 1731 | 1739 | Dysuria | Trimethoprim | 5329 | For MSU. |
| 28.05.98 | 19.12.81 | F | | 1726 | 1731 | Vaginal thrush | Diflucan | 5384 | She also has period pains, Rx. Paracetamol. |
| 22.05.98 | 25.06.62 | M | | 1005 | 1015 | For U/Es, Glucose, Cholesterol & FBC | | 5393 | |
| 26.05.98 | 26.06.62 | M | | 952 | 959 | BP 140/95 | If blood Glucose is okay, for Atenolol | 5393 | |
| 29.05.98 | 13.09.13 | F | Revisit | 1037 | 1041 | Still has giddiness | Referred to Neurologist | 5395 | |
| 27.05.98 | 18.04.63 | F | S/leave | 1030 | 1034 | Spondylosis | | 5415 | |
| 28.05.98 | 23.02.85 | F | Lump | 932 | 941 | Lump on fore-head | To observe | 543 | |

172

Result of a query that lists all consultations from the 22nd to the end of May 1998 (ConsultationsSeenFrom22ndTillEndOfMay1998)

| SurgeryDate | DateOfBirth | Sex | Diagnosis | TimeIn | TimeOut | Complaints | Treatments | NumbersID | Notes |
|---|---|---|---|---|---|---|---|---|---|
| 29.05.98 | 21.03.51 | F | Pain | 1012 | 1025 | Pain (L) lower abdomen | For MSU | 5479 | She is also depressed, referred to CPN. |
| 22.05.98 | 27.06.50 | M | | 1026 | 1029 | Hay fever | Clarityn | 559 | Nizoral shampoo script also given. |
| 26.05.98 | 22.03.67 | M | Pain | 1728 | 1731 | Back pain | Co-dydramol | 5596 | |
| 26.05.98 | 05.12.38 | M | | 1034 | 1040 | Diazepam script | | 5651 | |
| 26.05.98 | 17.07.97 | M | RTI | 1721 | 1727 | Cough | Amoxycillin | 5673 | |
| 29.05.98 | 20.05.30 | M | | 1129 | 1152 | Taxi Medical - 58.50 pounds paid | | 5728 | |
| 22.05.98 | 24.04.35 | F | RTI | 923 | 932 | Cough | Erythromycin | 5770 | Penicillin allergy. Sofradex ear drops, Calcichew D3 & Simple Linctus script also given. |
| 28.05.98 | 16.10.97 | M | RTI | 900 | 911 | Chesty cough | Amoxycillin & Salbutamol suspension | 5821 | |
| 28.05.98 | 16.08.50 | F | | 1643 | 1654 | Atenolol & Ferrous Sulphate script | | 583 | |
| 26.05.98 | 21.11.97 | M | RTI | 1654 | 1708 | Cough & vomiting | Referred to Paediatrician on call, Southend hospital | 5898 | |
| 29.05.98 | 13.08.97 | F | | 946 | 951 | Coughing again | Simple Linctus paediatric | 5910 | |
| 28.05.98 | 08.10.98 | F | Conjunctivitis | 1711 | 1719 | (L) eye discharging | Fucithalmic eye drops | 5948 | |

173

Result of a query that lists all consultations from the 22nd to the end of May 1998 (ConsultationsSeenFrom22ndTillEndOfMay1998)

| SurgeryDate | DateOfBirth | Sex | Diagnosis | TimeIn | TimeOut | Complaints | Treatments | NumbersID | Notes |
|---|---|---|---|---|---|---|---|---|---|
| 29.05.98 | 07.05.74 | M | Pain | 1110 | 1115 | Abdominal pain | Spasmonal & Colpermin | 5951 | |
| 28.05.98 | 23.03.26 | M | | 1019 | 1030 | No problems with coronary arteries | | 5954 | He saw the Cardiologist 2 weeks ago. |
| 26.05.98 | 13.02.47 | F | | 920 | 928 | Bowels irregular, ?IBS | Spasmonal | 5962 | |
| 27.05.98 | 13.02.72 | F | | 1007 | 1011 | Dizzy spells | For FBC | 5962 | |
| 29.05.98 | 17.12.31 | M | | 1115 | 1129 | Frank haematuria | Referred to Surgical Dr. on call, Basildon hospital | 5978 | |
| 27.05.98 | 29.08.43 | M | | 947 | 956 | Atenolol & Doxazosin script | | 5999 | |
| 22.05.98 | 24.05.29 | M | Pain | 1446 | 1505 | Painful & swollen (L) knee | Diclofenac & Flucloxacillin | 6 | Home visit. |
| 29.05.98 | 06.08.55 | F | S/leave | 929 | 938 | Breast cancer | | 6048 | |
| 22.05.98 | 06.04.33 | F | Revisit | 911 | 922 | Still has pains in her bowels | Referred to Gastroenterologist | 6056 | |
| 28.05.98 | 17.04.30 | M | RTI | 1030 | 1034 | Chesty cough | Amoxycillin & Salbutamol suspension | 6059 | |
| 22.05.98 | 09.07.66 | M | S/leave | 905 | 911 | Headaches | | 6061 | |
| 28.05.98 | 06.01.56 | M | Rash | 942 | 946 | Contact dermatitis (R) fingers | Fucidin-H ointment | 727 | |
| 28.05.98 | 21.09.98 | M | | 1744 | 1750 | Injury (L) little finger | For X-Ray | 785 | |
| 23.05.98 | 06.06.30 | M | URTI | 1004 | 1013 | Headaches, frontal sinuses are tender | Amoxycillin | 883 | For FBC & ESR. |

174

Result of a query that lists all consultations from the 22nd to the end of May 1998 (ConsultationsSeenFrom22ndTillEndOfMay1998)

| SurgeryDate | DateOfBirth | Sex | Diagnosis | TimeIn | TimeOut | Complaints | Treatments | NumbersID | Notes |
|---|---|---|---|---|---|---|---|---|---|
| 28.05.98 | 07.03.70 | M | Pain | 955 | 1002 | Pain (L) kidney area on micturition | For MSU | 899 | |
| 29.05.98 | 20.11.23 | M | RTI | 951 | 1000 | Cough | Ciprofloxacin | 916 | Diclofenac enteric coated script also given. |
| 26.05.98 | 25.05.50 | M | | 1709 | 1715 | Cholesterol level dropping | | 968 | |
| 26.05.98 | 20.09.34 | M | | 909 | 915 | Referred to Ophthalmologist | | Temp | He saw his optician 3/7 ago. |
| 27.05.98 | 08.08.33 | F | Pain | 1052 | 1058 | Low back pain | Diclofenac injection | Temp | |

Result of a query that lists all consultations from the 22nd to the end of May 1999 (ConsultationsSeenFrom22ndTillEndOfMay1999)

| SurgeryDate | DateOfBirth | Sex | Diagnosis | TimeIn | TimeOut | Complaints | Treatments | NumbersID | Notes |
|---|---|---|---|---|---|---|---|---|---|
| 26.05.99 | 04.07.16 | F | RTI | 1650 | 1652 | Cough | Amoxycillin | 1199 | |
| 27.05.99 | 03.08.33 | F | Pain | 1018 | 1029 | (R) sided lower abdominal pain | For USScan of the lower abdomen | 127 | |
| 28.05.99 | 23.12.52 | F | Rash | 1704 | 1709 | Itchy red rash on arms & legs | Fucidin-H cream | 136 | |
| 28.05.99 | 05.04.72 | M | | 904 | 912 | X-Ray (R) fingers: Fractured 5th Proximal phalanx | Advised to go to A/E | 1427 | |
| 28.05.99 | 15.04.51 | F | Rash | 1720 | 1725 | Sore & itchy rash around mouth | Fucidin-H cream | 1470 | |

Result of a query that lists all consultations from the 22nd to the end of May 1999 (ConsultationsSeenFrom22ndTillEndOfMay1999)

| SurgeryDate | DateOfBirth | Sex | Diagnosis | TimeIn | TimeOut | Complaints | Treatments | NumbersID | Notes |
|---|---|---|---|---|---|---|---|---|---|
| 25.05.99 | 22.07.39 | F | | 942 | 951 | Advised to be on Provera for at least 1 year | | 1546 | |
| 25.05.99 | 08.08.24 | F | | 1643 | 1657 | Slight PER VAGINA loss | On waiting list for TAH + BSO | 1559 | |
| 27.05.99 | 20.08.66 | F | RTI | 1741 | 1745 | Cough | Amoxycillin | 1602 | |
| 27.05.99 | 27.06.44 | M | | 1709 | 1719 | Awaiting letter from Physician | | 1673 | |
| 25.05.99 | 28.09.50 | F | Pain | 1724 | 1730 | Finger joints painful | Co-Proxamol & Diclofenac enteric coated | 1736 | |
| 24.05.99 | 01.10.51 | F | | 1727 | 1732 | Script for Ferrous Sulphate given | | 1769 | |
| 24.05.99 | 12.12.35 | M | Pain | 901 | 907 | ?Foreign body (L) heel | For X-Ray (L) heel | 1784 | |
| 26.05.99 | 20.06.38 | M | S/Leave | 923 | 925 | Craniotomy | | 1855 | |
| 27.05.99 | 16.09.49 | M | | 1745 | 1755 | Script for Atenolol & Co-Amilofruse given | | 1893 | |
| 26.05.99 | 30.12.62 | F | Hypertension | 943 | 956 | BP 160/100 | TenBen | 1900 | |
| 28.05.99 | 08.06.76 | M | Pain | 1006 | 1013 | Pain (R) upper back | Ibuprofen & Movelat cream | 2040 | New patient check done. |
| 24.05.99 | 19.12.57 | M | | 1843 | 1846 | LFTs normal | | 2267 | |
| 27.05.99 | 06.08.80 | F | Pain | 1800 | 1813 | Headaches | Co-dydramol | 2298 | She also has dizziness, for FBC. |
| 25.05.99 | 26.08.87 | F | Pain | 1730 | 1738 | Injury (R) little toe | For X-Ray | 2332 | |

## Result of a query that lists all consultations from the 22nd to the end of May 1999 (ConsultationsSeenFrom22ndTillEndOfMay1999)

| SurgeryDate | DateOfBirth | Sex | Diagnosis | TimeIn | TimeOut | Complaints | Treatments | NumbersID | Notes |
|---|---|---|---|---|---|---|---|---|---|
| 24.05.99 | 06.11.20 | M | RTI | 1048 | 1058 | Cough | Clarithromycin | 2423 | Script for Adalat LA 30 & Co-Amilofruse also given. |
| 27.05.99 | 06.11.20 | M | | 1755 | 1800 | Script for Adalat LA 20 & Co-Amilofruse | | 2423 | |
| 26.05.99 | 05.08.16 | F | | 1017 | 1031 | Alzheimer's disease | For Domiciliary visit by Psycho-geriatrician | 2424 | Daughter came to Surgery. |
| 28.05.99 | 26.03.87 | M | URTI | 1802 | 1806 | Sore throat | Amoxycillin | 2439 | |
| 25.05.99 | 06.12.61 | F | (L) Otitis Ext. | 1657 | 1703 | (L) ear ache | Amoxycillin & Otomize ear spray | 2467 | |
| 24.05.99 | 22.09.39 | F | | 959 | 1005 | Script for Co-Amoxiclav & Gliclazide given | | 2510 | |
| 24.05.99 | 04.04.38 | M | Pain | 1751 | 1802 | Pain (L) shoulder | For X-Ray (L) shoulder | 262 | |
| 28.05.99 | 19.03.25 | F | | 1754 | 1802 | Bilateral pedal oedema & itchy rash on legs | Fucidin-H cream, Clarithromycin & Bumetanide | 2634 | |
| 24.05.99 | 28.05.57 | F | | 1634 | 1641 | Script for Norethisterone given | | 2648 | |
| 28.05.99 | 10.02.24 | F | Hypertension | 1650 | 1704 | BP 200/98 | Bisoprolol | 2812 | |
| 26.05.99 | 18.02.68 | F | | 1250 | 1305 | Routine P/Natal visit | | 2901 | Home visit. |
| 27.05.99 | 17.01.39 | M | | 1652 | 1659 | Fever & Shivering | Amoxycillin | 2928 | |
| 25.05.99 | 15.10.25 | F | | 1030 | 1039 | Script for Co-Amilofruse given | | 2931 | |

Result of a query that lists all consultations from the 22nd to the end of May 1999 (ConsultationsSeenFrom22ndTillEndOfMay1999)

| SurgeryDate | DateOfBirth | Sex | Diagnosis | TimeIn | TimeOut | Complaints | Treatments | NumbersID | Notes |
|---|---|---|---|---|---|---|---|---|---|
| 26.05.99 | 05.05.53 | F | Revisit | 1752 | 1757 | Epigastric pain persists | Referred to Gastro-enterologist | 3000 | |
| 25.05.99 | 30.09.50 | M | | 906 | 915 | To continue on Omeprazole | | 3047 | |
| 25.05.99 | 06.12.52 | F | URTI | 1003 | 1010 | Sore throat | Amoxycillin | 3082 | |
| 25.05.99 | 14.03.85 | M | Pain | 1823 | 1831 | Kicked in the face & getting worse | Advised to go to A/E | 3144 | |
| 27.05.99 | 14.03.85 | M | Conjunctivitis | 1825 | 1827 | (R) eye red & sticky | Chloramphenicol eye drops | 3144 | |
| 24.05.99 | 10.12.30 | M | | 926 | 947 | Script for Atorvastatin given | | 328 | |
| 27.05.99 | 04.01.25 | M | | 1827 | 1835 | Cough | Ciprofloxacin | 333 | His daughter came to Surgery. For CXR. |
| 28.05.99 | 05.11.32 | F | Pain | 1013 | 1021 | Pain (L) side of chest, ?pleurisy | Amoxycillin & Paracetamol | 3380 | For MSU. |
| 26.05.99 | 19.07.52 | M | Rash | 956 | 1003 | Scaly weepy rash on feet | Flucloxacillin & Fucidin-H cream | 3430 | |
| 26.05.99 | 24.01.64 | M | S/Leave | 1714 | 1718 | Depression | | 3467 | |
| 24.05.99 | 11.04.21 | F | Pain | 1820 | 1843 | Severe colicky abdominal pain | Referred to Surgical Dr. on call | 3495 | |
| 25.05.99 | 09.08.89 | F | URTI | 1113 | 1126 | Sore throat | Amoxycillin | 3500 | |
| 25.05.99 | 14.02.24 | M | | 1711 | 1716 | Unwell & T.A.T.T. | For FBC, U/Es, LFTs, TFTs & Glucose | 3718 | |

**Result of a query that lists all consultations from the 22nd to the end of May 1999 (ConsultationsSeenFrom22ndTillEndOfMay1999)**

| SurgeryDate | DateOfBirth | Sex | Diagnosis | TimeIn | TimeOut | Complaints | Treatments | NumbersID | Notes |
|---|---|---|---|---|---|---|---|---|---|
| 28.05.99 | 14.02.24 | M | | 912 | 918 | Advised to take Solpadol, 2 tabs 4-6hrly prn | | 3718 | |
| 27.05.99 | 08.10.22 | M | | 1050 | 1103 | Bilateral inguinal hernia | Trusses | 373 | |
| 24.05.99 | 01.10.23 | F | Hypertension | 1736 | 1746 | BP 180/80 | TenBen | 3750 | Script for Paracetamol also given. |
| 24.05.99 | 24.09.41 | F | | 1812 | 1820 | Script for Detrusitol & Co-dydramol given | | 3760 | She also collapsed one week ago, for FBC & Glucose. |
| 28.05.99 | 26.01.61 | M | | 918 | 927 | For repeat U/Es & Creatinine Clearance test | | 3820 | |
| 28.05.99 | 30.10.50 | M | Pain | 1746 | 1754 | Pain (L) side of the head | Ibuprofen & Co-dydramol | 3829 | |
| 27.05.99 | 09.02.53 | F | Revisit | 1659 | 1706 | (R) ear is still sore | Referred to ENT Surgeon | 3852 | |
| 28.05.99 | 27.05.65 | F | | 1034 | 1042 | Bacterial vaginosis on smear | Metronidazole | 3920 | FP1001 (GMS4) form signed. |
| 26.05.99 | 31.03.86 | F | RTI | 1652 | 1700 | Cough | Amoxycillin | 4001 | Script for Chlorpheniramine also given. |
| 27.05.99 | 29.01.73 | F | Revisit | 934 | 944 | Itchy rash on face is still present | Referred to Dermatologist | 4063 | |

Result of a query that lists all consultations from the 22nd to the end of May 1999 (ConsultationsSeenFrom22ndTillEndOfMay1999)

| SurgeryDate | DateOfBirth | Sex | Diagnosis | TimeIn | TimeOut | Complaints | Treatments | NumbersID | Notes |
|---|---|---|---|---|---|---|---|---|---|
| 28.05.99 | 24.10.25 | F | | 927 | 950 | Deafness | Referred to ENT Surgeon | 4067 | Script for Ciprofloxacin suspension, Ibuprofen suspension & Amitriptyline suspension. |
| 25.05.99 | 10.08.67 | F | | 956 | 1003 | Inter-menstrual bleeding | Referred to Gynaecologist | 4075 | |
| 25.05.99 | 09.01.66 | F | Rash | 1703 | 1706 | Mole on (L) side of nose | Referred to Dermatologist | 4082 | |
| 25.05.99 | 17.10.89 | M | Rash | 1706 | 1711 | Itchy rash in between (L) toes | Terbinafine cream | 4094 | |
| 28.05.99 | 30.01.89 | M | Rash | 1643 | 1650 | Mole on the back bigger | Referred to Dermatologist | 4127 | |
| 24.05.99 | 29.07.54 | F | | 1017 | 1024 | Peri-menopausal | Premique cycle | 4197 | |
| 27.05.99 | 30.09.48 | F | Pain | 909 | 922 | Tender (R) Scaphoid bone | For X-Ray (R) wrist | 4237 | |
| 27.05.99 | 27.07.48 | M | Revisit | 1813 | 1816 | Psoriatic rash on legs & arms no better | Elocon cream | 4254 | |
| 28.05.99 | 19.05.89 | M | | 1629 | 1634 | Mum doesn't feel he needs to see the Psychiatrist any more | | 4257 | |
| 27.05.99 | 03.02.55 | M | | 1706 | 1709 | Script for Naproxen enteric coated given | | 4277 | |
| 25.05.99 | 30.10.47 | M | | 1758 | 1807 | Script for Trimethoprim given | | 431 | |

**Result of a query that lists all consultations from the 22nd to the end of May 1999 (ConsultationsSeenFrom22ndTillEndOfMay1999)**

| SurgeryDate | DateOfBirth | Sex | Diagnosis | TimeIn | TimeOut | Complaints | Treatments | NumbersID | Notes |
|---|---|---|---|---|---|---|---|---|---|
| 25.05.99 | 19.09.22 | F | | 924 | 942 | Patient informed that she has Salmonella poisoning | | 4371 | |
| 24.05.99 | 26.12.32 | F | | 1707 | 1718 | Script for Buscopan & Colpermin given | | 4437 | |
| 24.05.99 | 12.04.70 | M | | 1846 | 1850 | MSU - Calcium Oxalate present | | 4453 | |
| 24.05.99 | 06.01.69 | F | | 1708 | 1727 | Burst condom | Schering PC4 | 447 | |
| 28.05.99 | 31.12.22 | M | RTI | 950 | 959 | Cough | Amoxycillin | 4470 | Script for Paracetamol, Combivent nebules, Combivent inhaler, Simple Linctus & Prednisolone. |
| 27.05.99 | 08.04.93 | M | URTI | 1816 | 1825 | (R) ear ache | Paracetamol | 4476 | |
| 26.05.99 | 29.09.32 | F | Pain | 1320 | 1342 | Abdominal pain & fever | Referred to Surgical Dr. on call, SGH | 4487 | Home visit. |
| 26.05.99 | 03.04.69 | F | Pain | 1700 | 1706 | Abdominal pain | Omeprazole | 4508 | Penicillin allergy. |
| 24.05.99 | 06.03.92 | M | URTI | 1709 | 1718 | Sore throat & fever | Augmentin-Duo & Ibuprofen | 4515 | |
| 28.05.99 | 13.02.61 | F | Revisit | 959 | 1006 | Headaches persist | Referred to Neurologist | 4522 | |
| 25.05.99 | 01.02.59 | M | RTI | 1807 | 1817 | Cough | Amoxycillin | 4523 | Script for Tritace given. |
| 24.05.99 | 07.08.42 | F | | 1024 | 1029 | Due to have USScan of neck in August | | 4695 | |

## Result of a query that lists all consultations from the 22nd to the end of May 1999 (ConsultationsSeenFrom22ndTillEndOfMay1999)

| SurgeryDate | DateOfBirth | Sex | Diagnosis | TimeIn | TimeOut | Complaints | Treatments | NumbersID | Notes |
|---|---|---|---|---|---|---|---|---|---|
| 26.05.99 | 30.08.61 | M | | 1802 | 1812 | Snores & sleep apnoea | Referred to Physician | 4709 | |
| 26.05.99 | 21.05.35 | M | S/Leave | 1003 | 1017 | Cancer of Oesophagus | | 4788 | Script for Ranitidine suspension also given. |
| 24.05.99 | 08.01.29 | F | | 1225 | 1242 | Tired & lethargic | Ferrous Sulphate & Multivitamin | 4814 | Script for MST also given. Home visit. |
| 28.05.99 | 02.07.26 | M | | 1042 | 1044 | Ankle is swollen | See in 2 months | 4893 | |
| 25.05.99 | 01.02.30 | M | Deafness | 1754 | 1758 | Hard wax (R) ear | Referred to ENT Surgeon | 4905 | |
| 25.05.99 | 09.07.95 | M | | 951 | 956 | Script for Salbutamol & Chlorpheniramine suspensions | | 4924 | |
| 28.05.99 | 30.04.62 | M | URTI | 1742 | 1746 | Sore throat | Co-Amoxiclav | 5076 | |
| 24.05.99 | 09.02.65 | F | Pain | 1855 | 1709 | Abdominal pain | Cefadroxil & Mist Potassium Citrate | 5077 | For MSU. |
| 26.05.99 | 19.12.91 | F | RTI | 1646 | 1650 | Cough | Amoxycillin | 5107 | |
| 24.05.99 | 23.05.78 | F | | 1850 | 1855 | She wants T.O.P. | | 5204 | |
| 26.05.99 | 17.04.45 | F | | 930 | 934 | Pain (R) upper back | Diclofenac enteric coated | 5207 | |
| 26.05.99 | 06.06.78 | F | | 1743 | 1752 | Late period | For Pregnancy test | 5232 | |
| 27.05.99 | 20.04.55 | F | Pain | 1719 | 1724 | Neck ache | Ibuprofen & Co-dydramol | 5253 | |

Result of a query that lists all consultations from the 22nd to the end of May 1999 (ConsultationsSeenFrom22ndTillEndOfMay1999)

| SurgeryDate | DateOfBirth | Sex | Diagnosis | TimeIn | TimeOut | Complaints | Treatments | NumbersID | Notes |
|---|---|---|---|---|---|---|---|---|---|
| 27.05.99 | 04.12.57 | F |  | 926 | 934 | Script for Salbutamol inhaler & Fucibet cream given |  | 5288 |  |
| 26.05.99 | 01.06.93 | M | URTI | 1108 | 1111 | Sore throat | Amoxycillin | 5318 |  |
| 28.05.99 | 26.10.83 | M | Rash | 1730 | 1740 | Itchy rash on the legs | Fucidin-H cream & Loratadine | 5332 |  |
| 26.05.99 | 11.05.74 | F |  | 927 | 930 | Late period | For Pregnancy test | 5351 |  |
| 27.05.99 | 03.05.72 | F | URTI | 1029 | 1033 | Sore throat | Amoxycillin | 5373 | Script for Fluconazole also given. |
| 25.05.99 | 12.05.49 | F | RTI | 1721 | 1724 | Cough | Amoxycillin | 5549 |  |
| 24.05.99 | 27.12.59 | F |  | 1005 | 1013 | Patient has changed Epilim dose |  | 5609 |  |
| 28.05.99 | 10.06.97 | M | Rash | 1634 | 1643 | Red itchy rash on the legs | Aqueous cream & Fucidin-H cream | 5642 |  |
| 26.05.99 | 09.09.33 | F | RTI | 1735 | 1743 | Cough | Ciprofloxacin | 5754 |  |
| 25.05.99 | 24.04.35 | F | RTI | 1716 | 1721 | Cough | Amoxycillin | 5770 |  |
| 26.05.99 | 18.01.63 | M | Revisit | 1731 | 1735 | (R) knee is still sore | For Physiotherapy | 589 |  |
| 25.05.99 | 19.12.97 | M | RTI | 1817 | 1823 | Cough | Amoxycillin & Paracetamol | 5913 |  |
| 27.05.99 | 18.09.70 | M | S/Leave | 1733 | 1741 | Depression - Private & Med. 5 |  | 5926 |  |
| 24.05.99 | 29.07.51 | M |  | 913 | 926 | Script for Meloxicam & Omeprazole given |  | 5958 |  |
| 24.05.99 | 17.12.31 | M |  | 1013 | 1017 | To see P/Nurse in 6 months for U/Es |  | 5978 |  |

Result of a query that lists all consultations from the 22nd to the end of May 1999 (ConsultationsSeenFrom22ndTillEndOfMay1999)

| SurgeryDate | DateOfBirth | Sex | Diagnosis | TimeIn | TimeOut | Complaints | Treatments | NumbersID | Notes |
|---|---|---|---|---|---|---|---|---|---|
| 27.05.99 | 10.01.98 | F | RTI | 1033 | 1040 | Cough | Amoxycillin | 5984 | Script for Salbutamol suspension also given. |
| 25.05.99 | 31.08.70 | F | Pain | 1010 | 1023 | Abdominal pain | Referred to Surgeon (BUPA) | 6046 | |
| 25.05.99 | 13.11.85 | F | | 1039 | 1046 | T.A.T.T. | For FBC | 6067 | |
| 28.05.99 | 06.03.97 | F | URTI | 1048 | 1053 | (R) ear ache | Augmentin-Duo | 6090 | |
| 26.05.99 | 03.06.90 | M | | 905 | 923 | He has learning difficulties | | 6134 | |
| 28.05.99 | 03.06.90 | M | | 1725 | 1730 | (R) middle nail difficult to trim & sore | Referred to Chiropodist | 6134 | |
| 24.05.99 | 21.07.98 | F | Revisit | 1732 | 1736 | Bath oil not helping rash | Referred to Dermatologist | 6160 | |
| 24.05.99 | 22.07.17 | F | | 1802 | 1812 | Irritation all over | Hydroxyzine & Calamine lotion | 6182 | Script for Quinine Bisulphate also given. |
| 27.05.99 | 13.11.53 | F | Revisit | 1640 | 1652 | X-Ray (R) Shoulder normal | Inj. Depo-Medrone with Lidocaine | 6261 | |
| 24.05.99 | 07.11.94 | F | Rash | 1029 | 1039 | Itchy rash on trunk & fever | Calamine lotion, Loratadine, Paracetamol & Ibuprofen | 6279 | |
| 28.05.99 | 27.01.80 | F | Pain | 1044 | 1048 | Pain (R) side of head & nausea | Clotam Rapid | 6283 | Script for Elocon cream also given. |

## Result of a query that lists all consultations from the 22nd to the end of May 1999 (ConsultationsSeenFrom22ndTillEndOfMay1999)

| SurgeryDate | DateOfBirth | Sex | Diagnosis | TimeIn | TimeOut | Complaints | Treatments | NumbersID | Notes |
|---|---|---|---|---|---|---|---|---|---|
| 26.05.99 | 17.06.35 | F | | 1031 | 1037 | To continue on present medication | | 6286 | Her husband came to Surgery. |
| 27.05.99 | 04.07.71 | F | | 1232 | 1258 | Diarrhoea & Abdominal pain | Lomotil & Ciprofloxacin | 6291 | Home visit. |
| 28.05.99 | 28.11.84 | F | RTI | 1709 | 1720 | Cough | Amoxycillin | 6294 | |
| 27.05.99 | 20.08.74 | F | Pain | 1727 | 1733 | Neck ache | Ibuprofen & Co-dydramol | 6302 | She was involved in RTA & has not been to A/E. |
| 27.05.99 | 10.01.73 | F | Rash | 944 | 952 | Blisters around mouth | Fucidin cream | 6305 | |
| 24.05.99 | 29.09.34 | F | | 947 | 959 | For LFTs, CPK & fasting Cholesterol | | 6309 | |
| 26.05.99 | 11.05.76 | M | URTI | 925 | 927 | Sore throat | Amoxycillin | 6334 | |
| 28.05.99 | 17.10.97 | M | RTI | 1021 | 1027 | Cough & fever | Amoxycillin | 6338 | |
| 27.05.99 | 12.08.76 | M | | 1724 | 1727 | Script for Thioridazine given | | 6348 | |
| 26.05.99 | 20.06.30 | M | Pain | 1037 | 1044 | Pain (R) ankle | Ibuprofen | 6363 | |
| 26.05.99 | 06.07.55 | F | | 934 | 943 | LH & FSH results: probably Menopausal | | 6413 | |
| 25.05.99 | 15.12.65 | F | RTI | 1637 | 1643 | Cough | Amoxycillin | 6422 | She is 33 weeks gestation. |
| 24.05.99 | 09.01.62 | F | | 1746 | 1751 | T.A.T.T. | For FBC & TFTs | 78 | |
| 26.05.99 | 03.03.38 | F | | 1044 | 1105 | She needs artificial lower limbs | | 783 | |
| 27.05.99 | 05.10.74 | M | | 1040 | 1050 | Letter to Associate Neurologist regarding getting ENT appointment for him as planned | | 918 | |

### Result of a query that lists all consultations from the 22nd to the end of May 1999 (ConsultationsSeenFrom22ndTillEndOfMay1999)

| SurgeryDate | DateOfBirth | Sex | Diagnosis | TimeIn | TimeOut | Complaints | Treatments | NumbersID | Notes |
|---|---|---|---|---|---|---|---|---|---|
| 24.05.99 | 09.06.54 | F | | 1641 | 1707 | For USScan of pelvis & TFTs | | 927 | |
| 28.05.99 | 15.03.75 | F | | 1027 | 1034 | Script for Fluoxetine & Microgynon 30 given | | 934 | |
| 25.05.99 | 29.08.24 | M | | 1046 | 1058 | Feels congested | Amoxycillin & Rhinocort Aqua nasal spray | 955 | Script for Glandosane also given. |
| 25.05.99 | 12.09.26 | F | URTI | 1023 | 1030 | Sore throat | Amoxycillin | Temp | She also has hot flushes, Rx. Dixarit. |
| 25.05.99 | 24.03.75 | M | Rash | 1742 | 1754 | Reddish rash all over | Tetracycline | Temp | |
| 26.05.99 | 07.03.79 | F | URTI | 1815 | 1820 | Sore throat | Amoxycillin | Temp | |

### Result of a query that lists all consultations from the 22nd to the end of May 2000 (ConsultationsSeenFrom22ndTillEndOfMay2000)

| SurgeryDate | DateOfBirth | Sex | Diagnosis | TimeIn | TimeOut | Complaints | Treatments | NumbersID | Notes |
|---|---|---|---|---|---|---|---|---|---|
| 24.05.2000 | 31.12.1953 | F | | 1641 | 1646 | CXR - normal | | 1075 | |
| 24.05.2000 | 13.03.1954 | F | Hypertension | 944 | 1002 | BP 150/90 | Bendrofluazide | 1172 | |
| 23.05.2000 | 13.05.1914 | M | Revisit | 1026 | 1047 | Still unwell & pain (L) | Referred to Dr. on duty, Medical Assessment Unit | 1186 | |
| 24.05.2000 | 01.12.1934 | F | Pain | 1040 | 1052 | Pain (R) calf | Naftidrofuryl | 1371 | Penicillin allergy. |
| 23.05.2000 | 21.09.1924 | F | Pain | 1658 | 1709 | Multiple joint pains | Tramadol | 1419 | |

Result of a query that lists all consultations from the 22nd to the end of May 2000 (ConsultationsSeenFrom22ndTillEndOfMay2000)

| SurgeryDate | DateOfBirth | Sex | Diagnosis | TimeIn | TimeOut | Complaints | Treatments | NumbersID | Notes |
|---|---|---|---|---|---|---|---|---|---|
| 25.05.2000 | 05.01.1984 | M | Revisit | 1810 | 1814 | Wart on (R) hand is bigger & darker | Referred to Dermatologist (Basildon hospital) | 1504 | |
| 24.05.2000 | 04.03.1913 | F | | 1303 | 1315 | Dry flaky skin on the legs | Aqueous cream & Unguentum Merck | 1541 | Home visit. |
| 24.05.2000 | 08.08.1924 | F | | 1002 | 1028 | Script for Enlive & Senna given | | 1559 | |
| 25.05.2000 | 08.08.1924 | F | | 1235 | 1300 | Low back pain is worse | MST | 1559 | Home visit. |
| 25.05.2000 | 27.04.1968 | M | S/Leave | 1026 | 1033 | Diarrhoea & vomiting | | 1565 | |
| 23.05.2000 | 05.06.1980 | F | | 900 | 910 | Stomach swells up & constipated | Colpermin, Senna tablets & Lactulose | 1622 | Script for Ferrous Sulphate. |
| 25.05.2000 | 17.07.1970 | F | RTI | 904 | 914 | Cough | Amoxycillin | 1658 | Script for Fexofenadine given. |
| 26.05.2000 | 11.08.1962 | F | Conjunctivitis | 1710 | 1714 | Red, sore & sticky (L) eye | Chloramphenicol eye ointment | 1873 | FP1001 (GMS4) form signed. |
| 24.05.2000 | 04.01.1962 | F | | 1727 | 1733 | To discuss with Physician regarding U/Es results | | 1884 | |
| 30.05.2000 | 04.01.1962 | F | | 1633 | 1645 | Awaiting information from Physician | | 1884 | |
| 26.05.2000 | 16.09.1949 | M | | 1750 | 1805 | Script for Adalat LA 60 given | | 1893 | For Physiotherapy. |
| 25.05.2000 | 11.08.1926 | F | | 1048 | 1054 | Dizzy spells | Betahistine | 1907 | For FBC & TFTs. |

Result of a query that lists all consultations from the 22nd to the end of May 2000 (ConsultationsSeenFrom22ndTillEndOfMay2000)

| SurgeryDate | DateOfBirth | Sex | Diagnosis | TimeIn | TimeOut | Complaints | Treatments | NumbersID | Notes |
|---|---|---|---|---|---|---|---|---|---|
| 30.05.2000 | 22.10.1966 | M | S/Leave | 939 | 946 | Wife has medical problems post deliver - Private | | 1990 | Penicillin allergy. |
| 26.05.2000 | 22.09.1967 | F | | 1046 | 1049 | FP1001 (GMS4) form signed | | 2151 | |
| 26.05.2000 | 09.07.1940 | M | S/Leave | 905 | 910 | Pain (L) shoulder | Kapake | 2152 | |
| 26.05.2000 | 25.12.1958 | F | | 1805 | 1812 | Abscess (L) upper gum | Amoxycillin | 2205 | New Patient check done. |
| 25.05.2000 | 11.06.1968 | F | Pain | 951 | 959 | Low back pain | Ibuprofen | 2261 | For Lumbo-Sacral spine X-Ray & MSU. |
| 30.05.2000 | 06.11.1915 | M | RTI | 1645 | 1656 | Cough | Ciprofloxacin | 229 | Script for Chloramphenicol eye ointment, Acyclovir cream & Simple Linctus given. |
| 24.05.2000 | 08.05.1986 | F | Pain | 1646 | 1652 | Chest pain & haemoptysis | Referred to Paediatric Dr. on call, (Basildon hospital) | 2350 | |
| 24.05.2000 | 25.05.1925 | F | Hypertension | 1033 | 1040 | BP 160/110 | Bendrofluazide | 2414 | For U/Es, LFTs & Cholesterol. |
| 23.05.2000 | 06.11.1920 | M | | 910 | 918 | For fasting Blood Glucose | | 2423 | Septrin & Kapake allergy. |
| 26.05.2000 | 23.08.1956 | M | Pain | 915 | 929 | Pain (R) knee | Ibuprofen | 2484 | New Patient check done. For X-Ray (R) knee. |

188

Result of a query that lists all consultations from the 22nd to the end of May 2000 (ConsultationsSeenFrom22ndTillEndOfMay2000)

| SurgeryDate | DateOfBirth | Sex | Diagnosis | TimeIn | TimeOut | Complaints | Treatments | NumbersID | Notes |
|---|---|---|---|---|---|---|---|---|---|
| 26.05.2000 | 16.12.1984 | F | | 1100 | 1109 | Heavy per vagina bleeding & abdominal pain | Norethisterone & Buscopan | 2524 | |
| 25.05.2000 | 21.07.1986 | F | | 1656 | 1700 | (R) ear is sore | EarCalm | 2648 | |
| 25.05.2000 | 07.05.1978 | F | URTI | 1652 | 1656 | Sore throat | Amoxycillin | 2684 | |
| 25.05.2000 | 13.08.1934 | M | RTI | 1740 | 1749 | Cough | Amoxycillin | 2782 | |
| 22.05.2000 | 21.09.1919 | M | | 1020 | 1026 | Constipation | Senna, Co-danthramer & Glycerine suppositories | 2917 | |
| 30.05.2000 | 24.09.1970 | F | S/Leave | 1728 | 1735 | Abdominal pain | | 2935 | Script for Tylex given. |
| 23.05.2000 | 20.03.1919 | F | Pain | 1640 | 1653 | Back pain | Co-Proxamol, Senna & Didronel PMO | 2943 | For Physiotherapy. |
| 25.05.2000 | 31.10.1974 | M | RTI | 1730 | 1740 | Cough | Amoxycillin | 3120 | Abdominal pain, Rx. Ibuprofen & Co-dydramol. For MSU. |
| 22.05.2000 | 10.05.1968 | F | | 931 | 946 | Buzzing (R) ear | Betahistine | 3213 | Itchy rash in vulval area. Rx. Fucidin-H cream. |
| 22.05.2000 | 25.10.1968 | F | | 1729 | 1745 | Obesity | Referred to Endocrinologist | 3214 | |
| 23.05.2000 | 15.01.1957 | F | Depression | 928 | 941 | Unable to cope & suicidal | Referred to Psychiatric Dr. on call, SGH | 3262 | |
| 22.05.2000 | 02.12.1980 | M | | 1636 | 1640 | Hay fever | Loratadine | 3326 | |

**Result of a query that lists all consultations from the 22nd to the end of May 2000 (ConsultationsSeenFrom22ndTillEndOfMay2000)**

| SurgeryDate | DateOfBirth | Sex | Diagnosis | TimeIn | TimeOut | Complaints | Treatments | NumbersID | Notes |
|---|---|---|---|---|---|---|---|---|---|
| 25.05.2000 | 31.01.1987 | F | RTI | 1805 | 1810 | Cough | Amoxycillin | 3343 | |
| 30.05.2000 | 01.07.1979 | M | Lump | 1717 | 1728 | Swelling (L) testicle | For USScan of the testicles | 3369 | Penicillin allergy. |
| 22.05.2000 | 02.11.1991 | M | | 985 | 1002 | Script for Sotalol & Warfarin given | | 3445 | |
| 23.05.2000 | 19.02.1942 | F | URTI | 923 | 928 | Sinuses are tender | Amoxycillin | 3481 | |
| 22.05.2000 | 10.01.1992 | M | RTI | 1812 | 1817 | Cough | Erythromycin | 3492 | Penicillin allergy. |
| 22.05.2000 | 01.11.1954 | F | S/Leave | 1718 | 1723 | Hysteroscopy - Med. 5 | | 3520 | |
| 23.05.2000 | 02.11.1938 | M | URTI | 1726 | 1736 | (R) ear discharge | Amoxycillin & Otomize ear spray. | 3603 | |
| 22.05.2000 | 18.01.1958 | M | S/Leave | 1713 | 1718 | Chicken Pox | | 3654 | |
| 30.05.2000 | 13.07.1914 | M | | 954 | 1007 | Script for Digoxin & Multivitamins given | | 3714 | Aspirin allergy. |
| 22.05.2000 | 05.06.1924 | M | | 1745 | 1750 | Nostrils are sore & stuffy | Naseptin cream | 381 | |
| 24.05.2000 | 29.09.1923 | F | | 1028 | 1033 | For Direct Coomb's test, serum Ferritin, B12 & Folate | | 3868 | |
| 26.05.2000 | 06.02.1993 | F | Conjunctivitis | 1707 | 1710 | Redness & stickiness in both eyes | Chloramphenicol eye drops | 3893 | Diarrhoea, Rx. Dioralyte. |
| 30.05.2000 | 21.05.1974 | M | URTI | 1007 | 1015 | (L) ear ache | Amoxycillin & Otomize ear spray | 3911 | |
| 24.05.2000 | 11.06.1962 | F | Pain | 1052 | 1100 | Headaches | Ibuprofen | 4023 | |
| 26.05.2000 | 02.07.1991 | M | Conjunctivitis | 1737 | 1743 | (R) eye is red & swollen | Chloramphenicol eye drops | 4035 | |

## Result of a query that lists all consultations from the 22nd to the end of May 2000 (ConsultationsSeenFrom22ndTillEndOfMay2000)

| SurgeryDate | DateOfBirth | Sex | Diagnosis | TimeIn | TimeOut | Complaints | Treatments | NumbersID | Notes |
|---|---|---|---|---|---|---|---|---|---|
| 23.05.2000 | 21.01.1929 | F | URTI | 1716 | 1721 | Sinuses tender | Amoxycillin | 4116 | Zantac allergy. |
| 23.05.2000 | 20.10.1985 | M | Revisit | 1713 | 1716 | Lump in (R) breast is still present | Referred to Paediatrician (BUPA) | 4134 | |
| 30.05.2000 | 29.11.1962 | M | S/Leave | 1753 | 1802 | Low back pain - Private | | 4165 | |
| 30.05.2000 | 21.02.1916 | F | | 1656 | 1711 | Frequency, ?urgency | Tolterodine | 4178 | Penicillin allergy. |
| 25.05.2000 | 07.05.1923 | F | RTI | 924 | 946 | Cough & wheezy | Amoxycillin, Erythromycin, Frusemide, Seretide, Prednisolone & nebulizer | 4211 | |
| 24.05.2000 | 19.05.1989 | M | | 1757 | 1806 | (L) elbow movements following fracture is still reduced 9 months later | Referred to Orthopaedic Surgeon (Basildon hospital) | 4257 | |
| 23.05.2000 | 13.09.1992 | F | URTI | 1759 | 1805 | Infected rhinorrhoea | Amoxycillin | 4259 | |
| 26.05.2000 | 03.02.1955 | M | | 929 | 941 | Script for Bendrofluazide given | | 4277 | |
| 26.05.2000 | 24.06.1928 | M | | 1703 | 1707 | Indigestion | Lansoprazole | 4312 | |
| 25.05.2000 | 06.11.1968 | F | RTI | 1814 | 1822 | Cough again | Erythromycin | 4479 | Penicillin allergy. For CXR. |
| 22.05.2000 | 29.09.1932 | F | Revisit | 912 | 920 | X-Ray lumbar spine: Osteophytes D12, L1 & L2. Anterior spondylolisthesis L4 over L5 | For Physiotherapy | 4487 | |

Result of a query that lists all consultations from the 22nd to the end of May 2000 (ConsultationsSeenFrom22ndTillEndOfMay2000)

| SurgeryDate | DateOfBirth | Sex | Diagnosis | TimeIn | TimeOut | Complaints | Treatments | NumbersID | Notes |
|---|---|---|---|---|---|---|---|---|---|
| 23.05.2000 | 03.04.1969 | F | URTI | 1736 | 1740 | Sore throat | Amoxycillin | 4508 | ?Penicillin allergy. |
| 26.05.2000 | 31.01.1968 | F | Depression | 941 | 955 | Weepy & unable to cope | CPN | 4616 | |
| 23.05.2000 | 06.04.1978 | F | Pain | 1740 | 1748 | Pain (R) upper back | Diclofenac enteric coated | 4647 | Itchy & sticky (R) pierced ear, Rx. Erythromycin & Fucidin-H cream. Penicillin allergy. |
| 23.05.2000 | 20.09.1939 | M | | 1709 | 1713 | Private script for Viagra given | | 4817 | |
| 24.05.2000 | 26.06.1988 | M | URTI | 1100 | 1103 | Sore throat | Amoxycillin | 5073 | |
| 24.05.2000 | 30.04.1962 | M | S/Leave | 1737 | 1745 | (L) Inguinal hernia - Med. 3 & Med. 4 | | 5076 | |
| 26.05.2000 | 17.09.1975 | F | | 1714 | 1725 | Bruise on outer (L) upper thigh after being mugged on the train | | 5148 | |
| 26.05.2000 | 30.10.1920 | F | | 1031 | 1040 | Happy to continue with Ibuprofen | | 5160 | |
| 26.05.2000 | 16.10.1975 | F | | 1653 | 1657 | Vaginal thrush | Fluconazole | 5180 | |
| 22.05.2000 | 04.04.1996 | M | Rash | 1650 | 1703 | Itchy dry skin | Balneum Plus bath oil & Chlorpheniramine | 5282 | |
| 26.05.2000 | 04.04.1996 | M | | 1636 | 1647 | Letter to whom it may concern that due Medical reason he was unable to travel by bus | | 5282 | |
| 22.05.2000 | 15.07.1996 | F | Pain | 920 | 931 | Abdominal pain | Merbentyl | 5323 | |

Result of a query that lists all consultations from the 22nd to the end of May 2000 (ConsultationsSeenFrom22ndTillEndOfMay2000)

| SurgeryDate | DateOfBirth | Sex | Diagnosis | TimeIn | TimeOut | Complaints | Treatments | NumbersID | Notes |
|---|---|---|---|---|---|---|---|---|---|
| 22.05.2000 | 11.11.1969 | F | RTI | 1804 | 1812 | Cough | Amoxycillin | 5363 | |
| 26.05.2000 | 04.05.1945 | F | | 1812 | 1821 | Persistent cough | For CXR | 5416 | Script for Premique Cycle given. |
| 23.05.2000 | 15.11.1941 | F | Rash | 1000 | 1005 | Moles on back & above (L) upper eye lid | Referred to Dermatologist (Basildon) | 5438 | |
| 22.05.2000 | 25.04.1997 | F | | 1703 | 1713 | Still chesty despite antibiotics | Referred to Rapid Access clinic | 5575 | CXR - Persistent chest infection. |
| 22.05.2000 | 27.12.1959 | F | | 1640 | 1650 | Letter to whom it may concern regarding sitting arrangements on the plane in the hotel whilst on holidays | | 5609 | |
| 23.05.2000 | 21.07.1938 | M | | 1748 | 1754 | Wax in (R) ear | Waxsol | 5679 | |
| 24.05.2000 | 17.01.1956 | F | | 940 | 944 | Sepsis (R) index finger | Flucloxacillin | 5796 | Aspirin allergy. |
| 22.05.2000 | 31.01.1936 | M | Pain | 1757 | 1804 | Burning sensation & chest pain | GTN spray & Lansoprazole | 5797 | |
| 25.05.2000 | 21.08.1946 | F | Rash | 1642 | 1645 | Moles on upper back | Referred to Dermatologist (Basildon hospital) | 5902 | |
| 24.05.2000 | 08.01.1998 | F | | 1733 | 1737 | Script for Promethazine given | | 5948 | Penicillin allergy. |
| 26.05.2000 | 31.08.1970 | F | URTI | 1657 | 1703 | Sore throat | Amoxycillin | 6046 | |
| 23.05.2000 | 06.04.1933 | F | Pain | 1010 | 1020 | Pains in the fingers | Referred to Rheumatologist | 6056 | For RA Latex test. Script for Class 2 Thigh length stockings given. |

Result of a query that lists all consultations from the 22nd to the end of May 2000 (ConsultationsSeenFrom22ndTillEndOfMay2000)

| SurgeryDate | DateOfBirth | Sex | Diagnosis | TimeIn | TimeOut | Complaints | Treatments | NumbersID | Notes |
|---|---|---|---|---|---|---|---|---|---|
| 23.05.2000 | 23.07.1929 | M | Pain | 1020 | 1026 | Pain back of (L) calf on walking | Nafridrofuryl | 6057 | |
| 23.05.2000 | 19.09.1937 | M | | 1754 | 1759 | Advised to increase dietary salt intake | | 6104 | |
| 30.05.2000 | 20.04.1933 | F | | 902 | 913 | Hoarse voice | For TFTs | 6110 | For ESR. |
| 25.05.2000 | 21.03.1973 | M | Lump | 1759 | 1805 | Septic sebaceous cyst | Flucloxacillin | 6142 | Referred to Surgeon. |
| 23.05.2000 | 22.01.1944 | M | UTI | 1721 | 1726 | Dysuria | Trimethoprim | 6183 | Penicillin allergy. For MSU. |
| 23.05.2000 | 30.11.1908 | F | | 1005 | 1010 | Cataract both eyes | Referred to Ophthalmologist | 6194 | Vertigo, Rx. Betahistine. Penicillin allergy. |
| 23.05.2000 | 12.07.1955 | F | RTI | 918 | 923 | Cough | Amoxycillin | 6202 | |
| 25.05.2000 | 21.05.1958 | F | Revisit | 1635 | 1642 | Still coughing | Co-Amoxiclav | 6209 | |
| 24.05.2000 | 13.05.1982 | F | RTI | 927 | 932 | Cough | Amoxycillin | 6210 | |
| 30.05.2000 | 17.02.1977 | F | URTI | 1230 | 1245 | Sore throat | Amoxycillin & Paracetamol | 6212 | Home visit. |
| 22.05.2000 | 26.09.1998 | F | RTI | 1723 | 1729 | Cough | Amoxycillin | 6231 | Constipation, Rx. Lactulose. |
| 26.05.2000 | 24.02.1925 | M | Pain | 955 | 1007 | Pain (L) chest | Ibuprofen & Co-dydramol | 6239 | Script for Inj. Xylocaine given. |
| 24.05.2000 | 05.01.1995 | F | | 1717 | 1722 | Recurrent sore throats | Referred to ENT Surgeon | 6252 | |
| 23.05.2000 | 09.05.1997 | M | URTI | 956 | 1000 | Sore throat | Amoxycillin & Paracetamol | 6253 | |
| 26.05.2000 | 11.09.1976 | F | S/Leave | 1821 | 1828 | Fainting & dizzy spells | For FBC | 6263 | |

Result of a query that lists all consultations from the 22nd to the end of May 2000 (ConsultationsSeenFrom22ndTillEndOfMay2000)

| SurgeryDate | DateOfBirth | Sex | Diagnosis | TimeIn | TimeOut | Complaints | Treatments | NumbersID | Notes |
|---|---|---|---|---|---|---|---|---|---|
| 25.05.2000 | 01.11.1998 | M | | 1703 | 1710 | Sore penis | Trimethoprim | 6266 | |
| 25.05.2000 | 20.08.1974 | F | Pain | 914 | 924 | Low back pain | Ibuprofen & Co-dydramol | 6302 | For Lumbo-Sacral spine X-Ray. |
| 25.05.2000 | 05.03.1979 | F | | 1002 | 1014 | Referred to Physician (Basildon hospital) regarding her hypertension | | 6320 | |
| 23.05.2000 | 11.05.1976 | M | S/Leave | 1636 | 1640 | Back pain | | 6334 | |
| 26.05.2000 | 23.01.1999 | F | Conjunctivitis | 1049 | 1100 | Puffed up eyes & diarrhoea | Chloramphenicol eye drops & Dioralyte | 6346 | |
| 24.05.2000 | 09.05.1989 | F | Pain | 901 | 915 | Headaches | Paracetamol | 6347 | |
| 30.05.2000 | 28.03.1945 | M | | 1802 | 1807 | Script for Tetracycline given | | 6357 | |
| 24.05.2000 | 25.07.1968 | F | | 919 | 927 | T.A.T.T. | For FBC & TFTs | 6371 | |
| 25.05.2000 | 03.12.1970 | F | | 1020 | 1026 | Letter to expedite Dermatology clinic appointment | | 6457 | |
| 22.05.2000 | 02.11.1989 | M | URTI | 1008 | 1013 | Sore throat | Amoxycillin | 6572 | |
| 22.05.2000 | 06.01.1965 | F | URTI | 1013 | 1016 | Sore throat | Amoxycillin | 6573 | |
| 24.05.2000 | 29.08.1999 | F | | 1652 | 1657 | Vomiting | Metoclopramide | 6593 | |
| 25.05.2000 | 22.04.1954 | M | Pain | 1749 | 1759 | He still has chest pain | Atenolol | 6614 | |
| 26.05.2000 | 09.11.1978 | F | Revisit | 1647 | 1653 | She is still choking in the evenings & mornings | | 6622 | Referred to ENT Surgeon |
| 30.05.2000 | 14.10.1997 | F | RTI | 919 | 924 | Cough & fever | Augmentin-Duo | 6626 | |

195

Result of a query that lists all consultations from the 22nd to the end of May 2000 (ConsultationsSeenFrom22ndTillEndOfMay2000)

| SurgeryDate | DateOfBirth | Sex | Diagnosis | TimeIn | TimeOut | Complaints | Treatments | NumbersID | Notes |
|---|---|---|---|---|---|---|---|---|---|
| 30.05.2000 | 28.11.1978 | F | | 1735 | 1743 | Heartburn | Gaviscon | 6636 | Penicillin allergy. 18/40 gestation. |
| 24.05.2000 | 02.12.1994 | F | | 1714 | 1717 | Head lice | Full Marks | 6655 | |
| 24.05.2000 | 28.02.1960 | F | Pain | 1745 | 1757 | Pain (L) knee | Kapake | 6662 | |
| 24.05.2000 | 22.06.1962 | M | S/Leave | 1722 | 1727 | Facial scarring, Depressed skull fracture | | 6669 | |
| 25.05.2000 | 28.09.1998 | F | URTI | 1014 | 1020 | Infected rhinorrhoea | Amoxycillin & Paracetamol | 6702 | |
| 30.05.2000 | 23.02.1940 | M | RTI | 1711 | 1717 | Cough | Amoxycillin | 6704 | |
| 22.05.2000 | 08.10.1940 | F | Pain | 903 | 912 | Pain & reduced movement (R) shoulder | For Physiotherapy | 6705 | |
| 30.05.2000 | 05.10.1940 | F | | 913 | 919 | Referred to Psychiatrist | | 6707 | Home visit. |
| 22.05.2000 | 06.06.1978 | F | | 1125 | 1130 | Routine P/Natal check | | 6712 | |
| 22.05.2000 | 17.09.1943 | M | | 1817 | 1825 | Advised to stop driving for 1 month & to inform DVLA following his T.I.A. | | 6719 | |
| 23.05.2000 | 02.09.1994 | F | Conjunctivitis | 1653 | 1658 | Eyes sticky | Chloramphenicol eye drops | 6732 | Script for Oilatum Plus bath emollient given. |
| 23.05.2000 | 04.05.1937 | F | Pain | 941 | 956 | Injury (R) ankle | For X-Ray (R) ankle | | |

196

Result of a query that lists all consultations from the 22nd to the end of May 2000 (ConsultationsSeenFrom22ndTillEndOfMay2000)

| SurgeryDate | DateOfBirth | Sex | Diagnosis | TimeIn | TimeOut | Complaints | Treatments | NumbersID | Notes |
|---|---|---|---|---|---|---|---|---|---|
| 25.05.2000 | 20.04.1932 | M | Revisit | 959 | 1002 | Persistent sore throat | Referred to ENT Surgeon (Basildon hospital) | 6732 | |
| 25.05.2000 | 22.12.1921 | M | | 1033 | 1048 | Letter to whom it may concern that he cannot act for himself | | 6756 | Wife came to Surgery. |
| 26.05.2000 | 30.10.1967 | M | Pain | 1040 | 1046 | Pain in (R) leg | Movelar gel | 6783 | Dermoid cyst (L) side of upper lip, referred to Plastic Surgeon. Wax in ears, Rx. Waxsol. |
| 26.05.2000 | 23.11.1974 | F | URTI | 1109 | 1114 | Sore throat | Penicillin V | 6784 | |
| 26.05.2000 | 11.04.1952 | F | | 1743 | 1750 | LH 29.7 U/L & FSH 45.1 U/L | Premique Cycle | 755 | |
| 26.05.2000 | 28.08.1946 | F | Revisit | 1007 | 1017 | Occipital Lichen Simplex is worse | Referred to Dermatologist | 799 | Script for Arthrotec & Aqueous cream given. |
| 24.05.2000 | 04.04.1963 | M | | 1806 | 1822 | Taxi Medical done | | 848 | New Patient check done. Tetanus Toxoid Booster given. |
| 22.05.2000 | 17.04.1940 | F | Vertigo | 1750 | 1757 | Dizzy & light-headed | Prochlorperazine | 86 | |
| 26.05.2000 | 17.04.1940 | F | | 1725 | 1733 | Script for Cinnarizine given | | 86 | |
| 22.05.2000 | 05.09.1961 | F | Conjunctivitis | 955 | 958 | (R) eye is sore | Chloramphenicol eye ointment | 882 | |

### Result of a query that lists all consultations from the 22nd to the end of May 2000 (ConsultationsSeenFrom22ndTillEndOfMay2000)

| SurgeryDate | DateOfBirth | Sex | Diagnosis | TimeIn | TimeOut | Complaints | Treatments | NumbersID | Notes |
|---|---|---|---|---|---|---|---|---|---|
| 25.05.2000 | 16.10.1943 | F | | 1710 | 1730 | Script for Nafridrofuryl given | | 898 | New Patient check done. |
| 30.05.2000 | 05.10.1974 | M | S/Leave | 1743 | 1751 | Pain (R) shoulder - Med. 4 | | 918 | |
| 24.05.2000 | 23.10.1959 | M | | 1705 | 1714 | Lower gum sore & tender | Erythromycin | Temp | Penicillin allergy. |
| 26.05.2000 | 31.05.1991 | F | URTI | 1017 | 1031 | Sore throat | Amoxycillin & Paracetamol | Temp | Sticky (L) eye, Rx. Chloramphenicol eye drops. |

### Result of a query that lists all consultations from the 22nd to the end of May 2001 (ConsultationsSeenFrom22ndTillEndOfMay2001)

| SurgeryDate | DateOfBirth | Sex | Diagnosis | TimeIn | TimeOut | Complaints | Treatments | NumbersID | Notes |
|---|---|---|---|---|---|---|---|---|---|
| 23.05.2001 | 20.11.1946 | M | Pain | 1655 | 1659 | Injury (L) wrist & (L) thumb | For X-Ray | 1011 | |
| 24.05.2001 | 16.03.1947 | F | | 1011 | 1022 | Yellow spots at the back of the throat | Penicillin V | 107 | Heartburn, Rx. Lansoprazole. Depressed, Rx. Fluoxetine. For FBC & TFTs. |
| 30.05.2001 | 09.11.1976 | M | Rash | 1753 | 1803 | Flaky scalp | Ketoconazole shampoo | 108 | |
| 23.05.2001 | 20.07.1956 | M | | 1720 | 1723 | Itchy anus | Xyloproct ointment | 1126 | |
| 25.05.2001 | 18.05.1949 | M | S/Leave | 1138 | 1142 | Injury (R) shoulder | | 1160 | |

Result of a query that lists all consultations from the 22nd to the end of May 2001 (ConsultationsSeenFrom22ndTillEndOfMay2001)

| SurgeryDate | DateOfBirth | Sex | Diagnosis | TimeIn | TimeOut | Complaints | Treatments | NumbersID | Notes |
|---|---|---|---|---|---|---|---|---|---|
| 29.05.2001 | 30.07.1952 | F | | 937 | 949 | Wants her period delayed whilst on holidays | Norethisterone | 1170 | |
| 23.05.2001 | 17.09.1986 | F | | 1028 | 1034 | Her horse trod on her (R) foot | Advised to go to A/E | 1173 | |
| 25.05.2001 | 23.10.1969 | F | Rash | 1750 | 1754 | Itchy rash on arms & legs | Unguentum Merck & Loratadine | 1206 | Trimethoprim allergy. |
| 22.05.2001 | 24.10.1929 | F | Lump | 1128 | 1136 | Small lipoma on (L) thigh | For excision at minor surgery | 1255 | |
| 23.05.2001 | 27.08.1970 | M | S/Leave | 1122 | 1124 | Operation on (R) knee | | 1262 | |
| 22.05.2001 | 05.02.1946 | F | Revisit | 1148 | 1158 | Still has generalised itching & dry skin | Referred to Dermatologist | 1268 | |
| 29.05.2001 | 15.04.1951 | F | | 1047 | 1054 | Small boil in (L) axilla & (R) ear ache | Flucloxacillin, Fucidin-H cream & Otomize ear spray | 1470 | |
| 29.05.2001 | 28.07.1936 | M | Pain | 1022 | 1033 | Neck pain following RTA | Ibuprofen | 1508 | |
| 22.05.2001 | 17.09.1916 | F | | 1258 | 1328 | Depressed & chesty cough | Amoxycillin & Fluoxetine | 1531 | Home visit. Script for Losartan given. The Disabled Parking Badge form completed. |
| 24.05.2001 | 20.08.1966 | F | | 1805 | 1815 | 6 month check for the Accolate study | | 1602 | |

199

Result of a query that lists all consultations from the 22nd to the end of May 2001 (ConsultationsSeenFrom22ndTillEndOfMay2001)

| SurgeryDate | DateOfBirth | Sex | Diagnosis | TimeIn | TimeOut | Complaints | Treatments | NumbersID | Notes |
|---|---|---|---|---|---|---|---|---|---|
| 24.05.2001 | 17.07.1970 | F | | 1657 | 1712 | Nasal congestion from hay fever | Sodium Cromoglycate nasal spray | 1658 | 26/40 gestation. |
| 30.05.2001 | 19.08.1926 | F | | 1022 | 1028 | Script for Heli clear given | | 1907 | Pallor, for FBC. |
| 24.05.2001 | 11.12.1977 | M | | 1712 | 1719 | He wonders if he has STD | Referred to GUM clinic | 1922 | |
| 22.05.2001 | 12.02.1917 | M | | 1056 | 1108 | He would like to buy nebulizer | Advised to see P/ Nurse | 2006 | |
| 25.05.2001 | 06.07.1936 | F | | 1643 | 1651 | Dizziness & tinnitus | Betahistine | 2150 | Script for Multivitamins. |
| 22.05.2001 | 21.07.1919 | M | Pain | 1012 | 1026 | Pain (L) Tibia & (L) leg | Naftidrofuryl | 226 | For FBC & Fasting Cholesterol. |
| 30.05.2001 | 25.07.1988 | F | Rash | 1647 | 1653 | Itchy rash on the face & trunk | Loratadine, Balneum Plus bath oil & Unguentum Merck | 2336 | |
| 22.05.2001 | 23.04.1950 | F | S/Leave | 1742 | 1753 | Unwell after epidural injection | | 2369 | |
| 23.05.2001 | 28.03.1970 | F | S/Leave | 1011 | 1028 | Pain & numbness in (R) hand | | 2375 | |
| 25.05.2001 | 02.12.1948 | M | | 1805 | 1813 | Plasma Glucose 6.8 mmols/L | For modified GTT | 2380 | |
| 24.05.2001 | 07.02.1921 | M | Pain | 1640 | 1651 | Back pain | Paracetamol | 2381 | For Physiotherapy & for X-Ray Lumbar spine. |

Result of a query that lists all consultations from the 22nd to the end of May 2001 (ConsultationsSeenFrom22ndTillEndOfMay2001)

| SurgeryDate | DateOfBirth | Sex | Diagnosis | TimeIn | TimeOut | Complaints | Treatments | NumbersID | Notes |
|---|---|---|---|---|---|---|---|---|---|
| 29.05.2001 | 28.05.1957 | F | | 902 | 908 | Wants her period delayed whilst on holidays | Norethisterone | 2648 | |
| 23.05.2001 | 26.10.1965 | M | | 1806 | 1810 | Septic & itchy insect bites both knees | Flucloxacillin & Loratadine | 2769 | |
| 30.05.2001 | 11.08.1935 | F | | 927 | 929 | Late period | For Pregnancy test | 2836 | |
| 24.05.2001 | 13.04.1929 | F | | 1137 | 1149 | Deafness | Referred to ENT Surgeon (Basildon hospital) | 2873 | Pallor, for FBC. |
| 22.05.2001 | 05.07.1952 | F | | 1804 | 1812 | D&V | Electrolade | 2894 | |
| 24.05.2001 | 06.04.1924 | F | | 1108 | 1123 | Script for Gliclazide given | | 2909 | Penicillin allergy. |
| 25.05.2001 | 01.02.1931 | M | | 1119 | 1138 | He will see P/Nurse regarding getting appropriate spacer device | | 2965 | |
| 25.05.2001 | 26.06.1946 | M | S/Leave | 1110 | 1119 | Depression - Private | | 3025 | |
| 23.05.2001 | 15.02.1932 | F | Pain | 1751 | 1800 | Pain & swelling (R) knee | Inj. Depo-Medrone with Lidocaine | 3043 | Penicillin allergy. |
| 30.05.2001 | 15.02.1932 | F | | 1106 | 1123 | Inj. Depo-Medrone with Lidocaine to (R) knee | | 3043 | |
| 24.05.2001 | 16.11.1984 | F | URTI | 1103 | 1108 | Sore throat | Amoxycillin | 3338 | |

Result of a query that lists all consultations from the 22nd to the end of May 2001 (ConsultationsSeenFrom22ndTillEndOfMay2001)

| SurgeryDate | DateOfBirth | Sex | Diagnosis | TimeIn | TimeOut | Complaints | Treatments | NumbersID | Notes |
|---|---|---|---|---|---|---|---|---|---|
| 24.05.2001 | 18.07.1978 | F | | 1757 | 1805 | Requests abdominal paste for itchy stretch marks | Not known | 337 | 36/40 gestation. |
| 30.05.2001 | 28.01.1969 | M | Pain | 1041 | 1046 | Back Pain | Dihydrocodeine | 3471 | |
| 29.05.2001 | 19.05.1956 | F | S/Leave | 1642 | 1645 | Bilateral Chevron Osteotomy | | 3568 | |
| 30.05.2001 | 21.02.1992 | F | | 1102 | 1106 | Paronychia (R) thumb | Erythromycin & Fucidin cream | 3586 | Penicillin allergy. |
| 22.05.2001 | 27.02.1992 | M | RTI | 1753 | 1758 | Cough | Erythromycin | 3589 | Penicillin allergy. |
| 22.05.2001 | 17.03.1924 | M | | 1758 | 1804 | For repeat LFTs in 3 months | | 3592 | |
| 22.05.2001 | 14.12.1938 | F | | 1733 | 1742 | Fasting Cholesterol 7.5 mmols/L | Diet sheet given | 36 | |
| 25.05.2001 | 23.01.1950 | F | Revisit | 1739 | 1746 | Her heartburn is worse | Referred to Gastro-enterologist | 3645 | Script for Ranitidine given. |
| 30.05.2001 | 23.05.1927 | M | | 901 | 913 | Infected burn on the fore-head | Erythromycin & Fucidin-H gel | 3716 | Penicillin allergy. |
| 23.05.2001 | 23.07.1973 | M | S/Leave | 1001 | 1006 | Cellulitis | | 3725 | |
| 23.05.2001 | 29.08.1934 | F | Pain | 1126 | 1145 | Pain in (L) thigh & (L) buttock | Flucloxacillin, Amoxycillin, Diclofenac enteric coated & Dihydrocodeine | 3729 | |
| 25.05.2001 | 29.08.1934 | F | | 1142 | 1151 | Vomiting | Metoclopramide | 3729 | |
| 22.05.2001 | 30.10.1950 | M | | 1046 | 1056 | Script for Atorvastatin & Lansoprazole given | | 3829 | For FBC, TFTs & Fasting Cholesterol. |
| 25.05.2001 | 16.10.1959 | F | | 1707 | 1713 | Hypothyroidism | Thyroxine | 3929 | |

## Result of a query that lists all consultations from the 22nd to the end of May 2001 (ConsultationsSeenFrom22ndTillEndOfMay2001)

| SurgeryDate | DateOfBirth | Sex | Diagnosis | TimeIn | TimeOut | Complaints | Treatments | NumbersID | Notes |
|---|---|---|---|---|---|---|---|---|---|
| 22.05.2001 | 04.09.1952 | M | Revisit | 1026 | 1038 | Multiple joint pains is still bad | Flucloxacillin & Diclofenac enteric coated | 4128 | For FBC & ESR. Referred to Rheumatologist. |
| 24.05.2001 | 04.11.1947 | F | | 1733 | 1739 | Itchy legs | Hydroxyzine | 4165 | Penicillin & Klaricid allergy. |
| 29.05.2001 | 21.02.1916 | F | Revisit | 1033 | 1041 | Still has pain in (L) shoulder | Inj. Depo-Medrone with Lidocaine | 4178 | Penicillin allergy. |
| 22.05.2001 | 19.05.1989 | M | URTI | 1728 | 1733 | Bilateral ear ache | Amoxycillin | 4257 | |
| 25.05.2001 | 27.08.1990 | F | Rash | 1746 | 1750 | Weepy rash in the elbow creases | Fucidin-H cream | 4303 | Darkish moles on back of neck, referred to Dermatologist. |
| 29.05.2001 | 24.12.1972 | F | Rash | 1714 | 1724 | Finger nails & skin around the nails are itchy, sore & breaking off | Daktacort cream | 4373 | |
| 22.05.2001 | 12.08.1967 | F | | 1707 | 1714 | Offensive vaginal discharge again | Metronidazole | 4402 | |
| 30.05.2001 | 08.04.1944 | F | S/Leave | 1713 | 1720 | Food poisoning - Private | | 4465 | |
| 29.05.2001 | 29.09.1932 | F | Revisit | 908 | 924 | Pain (L) shoulder has persisted | Inj. Depo-Medrone with Lidocaine | 4487 | Script for Orlistat given. |
| 23.05.2001 | 25.05.1970 | M | | 1118 | 1122 | Weepy spots on the face | Flucloxacillin | 4592 | For FBC & Fasting Glucose. |
| 22.05.2001 | 22.11.1983 | F | URTI | 1659 | 1707 | Sore throat | Amoxycillin | 464 | |
| 24.05.2001 | 16.11.1962 | F | | 1725 | 1733 | Script for Zopiclone given | | 4655 | |

Result of a query that lists all consultations from the 22nd to the end of May 2001 (ConsultationsSeenFrom22ndTillEndOfMay2001)

| SurgeryDate | DateOfBirth | Sex | Diagnosis | TimeIn | TimeOut | Complaints | Treatments | NumbersID | Notes |
|---|---|---|---|---|---|---|---|---|---|
| 24.05.2001 | 02.07.1943 | M | | 1128 | 1137 | Script for Diclofenac enteric coated given | | 4667 | |
| 30.05.2001 | 11.08.1935 | F | Lump | 920 | 927 | Reddish hard lump on (L) foot | For X-Ray (L) foot | 4670 | For FBC & ESR. |
| 25.05.2001 | 29.11.1994 | F | URTI | 1713 | 1719 | Sore throat | Amoxycillin & Paracetamol | 4691 | |
| 22.05.2001 | 10.01.1995 | F | | 1141 | 1145 | Infected insect bite on (R) hand | Flucloxacillin & Loratadine | 4728 | |
| 22.05.2001 | 30.03.1986 | F | Pain | 1639 | 1650 | Pain (R) foot & (R) ankle | Ibuprofen | 4829 | For X-Ray. |
| 23.05.2001 | 10.03.1968 | M | | 1124 | 1126 | Abscess (R) upper gum | Amoxycillin | 4871 | |
| 30.05.2001 | 06.03.1963 | M | | 1814 | 1822 | Inclusion cyst (L) side of back | Referred to Surgeon | 4958 | |
| 24.05.2001 | 07.04.1949 | F | URTI | 1719 | 1725 | Itchy (R) ear | Otomize ear spray | 513 | |
| 25.05.2001 | 16.03.1978 | M | S/Leave | 1800 | 1805 | Injury (R) thumb | | 5202 | Penicillin allergy. |
| 29.05.2001 | 18.06.1946 | F | S/Leave | 1054 | 1059 | Laparoscopic Cholecystectomy - Med. 5 | | 5355 | |
| 29.05.2001 | 18.03.1969 | M | Pain | 1645 | 1651 | Pain & injury (R) big toe | For X-Ray (R) big toe & for serum Uric Acid | 5435 | |
| 23.05.2001 | 10.06.1969 | F | URTI | 1652 | 1655 | Sore throat | Amoxycillin | 5532 | |
| 24.05.2001 | 06.12.1947 | M | | 1034 | 1042 | Red, inflamed & sore (R) big toe | Diclofenac enteric coated & Flucloxacillin | 5551 | |

Result of a query that lists all consultations from the 22nd to the end of May 2001 (ConsultationsSeenFrom22ndTillEndOfMay2001)

| SurgeryDate | DateOfBirth | Sex | Diagnosis | TimeIn | TimeOut | Complaints | Treatments | NumbersID | Notes |
|---|---|---|---|---|---|---|---|---|---|
| 25.05.2001 | 17.01.1965 | F |  | 1731 | 1739 | Partner's blood sent for genotyping |  | 5571 | Patient has anti-Duffy antibodies. |
| 29.05.2001 | 17.01.1965 | F |  | 1655 | 1701 | Vaginal thrush | Clotrimazole pessary | 5571 | 15/40 gestation. |
| 30.05.2001 | 27.12.1959 | F | Depression | 950 | 1015 | Depressed & unable to cope | Citalopram | 5609 | Swollen glands, Rx. Ceporex. |
| 29.05.2001 | 09.07.1969 | M |  | 1729 | 1732 | Hay fever | Cetirizine | 563 |  |
| 24.05.2001 | 24.06.1933 | M | Rash | 1042 | 1048 | Raised multiple blood blisters on the trunk | Referred to Dermatologist | 5652 | Penicillin allergy. |
| 24.05.2001 | 17.01.1953 | M |  | 1048 | 1103 | Dog bite (R) thumb & (R) index finger | Co-Amoxiclav | 5680 | Tetanus toxoid Booster given. |
| 25.05.2001 | 12.01.1929 | M |  | 1034 | 1041 | Script for Diclofenac enteric coated & Lansoprazole given |  | 5703 |  |
| 23.05.2001 | 24.04.1935 | F | Revisit | 1659 | 1702 | (L) ear is still weepy | Erythromycin | 5770 |  |
| 23.05.2001 | 21.06.1933 | M | Pain | 1702 | 1707 | Pain (L) shoulder | Inj. Depo-Medrone with Lidocaine | 5771 |  |
| 25.05.2001 | 21.06.1933 | M |  | 1151 | 1201 | Inj; Depo-Medrone with Lidocaine given to (L) shoulder |  | 5771 |  |
| 25.05.2001 | 07.08.1996 | F | URTI | 1719 | 1723 | Infected rhinorrhoea | Amoxycillin | 5784 |  |
| 29.05.2001 | 16.08.1950 | F | Pain | 1701 | 1706 | Back ache | Co-dydramol | 583 | Penicillin allergy. For MSU & FBC. |
| 30.05.2001 | 08.08.1924 | F |  | 1028 | 1041 | Going to Spain for 2 weeks | General advice given | 5868 |  |
| 30.05.2001 | 22.03.1989 | M |  | 1709 | 1713 | Septic abrasion on face | Flucloxacillin & Fucidin-H gel | 5935 |  |

205

Result of a query that lists all consultations from the 22nd to the end of May 2001 (ConsultationsSeenFrom22ndTillEndOfMay2001)

| SurgeryDate | DateOfBirth | Sex | Diagnosis | TimeIn | TimeOut | Complaints | Treatments | NumbersID | Notes |
|---|---|---|---|---|---|---|---|---|---|
| 30.05.2001 | 14.08.1956 | M | Pain | 1701 | 1709 | Pain (R) shoulder | Ibuprofen | 5936 | |
| 23.05.2001 | 19.10.1953 | F | Pain | 1647 | 1652 | Back pain | Tramadol | 5957 | For MSU. |
| 29.05.2001 | 29.07.1951 | M | | 1633 | 1642 | Advised to continue Esomeprazole | | 5958 | |
| 22.05.2001 | 05.12.1920 | M | Pain | 1108 | 1128 | Neck pain | Movelat cream | 6015 | |
| 29.05.2001 | 08.02.1998 | M | | 1059 | 1119 | Swollen face post dog-bite | Augmentin-Duo & Ibuprofen | 6024 | |
| 24.05.2001 | 26.10.1997 | F | | 1123 | 1128 | Cough | Pholcodeine Paediatric | 6084 | |
| 29.05.2001 | 26.10.1997 | F | RTI | 1732 | 1736 | Cough | Erythromycin | 6084 | Oral thrush, Rx. Nystatin suspension. |
| 29.05.2001 | 13.05.1996 | F | URTI | 1803 | 1809 | Sore throat | Amoxycillin | 6103 | Referred to ENT Surgeon (Basildon hospital). |
| 25.05.2001 | 27.11.1958 | M | | 1723 | 1731 | Diarrhoea & scabs in the nostril | Loperamide & Naseptin cream | 6107 | |
| 29.05.2001 | 13.08.1998 | M | URTI | 1041 | 1047 | Infected rhinorrhoea | Erythromycin & Paracetamol | 6175 | |
| 23.05.2001 | 30.05.1936 | M | | 1054 | 1108 | Script for Felodipine & Diprosalic ointment given | | 6236 | |
| 25.05.2001 | 05.10.1995 | F | RTI | 1057 | 1100 | Cough | Amoxycillin | 6252 | |
| 25.05.2001 | 09.05.1997 | M | RTI | 1053 | 1057 | Cough | Amoxycillin & Pholcodine paediatric | 6253 | |

Result of a query that lists all consultations from the 22nd to the end of May 2001 (ConsultationsSeenFrom22ndTillEndOfMay2001)

| SurgeryDate | DateOfBirth | Sex | Diagnosis | TimeIn | TimeOut | Complaints | Treatments | NumbersID | Notes |
|---|---|---|---|---|---|---|---|---|---|
| 25.05.2001 | 01.11.1998 | M | | 1657 | 1707 | Limping since a fall | Advised to go to A/E | 6266 | |
| 22.05.2001 | 12.04.1952 | M | S/Leave | 1145 | 1148 | Pain (R) hip | | 6322 | Script for Tramadol given. |
| 29.05.2001 | 14.04.1946 | F | RTI | 1724 | 1729 | Cough | Amoxycillin | 6333 | |
| 24.05.2001 | 22.07.1968 | F | | 1007 | 1011 | Bleeding haemorrhoids | Referred to Surgeon (Basildon hospital) | 6339 | |
| 24.05.2001 | 10.03.1970 | M | Revisit | 1026 | 1034 | Still gets chest pain | Referred to Cardiologist (Basildon hospital) | 6343 | Penicillin allergy. |
| 25.05.2001 | 14.04.1978 | F | Pain | 1100 | 1110 | Neck pain after RTA | Diclofenac enteric coated & Co-dydramol | 6464 | |
| 30.05.2001 | 14.04.1978 | F | | 1803 | 1814 | Neck Pain - Private & Med. 5 | | 6464 | |
| 30.05.2001 | 29.03.1974 | M | | 1730 | 1738 | Hay fever | Loratadine | 6489 | For X-Ray (L) little toe. FP1001 (GMS4) form given. |
| 23.05.2001 | 03.02.1927 | M | | 1044 | 1050 | Glucose 6.1 mmols/L | For modified GTT | 6531 | |
| 25.05.2001 | 24.03.1940 | F | | 1023 | 1029 | Skin tags on neck | For Cryotherapy in Minor clinic | 6567 | Distalgesic allergy. |
| 23.05.2001 | 22.07.1920 | F | URTI | 1707 | 1720 | sore throat | Erythromycin & Simple Linctus | 6599 | Penicillin allergy. |

Result of a query that lists all consultations from the 22nd to the end of May 2001 (ConsultationsSeenFrom22ndTillEndOfMay2001)

| SurgeryDate | DateOfBirth | Sex | Diagnosis | TimeIn | TimeOut | Complaints | Treatments | NumbersID | Notes |
|---|---|---|---|---|---|---|---|---|---|
| 30.05.2001 | 31.05.1946 | F | | 1046 | 1050 | Script for Citalopram given | | 6615 | |
| 23.05.2001 | 20.11.1945 | M | | 1637 | 1644 | Blocked ears | Sodium Bicarbonate ear drops | 6617 | Penicillin allergy. |
| 30.05.2001 | 26.03.1947 | F | | 1720 | 1730 | Script for Orlistat & Bendrofluazide given | | 6634 | |
| 25.05.2001 | 18.10.1927 | F | | 1651 | 1657 | Giddy | Betahistine | 6641 | |
| 30.05.2001 | 08.05.1939 | F | | 1822 | 1851 | Patient & her son came regarding her Driving Licence | | 6643 | |
| 25.05.2001 | 24.04.1966 | M | Revisit | 1002 | 1023 | Still has bad headaches | For FBC & Fasting Glucose | 669 | |
| 30.05.2001 | 25.08.1990 | M | | 940 | 950 | Hay fever & running nose | Fluticasone nasal spray & Loratadine | 6718 | |
| 22.05.2001 | 25.06.1947 | F | | 1136 | 1141 | Advised to get her usual medication for 3 months | | 6733 | |
| 23.05.2001 | 11.01.1951 | F | Revisit | 1050 | 1054 | Neck pain is worse | Tramadol | 6735 | |
| 24.05.2001 | 20.12.1979 | F | | 1022 | 1026 | Late period | For Pregnancy test | 6746 | |
| 25.05.2001 | 21.06.1971 | F | | 1041 | 1053 | Offensive vaginal discharge after sex | Advised to contact the GUM clinic | 6757 | |
| 29.05.2001 | 20.09.1943 | F | | 1705 | 1714 | Cholesterol 6.2 mmols/L | Cerivastatin | 6781 | For LFTs. |

Result of a query that lists all consultations from the 22nd to the end of May 2001 (ConsultationsSeenFrom22ndTillEndOfMay2001)

| SurgeryDate | DateOfBirth | Sex | Diagnosis | TimeIn | TimeOut | Complaints | Treatments | NumbersID | Notes |
|---|---|---|---|---|---|---|---|---|---|
| 23.05.2001 | 28.12.1927 | M | Revisit | 1034 | 1044 | The abdominal pain has persisted | Referred to Surgeon (BUPA) | 6845 | Script for Fluocinolone cream given. |
| 22.05.2001 | 03.12.1989 | F | URTI | 1656 | 1659 | Sore throat | Erythromycin | 6882 | Penicillin allergy. |
| 29.05.2001 | 16.09.1960 | M | | 1759 | 1803 | Script for Lansoprazole given | | 6890 | Referred to Gastro-enterologist |
| 30.05.2001 | 19.10.1971 | M | | 1015 | 1022 | Infected insect bite (L) leg | Flucloxacillin & Fucidin-H cream | 6891 | |
| 29.05.2001 | 13.10.1965 | F | | 933 | 937 | Intermenstrual PER VAGINA discharge | Advised to observe | 6918 | |
| 30.05.2001 | 13.10.1965 | F | | 913 | 920 | Offensive PER VAGINA bleeding | Erythromycin & Norethisterone | 6918 | For FBC. |
| 30.05.2001 | 10.09.1950 | F | S/Leave | 1050 | 1102 | Depression - Med. 5 | | 6924 | |
| 25.05.2001 | 11.09.2000 | F | RTI | 1813 | 1818 | Cough | Amoxycillin | 6935 | |
| 29.05.2001 | 17.09.1966 | F | | 924 | 933 | Hay fever & streaming eyes | Nedocromil eye drops | 6939 | |
| 29.05.2001 | 05.01.1960 | F | | 1736 | 1743 | ?UTI | For MSU | 6958 | |
| 30.05.2001 | 24.01.1924 | M | | 929 | 940 | Pain (L) big toe | Ibuprofen & Flucloxacillin | 6985 | For Uric Acid. |
| 23.05.2001 | 08.08.1997 | F | RTI | 1800 | 1806 | Cough | Amoxycillin | 7018 | |
| 22.05.2001 | 14.04.1987 | M | Revisit | 1650 | 1656 | He still has abdominal pain & diarrhoea | Referred to Paediatrician (Basildon hospital) | 7022 | Hay fever, Rx. Loratadine & Beclomethasone nasal spray. |
| 30.05.2001 | 03.03.1925 | F | | 1744 | 1753 | Script for Ibuprofen, Co-dydramol & Calcichew D3 forte given | | 7036 | Penicillin allergy. |

209

Result of a query that lists all consultations from the 22nd to the end of May 2001 (ConsultationsSeenFrom22ndTillEndOfMay2001)

| SurgeryDate | DateOfBirth | Sex | Diagnosis | TimeIn | TimeOut | Complaints | Treatments | NumbersID | Notes |
|---|---|---|---|---|---|---|---|---|---|
| 29.05.2001 | 24.04.2000 | F | | 1000 | 1022 | ?Coeliac disease | Referred to Paediatrician (Basildon hospital) | 7043 | |
| 29.05.2001 | 17.02.2001 | M | | 1809 | 1817 | Blistered skin (L) cheek | Flucloxacillin & Fucidin cream | 7046 | Oral thrush, Rx. Nystatin suspension. |
| 22.05.2001 | 07.07.1980 | M | | 1038 | 1046 | He may want to be referred to Gastro-enterologist privately | | 7057 | |
| 25.05.2001 | 26.03.2001 | F | Rash | 1029 | 1034 | Itchy red rash on trunk | Aqueous cream & Unguentum Merck | 7058 | |
| 23.05.2001 | 29.09.1945 | F | | 1108 | 1118 | Advised to contact the London hospital to fax us the hospital letter | | 7075 | |
| 30.05.2001 | 02.10.1945 | F | | 1637 | 1647 | Depression since her husband died | Benfleet Open Door & Samaritans suggested | 7087 | |
| 30.05.2001 | 18.10.1920 | F | | 1653 | 1701 | Script for Atenolol, Paracetamol & Fucidin-H gel given | | 7088 | |
| 22.05.2001 | 01.04.1994 | F | Conjunctivitis | 1714 | 1718 | Pussy red (R) eye | Chloramphenicol eye drops | 7098 | |
| 24.05.2001 | 06.11.1981 | M | Pain | 1739 | 1757 | (R) ankle with abrasion | Flucloxacillin & Diclofenac enteric coated | 852 | |

## Result of a query that lists all consultations from the 22nd to the end of May 2001 (ConsultationsSeenFrom22ndTillEndOfMay2001)

| SurgeryDate | DateOfBirth | Sex | Diagnosis | TimeIn | TimeOut | Complaints | Treatments | NumbersID | Notes |
|---|---|---|---|---|---|---|---|---|---|
| 22.05.2001 | 09.06.1954 | F |  | 1718 | 1728 | Hot flushes | Conjugate Equine Oestrogens | 927 |  |
| 24.05.2001 | 04.04.1959 | M | Hypertension | 1651 | 1657 | BP 152/104 | Bendrofluazide | 969 |  |
| 29.05.2001 | 09.10.1928 | F | URTI | 1750 | 1759 | (L) ear ache | Amoxycillin & Otomize ear spray | Temp |  |

## Result of a query that lists all consultations from the 22nd to the end of May 2003 (ConsultationsSeenFrom22ndTillEndOfMay2003)

| SurgeryDate | DateOfBirth | Sex | Diagnosis | TimeIn | TimeOut | Complaints | Treatments | NumbersID | Notes |
|---|---|---|---|---|---|---|---|---|---|
| 23.05.2003 | 21.02.1962 | M |  | 1651 | 1701 | USScan of the gall bladder showed gall bladder stones or polyp | Referred to Surgeon (BUPA) | 101 | Penicillin allergy. |
| 30.05.2003 | 30.03.1923 | M | Rash | 1043 | 1051 | Red rash on trunk & both legs | Miconazole 2% + 1% Hydrocortisone cream | 1060 |  |
| 23.05.2003 | 07.01.1954 | F | Rash | 1751 | 1757 | Spots on face | Tetracycline | 1097 |  |
| 22.05.2003 | 17.09.1986 | F | Pain | 925 | 933 | Bose bleeds & headaches | Co-codamol & Ibuprofen | 1173 |  |
| 30.05.2003 | 17.09.1986 | F | Revisit | 1814 | 1837 | Still has headaches, tender sinuses & nose bleeds | Referred to ENT Surgeon | 1173 | Letter to whom it may concern that she cannot take GCSE exams. |

Result of a query that lists all consultations from the 22nd to the end of May 2003 (ConsultationsSeenFrom22ndTillEndOfMay2003)

| SurgeryDate | DateOfBirth | Sex | Diagnosis | TimeIn | TimeOut | Complaints | Treatments | NumbersID | Notes |
|---|---|---|---|---|---|---|---|---|---|
| 22.05.2003 | 27.10.1960 | F | Pain | 933 | 940 | Back Pain | Diclofenac enteric coated, Dihydrocodeine & Ranitidine | 1175 | |
| 30.05.2003 | 19.06.1959 | M | S/Leave | 1658 | 1706 | Chest infection | | 1191 | Script for Amoxycillin given. |
| 28.05.2003 | 19.01.1965 | F | S/Leave | 1029 | 1039 | Asthma attack & chest infection | | 1281 | |
| 28.05.2003 | 06.06.1947 | F | | 1039 | 1045 | Rectocele noted on vaginal examination | Referred to Gynaecologist | 1354 | |
| 28.05.2003 | 12.05.1963 | F | | 910 | 917 | To have HVS & Chlamydial swabs done with P/Nurse | | 1506 | |
| 23.05.2003 | 03.04.1987 | F | RTI | 1630 | 1642 | Chest cough | Amoxicillin | 1654 | FP1001 (GMS4) form signed. Script for Microgynon-30 given. |
| 30.05.2003 | 15.10.1923 | F | | 1712 | 1719 | To continue with Fucidin cream for her leg | | 1711 | |
| 28.05.2003 | 21.11.1954 | M | | 917 | 921 | Dysphagia & feeling of something lodged in his throat | Referred to ENT Surgeon (BUPA) | 2018 | |
| 22.05.2003 | 30.09.1967 | F | Rash | 1102 | 1110 | ?Viral rash | To use own analgesia | 2067 | |
| 23.05.2003 | 18.03.1985 | F | | 905 | 909 | Script for Microgynon-30 given | | 2199 | FP1001 (GMS4) form signed. |

Result of a query that lists all consultations from the 22nd to the end of May 2003 (ConsultationsSeenFrom22ndTillEndOfMay2003)

| SurgeryDate | DateOfBirth | Sex | Diagnosis | TimeIn | TimeOut | Complaints | Treatments | NumbersID | Notes |
|---|---|---|---|---|---|---|---|---|---|
| 22.05.2003 | 11.06.1968 | F | | 959 | 1019 | Script for Frusemide given | | 2261 | For U/Es & Fasting Cholesterol. |
| 30.05.2003 | 11.06.1968 | F | Hypertension | 1740 | 1758 | BP 137/106 | Bendrofluazide | 2261 | |
| 30.05.2003 | 15.06.1935 | F | RTI | 918 | 925 | Chesty cough | Amoxycillin | 227 | |
| 30.05.2003 | 23.04.1950 | F | | 1705 | 1712 | Head cold & flu | Amoxycillin | 2369 | |
| 30.05.2003 | 28.03.1970 | F | | 1140 | 1154 | Pain & tenderness (R) calf | Referred to DVT Clinic, SGH | 2375 | Routine P/Natal check. |
| 27.05.2003 | 13.11.1970 | F | | 1636 | 1654 | To go to A/E regarding injury to (L) ankle | | 2578 | |
| 29.05.2003 | 04.04.1938 | M | | 945 | 955 | Script for Esomeprazole given | | 262 | |
| 28.05.2003 | 19.03.1925 | F | Revisit | 921 | 926 | The area around the (L) breast is still red | Flucloxacillin | 2634 | |
| 29.05.2003 | 06.01.1943 | F | Revisit | 924 | 932 | (L) knee is still painful | Referred to Orthopaedic Surgeon (Basildon Hospital) | 2642 | |
| 27.05.2003 | 28.05.1957 | F | Rash | 915 | 921 | Shingles rash on (R) T9 | Famciclovir | 2648 | |
| 27.05.2003 | 12.06.1983 | M | URTI | 1750 | 1756 | Sore throat | Amoxycillin | 2719 | Recurrent infections, for FBC & Fasting Glucose. |
| 30.05.2003 | 12.06.1983 | M | S/Leave | 1758 | 1802 | Sore throat - Private | | 2719 | |
| 29.05.2003 | 08.04.1990 | M | Pain | 942 | 945 | Pain (L) knee, ?Osgood Schlatter's disease | Paracetamol | 2789 | Cefaclor allergy. |
| 27.05.2003 | 27.11.1947 | F | URTI | 1727 | 1734 | Infected rhinorrhoea | Amoxycillin | 2831 | |

213

Result of a query that lists all consultations from the 22nd to the end of May 2003 (ConsultationsSeenFrom22ndTillEndOfMay2003)

| SurgeryDate | DateOfBirth | Sex | Diagnosis | TimeIn | TimeOut | Complaints | Treatments | NumbersID | Notes |
|---|---|---|---|---|---|---|---|---|---|
| 22.05.2003 | 14.12.1971 | M | | 940 | 959 | To contact the Dermatologist at SGH when he comes back from holidays | | 2833 | |
| 28.05.2003 | 28.03.1926 | F | | 1710 | 1715 | Pedal oedema | Frusemide | 2837 | |
| 22.05.2003 | 05.01.1946 | F | | 1028 | 1048 | To see Surgery Counsellor regarding her alcoholic problems | | 3017 | For U/Es, FBC, LFTs & Fasting Glucose. |
| 29.05.2003 | 15.02.1932 | F | | 1019 | 1031 | Dizzy spells & neck pain | Prochlorperazine | 3043 | for Cervical X-Ray, FBC & Fasting Glucose. |
| 23.05.2003 | 13.02.1938 | M | Hypertension | 940 | 948 | BP 177/105 | Bendrofluazide & Atenolol | 3113 | |
| 23.05.2003 | 24.03.1985 | M | S/Leave | 1017 | 1023 | Appendicectomy | | 3144 | |
| 23.05.2003 | 12.05.1973 | M | Pain | 919 | 925 | Low back Pain & diarrhoea | Co-codamol & Loperamide | 3442 | For Lumbar spine X-Ray. Penicillin allergy. |
| 28.05.2003 | 15.07.1956 | M | S/Leave | 931 | 939 | Crohn's disease & pan proctocolectomy - Med. 5 | | 352 | |
| 30.05.2003 | 19.06.1966 | F | RTI | 1106 | 1120 | Chesty cough & asthma attack | Amoxycillin, Prednisolone enteric coated, Budesonide/ Formoterol 200/6 & Nebulizer | 3521 | |
| 29.05.2003 | 04.10.1947 | F | | 912 | 915 | She didn't like the HRT | | 3556 | |

Result of a query that lists all consultations from the 22nd to the end of May 2003 (ConsultationsSeenFrom22ndTillEndOfMay2003)

| SurgeryDate | DateOfBirth | Sex | Diagnosis | TimeIn | TimeOut | Complaints | Treatments | NumbersID | Notes |
|---|---|---|---|---|---|---|---|---|---|
| 28.05.2003 | 09.06.1953 | M | S/Leave | 952 | 1003 | Fractured (R) Humerus - Med. 5 |  | 3695 |  |
| 29.05.2003 | 07.07.1961 | F | Pain | 1031 | 1040 | Pain & swelling (L) knee | For X-Ray (L) knee | 3768 |  |
| 30.05.2003 | 28.06.1957 | M | URTI | 1723 | 1727 | Sore throat | Amoxycillin | 3923 |  |
| 22.05.2003 | 19.05.1964 | M |  | 911 | 916 | Script for Bendrofluazide given |  | 3995 |  |
| 28.05.2003 | 05.07.1931 | F | Pain | 1741 | 1747 | Acute gout | Etoricoxib | 4008 |  |
| 27.05.2003 | 07.10.1933 | M |  | 1009 | 1013 | Infected blisters on back of ankles | Flucloxacillin | 4055 | Script for Olanzapine given. |
| 28.05.2003 | 21.02.1916 | F | Pain | 941 | 952 | Pain & swollen (L) knee | For X-Ray | 4178 | Penicillin allergy. |
| 28.05.2003 | 02.02.1994 | M |  | 1715 | 1718 | Sore (R) nostril | Naseptin cream | 4319 |  |
| 27.05.2003 | 31.07.1972 | F |  | 1654 | 1703 | Routine A/Natal check |  | 4398 |  |
| 29.05.2003 | 10.08.1985 | F |  | 915 | 924 | Vaginal thrush | Fluconazole | 4429 |  |
| 28.05.2003 | 10.03.1936 | F |  | 1017 | 1025 | Wound on (L) breast | Flucloxacillin & Fusidic Acid cream | 4442 |  |
| 23.05.2003 | 06.11.1968 | F | RTI | 948 | 953 | Chest cough | Erythromycin | 4479 | Penicillin allergy. |
| 28.05.2003 | 06.11.1968 | F |  | 1718 | 1724 | Script for Salbutamol inhaler given |  | 4479 | Penicillin allergy. |
| 29.05.2003 | 06.11.1968 | F | Pain | 1044 | 1056 | Pain (R) loin & urine is dark | Trimethoprim & Co-codamol | 4479 | Penicillin allergy. |
| 27.05.2003 | 30.08.1977 | M |  | 1029 | 1034 | Septic insect bites on ankles | Flucloxacillin & Fusidic Acid cream | 450 |  |

215

Result of a query that lists all consultations from the 22nd to the end of May 2003 (ConsultationsSeenFrom22ndTillEndOfMay2003)

| SurgeryDate | DateOfBirth | Sex | Diagnosis | TimeIn | TimeOut | Complaints | Treatments | NumbersID | Notes |
|---|---|---|---|---|---|---|---|---|---|
| 23.05.2003 | 16.11.1962 | F | | 1819 | 1840 | Advised to go to Runwell hospital where she will probably get her medication | | 4655 | |
| 23.05.2003 | 13.03.1932 | M | | 1011 | 1017 | Injection Zoladex given | | 4699 | |
| 27.05.2003 | 29.06.1953 | F | UTI | 1721 | 1727 | Frequency of micturition & dysuria | Trimethoprim | 487 | For MSU. |
| 27.05.2003 | 28.11.1991 | M | Revisit | 1703 | 1705 | Still unable to retract his fore-skin fully | Referred to Surgeon | 5079 | |
| 30.05.2003 | 04.10.1968 | F | | 915 | 918 | For repeat TFTs in 6 months | | 511 | |
| 22.05.2003 | 07.04.1949 | F | | 1048 | 1102 | Tenderness around laparoscopic wound | Flucloxacillin | 513 | |
| 27.05.2003 | 17.02.1972 | F | | 909 | 915 | To book own appointment to see a Chiropractor regarding her painful neck | | 5279 | FP1001 (GMS4) form signed. Penicillin allergy. |
| 22.05.2003 | 24.06.1937 | M | | 905 | 911 | Script for Dihydrocodeine given | | 5437 | |
| 30.05.2003 | 10.06.1969 | F | | 1009 | 1022 | Injury (L) knee | Referred to Fracture Clinic (Basildon Hospital) | 5532 | |
| 29.05.2003 | 12.05.1949 | F | RTI | 1009 | 1013 | Cough | Amoxycillin | 5549 | For CXR. |

216

Result of a query that lists all consultations from the 22nd to the end of May 2003 (ConsultationsSeenFrom22ndTillEndOfMay2003)

| SurgeryDate | DateOfBirth | Sex | Diagnosis | TimeIn | TimeOut | Complaints | Treatments | NumbersID | Notes |
|---|---|---|---|---|---|---|---|---|---|
| 28.05.2003 | 24.04.1935 | F | | 1802 | 1812 | To increase salt intake | | 5770 | |
| 28.05.2003 | 22.05.1935 | M | | 1812 | 1815 | Script for Erythromycin given | | 5771 | Wife came to Surgery. |
| 23.05.2003 | 04.07.1973 | F | | 953 | 959 | Intermenstrual bleeding & offensive vaginal discharge | For HVS & Chlamydial swabs | 5950 | |
| 28.05.2003 | 22.02.1936 | F | Pain | 1006 | 1017 | Joint pains & neck ache | Erythromycin & Ranitidine | 5955 | For Cervical X-Ray. Penicillin allergy. |
| 30.05.2003 | 03.12.1955 | F | | 1727 | 1737 | Dizzy spells | For FBC, Ferritin & FSH | 614 | |
| 30.05.2003 | 03.05.1936 | M | | 1101 | 1106 | Injection Zoladex given | | 6236 | |
| 27.05.2003 | 20.12.1922 | F | | 1712 | 1716 | To continue with the cream for her thumb | | 6237 | |
| 27.05.2003 | 22.07.1968 | F | Rash | 951 | 1001 | Chicken Pox rash | Acyclovir | 6339 | |
| 27.05.2003 | 04.05.1961 | M | Revisit | 1001 | 1009 | Still coughing, tightness in the chest | Fexofenadine, Salbutamol easi-breathe inhaler & Galpseud | 6340 | Now owns budgerigars. Penicillin allergy. |
| 22.05.2003 | 01.08.1945 | F | Hypertension | 1019 | 1028 | BP 168/106 | Coracten XL | 6491 | |
| 23.05.2003 | 27.08.1948 | F | Rash | 1757 | 1806 | Pityriasis Versicolor rash | Itraconazole & Selsun shampoo | 6538 | |
| 29.05.2003 | 27.08.1948 | F | | 955 | 1009 | Script for Selsun Shampoo given | | 6538 | |
| 30.05.2003 | 14.11.1916 | F | | 1003 | 1009 | Tender septic spot on the lower lip | Flucloxacillin & Fusidic Acid cream | 6591 | |

Result of a query that lists all consultations from the 22nd to the end of May 2003 (ConsultationsSeenFrom22ndTillEndOfMay2003)

| SurgeryDate | DateOfBirth | Sex | Diagnosis | TimeIn | TimeOut | Complaints | Treatments | NumbersID | Notes |
|---|---|---|---|---|---|---|---|---|---|
| 29.05.2003 | 28.11.1978 | F | | 1315 | 1335 | Routine P/Natal visit | | 6636 | Home visit. |
| 30.05.2003 | 20.10.1983 | F | | 938 | 1003 | Recurrent asthma attacks | Referred to chest Physician (Basildon Hospital) | 6665 | FP1001 (GMS4) form signed. |
| 23.05.2003 | 06.03.1969 | F | | 1725 | 1730 | Script for Microgynon-30 given | | 6681 | |
| 23.05.2003 | 21.12.1991 | M | Pain | 1647 | 1651 | Tender 5$^{th}$ (R) metacarpal following injury | For X-Ray (R) hand | 6779 | |
| 30.05.2003 | 21.12.1991 | M | | 925 | 930 | X-Ray: Fractured (R) 5$^{th}$ metacarpal | Referred to Fracture Clinic | 6779 | |
| 23.05.2003 | 23.11.1946 | M | Conjunctivitis | 1710 | 1719 | Watery (R) eye | Chloramphenicol eye drops | 6822 | T.A.T.T, for FBC, TFTs & Fasting Glucose. |
| 30.05.2003 | 25.08.1957 | M | | 1706 | 1712 | Viagra - Private prescription | | 6876 | |
| 28.05.2003 | 01.01.1962 | M | | 1639 | 1647 | Anxiety - Med. 5 | | 6879 | |
| 27.05.2003 | 04.09.2000 | M | | 939 | 951 | Cold, chesty cough & wheezy | Amoxycillin, Salbutamol inhaler & Volumatic Space haler | 6921 | |
| 30.05.2003 | 03.03.1934 | M | | 1022 | 1035 | Dry mouth | Glandosane spray | 6984 | |
| 27.05.2003 | 09.03.1937 | F | Revisit | 921 | 933 | Still has (L) hip | For Physiotherapy | 7019 | |
| 23.05.2003 | 24.07.1976 | F | | 909 | 916 | Script for Microgynon-30 given | | 7034 | FP1001 (GMS4) form signed. |

218

Result of a query that lists all consultations from the 22nd to the end of May 2003 (ConsultationsSeenFrom22ndTillEndOfMay2003)

| SurgeryDate | DateOfBirth | Sex | Diagnosis | TimeIn | TimeOut | Complaints | Treatments | NumbersID | Notes |
|---|---|---|---|---|---|---|---|---|---|
| 23.05.2003 | 24.04.2000 | F | Rash | 959 | 1005 | Impetigo rash on face | Flucloxacillin & Mupirocin cream | 7043 | |
| 30.05.2003 | 07.07.1980 | M | | 1051 | 1101 | Mouth ulcers & small blisters on penis | Amoxycillin | 7057 | To go to GUM Clinic if blisters on the penis persist. |
| 29.05.2003 | 28.02.1975 | M | | 1013 | 1019 | FBC & TFTs - normal | | 7072 | |
| 28.05.2003 | 17.10.1980 | F | Pain | 1705 | 1710 | Multiple joints pain | For RA Latex test | 7117 | FP1001 (GMS4) form signed. |
| 28.05.2003 | 18.06.2001 | M | RTI | 1025 | 1029 | Cough | Amoxycillin | 7138 | |
| 27.05.2003 | 31.05.1972 | F | | 1734 | 1740 | Possible viral rash | | 7176 | |
| 30.05.2003 | 04.10.1937 | F | Pain | 908 | 915 | Pain on dorsi-flexing the (R) foot | Dihydrocodeine | 7206 | |
| 30.05.2003 | 09.09.1946 | M | Revisit | 1737 | 1740 | Spot on (R) leg is improving | Flucloxacillin | 7284 | |
| 28.05.2003 | 03.04.1937 | F | | 1656 | 1705 | Cyst in (R) cheek | Amoxycillin | 7307 | |
| 29.05.2003 | 04.01.2002 | M | | 1138 | 1143 | Septic insect bite marks on (R) ear, face & leg | Flucloxacillin & Fusidic Acid cream | 7328 | |
| 28.05.2003 | 06.02.1968 | F | Revisit | 1747 | 1750 | Still has (L) ear pain & sinus problems | Amoxycillin | 7343 | Recurrent (L) ear ache, referred to Surgeon (Basildon Hospital). |
| 28.05.2003 | 25.02.2002 | F | | 901 | 906 | It hurts her when she moves her bowels | Referred to Paediatrician | 7402 | |

Result of a query that lists all consultations from the 22nd to the end of May 2003 (ConsultationsSeenFrom22ndTillEndOfMay2003)

| SurgeryDate | DateOfBirth | Sex | Diagnosis | TimeIn | TimeOut | Complaints | Treatments | NumbersID | Notes |
|---|---|---|---|---|---|---|---|---|---|
| 22.05.2003 | 28.12.1921 | M | RTI | 1110 | 1120 | Cough, dyspnoea & discharging (R) ear | Amoxycillin, Galpseud, Otomize ear spray & Ipratropium bromide inhaler | 7407 | |
| 27.05.2003 | 04.08.1936 | M | Revisit | 933 | 939 | Hearing now goes up & down | Sodium bicarbonate ear drops | 7443 | To have ears syringed with P/ Nurse. |
| 28.05.2003 | 29.04.2002 | M | URTI | 1750 | 1755 | Pulling ears & fever | Amoxycillin | 7452 | |
| 27.05.2003 | 01.10.1991 | F | URTI | 1716 | 1721 | Sore throat | Erythromycin & Paracetamol | 7463 | Penicillin allergy. |
| 30.05.2003 | 04.11.1934 | M | | 1640 | 1649 | Script for Amitriptyline & Bendrofluazide given | | 7490 | Trimethoprim allergy. |
| 30.05.2003 | 27.09.1969 | F | S/Leave | 1632 | 1640 | Faint & dizzy - Private | | 7495 | Trimethoprim allergy. |
| 29.05.2003 | 19.09.1938 | F | URTI | 1040 | 1044 | Sore throat, ear ache & dizziness | Amoxycillin, Otomize ear spray & Prochlorperazine | 7513 | |
| 23.05.2003 | 11.01.1941 | F | UTI | 1642 | 1647 | Dysuria | For MSU | 7574 | |
| 27.05.2003 | 25.02.1934 | M | Revisit | 1740 | 1747 | Still unable to breathe | Salbutamol easi-breathe inhaler | 7599 | For CXR. |
| 23.05.2003 | 22.05.1920 | F | | 925 | 930 | Insomnia | Temazepam | 7601 | |
| 28.05.2003 | 17.07.1940 | F | | 1045 | 1052 | Sepsis around (L) mastectomy wound | Flucloxacillin | 7627 | Penicillin allergy. |
| 29.05.2003 | 12.08.1939 | F | Depression | 901 | 912 | Weepy, lost her partner 3 weeks ago | Fluoxetine | 7678 | To see P/ Counsellor. |

Result of a query that lists all consultations from the 22nd to the end of May 2003 (ConsultationsSeenFrom22ndTillEndOfMay2003)

| SurgeryDate | DateOfBirth | Sex | Diagnosis | TimeIn | TimeOut | Complaints | Treatments | NumbersID | Notes |
|---|---|---|---|---|---|---|---|---|---|
| 30.05.2003 | 04.01.1950 | F | | 1719 | 1723 | Dizziness | Prochlorperazine | 7685 | Back Pain, for MSU. Penicillin allergy. |
| 30.05.2003 | 26.04.1943 | M | | 904 | 908 | (R) Total hip replacement | | 7697 | Penicillin allergy. |
| 30.05.2003 | 07.01.1944 | M | | 1120 | 1133 | Dyspnoea with history of asbestos plaque | Referred to Chest Physician (Basildon Hospital) | 7714 | For CXR. |
| 23.05.2003 | 14.07.1965 | F | | 1800 | 1814 | Hay fever | Levocetirizine | 7716 | |
| 23.05.2003 | 13.04.1944 | M | Hypertension | 1701 | 1710 | BP 142/104 | Bendrofluazide | 7753 | For FBC, U/Es, Fasting Cholesterol & LFTs. |
| 28.05.2003 | 11.02.1949 | M | | 1724 | 1741 | The Parking Badge Scheme for Disabled People Medical Practitioner Report completed | | 7758 | |
| 30.05.2003 | 02.11.1954 | F | Pain | 1802 | 1814 | Mouth pain following dental operation | Dihydrocodeine, Diclofenac enteric coated & Ranitidine | 780 | Penicillin allergy. Script for Fusidic Acid 2% + 1% Hydrocortisone cream given. |
| 30.05.2003 | 18.12.1946 | M | | 1035 | 1043 | Rheumatoid Factor 8 iu/ml | | 7800 | |
| 30.05.2003 | 03.03.1938 | F | RTI | 1649 | 1658 | Chesty cough | Erythromycin & Salbutamol inhaler | 783 | For CXR. |

221

## Result of a query that lists all consultations from the 22nd to the end of May 2003 (ConsultationsSeenFrom22ndTillEndOfMay2003)

| SurgeryDate | DateOfBirth | Sex | Diagnosis | TimeIn | TimeOut | Complaints | Treatments | NumbersID | Notes |
|---|---|---|---|---|---|---|---|---|---|
| 28.05.2003 | 25.10.1966 | M | | 906 | 910 | Script for Sibutramine given | | 800 | |
| 29.05.2003 | 13.09.1918 | M | Revisit | 932 | 942 | The tingling in the fingers are getting worse | Referred to Orthopaedic Surgeon | 841 | |
| 28.05.2003 | 05.07.1950 | M | | 1003 | 1006 | Unwell & hot sweats | Erythromycin | 877 | |
| 28.05.2003 | 15.04.1973 | F | Anaemia | 1647 | 1656 | Hb 11.4 g/dl | For B12, Folate & Ferritin | 942 | |
| 28.05.2003 | 16.07.1983 | F | | 1755 | 1802 | Script for Venlafaxine given | | 967 | |

## Result of a query that lists all consultations from the 22nd to the end of May 2004 (ConsultationsSeenFrom22ndTillEndOfMay2004)

| SurgeryDate | DateOfBirth | Sex | Diagnosis | TimeIn | TimeOut | Complaints | Treatments | NumbersID | Notes |
|---|---|---|---|---|---|---|---|---|---|
| 24.05.2004 | 13.03.1954 | F | | 1705 | 1714 | Script for Atenolol given | | 1172 | Penicillin allergy. |
| 27.05.2004 | 20.02.1930 | M | Revisit | 924 | 931 | Still has raw feeling in the throat | Referred to ENT Surgeon | 1254 | Penicillin & Erythromycin allergy. |
| 25.05.2004 | 26.11.1935 | M | Pain | 1705 | 1720 | Multiple joints pains | Referred to Rheumatologist | 1276 | |
| 25.05.2004 | 08.10.1961 | M | S/Leave | 905 | 914 | Fracture 4th (L) toe - Med. 5 | | 1280 | Referred to Fracture clinic. |
| 24.05.2004 | 15.09.1976 | M | | 1653 | 1701 | Scars on legs are healing well | | 137 | |

Result of a query that lists all consultations from the 22nd to the end of May 2004 (ConsultationsSeenFrom22ndTillEndOfMay2004)

| SurgeryDate | DateOfBirth | Sex | Diagnosis | TimeIn | TimeOut | Complaints | Treatments | NumbersID | Notes |
|---|---|---|---|---|---|---|---|---|---|
| 27.05.2004 | 04.09.1963 | F | | 1020 | 1027 | To attend FP Clinic for the removal of her IUCD for her abdominal pain | | 1722 | FP1001 (GMS4) form signed. |
| 27.05.2004 | 23.07.1923 | M | | 931 | 936 | Bilateral pedal oedema | Frusemide | 175 | |
| 24.05.2004 | 20.05.1938 | F | | 1728 | 1739 | Script for Aspirin e/c given | | 1869 | |
| 28.05.2004 | 04.01.1962 | F | RTI | 1000 | 1004 | Chesty cough | Amoxycillin | 1884 | Trimethoprim allergy. |
| 28.05.2004 | 16.09.1949 | M | Hypertension | 1746 | 1801 | BP 150/104 | Bendrofluazide | 1893 | Script for Simvastatin given. Mole on the (L) arm that has gone bigger, Referred to Dermatologist (Basildon Hospital). |
| 25.05.2004 | 06.07.1936 | F | | 1730 | 1742 | Losing her hair | Referred to Dermatologist (Basildon Hospital) | 2150 | Penicillin allergy. |
| 24.05.2004 | 10.08.1931 | M | | 904 | 909 | Script for Co-codamol given | | 2182 | Aspirin allergy. |
| 28.05.2004 | 28.03.1970 | F | | 900 | 907 | Vaginal thrush | Fluconazole | 2375 | |
| 25.05.2004 | 13.11.1952 | F | | 1038 | 1044 | For FBC | | 2474 | |
| 28.05.2004 | 22.09.1939 | F | RTI | 955 | 1000 | Chesty cough | Amoxycillin | 2510 | |
| 26.05.2004 | 24.03.1973 | M | S/Leave | 1040 | 1045 | Throat infection | | 2784 | Script for Erythromycin given. |

Result of a query that lists all consultations from the 22nd to the end of May 2004 (ConsultationsSeenFrom22ndTillEndOfMay2004)

| SurgeryDate | DateOfBirth | Sex | Diagnosis | TimeIn | TimeOut | Complaints | Treatments | NumbersID | Notes |
|---|---|---|---|---|---|---|---|---|---|
| 25.05.2004 | 25.05.1976 | F | | 1018 | 1028 | For U/Es, Fasting Glucose, FBC & TFTs | | 2797 | |
| 24.05.2004 | 06.04.1924 | F | | 909 | 917 | For Echocardiography | | 2909 | Penicillin allergy. |
| 28.05.2004 | 15.03.1946 | F | | 1634 | 1649 | Hyperkalaemia | Calcium Polystyrene sulphate | 2975 | |
| 25.05.2004 | 15.06.1980 | M | | 1044 | 1100 | Script for Mefloquine given | | 3074 | |
| 26.05.2004 | 02.11.1953 | F | | 1029 | 1033 | Script for Salbutamol inhaler given | | 3182 | Penicillin allergy. |
| 24.05.2004 | 15.04.1953 | M | | 1701 | 1705 | He will see the Cardiologist to get the prescription privately | | 3228 | |
| 27.05.2004 | 20.11.1965 | M | | 1035 | 1045 | Cold sores on the lower lips | Acyclovir | 3254 | |
| 27.05.2004 | 25.06.1938 | F | | 958 | 1014 | To keep her feet elevated | | 3415 | |
| 24.05.2004 | 19.07.1952 | M | | 1010 | 1015 | For X-Ray (L) knee | | 3430 | |
| 28.05.2004 | 19.07.1952 | M | | 1808 | 1816 | To try OTC Co-codamol for his painful (L) knee swelling | | 3430 | |
| 26.05.2004 | 12.08.1944 | M | | 922 | 930 | Script for Dihydrocodeine given | | 364 | |
| 27.05.2004 | 14.06.1957 | F | RTI | 936 | 943 | Chesty cough | Amoxycillin | 3661 | Septrin allergy. |
| 25.05.2004 | 06.08.1966 | F | | 1647 | 1654 | HVS - Candidiasis | Fluconazole | 3747 | Penicillin allergy. |

Result of a query that lists all consultations from the 22nd to the end of May 2004 (ConsultationsSeenFrom22ndTillEndOfMay2004)

| SurgeryDate | DateOfBirth | Sex | Diagnosis | TimeIn | TimeOut | Complaints | Treatments | NumbersID | Notes |
|---|---|---|---|---|---|---|---|---|---|
| 27.05.2004 | 29.09.1992 | M | Pain | 908 | 914 | Pain (L) ankle | Referred to Orthopaedic Surgeon | 3751 | |
| 24.05.2004 | 10.06.1928 | F | RTI | 1640 | 1648 | Chesty cough | Erythromycin | 3884 | Script for Frusemide & Bendrofluazide given. Penicillin allergy. |
| 25.05.2004 | 16.12.1949 | M | Revisit | 1755 | 1806 | Still feels very dizzy & unwell | Referred to General Physician (BUPA) | 3960 | Penicillin allergy. |
| 25.05.2004 | 17.01.1977 | F | URTI | 1806 | 1811 | Ears & sinuses feel blocked | Amoxycillin | 403 | |
| 28.05.2004 | 15.09.1964 | F | | 1801 | 1808 | For Fasting Blood Glucose | | 4133 | |
| 26.05.2004 | 03.07.1940 | F | | 1002 | 1015 | Script for Bendrofluazide given | | 4223 | |
| 24.05.2004 | 13.07.1924 | F | | 941 | 954 | Script for Simvastatin & Lisinopril given | | 4244 | |
| 24.05.2004 | 30.10.1947 | M | | 1754 | 1801 | For FBC, Fasting Glucose & TFTs | | 431 | Scoline sensitive. |
| 25.05.2004 | 06.01.1969 | F | | 1654 | 1705 | To keep a menstrual chart | | 447 | |
| 24.05.2004 | 31.12.1922 | M | | 1635 | 1640 | Script for Prednisolone & Bumetanide given | | 4470 | |
| 27.05.2004 | 06.11.1968 | F | | 1045 | 1054 | Unprotected sexual intercourse | Levonorgestrel 750mcg | 4479 | Penicillin allergy. |

Result of a query that lists all consultations from the 22nd to the end of May 2004 (ConsultationsSeenFrom22ndTillEndOfMay2004)

| SurgeryDate | DateOfBirth | Sex | Diagnosis | TimeIn | TimeOut | Complaints | Treatments | NumbersID | Notes |
|---|---|---|---|---|---|---|---|---|---|
| 28.05.2004 | 09.04.1938 | M | | 1022 | 1031 | Script for Perindopril given | | 4519 | Tetracycline allergy. |
| 25.05.2004 | 28.02.1927 | M | | 956 | 1018 | PSA = 2389.00 ng/ml, grossly elevated | Referred to Urologist (cancer referral) | 4838 | |
| 26.05.2004 | 27.11.1992 | F | Pain | 905 | 912 | Pain (R) ankle | Ibuprofen | 4913 | |
| 28.05.2004 | 31.01.1964 | F | | 1726 | 1735 | For Fasting Cholesterol with P/Nurse in 6 months | | 5334 | |
| 24.05.2004 | 03.04.1997 | M | Conjunctivitis | 1718 | 1724 | Itchy & red (L) eye | Chloramphenicol eye drops | 5566 | Penicillin allergy. |
| 24.05.2004 | 06.05.1997 | M | | 858 | 9004 | Hay fever | Loratadine | 5645 | Penicillin allergy. |
| 28.05.2004 | 24.04.1935 | F | Pain | 1711 | 1718 | Chesty pain on swallowing solids & tablets | Lansoprazole orodispersible | 5770 | |
| 24.05.2004 | 23.03.1926 | M | | 1744 | 1748 | No bony abnormality on cervical X-Ray | | 5954 | |
| 28.05.2004 | 02.02.1998 | F | | 923 | 927 | Rash on upper lip, infected | Flucloxacillin | 5967 | |
| 26.05.2004 | 17.12.1931 | M | | 901 | 905 | To see P/Nurse fro ear syringing | | 5978 | |
| 25.05.2004 | 30.01.1931 | F | | 1630 | 1647 | For repeat ESR in 2 weeks | | 600 | |
| 25.05.2004 | 05.12.1920 | M | | 1742 | 1755 | Spurious diarrhoea due to chronic constipation | Macrogol compound npf oral powder | 6015 | |
| 25.05.2004 | 20.04.1936 | F | | 914 | 920 | Script for Etodolac given | | 6147 | |

226

## Result of a query that lists all consultations from the 22nd to the end of May 2004 (ConsultationsSeenFrom22ndTillEndOfMay2004)

| SurgeryDate | DateOfBirth | Sex | Diagnosis | TimeIn | TimeOut | Complaints | Treatments | NumbersID | Notes |
|---|---|---|---|---|---|---|---|---|---|
| 28.05.2004 | 12.12.1989 | M | | 1704 | 1711 | Polyuria & polydipsia | For FBC, U/Es, Fasting Glucose & MSU | 6326 | |
| 25.05.2004 | 07.03.1999 | F | | 1811 | 1821 | Abdominal pain & vomiting | Amoxycillin & Metoclopramide | 6381 | |
| 24.05.2004 | 03.07.1914 | M | | 1300 | 1308 | To continue with own Co-Proxamol for his chest pain | | 6546 | Home visit. |
| 24.05.2004 | 19.09.1925 | F | | 933 | 941 | For X-Rays of the knees | | 665 | Penicillin allergy. |
| 24.05.2004 | 17.09.1943 | M | | 1748 | 1754 | Script for Bisoprolol & Spironolactone given | | 6712 | |
| 28.05.2004 | 17.09.1943 | M | Pain | 1649 | 1658 | Pain (L) loin & constipation | Glycerol suppositories, Amoxycillin & Macrogol compound npf oral powder 6.9g | 6712 | For MSU. |
| 24.05.2004 | 04.05.1937 | F | | 1232 | 1250 | Diarrhoea & abdominal pain | Loperamide & Paracetamol | 6723 | Home visit. |
| 24.05.2004 | 21.06.1975 | F | | 1015 | 1021 | Area bitten by a dog is sore | | 679 | |
| 26.05.2004 | 16.01.1998 | F | URTI | 1051 | 1100 | Sore throat | Erythromycin | 6809 | |
| 25.05.2004 | 23.11.1946 | M | | 928 | 930 | He has brought in forms to be completed | | 6822 | |
| 25.05.2004 | 17.09.1966 | F | | 1720 | 1730 | To use OTC Nurofen for her finger pain | | 6939 | |

227

Result of a query that lists all consultations from the 22nd to the end of May 2004 (ConsultationsSeenFrom22ndTillEndOfMay2004)

| SurgeryDate | DateOfBirth | Sex | Diagnosis | TimeIn | TimeOut | Complaints | Treatments | NumbersID | Notes |
|---|---|---|---|---|---|---|---|---|---|
| 27.05.2004 | 24.07.1976 | F | | 946 | 951 | To take own Piriton for her hay fever | | 7034 | |
| 26.05.2004 | 07.07.1980 | M | S/Leave | 930 | 945 | Anxiety & Tourette syndrome | | 7057 | |
| 26.05.2004 | 08.07.2000 | M | | 1025 | 1029 | Dysuria | For MSU | 7081 | |
| 24.05.2004 | 03.07.1939 | M | | 954 | 1002 | Script for Metformin given | | 7144 | |
| 28.05.2004 | 19.01.2001 | M | | 1016 | 1022 | Coughing | Salbutamol inhaler & Volumatic | 7256 | |
| 24.05.2004 | 23.11.1968 | M | | 917 | 929 | Awaiting stool culture result | | 7360 | |
| 28.05.2004 | 08.10.1963 | M | Revisit | 1742 | 1746 | Still coughing | Erythromycin & Salbutamol | 7400 | |
| 24.05.2004 | 06.09.1974 | M | | 1021 | 1030 | Script for Diclofenac e/c & Cetirizine given | | 7436 | |
| 28.05.2004 | 04.04.1953 | M | | 1718 | 1726 | Hay fever | Fexofenadine | 7467 | |
| 25.05.2004 | 28.03.1960 | F | RTI | 1826 | 1834 | Chesty cough | Amoxycillin | 7518 | |
| 24.05.2004 | 20.08.1945 | M | | 1724 | 1728 | To take OTC Co-codamol for the ache in his (L) loin | | 7531 | |
| 26.05.2004 | 11.01.1941 | F | | 1015 | 1025 | Script for Tolterodine given | | 7574 | |
| 27.05.2004 | 26.07.1960 | F | | 919 | 924 | Script for Amitriptyline given | | 7591 | |

Result of a query that lists all consultations from the 22nd to the end of May 2004 (ConsultationsSeenFrom22ndTillEndOfMay2004)

| SurgeryDate | DateOfBirth | Sex | Diagnosis | TimeIn | TimeOut | Complaints | Treatments | NumbersID | Notes |
|---|---|---|---|---|---|---|---|---|---|
| 28.05.2004 | 22.05.1920 | F | | 913 | 918 | Her toes which she had done at Hadleigh seem okay | | 7601 | Penicillin allergy. |
| 25.05.2004 | 07.08.1969 | F | URTI | 920 | 928 | Sore throat | Amoxycillin | 7622 | |
| 26.05.2004 | 07.02.1948 | M | | 945 | 1002 | Script for Flucloxacillin, Fusidic Acid cream, Macrogol compound npf oral powder & Levothyroxine given | | 7684 | Referred to Dermatologist (Basildon Hospital). |
| 24.05.2004 | 25.09.1987 | M | | 1648 | 1653 | Script for Miconazole 2% + 1% Hydrocortisone given | | 7781 | |
| 25.05.2004 | 03.03.1938 | F | Rash | 1313 | 1330 | Itchy rash under breasts & in the groin | Miconazole 2% + 1% Hydrocortisone cream | 783 | Home visit. |
| 26.05.2004 | 06.10.1952 | M | S/Leave | 1033 | 1040 | Back Pain - Med. 5 | | 7843 | |
| 24.05.2004 | 01.12.1942 | M | | 1801 | 1815 | Injection Depo-Medrone with Lidocaine 2mls given to (R) Shoulder | | 7845 | |
| 28.05.2004 | 05.10.1975 | M | | 907 | 913 | To contact diving organization regarding medical for his diving course in Greece | | 7848 | |

229

Result of a query that lists all consultations from the 22nd to the end of May 2004 (ConsultationsSeenFrom22ndTillEndOfMay2004)

| SurgeryDate | DateOfBirth | Sex | Diagnosis | TimeIn | TimeOut | Complaints | Treatments | NumbersID | Notes |
|---|---|---|---|---|---|---|---|---|---|
| 25.05.2004 | 22.07.2003 | M | | 1028 | 1038 | Script for Fusidic Acid 2% + 1% Hydrocortisone cream, Salbutamol inhaler & Volumatic given | | 7855 | |
| 25.05.2004 | 23.10.1947 | F | URTI | 953 | 956 | (R) ear ache | Amoxycillin | 7877 | |
| 25.05.2004 | 19.05.1935 | F | | 936 | 946 | For serum Cholesterol | | 7889 | |
| 27.05.2004 | 19.05.1935 | F | UTI | 914 | 919 | Frequency of micturition | Amoxycillin | 7889 | For MSU. |
| 25.05.2004 | 06.10.1933 | M | | 930 | 936 | Script for Simvastatin & Bendrofluazide given | | 7890 | |
| 26.05.2004 | 02.11.1946 | M | | 915 | 922 | For B12, Folate & Ferritin | | 7895 | Diclofenac & Misoprostol allergy. |
| 28.05.2004 | 26.06.1945 | F | UTI | 1004 | 1016 | Dysuria | Amoxycillin | 939 | For MSU. |
| 25.05.2004 | 27.05.1951 | F | S/Leave | 946 | 953 | Tingling & dull ache in fingers | | NP (BH) | |
| 24.05.2004 | 02.06.1944 | F | | 929 | 933 | She cannot swallow Coracten capsules | | NP (GJ) | Penicillin allergy. |
| 28.05.2004 | 03.03.1937 | M | | 1658 | 1704 | To continue with his present medication | | NP (JEC) | |
| 28.05.2004 | 16.03.1960 | M | RTI | 918 | 923 | Chesty cough | Amoxycillin | NP (JFS) | |
| 26.05.2004 | 19.02.1975 | F | Pain | 1045 | 1051 | Epigastric pain & vomiting | Omeprazole & Metoclopramide | NP (JM) | Penicillin allergy. |
| 27.05.2004 | 29.08.1970 | F | S/Leave | 1027 | 1035 | Depression | | NP (JNF) | Script for Amitriptyline given. |

### Result of a query that lists all consultations from the 22nd to the end of May 2004 (ConsultationsSeenFrom22ndTillEndOfMay2004)

| SurgeryDate | DateOfBirth | Sex | Diagnosis | TimeIn | TimeOut | Complaints | Treatments | NumbersID | Notes |
|---|---|---|---|---|---|---|---|---|---|
| 24.05.2004 | 03.01.1995 | F | Revisit | 1739 | 1744 | Still has dysuria despite MSU being normal | Referred to Paediatrician | NP (JT) | |
| 24.05.2004 | 05.01.1922 | F | RTI | 1002 | 1010 | Chesty cough | Amoxycillin | NP (MP) | Script for Simvastatin given. |
| 25.05.2004 | 07.02.1972 | F | | 1821 | 1826 | Pain lower abdomen | For MSU | NP (SR) | |
| 28.05.2004 | 23.06.1978 | F | RTI | 947 | 955 | Chesty cough | Amoxycillin | NP NS) | |

### Result of a query that lists all consultations from the 22nd to the end of May 2005 (ConsultationsSeenFrom22ndTillEndOfMay2005)

| SurgeryDate | DateOfBirth | Sex | Diagnosis | TimeIn | TimeOut | Complaints | Treatments | NumbersID | Notes |
|---|---|---|---|---|---|---|---|---|---|
| 24.05.2005 | 08.11.1931 | F | | 1656 | 1702 | Script for Atenolol & Gaviscon given | | 312 | |
| 27.05.2005 | 21.10.1929 | F | | 1806 | 1810 | Hot rash on leg like phlebitis | Erythromycin & Fusidic Acid cream | 1129 | Penicillin allergy. |
| 24.05.2005 | 22.05.1931 | F | | 1035 | 1038 | Bad diarrhoea, now clearing | Stool for C&S | 1183 | |
| 24.05.2005 | 20.01.1943 | M | | 1808 | 1818 | Loss of taste & dry cough | Referred to ENT Surgeon | 1208 | |
| 24.05.2005 | 15.06.1974 | F | Pain | 1647 | 1656 | Headaches | Propranolol | 1219 | Dalacin allergy. |
| 26.05.2005 | 27.06.1986 | M | | 933 | 939 | Dizzy, hot & sweaty | Erythromycin & Prochlorperazine | 1267 | Penicillin allergy. |
| 27.05.2005 | 09.10.1924 | F | | 1729 | 1735 | Sore (L) ear lobe | Flucloxacillin & Fusidic Acid cream | 1477 | |

## Result of a query that lists all consultations from the 22nd to the end of May 2005 (ConsultationsSeenFrom22ndTillEndOfMay2005)

| SurgeryDate | DateOfBirth | Sex | Diagnosis | TimeIn | TimeOut | Complaints | Treatments | NumbersID | Notes |
|---|---|---|---|---|---|---|---|---|---|
| 27.05.2005 | 05.08.1942 | M | | 911 | 922 | For Physiotherapy for his (R) knee pain | | 1573 | |
| 23.05.2005 | 03.05.1951 | F | RTI | 1649 | 1656 | Chesty cough | Amoxycillin | 162 | Cefaclor allergy. |
| 23.05.2005 | 30.05.1916 | M | | 1353 | 1405 | Vertigo | Prochlorperazine | 1712 | Home visit. |
| 23.05.2005 | 11.10.1938 | F | | 1040 | 1054 | Diabetic Clinic check | | 1832 | |
| 26.05.2005 | 20.05.1938 | F | | 1017 | 1038 | Script for Lisinopril & Ezetimibe given | | 1869 | |
| 27.05.2005 | 25.09.1987 | F | URTI | 1707 | 1710 | Sore throat | Phenoxymethylpenicillin | 1968 | |
| 24.05.2005 | 11.11.1927 | M | Hypertension | 1038 | 1049 | BP 169/95 | Nifedipine m/r tablet & Bendrofluazide | 2105 | |
| 26.05.2005 | 06.07.1936 | F | | 1001 | 1017 | Cold sores | Acyclovir tablets | 2150 | Penicillin allergy. |
| 23.05.2005 | 16.01.1952 | F | Pain | 905 | 919 | Back Pain | Co-codamol | 2220 | For X-Ray Lumbar Spine. Penicillin allergy. Referred to Gynaecologist (Basildon Hospital). |
| 26.05.2005 | 21.08.1933 | M | | 1755 | 1805 | Script for Amoxycillin given | | 230 | |
| 26.05.2005 | 11.05.1959 | F | URTI | 1751 | 1755 | Sore throat | Erythromycin | 2351 | Penicillin & Septrin allergy. |
| 26.05.2005 | 10.10.1964 | F | | 1637 | 1641 | Vaginal thrush | Clotrimazole pessary | 2355 | |
| 25.05.2005 | 24.03.1959 | F | S/Leave | 1652 | 1655 | Fractured ribs - Med. 5 | | 2580 | |
| 25.05.2005 | 15.08.1953 | F | | 1710 | 1718 | Script for Co-codamol given | | 2625 | |

Result of a query that lists all consultations from the 22nd to the end of May 2005 (ConsultationsSeenFrom22ndTillEndOfMay2005)

| SurgeryDate | DateOfBirth | Sex | Diagnosis | TimeIn | TimeOut | Complaints | Treatments | NumbersID | Notes |
|---|---|---|---|---|---|---|---|---|---|
| 26.05.2005 | 20.03.1959 | F | Pain | 939 | 951 | Pain in knees | Referred to Physiotherapy | 3166 | Septrin allergy. |
| 24.05.2005 | 31.05.1947 | F | Pain | 913 | 918 | Painful 4th (R) toe | For X-Ray | 3316 | Penicillin allergy. |
| 24.05.2005 | 18.07.1978 | F | URTI | 1753 | 1757 | (L) ear infection | Amoxycillin | 337 | |
| 24.05.2005 | 19.07.1952 | M | | 925 | 934 | Advised to contact the hospital regarding his next sigmoidoscopy appointment | | 3430 | |
| 26.05.2005 | 12.04.1938 | M | | 1701 | 1705 | Arthritis pain in hands & neck | Diclofenac e/c, Omeprazole & Co-codamol | 3480 | |
| 24.05.2005 | 19.02.1942 | F | | 1702 | 1712 | Script for Nicotine patch '10' given | | 3481 | |
| 25.05.2005 | 14.04.1957 | F | | 1718 | 1722 | Plaster cast on (R) leg due out tomorrow | | 3661 | |
| 24.05.2005 | 10.06.1928 | F | | 1011 | 1020 | To continue with the present doses of her medication | | 3884 | Penicillin allergy. |
| 25.05.2005 | 12.09.1947 | F | | 1028 | 1044 | Letter to whom it may concern that she is our patient & that she resides at her address | | 3908 | |
| 23.05.2005 | 20.12.1931 | M | | 959 | 1008 | (R) ear lobe infection | Flucloxacillin | 4020 | |
| 24.05.2005 | 09.06.1993 | F | | 1742 | 1753 | Naughty & disruptive at school & at home | Referred to Child Psychiatrist | 4039 | |
| 25.05.2005 | 12.08.1993 | F | Pain | 1751 | 1755 | Pain in (R) knee anteriorly | Paracetamol | 4115 | |

233

## Result of a query that lists all consultations from the 22nd to the end of May 2005 (ConsultationsSeenFrom22ndTillEndOfMay2005)

| SurgeryDate | DateOfBirth | Sex | Diagnosis | TimeIn | TimeOut | Complaints | Treatments | NumbersID | Notes |
|---|---|---|---|---|---|---|---|---|---|
| 27.05.2005 | 23.09.1993 | M | Rash | 1758 | 1801 | Moles on back which has got bigger & darker | Referred to Dermatologist (Basildon Hospital) | 4185 | |
| 27.05.2005 | 27.02.1950 | M | | 1109 | 1114 | Giddy & nausea | Prochlorperazine | 4348 | |
| 27.05.2005 | 03.10.1926 | M | | 1710 | 1715 | For B12, Ferritin & Folate | | 4399 | |
| 25.05.2005 | 21.02.1976 | F | S/Leave | 954 | 1000 | Stress - Med. 5 | | 4585 | |
| 24.05.2005 | 28.08.1984 | M | Rash | 1739 | 1742 | Scab on scalp | Referred to Dermatologist (Basildon Hospital) | 4862 | |
| 25.05.2005 | 03.01.1914 | F | | 908 | 916 | Pain (R) foot | For X-Ray | 4877 | Lederfen allergy. |
| 27.05.2005 | 03.01.1914 | F | UTI | 1742 | 1754 | Urine smells | Trimethoprim | 4877 | Script for Paracetamol given. For MSU & FBC. |
| 23.05.2005 | 02.05.1962 | F | Pain | 1812 | 1821 | Back ache bad again | Referred to Orthopaedic Surgeon (Basildon Hospital) | 4887 | |
| 24.05.2005 | 27.09.1986 | M | | 1757 | 1802 | Unable to hear well | To try OTC Otocalm | 4993 | |
| 27.05.2005 | 09.02.1965 | F | URTI | 1103 | 1109 | Dizzy, nausea & sore throat | Amoxycillin & Prochlorperazine | 5077 | |
| 27.05.2005 | 02.05.1985 | F | Pain | 958 | 1011 | Abdominal pain | Dihydrocodeine & Lactulose | 5114 | |

234

Result of a query that lists all consultations from the 22nd to the end of May 2005 (ConsultationsSeenFrom22ndTillEndOfMay2005)

| SurgeryDate | DateOfBirth | Sex | Diagnosis | TimeIn | TimeOut | Complaints | Treatments | NumbersID | Notes |
|---|---|---|---|---|---|---|---|---|---|
| 26.05.2005 | 07.10.1944 | M | | 919 | 933 | Advised to see DSS about returning to work after being made incapable of working by the DSS | | 5141 | |
| 27.05.2005 | 25.06.1996 | F | Rash | 1722 | 1729 | Eczema on neck & back worse | Referred to Dermatologist (Basildon Hospital) | 5304 | Script for Loratadine given. |
| 25.05.2005 | 26.10.1960 | F | Pain | 1734 | 1739 | Back Pain | Referred to Orthopaedic Surgeon (BUPA) | 5319 | |
| 27.05.2005 | 08.06.1996 | M | Rash | 1754 | 1758 | Moles on body getting bigger | Referred to Dermatologist (Basildon Hospital) | 5324 | |
| 25.05.2005 | 31.01.1964 | F | URTI | 1655 | 1659 | Sore throat | Amoxycillin | 5334 | |
| 27.05.2005 | 03.04.1997 | M | | 1011 | 1020 | Pyrexial & unwell | Erythromycin | 5566 | Penicillin allergy. |
| 26.05.2005 | 19.05.1988 | F | URTI | 1655 | 1701 | (R) ear ache | Amoxycillin | 5579 | Script for Loratadine given |
| 25.05.2005 | 24.04.1935 | F | RTI | 1012 | 1028 | Chesty cough | Amoxycillin | 5770 | Script for Artificial salive spray given. |
| 24.05.2005 | 31.01.1936 | M | RTI | 1020 | 1028 | Chesty cough | Amoxycillin | 5797 | |
| 25.05.2005 | 20.02.1937 | F | | 1635 | 1652 | Script for Dihydrocodeine given | | 5798 | |
| 25.05.2005 | 03.03.1946 | M | | 903 | 908 | Script for Simvastatin given | | 5845 | |

Result of a query that lists all consultations from the 22nd to the end of May 2005 (ConsultationsSeenFrom22ndTillEndOfMay2005)

| SurgeryDate | DateOfBirth | Sex | Diagnosis | TimeIn | TimeOut | Complaints | Treatments | NumbersID | Notes |
|---|---|---|---|---|---|---|---|---|---|
| 27.05.2005 | 07.05.1974 | M | | 1801 | 1806 | Script for Dihydrocodeine given | | 5951 | |
| 26.05.2005 | 13.10.1989 | F | | 1116 | 1124 | Dizziness & nausea | Prochlorperazine | 6195 | |
| 26.05.2005 | 14.01.1934 | F | Pain | 908 | 919 | Back Pain | Co-codamol & Erodolac capsules | 6234 | |
| 25.05.2005 | 01.01.1924 | M | | 1722 | 1728 | Script for Dipyridamole m/r & Aspirin dispersible given | | 6353 | |
| 25.05.2005 | 09.12.1945 | F | | 920 | 924 | To reduce Spironolactone to 50mg daily | | 6467 | |
| 26.05.2005 | 06.12.1985 | F | | 1821 | 1830 | Pregnancy test positive | | 6587 | |
| 23.05.2005 | 09.04.1944 | F | | 1821 | 1834 | Injection Depo-Medrone with Lidocaine given to the (R) knee | | 6592 | |
| 24.05.2005 | 20.10.1983 | F | | 1001 | 1011 | Small sore lump (R) lower eye lid | Chloramphenicol eye ointment | 6665 | |
| 26.05.2005 | 04.05.1937 | F | | 1709 | 1722 | To see own Optician regarding what is growing in her (R) eye | | 6723 | |
| 25.05.2005 | 19.12.1974 | F | | 1054 | 1110 | Routine P/Natal with baby check in Surgery | | 6729 | |
| 26.05.2005 | 16.07.1969 | F | Revisit | 1038 | 1046 | Still has horrible taste in mouth | Referred to ENT Surgeon (Basildon Hospital) | 6747 | |

Result of a query that lists all consultations from the 22nd to the end of May 2005 (ConsultationsSeenFrom22ndTillEndOfMay2005)

| SurgeryDate | DateOfBirth | Sex | Diagnosis | TimeIn | TimeOut | Complaints | Treatments | NumbersID | Notes |
|---|---|---|---|---|---|---|---|---|---|
| 25.05.2005 | 16.09.1936 | M | | 916 | 920 | Private script for Viagra given | | 693 | |
| 23.05.2005 | 31.05.1969 | F | | 952 | 959 | Pregnancy test positive | | 6949 | |
| 27.05.2005 | 01.01.1968 | F | S/Leave | 1054 | 1103 | Vaginal hysterectomy - Med. 5 | | 7021 | |
| 26.05.2005 | 05.02.1943 | F | | 1722 | 1735 | For repeat Cholesterol in 6 months | | 7066 | |
| 26.05.2005 | 15.03.1922 | F | | 1648 | 1655 | Ulcers on lower eye lids | Erythromycin & Chloramphenicol eye drops | 7229 | |
| 24.05.2005 | 14.07.1952 | M | URTI | 1802 | 1808 | Bilateral ear ache | Amoxycillin | 7298 | |
| 24.05.2005 | 25.04.1998 | F | | 1028 | 1035 | Recurrent bilateral ear infections | Erythromycin | 7299 | Referred to ENT Surgeon. |
| 23.05.2005 | 28.09.1978 | F | | 1802 | 1812 | Heavy periods | Microgynon 30 | 7308 | |
| 25.05.2005 | 03.07.1950 | F | | 944 | 954 | Referred to Occupational therapist for splinting fitting for the pains in her (R) hand especially | | 7468 | |
| 24.05.2005 | 06.03.1957 | F | | 934 | 939 | To observe the small lump on her (R) upper arm | | 7478 | |

Result of a query that lists all consultations from the 22nd to the end of May 2005 (ConsultationsSeenFrom22ndTillEndOfMay2005)

| SurgeryDate | DateOfBirth | Sex | Diagnosis | TimeIn | TimeOut | Complaints | Treatments | NumbersID | Notes |
|---|---|---|---|---|---|---|---|---|---|
| 25.05.2005 | 27.04.1925 | M | | 924 | 935 | Letter written to Nephrologist regarding his abnormal urine micro-albumin screen result | | 751 | |
| 27.05.2005 | 31.01.1959 | M | | 922 | 930 | For Cholesterol & HBA1c | | 7513 | |
| 27.05.2005 | 19.09.1938 | F | | 930 | 940 | For CXR & For MSU | | 7513 | |
| 24.05.2005 | 20.02.1953 | F | Revisit | 918 | 925 | Twisted (R) ankle is still quite painful | Referred to Orthopaedic Surgeon (Basildon Hospital) | 7559 | |
| 24.05.2005 | 22.06.1974 | F | | 1635 | 1643 | To think of changing to an alternative contraception to Dianette | | 7596 | |
| 27.05.2005 | 22.05.1920 | F | URTI | 1646 | 1655 | Pain in (R) ear | Erythromycin | 7601 | Penicillin allergy. |
| 24.05.2005 | 16.04.1938 | M | | 1712 | 1724 | Redness of (L) big toe | Etoricoxib & Flucloxacillin | 7626 | For X-Ray. |
| 23.05.2005 | 09.10.1966 | F | | 919 | 924 | For FBC & TFTs | | 7710 | |
| 23.05.2005 | 01.08.1950 | M | | 1008 | 1011 | To put in a self-certificate | | 7763 | |
| 26.05.2005 | 31.03.1939 | M | | 1805 | 1821 | The Parking Badge Scheme for Disabled People Medical Practitioner Report completed | | 7829 | |

238

Result of a query that lists all consultations from the 22nd to the end of May 2005 (ConsultationsSeenFrom22ndTillEndOfMay2005)

| SurgeryDate | DateOfBirth | Sex | Diagnosis | TimeIn | TimeOut | Complaints | Treatments | NumbersID | Notes |
|---|---|---|---|---|---|---|---|---|---|
| 23.05.2005 | 29.01.1941 | M | | 928 | 952 | Persistent dysuria & urine seems like faeces | Referred to Urologist (Basildon Hospital Urgent) | 7839 | |
| 23.05.2005 | 12.08.1970 | F | | 1728 | 1738 | Recurrent sore throats | Phenoxymethylpenicillin | 7856 | Referred to ENT Surgeon. |
| 24.05.2005 | 10.04.1920 | M | | 939 | 952 | Quite itchy rash all over | Fexofenadine | 7910 | |
| 23.05.2005 | 26.08.2003 | F | Revisit | 1711 | 1719 | Still has sticky eyes | Fusidic Acid eye drops | 7917 | |
| 25.05.2005 | 05.12.1973 | F | Pain | 1044 | 1054 | Abdominal pain & vomiting | Metoclopramide | 7922 | For MSU. |
| 25.05.2005 | 21.07.1963 | F | | 1659 | 1710 | Script for Fluoxetine given | | 835 | |
| 24.05.2005 | 01.07.1927 | F | URTI | 1340 | 1350 | Sore throat | Amoxycillin | 911 | Home visit. |
| 24.05.2005 | 20.11.1923 | M | RTI | 1350 | 1400 | Cough | Amoxycillin | 916 | Home visit. Script for Salbutamol inhaler given. |
| 23.05.2005 | 05.10.1974 | M | | 1749 | 1802 | For GTT | | 918 | Asthma check done. |
| 23.05.2005 | 07.12.1986 | F | | 1738 | 1749 | Burst condom | Levonorgestrel | 95 | |
| 26.05.2005 | 08.12.1962 | F | | 1735 | 1751 | Script for Ferrous Sulphate & Norethisterone given | | 981 | Penicillin allergy. |
| 24.05.2005 | 12.05.1936 | M | | 1724 | 1739 | Awaiting MRI scan results | | NP (AM) | |
| 24.05.2005 | 13.11.1932 | M | | 1430 | 1440 | Bilateral pedal oedema & depressed | Fluoxetine & Frusemide | NP (AP) | Home visit. |

Result of a query that lists all consultations from the 22nd to the end of May 2005 (ConsultationsSeenFrom22ndTillEndOfMay2005)

| SurgeryDate | DateOfBirth | Sex | Diagnosis | TimeIn | TimeOut | Complaints | Treatments | NumbersID | Notes |
|---|---|---|---|---|---|---|---|---|---|
| 24.05.2005 | 20.12.2004 | F | | 1643 | 1647 | To use Normal Saline drops for her snuffles at night | | NP (AP) | |
| 23.05.2005 | 11.02.1986 | F | | 1642 | 1649 | Late Period | For Pregnancy test | NP (CC) | |
| 27.05.2005 | 23.08.1968 | F | Pain | 1715 | 1722 | Pain (L) leg with bruises & prominent varicose veins | Referred to Vascular Surgeon | NP (DH) | |
| 24.05.2005 | 03.03.1937 | M | | 952 | 1001 | To go back on the Pizotifen | | NP (EJC) | |
| 24.05.2005 | 15.05.1920 | F | | 1410 | 1420 | Insomnia | Temazepam | NP (GN) | Home visit. Script for Chlorpromazine given. |
| 27.05.2005 | 11.12.1944 | F | Pain | 1735 | 1742 | (L) upper abdominal pain | For USScan of the abdomen | NP (GW) | Codeine allergy. |
| 27.05.2005 | 27.08.1933 | M | Rash | 1655 | 1707 | Mole on upper back | Referred to Dermatologist (Basildon Hospital) | NP (HA) | |
| 27.05.2005 | 17.08.1912 | F | | 940 | 958 | To go to A/E for injury to his (R) hand | | NP (IA) | The Parking Badge Scheme for Disabled People Medical Practitioner Report completed. |
| 26.05.2005 | 12.04.1932 | F | | 1124 | 1142 | Script for Pravastatin & Perindopril given | | NP (JA) | |
| 27.05.2005 | 18.07.1929 | F | | 904 | 911 | Dizziness | For FBC | NP (JG) | |
| 23.05.2005 | 20.05.2003 | M | RTI | 1719 | 1728 | Chesty cough | Amoxycillin | NP (JR) | Penicillin allergy. |

Result of a query that lists all consultations from the 22nd to the end of May 2005 (ConsultationsSeenFrom22ndTillEndOfMay2005)

| SurgeryDate | DateOfBirth | Sex | Diagnosis | TimeIn | TimeOut | Complaints | Treatments | NumbersID | Notes |
|---|---|---|---|---|---|---|---|---|---|
| 26.05.2005 | 21.02.1941 | M | | 1046 | 1116 | Script for Co-codamol & Amitriptyline given | | NP (LS) | |
| 27.05.2005 | 05.06.1955 | M | | 1038 | 1054 | For Oral GTT | | NP (MAM) | Referred to General Surgeon regarding his rectal bleeding. |
| 27.05.2005 | 06.03.1926 | F | | 1020 | 1038 | Script for Atenolol given | | NP (MT) | |
| 25.05.2005 | 23.06.1978 | F | | 1728 | 1734 | She will like her period postponed whilst on holidays | Norethisterone | NP (NS) | |
| 23.05.2005 | 13.03.1947 | F | S/Leave | 1027 | 1040 | (L) Renal stone operation | | NP (PR) | Diabetic Clinic check. |
| 26.05.2005 | 12.08.1938 | M | | 1705 | 1709 | To see Practice Counsellor | | NP (SM) | Penicillin allergy. |
| 25.05.2005 | 28.02.1941 | F | | 1000 | 1012 | To reduce the dose of Gliclazide to 40mg daily | | NP (SW) | Septrin allergy. |
| 25.05.2005 | 18.06.1960 | F | Depression | 1739 | 1751 | Flood of tears | To see the Practice Counsellor | NP AF) | |
| 25.05.2005 | 29.10.1974 | F | | 1755 | 1802 | Script for Cilest given | | Temp | |
| 26.05.2005 | 27.07.1970 | F | UTI | 951 | 1001 | Dysuria | Trimethoprim | Temp | Penicillin allergy. For MSU. |

Result of a query that lists all consultations from the 22nd to the end of May 2006 (ConsultationsSeenFrom22ndTillEndOfMay2006)

| SurgeryDate | DateOfBirth | Sex | Diagnosis | TimeIn | TimeOut | Complaints | Treatments | Initials | Notes |
|---|---|---|---|---|---|---|---|---|---|
| 22.05.2006 | 14.08.1935 | M | | 938 | 950 | Yearly Diabetic Monitoring Done | | RAT | |
| 22.05.2006 | 28.06.1959 | F | Pain | 1010 | 1022 | Bilateral knee pain | For X-Ray | PIS | Script for Orlistat given. |
| 22.05.2006 | 06.01.1943 | F | | 1022 | 1039 | Yearly Diabetic Monitoring Done | | PC | |
| 22.05.2006 | 25.02.1941 | F | RTI | 1039 | 1049 | Chesty cough | Amoxycillin | SJW | |
| 22.05.2006 | 26.03.1980 | F | | 1049 | 1056 | Script for Cilest given | | TM | |
| 22.05.2006 | 27.08.1952 | F | | 1056 | 1107 | Script for Ciprofloxacin & Simvastatin given | | KLB | |
| 22.05.2006 | 20.09.1965 | M | S/Leave | 1107 | 1114 | Urinary Tract Infection | | VJC | Referred to Practice Counsellor for feeling low & depressed. |
| 22.05.2006 | 27.04.1925 | M | | 1114 | 1121 | Patient should not go on ACE Inhibitors etc. | | RWF | |
| 22.05.2006 | 04.11.1934 | M | | 1121 | 1129 | Script for Co-codamol & Trimethoprim given | | TEC | |
| 22.05.2006 | 08.04.2005 | M | RTI | 1129 | 1136 | Cough | Amoxycillin | CPE | Script for Chloramphenicol eye drops & Salbutamol solution given. |
| 22.05.2006 | 19.01.1964 | F | RTI | 1139 | 1144 | Chesty cough | Ciprofloxacin | NAB | |

Result of a query that lists all consultations from the 22nd to the end of May 2006 (ConsultationsSeenFrom22ndTillEndOfMay2006)

| SurgeryDate | DateOfBirth | Sex | Diagnosis | TimeIn | TimeOut | Complaints | Treatments | Initials | Notes |
|---|---|---|---|---|---|---|---|---|---|
| 22.05.2006 | 30.07.1953 | F | | 1144 | 1154 | Script for Loratadine & Chloramphenicol eye ointment given | | SS | |
| 22.05.2006 | 04.09.1958 | F | | 1644 | 1654 | Dizzy spells are a lot better | | LKW | |
| 22.05.2006 | 14.08.1947 | F | S/Leave | 1709 | 1719 | Burns to (L) fingers | | PJH | |
| 22.05.2006 | 25.02.1950 | F | | 1730 | 1736 | Script for Amoxycillin & Dihydrocodeine given | | CAS | |
| 22.05.2006 | 23.07.1984 | F | | 1736 | 1745 | Script for Citalopram, Flucloxacillin & Fusidic acid with Hydrocortisone given | | MNW | |
| 22.05.2006 | 05.12.1934 | F | | 1745 | 1750 | Script for Chloramphenicol eye drops & Loratadine given | | JS | |
| 22.05.2006 | 13.02.1963 | F | | 1750 | 1755 | Chesty cough | Amoxycillin | VN | |
| 22.05.2006 | 30.03.1943 | M | | 1813 | 1825 | Script for Dihydrocodeine & Omeprazole given | | BW | |
| 22.05.2006 | 02.03.1918 | F | | 1825 | 1835 | Script for Amoxycillin & Fusidic acid eye drops given | | YV | |
| 22.05.2006 | 10.02.1937 | F | | 1835 | 1850 | Script for Vitamin bpc capsules given | | MC | |
| 23.05.2006 | 29.01.1941 | M | | 940 | 1005 | Script for Ferrous Sulphate given | | AD | |

Result of a query that lists all consultations from the 22nd to the end of May 2006 (ConsultationsSeenFrom22ndTillEndOfMay2006)

| SurgeryDate | DateOfBirth | Sex | Diagnosis | TimeIn | TimeOut | Complaints | Treatments | Initials | Notes |
|---|---|---|---|---|---|---|---|---|---|
| 23.05.2006 | 10.12.1986 | F | | 1005 | 1011 | Pregnancy test positive | | HEB | |
| 23.05.2006 | 18.07.1978 | F | | 1011 | 1018 | Script for Microgynon given | | TJS | |
| 23.05.2006 | 24.04.1931 | F | RTI | 1018 | 1027 | Chesty cough | Erythromycin | JWB | |
| 23.05.2006 | 14.05.1971 | M | | 1027 | 1033 | Boil in (R) axilla | Flucloxacillin & Fusidic acid cream | NJF | |
| 23.05.2006 | 27.04.1928 | M | | 1033 | 1038 | Hay fever with nasal blockage | Beclomethasone aqueous nasal spray & Loratadine | RFU | Script for Beclomethasone inhaler given. |
| 23.05.2006 | 09.07.1964 | F | RTI | 1045 | 1050 | Chesty cough | Amoxycillin | JR | |
| 23.05.2006 | 18.07.1965 | F | | 1050 | 1058 | Paronychia (R) thumb | Flucloxacillin & Fusidic acid cream | LSC | |
| 23.05.2006 | 27.11.1952 | F | | 1106 | 1121 | To stop Atenolol to which she had adverse reaction | | JD | |
| 23.05.2006 | 10.11.2001 | F | RTI | 1121 | 1125 | Chesty cough | Amoxycillin | GLB | |
| 23.05.2006 | 13.10.1989 | F | URTI | 1125 | 1130 | Weepy (R) ear ache | Amoxycillin | RLB | |
| 23.05.2006 | 24.02.1921 | F | Pain | 1130 | 1136 | Pain both knees | Injection Depo-Medrone with Lidocaine | EIW | |

Result of a query that lists all consultations from the 22nd to the end of May 2006 (ConsultationsSeenFrom22ndTillEndOfMay2006)

| SurgeryDate | DateOfBirth | Sex | Diagnosis | TimeIn | TimeOut | Complaints | Treatments | Initials | Notes |
|---|---|---|---|---|---|---|---|---|---|
| 23.05.2006 | 17.03.1924 | M | | 1136 | 1156 | Injection Depo-Medrone with Lidocaine given to the (R) shoulder | | JHB | |
| 23.05.2006 | 24.02.1921 | F | | 1156 | 1214 | Injection Depo-Medrone with Lidocaine given to the (R) knee | | EIW | |
| 24.05.2006 | 28.07.1957 | F | | 946 | 954 | Script for Rizatriptan wafer given | | MES | |
| 24.05.2006 | 25.08.1957 | M | S/Leave | 956 | 1003 | Back Pain - Med. 5 | | GC | |
| 24.05.2006 | 08.12.1930 | M | RTI | 1003 | 1014 | Chesty cough | Ciprofloxacin | FSR | Wife came to Surgery. |
| 24.05.2006 | 27.11.2004 | F | URTI | 1014 | 1017 | Infected rhinorrhoea | Amoxycillin | JLR | |
| 24.05.2006 | 07.02.1972 | F | RTI | 1017 | 1020 | Chesty cough | Amoxycillin | SVR | |
| 24.05.2006 | 07.05.1978 | F | | 1020 | 1027 | For FBC, TFTs, Fasting Cholesterol & Fasting Glucose | | NA | |
| 24.05.2006 | 29.04.1935 | F | | 1027 | 1043 | I explained to her that it is better to come in with her son to discuss about him | | CM | |
| 24.05.2006 | 22.04.1942 | F | RTI | 1043 | 1047 | Chesty cough | Amoxycillin | JS | |
| 24.05.2006 | 22.03.1933 | F | RTI | 1047 | 1057 | Chesty cough | Erythromycin | LLW | |
| 24.05.2006 | 06.02.1968 | F | | 1057 | 1106 | Script for Loratadine given | | TW | |
| 24.05.2006 | 12.08.1931 | F | | 1106 | 1116 | Script for Paracetamol given | | PT | |

Result of a query that lists all consultations from the 22nd to the end of May 2006 (ConsultationsSeenFrom22ndTillEndOfMay2006)

| SurgeryDate | DateOfBirth | Sex | Diagnosis | TimeIn | TimeOut | Complaints | Treatments | Initials | Notes |
|---|---|---|---|---|---|---|---|---|---|
| 24.05.2006 | 25.12.1948 | M | | 1116 | 1130 | BP 122/82 | | CGB | |
| 24.05.2006 | 10.10.1964 | F | URTI | 1130 | 1135 | Sore throat | Amoxycillin | KF | |
| 24.05.2006 | 11.04.1982 | F | URTI | 1137 | 1147 | Sore throat | Amoxycillin | JLS | |
| 24.05.2006 | 28.02.1927 | M | | 1335 | 1350 | Redness both legs | Penicillin V & Fusidic acid cream | WE | Home visit. |
| 24.05.2006 | 15.02.1932 | F | | 1636 | 1656 | Script for Clopidogrel given | | JS | |
| 24.05.2006 | 20.04.1945 | F | | 1656 | 1706 | Script for Omeprazole & Vitamin bpc given | | KCY | For X-Ray (R) hand. |
| 24.05.2006 | 13.09.1992 | F | Pain | 1706 | 1712 | Back Pain | Ibuprofen | MRW | |
| 24.05.2006 | 24.04.1935 | F | | 1712 | 1719 | X-Ray Lumbar Spine showed osteoporosis | | DAS | |
| 24.05.2006 | 16.07.1967 | F | | 1721 | 1730 | For repeat FBC in 6 months | | MJN | |
| 24.05.2006 | 05.08.2005 | M | | 1730 | 1736 | Script for Flucloxacillin, Oilatum Plus & E45 cream given | | JMMO | |
| 24.05.2006 | 06.07.1968 | F | | 1738 | 1744 | Script for Citalopram given | | TEM | |
| 24.05.2006 | 19.01.1964 | F | S/Leave | 1747 | 1754 | Flu symptoms - Med. 5 | | NAB | |
| 24.05.2006 | 08.05.1974 | M | | 1754 | 1808 | Script for Acyclovir tablets & Fusidic acid with hydrocortisone cream given | | TW | |

Result of a query that lists all consultations from the 22nd to the end of May 2006 (ConsultationsSeenFrom22ndTillEndOfMay2006)

| SurgeryDate | DateOfBirth | Sex | Diagnosis | TimeIn | TimeOut | Complaints | Treatments | Initials | Notes |
|---|---|---|---|---|---|---|---|---|---|
| 24.05.2006 | 09.07.1959 | F |  | 1814 | 1824 | To continue with Omeprazole |  | LH |  |
| 24.05.2006 | 03.07.1989 | M |  | 1826 | 1834 | For FBC, Fasting Glucose & TFTs |  | WDH |  |
| 25.05.2006 | 03.10.2003 | M |  | 945 | 953 | To use own Talc powder for the prickly heat rash on chest wall |  | BTA |  |
| 25.05.2006 | 27.11.1992 | F | Conjunctivitis | 955 | 1001 | Sticky eyes | Chloramphenicol eye drops | CJK |  |
| 25.05.2006 | 27.08.1922 | M | Lump | 1001 | 1013 | Inflamed (R) Olecranon bursa | Flucloxacillin & Co-dydramol | AC | For aspiration. |
| 25.05.2006 | 26.09.1973 | F | RTI | 1013 | 1020 | Chesty cough | Amoxycillin | SJS |  |
| 25.05.2006 | 06.01.1955 | M |  | 1025 | 1032 | Vertigo | Prochlorperazine | MAS |  |
| 25.05.2006 | 21.06.1959 | M | Pain | 1032 | 1043 | Back Pain | Diclofenac e/c | SJW |  |
| 25.05.2006 | 25.08.1963 | M | Rash | 1043 | 1052 | Urticarial rash | Fexofenadine | PW |  |
| 25.05.2006 | 24.12.1972 | F |  | 1052 | 1104 | Script for Diclofenac e/c & Dihydrocodeine given |  | GM |  |
| 25.05.2006 | 14.05.1923 | M |  | 1104 | 1114 | Yearly Diabetic Monitoring Done |  | AM |  |
| 25.05.2006 | 25.09.1984 | M |  | 1114 | 1125 | Script for Fusidic acid with betamethasone cream, Miconazole with hydrocortisone cream & Soya with Lauromacrogols bath oil given |  | JW |  |

247

Result of a query that lists all consultations from the 22nd to the end of May 2006 (ConsultationsSeenFrom22ndTillEndOfMay2006)

| SurgeryDate | DateOfBirth | Sex | Diagnosis | TimeIn | TimeOut | Complaints | Treatments | Initials | Notes |
|---|---|---|---|---|---|---|---|---|---|
| 25.05.2006 | 27.08.1922 | M | | 1125 | 1149 | (R) Olecranon bursa aspirated | | AC | |
| 25.05.2006 | 01.01.1924 | M | | 1149 | 1158 | For B12, Folate & Ferritin | | HAB | |
| 25.05.2006 | 25.08.1936 | M | | 1158 | 1205 | For B12, Folate & Ferritin | | CAJ | Script for Simvastatin given. |
| 25.05.2006 | 22.02.1933 | F | | 1205 | 1215 | No abnormality noted on rectal examination | | LLW | |
| 25.05.2006 | 16.03.1955 | F | | 1225 | 1235 | Jaundiced, feels itchy & tired | Referred to Hepatology clinic, Kings College Hospital | SJC | |
| 25.05.2006 | 24.02.1944 | F | | 1640 | 1659 | Script for Ezetimibe given | | IEA | |
| 25.05.2006 | 12.11.2000 | M | | 1656 | 1703 | Script for Piperazine given | | JLW | |
| 25.05.2006 | 11.01.1986 | F | | 1707 | 1714 | Script for Microgynon 30 & Flucloxacillin given | | SJW | |
| 25.05.2006 | 06.06.1959 | M | Pain | 1714 | 1721 | Whiplash injury | Co-codamol & Diclofenac e/c | TJS | |
| 25.05.2006 | 05.12.1956 | M | | 1721 | 1727 | To avoid taking Diazepam as they are addictive | | DTB | |
| 25.05.2006 | 06.04.1937 | M | | 1727 | 1738 | Script for Diazepam, Amoxycillin & Omeprazole given | | GWH | |

Result of a query that lists all consultations from the 22nd to the end of May 2006 (ConsultationsSeenFrom22ndTillEndOfMay2006)

| SurgeryDate | DateOfBirth | Sex | Diagnosis | TimeIn | TimeOut | Complaints | Treatments | Initials | Notes |
|---|---|---|---|---|---|---|---|---|---|
| 25.05.2006 | 01.05.1987 | F | | 1748 | 1803 | Persistent per vagina loss post delivery | Erythromycin | JED | |
| 25.05.2006 | 06.09.1964 | F | | 1803 | 1812 | For FBC, Fasting Glucose, Fasting Cholesterol, U/Es, LFTs & TFTs | | ELB | |
| 25.05.2006 | 24.01.1952 | F | | 1812 | 1830 | Referred to ENT Surgeon regarding lump to (L) of his uvula | | BDG | |
| 26.05.2006 | 29.08.1981 | F | | 948 | 953 | Pregnancy test positive | | CC | |
| 26.05.2006 | 26.12.1947 | M | S/Leave | 953 | 959 | Radical (L) Nephrectomy | | RDG | |
| 26.05.2006 | 25.12.1942 | M | | 959 | 1004 | Script for Nystatin given | | RFL | |
| 26.05.2006 | 28.12.1962 | M | URTI | 1004 | 1009 | (L) ear ache & discharge | Amoxycillin | KF | |
| 26.05.2006 | 29.04.1925 | M | | 1009 | 1017 | Referred to Orthopaedic Surgeon regarding pain in the (R) hip | | ADR | |
| 26.05.2006 | 11.12.1944 | F | | 1027 | 1041 | Script for Sodium Valproate & Co-megaldrox given | | GNW | |
| 26.05.2006 | 26.04.1944 | F | RTI | 1041 | 1052 | Chesty cough | Amoxycillin | AW | |

249

Result of a query that lists all consultations from the 22nd to the end of May 2006 (ConsultationsSeenFrom22ndTillEndOfMay2006)

| SurgeryDate | DateOfBirth | Sex | Diagnosis | TimeIn | TimeOut | Complaints | Treatments | Initials | Notes |
|---|---|---|---|---|---|---|---|---|---|
| 26.05.2006 | 22.03.1936 | F |  | 1052 | 1059 | To see nurse in 5 months for repeat HBA1c |  | ME |  |
| 26.05.2006 | 02.07.1924 | M |  | 1059 | 1109 | Bilateral pedal oedema | Frusemide | TCC |  |
| 26.05.2006 | 23.10.1947 | F | RTI | 1109 | 1120 | Chesty cough & wheezy | Amoxycillin & Prednisolone e/c | EEV |  |
| 26.05.2006 | 05.07.1950 | M |  | 1132 | 1153 | Script for Omeprazole & Prochlorperazine given |  | JMG |  |
| 26.05.2006 | 25.06.1938 | M |  | 1310 | 1322 | Diarrhoea | Co-Phenotrope, Ciprofloxacin & Electrolade | JEL | Home visit. |
| 26.05.2006 | 26.05.1979 | F |  | 1645 | 1652 | Script for Microgynon 30 given |  | WEE |  |
| 26.05.2006 | 29.12.2005 | M | RTI | 1652 | 1657 | Cough | Amoxycillin | HAP |  |
| 26.05.2006 | 12.01.1929 | M |  | 1701 | 1719 | Script for Fusidic acid with hydrocortisone & Hydroxocobalamin injection given |  | KJM |  |
| 26.05.2006 | 22.04.2006 | M | Rash | 1719 | 1724 | Nappy rash | Timodine | AJW |  |
| 26.05.2006 | 18.02.1992 | F | Rash | 1733 | 1739 | Septic insect bite on back | Flucloxacillin | 43070 |  |
| 26.05.2006 | 10.01.1973 | F |  | 1739 | 1749 | Script for Clotrimazole cream & pessary, Citalopram & Flucloxacillin given |  | NO |  |
| 26.05.2006 | 05.07.1947 | M | RTI | 1749 | 1754 | Cough | Amoxycillin | LW |  |

250

Result of a query that lists all consultations from the 22nd to the end of May 2006 (ConsultationsSeenFrom22ndTillEndOfMay2006)

| SurgeryDate | DateOfBirth | Sex | Diagnosis | TimeIn | TimeOut | Complaints | Treatments | Initials | Notes |
|---|---|---|---|---|---|---|---|---|---|
| 26.05.2006 | 07.10.1981 | M | Rash | 1808 | 1814 | Itchy rash on shoulders | Loratadine | JPB | |
| 30.05.2006 | 08.09.1957 | M | | 943 | 956 | Yearly Diabetic Monitoring Done | | TJG | |
| 30.05.2006 | 26.05.1926 | M | | 956 | 1006 | Script for Amoxycillin & Ferrous Sulphate given | | JKS | |
| 30.05.2006 | 23.09.1990 | F | | 1006 | 1016 | To see nurse for Depo-Provera or preferable to go to FP Clinic | | LET | |
| 30.05.2006 | 25.08.1963 | M | S/Leave | 1016 | 1022 | (L) thigh injury - Med. 5 | | PW | |
| 30.05.2006 | 17.09.1965 | F | Conjunctivitis | 1022 | 1028 | Sore & discharging eye | Chloramphenicol eye drops | PAE | |
| 30.05.2006 | 23.08.1975 | M | | 1028 | 1032 | (L) Dental abscess | Amoxycillin | IMER | |
| 30.05.2006 | 27.08.1935 | M | | 1032 | 1040 | To see nurse in 3 to 6 months for a repeat FBC | | AAS | |
| 30.05.2006 | 19.09.1938 | F | | 1040 | 1047 | Script for GTN spray given | | MPS | |
| 30.05.2006 | 25.06.1921 | M | | 1056 | 1109 | Script for Co-codamol given | | HRP | |
| 30.05.2006 | 22.01.1986 | F | | 1122 | 1132 | For X-Ray of (L) knee | | LM | |
| 30.05.2006 | 06.08.1921 | F | | 1132 | 1141 | For X-Ray of (R) shoulder | | EE | Script for Dihydrocodeine given. |

Result of a query that lists all consultations from the 22nd to the end of May 2006 (ConsultationsSeenFrom22ndTillEndOfMay2006)

| SurgeryDate | DateOfBirth | Sex | Diagnosis | TimeIn | TimeOut | Complaints | Treatments | Initials | Notes |
|---|---|---|---|---|---|---|---|---|---|
| 30.05.2006 | 31.01.1964 | F | | 1141 | 1149 | For X-Ray of (R) hip | | DH | Script for Co-codamol given. |
| 30.05.2006 | 03.01.1914 | F | | 1400 | 1410 | Script for Enlive Plus & Prochlorperazine given | | LG | Home visit. |
| 30.05.2006 | 20.12.1922 | F | Rash | 1646 | 1657 | Contact Dermatitis both hands | Betamethasone cream 0.1% | DEA | Script for Fusidic acid eye drops given. |
| 30.05.2006 | 04.12.1957 | F | RTI | 1657 | 1703 | Chesty cough | Amoxycillin | TA | |
| 30.05.2006 | 17.03.1967 | F | | 1708 | 1717 | Dizzy spells | Prochlorperazine | SOOS | |
| 30.05.2006 | 22.06.1973 | F | S/Leave | 1717 | 1732 | Back Pain - Private | | JAP | Script for Co-codamol & Diclofenac e/c. |
| 30.05.2006 | 04.05.1937 | F | | 1732 | 1744 | Script for Amoxycillin given | | DMB | For MSU. |
| 30.05.2006 | 16.03.1955 | F | | 1744 | 1751 | Generalised pruritus | Levocetirizine | SJL | |
| 30.05.2006 | 14.06.1945 | M | Pain | 1751 | 1802 | Pain, redness & swelling (L) foot | Flucloxacillin, diclofenac e/c & Co-codamol | BL | |
| 30.05.2006 | 07.07.1961 | F | | 1802 | 1810 | Script for Trimethoprim given | | SSO | For MSU. |
| 30.05.2006 | 10.04.1958 | F | S/Leave | 1810 | 1816 | Kidney infection | | DAB | |
| 30.05.2006 | 08.09.1964 | F | | 1816 | 1825 | Bilateral pedal oedema | Frusemide | DMB | For serum BNP. |
| 30.05.2006 | 20.02.1954 | F | S/Leave | 1825 | 1838 | Depression - Private | | VB | Referred to Practice Counsellor. |
| 30.05.2006 | 16.12.1997 | F | URTI | 1838 | 1844 | Sore throat (R) ear ache | Amoxycillin | JEH | |

Result of a query that lists all consultations from the 22nd to the end of May 2007 (ConsultationsSeenFrom22ndTillEndOfMay2007)

| SurgeryDate | DateOfBirth | Sex | Diagnosis | TimeIn | TimeOut | Complaints | Treatments | Initials | Notes |
|---|---|---|---|---|---|---|---|---|---|
| 22.05.2007 | 23.02.1941 | M | | 942 | 956 | Script for Ciprofloxacin given | | RWM | |
| 22.05.2007 | 02.05.1962 | F | | 956 | 1007 | Script for Ferrous Sulphate & Folic acid given | | DP | |
| 22.05.2007 | 08.11.1960 | F | RTI | 1007 | 1015 | Chesty cough | Amoxycillin | EI | |
| 22.05.2007 | 06.08.1930 | F | | 1015 | 1021 | Script for Co-codamol given | | LP | |
| 22.05.2007 | 16.04.1995 | F | | 1021 | 1027 | Threadworms | Mebendazole | SMG | |
| 22.05.2007 | 17.10.1933 | M | | 1027 | 1031 | Script for Olanzapine given | | FDF | |
| 22.05.2007 | 16.12.1959 | F | | 1051 | 1059 | Script for Amoxycillin given | | SLC | |
| 22.05.2007 | 03.04.1920 | F | | 1059 | 1123 | Referred to General Physician regarding her dizziness | | JA | Script for Prochlorperazine given. |
| 22.05.2007 | 08.10.1940 | M | | 1123 | 1135 | The Parking Badge Scheme for Disabled People Medical Practitioner form completed with the patient | | GAFM | |
| 22.05.2007 | 03.05.1978 | M | | 1135 | 1146 | Referred to Dermatologist regarding fibromas on his head & neck | | DCL | Script for Omeprazole given. |
| 22.05.2007 | 09.07.1959 | F | | 1644 | 1658 | For repeat U/Es & serum cholesterol in 6 months with the nurse | | LH | |

253

Result of a query that lists all consultations from the 22nd to the end of May 2007 (ConsultationsSeenFrom22ndTillEndOfMay2007)

| SurgeryDate | DateOfBirth | Sex | Diagnosis | TimeIn | TimeOut | Complaints | Treatments | Initials | Notes |
|---|---|---|---|---|---|---|---|---|---|
| 22.05.2007 | 23.09.1944 | M | | 1658 | 1707 | For repeat LFTs & serum cholesterol in 6 months with the nurse | | VRE | |
| 22.05.2007 | 10.08.1985 | F | URTI | 1707 | 1716 | Sore throat | Amoxycillin | HNB | Script for Fusidic acid cream given. |
| 22.05.2007 | 16.05.1964 | M | URTI | 1716 | 1720 | (R) ear ache | Amoxycillin | GDC | |
| 22.05.2007 | 20.08.1939 | F | | 1720 | 1727 | Script for Levothyroxine given | | SLT | |
| 22.05.2007 | 21.07.1919 | M | | 1727 | 1741 | Script for Loperamide given | | SEB | Stool for C&S. |
| 22.05.2007 | 04.09.1958 | F | | 1741 | 1752 | Referred to Neurologist regarding heaviness in the head & nausea feeling recurrently | | LKW | |
| 22.05.2007 | 14.08.1947 | F | | 1755 | 1802 | Added on the X-Ray form that she will be having X-Ray of the (L) thigh | | PJH | |
| 22.05.2007 | 28.06.1959 | M | | 1802 | 1812 | BP 155/97 | | SCU | |
| 23.05.2007 | 07.03.1955 | F | | 942 | 1000 | Script for Folic acid given | | DN | |
| 23.05.2007 | 05.07.1931 | F | | 1000 | 1014 | To see the nurse for urinalysis for proteinuria | | AVD | |
| 23.05.2007 | 22.08.1980 | F | | 1014 | 1031 | For FBC, TFTs, LFTs & Fasting Cholesterol | | CJW | |

Result of a query that lists all consultations from the 22nd to the end of May 2007 (ConsultationsSeenFrom22ndTillEndOfMay2007)

| SurgeryDate | DateOfBirth | Sex | Diagnosis | TimeIn | TimeOut | Complaints | Treatments | Initials | Notes |
|---|---|---|---|---|---|---|---|---|---|
| 23.05.2007 | 31.08.1963 | M | | 1031 | 1040 | Referred to Neurologist regarding loss of memory & lack of concentration since being knocked down by car in Benfleet | | JR | |
| 23.05.2007 | 08.06.1976 | M | | 1040 | 1048 | Script for Dihydrocodeine given | | LDN | |
| 23.05.2007 | 10.08.1931 | M | | 1048 | 1056 | Script for Injection MethylPrednisolone with Lidocaine 2mls given | | REW | |
| 23.05.2007 | 18.09.1943 | F | | 1056 | 1112 | Referred to Practice Counsellor regarding family & marriage problems | | DAP | |
| 23.05.2007 | 20.10.1935 | F | | 1112 | 1120 | Script for Erythromycin given | | MM | Penicillin allergy. |
| 23.05.2007 | 29.11.1946 | F | | 1120 | 1127 | Script for Lisinopril given | | CMT | |
| 23.05.2007 | 03.03.1946 | M | | 1127 | 1137 | Script for Omeprazole given | | SP | |
| 23.05.2007 | 12.04.1952 | M | | 1137 | 1146 | Script for Dihydrocodeine, Diprobase cream & Soya with Lauromacrogols bath oil given | | RDC | |

Result of a query that lists all consultations from the 22nd to the end of May 2007 (ConsultationsSeenFrom22ndTillEndOfMay2007)

| SurgeryDate | DateOfBirth | Sex | Diagnosis | TimeIn | TimeOut | Complaints | Treatments | Initials | Notes |
|---|---|---|---|---|---|---|---|---|---|
| 23.05.2007 | 13.09.1918 | M | | 1152 | 1200 | Script for Tramadol m/r given | | EJG | |
| 23.05.2007 | 03.05.1946 | F | | 1200 | 1214 | Injection Depo-Medrone with Lidocaine given to the (R) shoulder | | JP | |
| 23.05.2007 | 21.07.1919 | M | | 1350 | 1405 | Script for Co-codamol, Electrolade & Erythromycin given | | SB | Home visit. |
| 23.05.2007 | 25.08.1933 | F | | 1645 | 1653 | Referred to ENT Surgeon regarding deafness both ears | | PCH | |
| 23.05.2007 | 12.10.1948 | F | | 1653 | 1706 | Script for Omeprazole given | | SFC | For Lumbar Spine X-Ray. |
| 23.05.2007 | 15.06.1954 | F | UTI | 1706 | 1713 | Dysuria & haematuria | Amoxycillin | PMB | For MSU. |
| 23.05.2007 | 18.02.1992 | F | | 1713 | 1719 | For repeat MSU | | 43070 | |
| 23.05.2007 | 03.10.1969 | F | | 1719 | 1730 | Cancer care review | | LJW | |
| 23.05.2007 | 11.08.1980 | F | | 1732 | 1742 | For Urine Pregnancy test | | MD | |
| 23.05.2007 | 03.05.1944 | F | | 1742 | 1752 | Medication review done | | JM | |
| 23.05.2007 | 10.03.2004 | M | URTI | 1752 | 1757 | (R) ear ache | Amoxycillin | DFJB | |
| 23.05.2007 | 13.07.1971 | M | | 1829 | 1838 | Script for Clotrimazole cream 2%, Diprobase cream, Fluconazole capsules & Soya with Lauromacrogols bath oil | | MB | |

Result of a query that lists all consultations from the 22nd to the end of May 2007 (ConsultationsSeenFrom22ndTillEndOfMay2007)

| SurgeryDate | DateOfBirth | Sex | Diagnosis | TimeIn | TimeOut | Complaints | Treatments | Initials | Notes |
|---|---|---|---|---|---|---|---|---|---|
| 24.05.2007 | 12.11.1968 | F | | 944 | 950 | Script for Amoxycillin given | | SEL | |
| 24.05.2007 | 18.03.1987 | F | | 956 | 1007 | Script for Amoxycillin, Co-codamol & Ibuprofen given | | LP | |
| 24.05.2007 | 12.09.1931 | F | | 1007 | 1016 | Script for Co-codamol given | | PRT | |
| 24.05.2007 | 23.02.1940 | M | | 1016 | 1024 | Script for Loratadine & Fusidic acid with hydrocortisone cream given | | BWH | |
| 24.05.2007 | 05.04.1991 | F | | 1024 | 1035 | Script for Microgynon 30 given | | LSR | |
| 24.05.2007 | 14.05.1951 | M | | 1033 | 1039 | Referred to Dermatologist regarding possible fungal nails infection | | DKW | |
| 24.05.2007 | 08.04.1948 | M | | 1053 | 1118 | Referred to Ophthalmologist regarding seeing cotton wool in the (R) eye | | WRT | Script for Lisinopril given. |
| 24.05.2007 | 11.11.1934 | M | | 1118 | 1128 | Script for Amoxycillin given | | VRB | |
| 24.05.2007 | 07.05.1938 | F | RTI | 1128 | 1135 | Script for Ciprofloxacin & Salbutamol inhaler given | | ILB | |

Result of a query that lists all consultations from the 22nd to the end of May 2007 (ConsultationsSeenFrom22ndTillEndOfMay2007)

| SurgeryDate | DateOfBirth | Sex | Diagnosis | TimeIn | TimeOut | Complaints | Treatments | Initials | Notes |
|---|---|---|---|---|---|---|---|---|---|
| 24.05.2007 | 04.12.1957 | F | | 1135 | 1145 | Script for Clobetasol cream & Salbutamol inhaler given | | TA | |
| 24.05.2007 | 09.04.1938 | M | | 1646 | 1700 | Referred to Dermatologist regarding red rash & itchy scalp | | NWH | |
| 24.05.2007 | 29.04.1925 | M | | 1700 | 1710 | Referred to Orthopaedic Surgeon regarding pain in the (R) hip | | ADR | |
| 24.05.2007 | 18.05.1971 | M | S/Leave | 1710 | 1718 | Arthroscopy & Lateral release - Med. 5 | | MJR | |
| 24.05.2007 | 16.08.1927 | F | URTI | 1718 | 1722 | Sore throat | Amoxycillin | EFM | |
| 24.05.2007 | 12.11.1950 | M | | 1726 | 1735 | To see the nurse for Hepatitis B booster | | MJP | |
| 24.05.2007 | 17.07.1993 | F | | 1735 | 1742 | To reduce the dose of the Sodium Valproate as she is getting side-effects from the higher dose | | JHM | |
| 24.05.2007 | 17.03.1967 | F | | 1742 | 1748 | Script for Flucloxacillin given | | SOSP | |
| 24.05.2007 | 06.10.1952 | M | | 1748 | 1754 | Script for Clarithromycin & Salbutamol inhaler given | | CJG | |

Result of a query that lists all consultations from the 22nd to the end of May 2007 (ConsultationsSeenFrom22ndTillEndOfMay2007)

| SurgeryDate | DateOfBirth | Sex | Diagnosis | TimeIn | TimeOut | Complaints | Treatments | Initials | Notes |
|---|---|---|---|---|---|---|---|---|---|
| 24.05.2007 | 13.09.1969 | M | | 1754 | 1806 | Counselled regarding the fact that he has anti-thrombin III deficiency & how to take preventative measures | | KDA | |
| 24.05.2007 | 28.03.1926 | F | | 1806 | 1817 | Script for Clarithromycin & Salbutamol inhaler given | | JD | |
| 25.05.2007 | 30.03.1943 | M | | 942 | 955 | Referred to ENT Surgeon regarding bilateral deafness | | BWF | Referred to Chest Physician regarding cough & wheezing. |
| 25.05.2007 | 28.02.1941 | F | | 955 | 1010 | BP 131/60 | | SJW | |
| 25.05.2007 | 21.05.1953 | F | | 1010 | 1018 | Script for Docusate Sodium, Erythromycin & Hyoscine butylbromide | | CB | |
| 25.05.2007 | 13.03.2006 | F | URTI | 1018 | 1023 | Infected rhinorrhoea | Amoxycillin | JSK | |
| 25.05.2007 | 06.02.1946 | F | | 1023 | 1032 | Migraine headaches | Pizotifen & Sumatriptan | KMT | |
| 25.05.2007 | 15.04.1956 | M | RTI | 1035 | 1044 | Chesty cough | Amoxycillin | MAO | |
| 25.05.2007 | 05.08.2005 | M | URTI | 1044 | 1056 | Infected rhinorrhoea | Amoxycillin | JMA | Script for Fusidic acid with hydrocortisone cream given. |
| 25.05.2007 | 12.05.1936 | M | | 1056 | 1104 | Script for Dihydrocodeine given | | AM | |

Result of a query that lists all consultations from the 22nd to the end of May 2007 (ConsultationsSeenFrom22ndTillEndOfMay2007)

| SurgeryDate | DateOfBirth | Sex | Diagnosis | TimeIn | TimeOut | Complaints | Treatments | Initials | Notes |
|---|---|---|---|---|---|---|---|---|---|
| 25.05.2007 | 06.03.1926 | F | | 1104 | 1114 | Script for Paracetamol given | | MHT | |
| 25.05.2007 | 02.02.1949 | F | URTI | 1114 | 1118 | Bilateral ear infection | Amoxycillin | LL | |
| 25.05.2007 | 04.05.1956 | M | | 1118 | 1129 | Script for Temazepam given | | JAP | Referred to Practice Counsellor regarding stress & nightmares following RTA with fatality (man died). |
| 25.05.2007 | 15.10.1923 | F | URTI | 1129 | 1136 | Head cold & sinusitis | Amoxycillin | DWP | |
| 25.05.2007 | 10.08.1931 | F | | 1136 | 1150 | Injection Depo-Medrone with Lidocaine given to the (R) shoulder | | REW | |
| 25.05.2007 | 13.11.1970 | F | | 1150 | 1200 | Script for Noriday given | | SD | |
| 29.05.2007 | 23.03.1926 | M | | 946 | 956 | Script for Amitriptyline & Sodium bicarbonate ear drops given | | JWH | |
| 29.05.2007 | 29.09.1932 | F | | 956 | 1006 | Script for Co-Amoxiclav & Lisinopril given | | SMD | |
| 29.05.2007 | 16.12.1959 | F | S/Leave | 1006 | 1021 | Sinusitis - Private & Med. 5 | | SLC | |
| 29.05.2007 | 29.01.1941 | M | | 1021 | 1029 | Script for Penicillin V given | | AD | |

Result of a query that lists all consultations from the 22nd to the end of May 2007 (ConsultationsSeenFrom22ndTillEndOfMay2007)

| SurgeryDate | DateOfBirth | Sex | Diagnosis | TimeIn | TimeOut | Complaints | Treatments | Initials | Notes |
|---|---|---|---|---|---|---|---|---|---|
| 29.05.2007 | 25.07.1939 | F | | 1029 | 1036 | To reduce the Gliclazide tablets from 1.5 to 1 tablet daily | | JLB | |
| 29.05.2007 | 02.03.1918 | F | | 1036 | 1048 | Script for Salbutamol inhaler given | | YV | |
| 29.05.2007 | 29.09.2003 | M | RTI | 1048 | 1054 | Chesty cough | Amoxycillin | CDL | Script for Chloramphenicol eye drops given. |
| 29.05.2007 | 27.07.2006 | F | RTI | 1054 | 1059 | Chesty cough | Amoxycillin | MEL | Script for Chloramphenicol eye drops given. |
| 29.05.2007 | 29.06.1933 | M | | 1059 | 1108 | Script for Calcipotriol with betamethasone ointment given | | BAT | |
| 29.05.2007 | 23.07.1934 | F | | 1108 | 1118 | Referred to Dermatologist regarding fibroma on her face | | MAH | |
| 29.05.2007 | 20.10.1925 | F | | 1240 | 1315 | Referred to Surgical Dr. on call, SGH, SAU regarding heavy rectal bleeding and abdominal pain | | MDH | Home visit. |
| 29.05.2007 | 08.06.1974 | M | | 1645 | 1656 | The requirements on the GP Report Insurance form discussed | | SWM | |
| 29.05.2007 | 18.09.1946 | F | | 1656 | 1704 | Script for Amorolfine nail lacquer 5% given | | SL | |

Result of a query that lists all consultations from the 22nd to the end of May 2007 (ConsultationsSeenFrom22ndTillEndOfMay2007)

| SurgeryDate | DateOfBirth | Sex | Diagnosis | TimeIn | TimeOut | Complaints | Treatments | Initials | Notes |
|---|---|---|---|---|---|---|---|---|---|
| 29.05.2007 | 22.01.1932 | M | | 1712 | 1720 | Patient informed about what happened during the arthroscopy | | JBW | |
| 29.05.2007 | 09.05.1937 | F | | 1720 | 1728 | To see the nurse for repeat FBC in 3 months | | KMN | |
| 29.05.2007 | 03.09.1980 | F | | 1728 | 1741 | Script for Erythromycin given | | KCS | Referred to ENT Surgeon regarding her epistaxes. |
| 29.05.2007 | 24.12.1929 | F | | 1741 | 1749 | She feels well in herself | | ECH | |
| 29.05.2007 | 19.01.1964 | F | | 1800 | 1806 | To have repeat FBC & serum Ferritin with nurse in 6 months | | NAB | |
| 29.05.2007 | 26.08.1982 | M | | 1812 | 1820 | Referred to Dermatologist regarding moles on his back | | BLS | |
| 29.05.2007 | 18.02.1961 | M | RTI | 1847 | 1852 | Chesty cough | Amoxycillin | MMA | |
| 30.05.2007 | 27.08.1935 | M | | 939 | 1002 | Script for Amoxycillin & Chloramphenicol eye drops given | | AAS | |
| 30.05.2007 | 20.04.1927 | F | | 1002 | 1008 | Script for Co-codamol given | | MW | |
| 30.05.2007 | 11.06.1951 | F | | 1008 | 1020 | Script for Amoxycillin given | | PAP | |
| 30.05.2007 | 12.04.1932 | F | | 1020 | 1029 | Script for Ezetimibe with Simvastatin given | | JMA | |

Result of a query that lists all consultations from the 22nd to the end of May 2007 (ConsultationsSeenFrom22ndTillEndOfMay2007)

| SurgeryDate | DateOfBirth | Sex | Diagnosis | TimeIn | TimeOut | Complaints | Treatments | Initials | Notes |
|---|---|---|---|---|---|---|---|---|---|
| 30.05.2007 | 29.07.1938 | M | RTI | 1031 | 1035 | Chesty cough | Amoxycillin | CD | |
| 30.05.2007 | 24.03.1935 | F | URTI | 1035 | 1040 | Sore throat | Amoxycillin | PW | |
| 30.05.2007 | 11.05.1962 | F | | 1040 | 1051 | For X-Rays (L) knee | | JAB | |
| 30.05.2007 | 12.11.1993 | F | RTI | 1051 | 1058 | Chesty cough | Amoxycillin | MB | Script for Desmopressin tablets given. |
| 30.05.2007 | 28.12.1962 | M | S/Leave | 1058 | 1105 | Pain (L) hip - Med. 4 | | KF | |
| 30.05.2007 | 05.04.2005 | F | | 1114 | 1120 | Script for Fusidic acid with hydrocortisone cream given | | TJB | |
| 30.05.2007 | 31.01.1938 | F | RTI | 1125 | 1132 | Chesty cough | Amoxycillin | JMS | |
| 30.05.2007 | 04.10.2004 | F | | 1132 | 1140 | Referred to ENT Surgeon regarding recurrent tonsillitis | | MY | Script for Erythromycin given. |
| 30.05.2007 | 27.08.1922 | M | | 1644 | 1649 | Chesty cough | Amoxycillin | AC | |
| 30.05.2007 | 01.06.1932 | M | | 1702 | 1711 | For B12, Folate & Ferritin | | IGH | |
| 30.05.2007 | 13.12.1986 | F | S/Leave | 1711 | 1721 | Back Pain - Med. 5 | | SAP | |
| 30.05.2007 | 17.05.1943 | M | | 1721 | 1730 | Referred to Dermatologist regarding red blotches on (L) foot & skin tags in the (L) axilla | | PJC | Referred to Practice Counsellor regarding feeling low. |
| 30.05.2007 | 06.06.1961 | M | | 1730 | 1735 | Epigastric discomfort | Omeprazole | LG | |
| 30.05.2007 | 21.09.1924 | F | | 1741 | 1749 | Script for Furosemide given | | GPM | |

Result of a query that lists all consultations from the 22nd to the end of May 2007 (ConsultationsSeenFrom22ndTillEndOfMay2007)

| SurgeryDate | DateOfBirth | Sex | Diagnosis | TimeIn | TimeOut | Complaints | Treatments | Initials | Notes |
|---|---|---|---|---|---|---|---|---|---|
| 30.05.2007 | 05.03.1985 | M | | 1749 | 1756 | Script for Omeprazole & Haloperidol given | | CJG | |
| 30.05.2007 | 06.09.1988 | F | | 1756 | 1805 | To stop the Depo-Provera & to see if the abdominal pain improves | | KAH | |
| 30.05.2007 | 03.05.1951 | F | | 1805 | 1815 | Due to be seen later by the Neurologist regarding her EEG result | | GAG | |
| 30.05.2007 | 23.07.1953 | M | S/Leave | 1815 | 1823 | Chest infection - Med. 5 | | THM | Script for Amoxycillin given. Referred to Chest Physician regarding persistent cough. |
| 30.05.2007 | 23.06.1941 | M | | 1835 | 1905 | HGV Medical done | | RWS | |

Result of a query that lists all consultations from the 22nd to the end of May 2008 (ConsultationsSeenFrom22ndTillEndOfMay2008)

| SurgeryDate | DateOfBirth | Sex | Diagnosis | TimeIn | TimeOut | Complaints | Treatments | Initials | Notes |
|---|---|---|---|---|---|---|---|---|---|
| 22.05.2008 | 23.02.1969 | M | | 943 | 952 | For Fasting Glucose, FBC & U/Es | | DJP | |
| 22.05.2008 | 16.05.1944 | F | | 952 | 1000 | Script for Omeprazole given | | JRL | |
| 22.05.2008 | 11.06.1962 | F | | 1013 | 1022 | Whiplash injury | Co-codamol & Diclofenac e/c | KLB | Aware of BMA RTA fee. |

Result of a query that lists all consultations from the 22$^{nd}$ to the end of May 2008 (ConsultationsSeenFrom22ndTillEndOfMay2008)

| SurgeryDate | DateOfBirth | Sex | Diagnosis | TimeIn | TimeOut | Complaints | Treatments | Initials | Notes |
|---|---|---|---|---|---|---|---|---|---|
| 22.05.2008 | 30.11.1945 | F | RTI | 1022 | 1032 | Chesty cough | Amoxycillin | JBJ | |
| 22.05.2008 | 01.01.1976 | M | | 1032 | 1037 | Referred to Dermatologist regarding mole on the lower back | | JJH | |
| 22.05.2008 | 14.01.1976 | M | | 1037 | 1046 | Referred to Paediatrician regarding his (R) hydrocele | | JJH | |
| 22.05.2008 | 11.02.1938 | M | RTI | 1046 | 1053 | Chesty cough | Amoxycillin | RJH | Script for Fusidic acid with Hydrocortisone cream given. |
| 22.05.2008 | 11.12.1943 | F | RTI | 1053 | 1056 | Chesty cough | Amoxycillin | PAH | |
| 22.05.2008 | 15.01.1959 | M | | 1056 | 1104 | Script for Flucloxacillin given | | ROW | |
| 22.05.2008 | 12.10.1946 | F | Pain | 1104 | 1112 | (R) shoulder pain | Co-dydramol | CPS | |
| 22.05.2008 | 10.08.1931 | M | | 1112 | 1120 | Script for Lactulose & Omeprazole given | | REW | |
| 22.05.2008 | 28.06.2007 | M | RTI | 1120 | 1128 | Chesty cough | Amoxycillin | SS | |
| 22.05.2008 | 28.09.1978 | F | | 1136 | 1147 | Routine mum & baby 6 weeks post-natal check done | | TLW | |
| 22.05.2008 | 08.04.1948 | M | | 1642 | 1649 | For repeat MSU in one month | | WRT | |
| 22.05.2008 | 21.09.1947 | M | | 1649 | 1655 | Bilateral plantar warts | Salicylic acid topical solution 26% | DL | |

265

Result of a query that lists all consultations from the 22nd to the end of May 2008 (ConsultationsSeenFrom22ndTillEndOfMay2008)

| SurgeryDate | DateOfBirth | Sex | Diagnosis | TimeIn | TimeOut | Complaints | Treatments | Initials | Notes |
|---|---|---|---|---|---|---|---|---|---|
| 22.05.2008 | 20.01.1987 | F | | 1655 | 1701 | Medication Review Done | | DLG | |
| 22.05.2008 | 02.06.1994 | F | Conjunctivitis | 1701 | 1706 | Discharge from the (R) eye | Chloramphenicol eye drops | EPB | |
| 22.05.2008 | 26.06.1951 | M | | 1712 | 1720 | For MSU, Fasting Glucose & PSA | | CLD | |
| 22.05.2008 | 28.03.1970 | F | URTI | 1720 | 1735 | (L) ear ache | Amoxycillin & Otomize ear spray | LJ | Referred to Endocrinologist regarding her PCOS. |
| 22.05.2008 | 10.08.1952 | F | Conjunctivitis | 1735 | 1745 | Bilateral sticky red eyes | Chloramphenicol eye drops | SAG | |
| 22.05.2008 | 21.06.1975 | F | RTI | 1745 | 1753 | Chesty cough | Amoxycillin | AKE | |
| 22.05.2008 | 15.07.1955 | F | RTI | 1753 | 1805 | Chesty cough | Amoxycillin | JDU | Referred to Dermatologist regarding round patches of rash on her arms, legs & abdomen. |
| 22.05.2008 | 09.08.1987 | F | URTI | 1805 | 1813 | (L) ear ache | Amoxycillin & Otomize ear spray | RJM | Referred to Dermatologist regarding itchy whitish patches on her arms & legs. |
| 22.05.2008 | 30.03.1985 | M | S/Leave | 1813 | 1825 | Chest Infection - Private | | JD | Script for Erythromycin given. Penicillin allergy. |

Result of a query that lists all consultations from the 22nd to the end of May 2008 (ConsultationsSeenFrom22ndTillEndOfMay2008)

| SurgeryDate | DateOfBirth | Sex | Diagnosis | TimeIn | TimeOut | Complaints | Treatments | Initials | Notes |
|---|---|---|---|---|---|---|---|---|---|
| 23.05.2008 | 01.02.1931 | M | | 926 | 934 | Script for Furosemide given | | MDS | For serum BNP. |
| 23.05.2008 | 15.01.1948 | F | | 934 | 940 | Referred to ENT Surgeon regarding persistent (R) ear ache | | EAW | |
| 23.05.2008 | 28.09.1939 | F | | 940 | 949 | Referred to Breast Surgeon regarding lump in the (R) axilla following operation for breast cancer | | LR | |
| 23.05.2008 | 16.07.1952 | F | | 949 | 1000 | Script for Amitriptyline given | | KAM | |
| 23.05.2008 | 23.03.1926 | M | | 1000 | 1014 | Script for Clotrimazole cream given | | JWH | |
| 23.05.2008 | 28.07.1990 | M | | 1023 | 1029 | Referred to Dermatologist regarding mole on neck | | KW | |
| 23.05.2008 | 09.09.1962 | F | | 1043 | 1050 | Referred to Orthopaedic Surgeon regarding pain in the (R) heel | | MLF | |
| 23.05.2008 | 03.10.1926 | M | | 1050 | 1100 | Script for Ferrous Sulphate & Folic acid given | | JAF | For USScan of the abdomen. |
| 23.05.2008 | 16.02.1931 | M | | 1100 | 1113 | For B12, Folate & Ferritin | | CHH | |

Result of a query that lists all consultations from the 22nd to the end of May 2008 (ConsultationsSeenFrom22ndTillEndOfMay2008)

| SurgeryDate | DateOfBirth | Sex | Diagnosis | TimeIn | TimeOut | Complaints | Treatments | Initials | Notes |
|---|---|---|---|---|---|---|---|---|---|
| 23.05.2008 | 27.03.1940 | F | | 1113 | 1120 | Script for Glucosamine & Co-codamol given | | MAD | |
| 23.05.2008 | 15.04.1973 | F | URTI | 1120 | 1129 | Sore throat | Amoxycillin | LJB | |
| 23.05.2008 | 15.10.1923 | F | | 1129 | 1147 | Script for Flucloxacillin & Fusidic acid cream given | | DWR | |
| 23.05.2008 | 29.08.1981 | F | | 1435 | 1500 | Routine immediate mum & baby check done at home following home delivery | | CC | |
| 27.05.2008 | 16.12.1959 | F | S/Leave | 954 | 958 | Sinus Infection - Med. 5 | | SLC | Script for Amoxycillin given. |
| 27.05.2008 | 09.11.1941 | F | | 958 | 1006 | She says her cough has improved since stopping Simvastatin | | LMD | |
| 27.05.2008 | 10.09.1919 | F | | 1006 | 1013 | For B12, Folate & Ferritin | | ALG | |
| 27.05.2008 | 21.11.1923 | M | RTI | 1013 | 1023 | Chesty cough | Amoxycillin | RU | |
| 27.05.2008 | 11.04.1968 | F | | 1025 | 1041 | Script for Ferrous Sulphate given | | TVC | Script for Co-codamol given. |
| 27.05.2008 | 17.08.1951 | M | | 1046 | 1100 | Script for Lisinopril & Simvastatin given | | 43070 | |
| 27.05.2008 | 17.03.1940 | F | | 1100 | 1116 | Script for Erythromycin given | | MER | Penicillin allergy. |

Result of a query that lists all consultations from the 22nd to the end of May 2008 (ConsultationsSeenFrom22ndTillEndOfMay2008)

| SurgeryDate | DateOfBirth | Sex | Diagnosis | TimeIn | TimeOut | Complaints | Treatments | Initials | Notes |
|---|---|---|---|---|---|---|---|---|---|
| 27.05.2008 | 28.10.1960 | M | | 1116 | 1126 | Script for Fexofenadine given | | JJK | Referred to Dermatologist regarding itchy scrotal & perineal rash. |
| 27.05.2008 | 21.12.1945 | F | | 1126 | 1133 | Septic insect bite on leg | Flucloxacillin | JAL | |
| 27.05.2008 | 03.05.1990 | F | | 1648 | 1654 | For repeat Pregnancy test in 3 weeks | | HLW | |
| 27.05.2008 | 06.09.1924 | M | | 1654 | 1700 | Script for Lamisil AT cream given | | FE | |
| 27.05.2008 | 08.05.1956 | F | | 1700 | 1706 | For X-Rays of the cervical & the thoracic spine | | SH | |
| 27.05.2008 | 26.03.1935 | F | | 1708 | 1718 | Referred to Chest Physician regarding her persistent breathlessness | | RJ | |
| 27.05.2008 | 18.02.1986 | M | | 1718 | 1722 | To continue with own Ibuprofen & analgesia following RTA as advised from SGH A/E | | ASB | |
| 27.05.2008 | 28.02.1941 | F | | 1728 | 1734 | Referred to Dermatologist regarding her toe nails going crumbling | | SJW | |
| 27.05.2008 | 28.12.1962 | F | | 1734 | 1739 | Script for Flucloxacillin given | | KF | |

Result of a query that lists all consultations from the 22nd to the end of May 2008 (ConsultationsSeenFrom22ndTillEndOfMay2008)

| SurgeryDate | DateOfBirth | Sex | Diagnosis | TimeIn | TimeOut | Complaints | Treatments | Initials | Notes |
|---|---|---|---|---|---|---|---|---|---|
| 27.05.2008 | 31.03.1967 | F |  | 1739 | 1745 | Script for Diclofenac e/c, Prednisolone & Salbutamol inhaler given |  | LJS |  |
| 27.05.2008 | 28.03.1970 | F |  | 1745 | 1752 | Referred to ENT Surgeon regarding persistent throat discomfort & (L) ear ache |  | LJ |  |
| 27.05.2008 | 23.06.1980 | M | Rash | 1753 | 1802 | Itchy rash on both feet | Fucidin H cream | CS |  |
| 27.05.2008 | 11.01.1969 | M |  | 1807 | 1815 | Referred to Practice Counsellor regarding feeling low & mood swings |  | RP | Script for Levitra given. |
| 27.05.2008 | 26.11.1959 | M |  | 1815 | 1821 | Referred to Dermatologist regarding changing mole on the (L) side of his face |  | BJW |  |
| 28.05.2008 | 16.05.1958 | M |  | 940 | 952 | Script for Rosiglitazone with Metformin & Simvastatin given |  | SOS | Referred for vasectomy. |
| 28.05.2008 | 25.08.1936 | M |  | 952 | 1003 | Script for Amoxycillin given |  | CAJ |  |
| 28.05.2008 | 10.09.1945 | F |  | 1003 | 1012 | For LFTs |  | JP |  |
| 28.05.2008 | 22.10.2004 | F |  | 1019 | 1026 | To see own optician regarding pain in her eyes |  | ELHH |  |

Result of a query that lists all consultations from the 22nd to the end of May 2008 (ConsultationsSeenFrom22ndTillEndOfMay2008)

| SurgeryDate | DateOfBirth | Sex | Diagnosis | TimeIn | TimeOut | Complaints | Treatments | Initials | Notes |
|---|---|---|---|---|---|---|---|---|---|
| 28.05.2008 | 05.08.1983 | F | S/Leave | 1035 | 1040 | Stress in Pregnancy - Med. 5 | | CLM | |
| 28.05.2008 | 01.04.1988 | F | | 1040 | 1047 | Script for Amoxycillin given | | KRW | |
| 28.05.2008 | 15.09.1939 | M | | 1047 | 1058 | Script for Omeprazole given | | WJS | |
| 28.05.2008 | 13.01.1957 | F | | 1058 | 1105 | Script for Amoxycillin given | | PAW | |
| 28.05.2008 | 02.02.1930 | M | | 1105 | 1124 | The result of the MRI scan explained to the patient | | KRC | |
| 28.05.2008 | 24.10.1940 | F | | 1124 | 1144 | To take OTC Aspirin dispersible | | JIB | |
| 28.05.2008 | 09.10.1974 | F | | 1645 | 1656 | Pregnancy test positive | | MJ | |
| 28.05.2008 | 17.01.1977 | F | | 1656 | 1702 | Script for Amoxycillin given | | MC | |
| 28.05.2008 | 21.01.1959 | F | | 1702 | 1708 | Referred to Dermatologist regarding solitary roughened lesion on the (L) leg | | KH | |
| 28.05.2008 | 05.04.1952 | M | | 1708 | 1715 | Awaiting result of the MRI scan arranged by the ENT Surgeon | | LFC | |
| 28.05.2008 | 14.08.1935 | M | | 1718 | 1730 | Script for Flucloxacillin given | | RAT | For serum Uric acid. |

Result of a query that lists all consultations from the 22nd to the end of May 2008 (ConsultationsSeenFrom22ndTillEndOfMay2008)

| SurgeryDate | DateOfBirth | Sex | Diagnosis | TimeIn | TimeOut | Complaints | Treatments | Initials | Notes |
|---|---|---|---|---|---|---|---|---|---|
| 28.05.2008 | 27.08.1922 | M | | 1738 | 1752 | Script for Co-codamol & Prednisolone e/c given | | AC | |
| 28.05.2008 | 06.09.1964 | F | | 1755 | 1801 | Script for Fluoxetine given | | ELB | |
| 28.05.2008 | 02.03.1957 | F | RTI | 1801 | 1806 | Chesty cough | Amoxycillin | EPS | |
| 28.05.2008 | 30.12.1952 | M | RTI | 1806 | 1811 | Chesty cough | Cefalexin | PBS | |
| 29.05.2008 | 25.03.1947 | F | | 942 | 953 | Script for Quinine Sulphate | | HER | |
| 29.05.2008 | 27.01.1934 | F | | 953 | 1016 | Script for Sodium chloride capsules | | JWC | |
| 29.05.2008 | 26.11.1929 | F | | 1016 | 1026 | Script for Carbomer 980 liquid eye drop gel & Prochlorperazine | | DEG | |
| 29.05.2008 | 08.03.1959 | F | | 1026 | 1032 | Referred to Rheumatologist regarding pain in both heels | | DM | |
| 29.05.2008 | 07.11.1968 | F | S/Leave | 1032 | 1038 | Stress - Med. 5 | | RGG | |
| 29.05.2008 | 09.03.1966 | M | | 1044 | 1052 | Referred to Oral Surgeon regarding the raised line in his mouth | | DM | |
| 29.05.2008 | 05.11.1924 | F | | 1100 | 1110 | Script for Co-codamol given | | BM | |

Result of a query that lists all consultations from the 22nd to the end of May 2008 (ConsultationsSeenFrom22ndTillEndOfMay2008)

| SurgeryDate | DateOfBirth | Sex | Diagnosis | TimeIn | TimeOut | Complaints | Treatments | Initials | Notes |
|---|---|---|---|---|---|---|---|---|---|
| 29.05.2008 | 25.01.1988 | F | RTI | 1110 | 1124 | Chesty cough | Amoxycillin | LB | Referred to Physiotherapist regarding back pain following RTA. |
| 29.05.2008 | 24.10.1990 | M | | 1124 | 1133 | Script for Amoxycillin & Metoclopramide given | | DKR | |
| 29.05.2008 | 03.04.1987 | F | | 1646 | 1654 | She brought in a Health Questionnaire to be completed (Lighter Life) | | LJP | |
| 29.05.2008 | 04.10.2002 | F | URTI | 1654 | 1659 | (R) ear ache | Erythromycin | TMM | Penicillin allergy. |
| 29.05.2008 | 21.10.1929 | F | | 1659 | 1703 | She had red rash on the legs which have now disappeared | | PMJ | |
| 29.05.2008 | 03.05.1944 | F | | 1703 | 1707 | Script for Tramadol capsules given | | JM | |
| 29.05.2008 | 09.08.1971 | M | | 1730 | 1738 | To take own Ibuprofen & analgesia for his coccyx pain | | JCW | |
| 29.05.2008 | 31.07.2006 | F | | 1743 | 1749 | Script for Fusidic acid with Hydrocortisone cream given | | MC | |
| 29.05.2008 | 03.03.1984 | M | | 1758 | 1810 | Script for Fusidic acid with Hydrocortisone cream given | | PWK | |
| 29.05.2008 | 15.06.1988 | M | | 1810 | 1827 | Script for Omeprazole given | | SK | Referred for Direct Access Gastroscopy. |

Result of a query that lists all consultations from the 22nd to the end of May 2008 (ConsultationsSeenFrom22ndTillEndOfMay2008)

| SurgeryDate | DateOfBirth | Sex | Diagnosis | TimeIn | TimeOut | Complaints | Treatments | Initials | Notes |
|---|---|---|---|---|---|---|---|---|---|
| 30.05.2008 | 01.04.1962 | F |  | 936 | 951 | Script for Hyoscine butylbromide given |  | TKC |  |
| 30.05.2008 | 04.09.1952 | M |  | 951 | 957 | Script for Flucloxacillin & Miconazole cream given |  | DJB |  |
| 30.05.2008 | 15.12.1972 | M |  | 957 | 1002 | For FBC & for CXR |  | LBJ |  |
| 30.05.2008 | 31.01.1941 | F |  | 1002 | 1011 | Referred to General Surgeon regarding her gall bladder stones |  | BFL |  |
| 30.05.2008 | 23.03.1926 | M |  | 1011 | 1029 | He brought in Alzheimer's helpline leaflet with view to being referred there which I explained to him was unlikely to be possible |  | JWH |  |
| 30.05.2008 | 29.12.1954 | F |  | 1029 | 1036 | To take own analgesia whilst waiting for the Physio. appointment for her back pain |  | PAK |  |
| 30.05.2008 | 19.06.1943 | M |  | 1036 | 1056 | Script for Oxybutynin given |  | BFS | For MSU, FBC, HbA1c, U/Es, LFTs, TFTs, Urine microalbumin screen & serum cholesterol. |
| 30.05.2008 | 24.08.1966 | M |  | 1056 | 1106 | He will come back later for his sick leave extension |  | IDG |  |

274

Result of a query that lists all consultations from the 22nd to the end of May 2008 (ConsultationsSeenFrom22ndTillEndOfMay2008)

| SurgeryDate | DateOfBirth | Sex | Diagnosis | TimeIn | TimeOut | Complaints | Treatments | Initials | Notes |
|---|---|---|---|---|---|---|---|---|---|
| 30.05.2008 | 07.11.1980 | M | URTI | 1106 | 1112 | (R) ear ache | Amoxycillin | DMB | |
| 30.05.2008 | 08.08.1918 | M | | 1112 | 1124 | Script for Furosemide given | | VHS | For CXR & for serum BNP. |
| 30.05.2008 | 11.12.1943 | F | | 1124 | 1150 | Script for Amoxycillin & Prednisolone e/c given | | PAH | |
| 30.05.2008 | 07.01.1944 | M | | 1524 | 1534 | Script for Lisinopril given | | JKC | Home visit. |

Result of a query that lists all consultations from the 22nd to the end of May 2009 (ConsultationsSeenFrom22ndTillEndOfMay2009)

| SurgeryDate | DateOfBirth | Sex | Diagnosis | TimeIn | TimeOut | Complaints | Treatments | Initials | Notes |
|---|---|---|---|---|---|---|---|---|---|
| 22.05.2009 | 22.03.1926 | M | | 928 | 958 | BP 138/68 | | JWH | |
| 22.05.2009 | 02.07.1937 | M | | 958 | 1002 | To see the nurse in 6 months for repeat serum Ferritin | | GG | |
| 22.05.2009 | 24.12.1962 | F | S/Leave | 1002 | 1012 | Medication Review Done | | CAW | |
| 22.05.2009 | 02.05.1949 | M | | 1012 | 1025 | Bilateral Hydrocele repair | | RB | Script for Bendroflumethiazide given. |
| 22.05.2009 | 07.09.1928 | M | | 1025 | 1030 | Medication Review Done | | LW | |
| 22.05.2009 | 05.03.1924 | M | | 1030 | 1039 | Script for Sildenafil "SLS" given | | CHD | |

**Result of a query that lists all consultations from the 22$^{nd}$ to the end of May 2009 (ConsultationsSeenFrom22ndTillEndOfMay2009)**

| SurgeryDate | DateOfBirth | Sex | Diagnosis | TimeIn | TimeOut | Complaints | Treatments | Initials | Notes |
|---|---|---|---|---|---|---|---|---|---|
| 22.05.2009 | 14.09.1962 | M | | 1039 | 1047 | Script for Omeprazole given | | SR | |
| 22.05.2009 | 10.05.1972 | F | | 1047 | 1058 | Her pelvic USScan was normal | | AC | |
| 22.05.2009 | 05.09.1933 | F | RTI | 1058 | 1111 | Chesty cough | Erythromycin | SMS | Script for Nystatin oral suspension given. Penicillin allergy. |

**Result of a query that lists all consultations from the 22$^{nd}$ to the end of May 2010 (ConsultationsSeenFrom22ndTillEndOfMay2010)**

| SurgeryDate | DateOfBirth | Sex | Diagnosis | TimeIn | TimeOut | Complaints | Treatments | Initials | Notes |
|---|---|---|---|---|---|---|---|---|---|
| 24.05.2010 | 08.04.1943 | M | RTI | 953 | 958 | Chesty cough | Amoxycillin | GM | Script for Otomize ear spray given. |
| 24.05.2010 | 05.06.1930 | F | | 958 | 1011 | Script for Betnovate cream, Quinine bisulphate & Sofradex eye drops given | | JMF | |
| 24.05.2010 | 08.04.1945 | M | | 1011 | 1020 | For X-Rays of the (L) shoulder | | GTW | |
| 24.05.2010 | 18.02.1956 | F | S/Leave | 1020 | 1041 | Med. 3 04/10 given for Hypertension from 21.05.10 for one week | | CJF | |
| 24.05.2010 | 25.01.1948 | F | | 1041 | 1052 | Script for Simvastatin given | | JW | |

Result of a query that lists all consultations from the 22nd to the end of May 2010 (ConsultationsSeenFrom22ndTillEndOfMay2010)

| SurgeryDate | DateOfBirth | Sex | Diagnosis | TimeIn | TimeOut | Complaints | Treatments | Initials | Notes |
|---|---|---|---|---|---|---|---|---|---|
| 24.05.2010 | 04.01.1967 | F | | 1052 | 1057 | Referred to Cardiologist for ECG as requested by the Neurologist | | MC | |
| 24.05.2010 | 15.12.1939 | M | | 1057 | 1103 | Medication Review Done | | ERC | |
| 24.05.2010 | 09.09.1993 | M | | 1103 | 1114 | Script for Amoxycillin given | | MPC | For FBC, U/Es & CRP. |
| 24.05.2010 | 02.12.1954 | M | | 1114 | 1142 | Referred to Endocrinologist (urgent) regarding his mild hyperthyroidism | | OAK | For Thyroid antibodies, PSA & USScan of the neck (urgent). |
| 24.05.2010 | 20.12.2009 | F | | 1142 | 1152 | Referred to Paediatric Dr. on call, SGH regarding her incessant screaming | | KL | |
| 24.05.2010 | 26.12.1947 | M | | 1152 | 1159 | Infected insect bit on his upper back | Flucloxacillin | RDG | |
| 24.05.2010 | 01.01.1953 | M | | 1646 | 1653 | Private script for Cialis given | | TPH | |
| 24.05.2010 | 23.08.1925 | F | | 1653 | 1705 | Medication Review Done | | REP | |
| 24.05.2010 | 17.07.1993 | F | | 1705 | 1715 | Script for Cetirizine given | | JHM | For Chest X-Rays. |
| 24.05.2010 | 29.09.1995 | M | | 1715 | 1720 | May need ENT Surgical future referral if he continues to cough up blood | | JSC | |

Result of a query that lists all consultations from the 22nd to the end of May 2010 (ConsultationsSeenFrom22ndTillEndOfMay2010)

| SurgeryDate | DateOfBirth | Sex | Diagnosis | TimeIn | TimeOut | Complaints | Treatments | Initials | Notes |
|---|---|---|---|---|---|---|---|---|---|
| 24.05.2010 | 11.09.1947 | M | | 1730 | 1736 | Script for Tramadol capsules given | | TSN | |
| 24.05.2010 | 18.11.1946 | F | | 1739 | 1750 | Referred to Orthopaedic Surgeon regarding pain at the back of the (L) knee | | JML | |
| 24.05.2010 | 23.06.1978 | F | | 1751 | 1811 | For X-Rays of the (R) wrist with Scaphoid views & for USScan of the pelvis (intravaginal) | | NPS | |
| 24.05.2010 | 31.08.1964 | M | | 1811 | 1815 | Script for Dihydrocodeine given | | CJW | |
| 25.05.2010 | 26.09.1937 | M | | 949 | 955 | For X-Rays of the Lumbar Spine & hips | | DJD | |
| 25.05.2010 | 06.05.1997 | M | RTI | 955 | 1001 | Barking cough | Erythromycin | DB | Penicillin allergy. |
| 25.05.2010 | 27.04.1928 | M | | 1001 | 1028 | Script for Citalopram & Macrogol compound half-strength oral powder sachets | | RFV | |
| 25.05.2010 | 17.08.1947 | F | | 1028 | 1036 | Referred to ENT Surgeon regarding her worsening hoarse voice | | SAA | |
| 25.05.2010 | 25.02.1920 | F | | 1036 | 1050 | Script for Co-phenotrope & Hyoscine butylbromide given | | RVC | |

Result of a query that lists all consultations from the 22nd to the end of May 2010 (ConsultationsSeenFrom22ndTillEndOfMay2010)

| SurgeryDate | DateOfBirth | Sex | Diagnosis | TimeIn | TimeOut | Complaints | Treatments | Initials | Notes |
|---|---|---|---|---|---|---|---|---|---|
| 25.05.2010 | 23.05.1952 | F |  | 1050 | 1054 | Medication Review Done |  | MEH |  |
| 25.05.2010 | 29.08.1924 | M |  | 1054 | 1104 | Medication Review Done |  | JFL |  |
| 25.05.2010 | 17.07.1981 | M | RTI | 1104 | 1109 | Chesty cough | Amoxycillin | BLW |  |
| 25.05.2010 | 30.03.1923 | M | RTI | 1134 | 1150 | Cough & has lost his voice | Ciprofloxacin | PGH | Home visit. |
| 25.05.2010 | 27.05.1941 | F |  | 1647 | 1652 | Script for Diclofenac e/c & Omeprazole given |  | MDR |  |
| 25.05.2010 | 08.08.1956 | M | S/Leave | 1652 | 1702 | Med. 3 04/10 given for Chest Infection for 2 weeks from 25.05.10 |  | JR |  |
| 25.05.2010 | 28.09.1959 | F |  | 1702 | 1708 | Referred to Rheumatologist regarding her multiple joints pains |  | CAS |  |
| 25.05.2010 | 26.03.1988 | M | S/Leave | 1708 | 1719 | Med. 3 04/10 given for Allergic Reaction to Zyban from 24.05.10 for one week |  | SL |  |
| 25.05.2010 | 01.12.1942 | M |  | 1719 | 1726 | Script for Prochlorperazine & Salbutamol inhaler given |  | MP |  |
| 25.05.2010 | 09.10.1949 | M |  | 1726 | 1746 | Medication Review Done |  | DS |  |
| 25.05.2010 | 17.04.1936 | M | RTI | 1746 | 1751 | Chesty cough | Ciprofloxacin | RB | Penicillin allergy. |

Result of a query that lists all consultations from the 22nd to the end of May 2010 (ConsultationsSeenFrom22ndTillEndOfMay2010)

| SurgeryDate | DateOfBirth | Sex | Diagnosis | TimeIn | TimeOut | Complaints | Treatments | Initials | Notes |
|---|---|---|---|---|---|---|---|---|---|
| 25.05.2010 | 26.08.1982 | M | S/Leave | 1751 | 1759 | Med. 3 04/10 given for Stress from 25.05.10 for 6 months | | BLS | |
| 25.05.2010 | 14.11.1963 | F | | 1759 | 1805 | Vomiting | Buccastem | SJK | |
| 25.05.2010 | 08.12.2000 | F | | 1805 | 1810 | To apply Calamine lotion for her rash | | EL | |
| 26.05.2010 | 23.12.1942 | F | | 942 | 957 | Referred to General Surgeon regarding possible epigastric incisional hernia | | JAP | Script for Amoxycillin given. |
| 26.05.2010 | 28.07.1957 | F | | 957 | 1007 | Script for Baclofen given | | MES | |
| 26.05.2010 | 07.10.1933 | M | | 1007 | 1010 | Script for Olanzapine given | | FDF | |
| 26.05.2010 | 25.04.1951 | F | | 1010 | 1029 | Script for Amorolfine 5% paint, Gliclazide & Lisinopril given | | SM | |
| 26.05.2010 | 21.08.1946 | F | | 1029 | 1034 | Referred to ENT Surgeon regarding recurrent throat infections | | JK | Script for Prochlorperazine given. |
| 26.05.2010 | 06.06.1961 | M | | 1034 | 1041 | Script for Citalopram given | | LG | |
| 26.05.2010 | 15.01.1935 | F | | 1041 | 1046 | Infected insect bite on the (R) lower leg | Flucloxacillin | JRS | |
| 26.05.2010 | 29.03.1930 | M | | 1049 | 1101 | Script for Co-codamol given | | EDT | |

Result of a query that lists all consultations from the 22nd to the end of May 2010 (ConsultationsSeenFrom22ndTillEndOfMay2010)

| SurgeryDate | DateOfBirth | Sex | Diagnosis | TimeIn | TimeOut | Complaints | Treatments | Initials | Notes |
|---|---|---|---|---|---|---|---|---|---|
| 26.05.2010 | 23.04.1923 | F | | 1101 | 1112 | Script for Doxepin & Temazepam given | | JD | |
| 26.05.2010 | 20.02.2004 | M | Conjunctivitis | 1112 | 1116 | Sticky eyes | Chloramphenicol eye drops | BJW | |
| 26.05.2010 | 12.10.2000 | M | | 1646 | 1655 | Script for Loratadine given | | LJDL | |
| 26.05.2010 | 23.04.2007 | M | | 1655 | 1703 | Referred to Paediatrician regarding pain in his penis & scrotal area | | HB | |
| 26.05.2010 | 20.11.1965 | M | | 1709 | 1718 | To have the testicular scan as arranged | | PJJ | |
| 26.05.2010 | 28.12.1962 | M | URTI | 1718 | 1728 | (L) ear ache | Amoxycillin & Otomize ear spray | KF | Script for Chloramphenicol eye drops given. |
| 26.05.2010 | 25.02.1975 | M | | 1728 | 1737 | Referred to Dermatologist regarding red bleeding spot on the (R) side of the chest | | GHD | Referred to Orthopaedic Surgeon regarding ganglion on the (R) wrist. For USScan of the upper abdomen. |
| 26.05.2010 | 23.04.1950 | F | | 1744 | 1749 | For X-Rays of the (R) shoulder | | PEH | |
| 26.05.2010 | 06.02.1944 | M | | 1749 | 1759 | To contact the Microbiology lab. regarding the result of his Hepatitis B status | | AMC | |

Result of a query that lists all consultations from the 22nd to the end of May 2010 (ConsultationsSeenFrom22ndTillEndOfMay2010)

| SurgeryDate | DateOfBirth | Sex | Diagnosis | TimeIn | TimeOut | Complaints | Treatments | Initials | Notes |
|---|---|---|---|---|---|---|---|---|---|
| 26.05.2010 | 02.06.1994 | F | | 1759 | 1804 | Referred to Podiatrist regarding her bilateral bunions | | EPB | |
| 27.05.2010 | 18.07.1978 | F | | 948 | 953 | Script for Norethisterone given | | TJS | |
| 27.05.2010 | 28.08.1946 | F | | 953 | 1001 | Referred to Dermatologist regarding multiple moles & blemishes on her skin | | VAG | |
| 27.05.2010 | 06.01.1955 | M | | 1001 | 1007 | Private script for Viagra given | | MAS | |
| 27.05.2010 | 03.08.1935 | M | | 1007 | 1019 | Script for Folic acid given | | RH | |
| 27.05.2010 | 14.04.2007 | M | RTI | 1019 | 1024 | Chesty cough | Amoxycillin | JJH | |
| 27.05.2010 | 23.05.1932 | M | | 1027 | 1037 | Script for Amitriptyline given | | EB | |
| 27.05.2010 | 01.01.1924 | M | | 1052 | 1102 | Referred to Haematologist regarding his persistently abnormal FBC results | | HAJB | |
| 27.05.2010 | 20.04.1927 | F | | 1102 | 1127 | Referred to Nephrologist regarding abnormal U/Es, Stage 4 CKD | | MW | Script for Allopurinol, Ibuprofen & Omeprazole given. |
| 27.05.2010 | 13.04.1942 | M | | 1127 | 1150 | Script for Otomize ear spray given | | HJM | For U/Es, B12, Folate & Ferritin. |

Result of a query that lists all consultations from the 22nd to the end of May 2010 (ConsultationsSeenFrom22ndTillEndOfMay2010)

| SurgeryDate | DateOfBirth | Sex | Diagnosis | TimeIn | TimeOut | Complaints | Treatments | Initials | Notes |
|---|---|---|---|---|---|---|---|---|---|
| 27.05.2010 | 31.10.1915 | F | | 1403 | 1422 | Script for BuTrans patches given | | MEC | Home visit. |
| 27.05.2010 | 26.10.1961 | M | | 1650 | 1707 | Referred to Cardiologist regarding his collapse & atrial fibrillation noted on his ECG | | CB | For Chest X-Rays, FBC, U/Es, Fasting Glucose, Fasting Lipids, CRP, TFTs & LFTs. |
| 27.05.2010 | 15.12.1935 | F | | 1707 | 1716 | For FBC, U/Es, TFTs, Cholesterol, LFTs & Fasting Glucose | | DL | |
| 27.05.2010 | 01.01.1936 | F | | 1716 | 1729 | Script for Folic acid & Omeprazole given | | ALC | |
| 27.05.2010 | 10.08.1952 | F | | 1729 | 1740 | Script for Metformin & Quinine Sulphate given | | SAG | |
| 27.05.2010 | 15.01.2001 | F | | 1740 | 1748 | Possible scabies rash on the legs | Lyclear Dermal cream | HLA | |
| 27.05.2010 | 15.09.1964 | F | | 1748 | 1758 | Script for Hyoscine butylbromide given | | TP | For USScan of the abdomen & Pelvis. |
| 27.05.2010 | 20.10.1953 | M | | 1758 | 1804 | Script for Flucloxacillin given | | PJH | |
| 27.05.2010 | 04.03.1963 | M | | 1804 | 1809 | For X-Rays of the (R) knee | | NDC | |
| 27.05.2010 | 20.12.2009 | F | | 1809 | 1818 | Script for Erythromycin given | | KL | Penicillin allergy. |
| 27.05.2010 | 17.03.1967 | M | | 1818 | 1830 | For X-Rays of the (R) shoulder | | TCS | Referred to Physiotherapist regarding pain in the (R) shoulder. |

Result of a query that lists all consultations from the 22nd to the end of May 2010 (ConsultationsSeenFrom22ndTillEndOfMay2010)

| SurgeryDate | DateOfBirth | Sex | Diagnosis | TimeIn | TimeOut | Complaints | Treatments | Initials | Notes |
|---|---|---|---|---|---|---|---|---|---|
| 28.05.2010 | 12.08.1936 | M | | 928 | 938 | Referred to Ophthalmologist regarding the wavy vision in his (R) eye when he closes his (L) eye | | RHP | |
| 28.05.2010 | 29.08.1939 | M | | 938 | 1004 | General discussion around him developing hypothyroidism & what to do about it explained to him | | JFP | |
| 28.05.2010 | 09.09.1993 | M | | 1004 | 1014 | For letter to whom it may concern regarding his recent neck swelling | | MPC | |
| 28.05.2010 | 22.04.1957 | M | S/Leave | 1014 | 1023 | Med. 3 04/10 given for Injury to the (R) knee from 28.05.10 for 3 months | | PJT | |
| 28.05.2010 | 01.10.1937 | F | | 1023 | 1034 | Medication Review Done | | SGE | |
| 28.05.2010 | 28.10.1930 | F | | 1034 | 1041 | Script for Erythromycin & Sodium Cromoglicate eye drops given | | KBC | |
| 28.05.2010 | 23.05.1927 | M | | 1041 | 1054 | Script for Oral rehydration salts oral powder given | | JM | Stool for C&S. |

## Result of a query that lists all consultations from the 22nd to the end of May 2010 (ConsultationsSeenFrom22ndTillEndOfMay2010)

| SurgeryDate | DateOfBirth | Sex | Diagnosis | TimeIn | TimeOut | Complaints | Treatments | Initials | Notes |
|---|---|---|---|---|---|---|---|---|---|
| 28.05.2010 | 31.10.1951 | F | | 1054 | 1100 | Script for Amoxycillin & Prochlorperazine given | | BAL | |
| 28.05.2010 | 31.01.2006 | M | | 1100 | 1106 | Balanitis | Trimethoprim | EWD | |

## Result of a query that lists all consultations from the 22nd to the end of May 2011 (ConsultationsSeenFrom22ndTillEndOfMay2011)

| SurgeryDate | DateOfBirth | Sex | Diagnosis | TimeIn | TimeOut | Complaints | Treatments | Initials | Notes |
|---|---|---|---|---|---|---|---|---|---|
| 23.05.2011 | 03.05.1946 | F | | 944 | 952 | Medication Review Done | | JP | |
| 23.05.2011 | 13.01.1957 | F | | 952 | 1005 | Script for Chloramphenicol eye drops, Mycophenolate, Oramorph, Paracetamol, Prednisolone e/c & Zopiclone given | | PAW | |
| 23.05.2011 | 11.08.1935 | F | | 1005 | 1019 | Script for Adcal-D3 Dissolve & Alendronic acid given | | CH | |
| 23.05.2011 | 27.04.1925 | M | | 1019 | 1031 | Medication Review Done | | RWF | |
| 23.05.2011 | 25.11.1949 | M | | 1031 | 1041 | Referred to Rheumatologist regarding pain in the base of both thumbs | | GJD | |

Result of a query that lists all consultations from the 22nd to the end of May 2011 (ConsultationsSeenFrom22ndTillEndOfMay2011)

| SurgeryDate | DateOfBirth | Sex | Diagnosis | TimeIn | TimeOut | Complaints | Treatments | Initials | Notes |
|---|---|---|---|---|---|---|---|---|---|
| 23.05.2011 | 06.01.1943 | F | | 1041 | 1051 | Script for Levothyroxine given | | PC | |
| 23.05.2011 | 27.01.1934 | F | | 1051 | 1058 | Medication Review Done | | JWC | |
| 23.05.2011 | 23.03.1926 | M | | 1058 | 1115 | Medication Review Done | | JWH | |
| 23.05.2011 | 12.06.1943 | M | | 1643 | 1652 | Script for Ferrous Fumarate given | | PB | |
| 23.05.2011 | 03.05.1981 | F | | 1652 | 1657 | Medication Review Done | | KLS | |
| 23.05.2011 | 09.07.1940 | M | | 1712 | 1740 | Medication Review Done | | WW | |
| 23.05.2011 | 26.09.2003 | F | | 1740 | 1746 | Stool for C&S | | ENF | |
| 23.05.2011 | 04.04.1938 | M | | 1746 | 1751 | Medication Review Done | | DB | |
| 23.05.2011 | 29.04.1937 | M | | 1751 | 1800 | Referred to Cardiologist regarding fainting episodes | | PGS | |
| 23.05.2011 | 20.04.1945 | F | | 1800 | 1808 | Script for Amoxycillin & Paracetamol given | | KCY | |
| 23.05.2011 | 05.03.1972 | M | S/Leave | 1808 | 1823 | Med. 3 04/10 given for Abdominal Pain & Depression from 20.05.11 for 3 months | | WDJGW | Script for Mirtazapine given |
| 23.05.2011 | 07.02.1911 | M | | 1823 | 1836 | Referred to Paediatrician regarding his grossly enlarging head circumference | | NDM | |

Result of a query that lists all consultations from the 22nd to the end of May 2011 (ConsultationsSeenFrom22ndTillEndOfMay2011)

| SurgeryDate | DateOfBirth | Sex | Diagnosis | TimeIn | TimeOut | Complaints | Treatments | Initials | Notes |
|---|---|---|---|---|---|---|---|---|---|
| 24.05.2011 | 17.03.1958 | M | | 944 | 1005 | Script for Candesartan & Co-codamol given | | KEW | |
| 24.05.2011 | 12.08.1936 | M | | 1005 | 1012 | Referred to Urologist regarding the large simple cyst noted on the lower pole of the (L) kidney on USScan of the abdomen | | RHP | |
| 24.05.2011 | 02.02.1975 | F | | 1012 | 1024 | Referred to Gynaecologist regarding the persistent (R) sided pelvic lower abdominal pain | | SAB | |
| 24.05.2011 | 14.02.1952 | M | S/Leave | 1024 | 1032 | Med. 3 04/10 given for (R) Shoulder & (R) carpal tunnel decompressions from 24.05.2011 for one month | | BHCH | |
| 24.05.2011 | 24.05.1976 | F | RTI | 1032 | 1038 | Chesty cough | Amoxycillin | HCLE | |
| 24.05.2011 | 07.10.1933 | M | | 1038 | 1044 | Script for Ferrous sulphate given | | FDF | For FBC & serum Ferritin. |
| 24.05.2011 | 06.04.1924 | F | | 1044 | 1051 | Medication Review Done | | EAS | |

Result of a query that lists all consultations from the 22nd to the end of May 2011 (ConsultationsSeenFrom22ndTillEndOfMay2011)

| SurgeryDate | DateOfBirth | Sex | Diagnosis | TimeIn | TimeOut | Complaints | Treatments | Initials | Notes |
|---|---|---|---|---|---|---|---|---|---|
| 24.05.2011 | 01.06.1947 | F | | 1051 | 1058 | Referred to Orthopaedic Surgeon regarding consideration for (L) THR as advised by the Orthopaedic surgeon | | VP | |
| 24.05.2011 | 13.11.2004 | F | | 1058 | 1108 | Referred to Orthopaedic Surgeon regarding pain on plantar flexing the (R) foot after injury on a trampoline | | EP | |
| 24.05.2011 | 11.03.1968 | F | | 1645 | 1703 | Script for Oxybutynin given | | EJA | For Pelvic USScan. |
| 24.05.2011 | 17.10.1997 | M | | 1703 | 1709 | For X-Rays of the (R) knee | | ORAG | |
| 24.05.2011 | 15.03.1984 | F | | 1709 | 1719 | Medication Review Done | | SLL | |
| 24.05.2011 | 12.02.1996 | M | | 1719 | 1724 | Script for Amoxycillin given | | JW | Referred to ENT Surgeon regarding his recurrent congested sinuses. |
| 24.05.2011 | 23.03.1967 | F | | 1724 | 1732 | Script for Amoxycillin & Neomycin/ chlorhexidine cream given | | TPW | |
| 24.05.2011 | 15.07.1956 | M | | 1732 | 1738 | Infected insect bite on (R) fore-arm | Flucloxacillin | DHC | |

Result of a query that lists all consultations from the 22nd to the end of May 2011 (ConsultationsSeenFrom22ndTillEndOfMay2011)

| SurgeryDate | DateOfBirth | Sex | Diagnosis | TimeIn | TimeOut | Complaints | Treatments | Initials | Notes |
|---|---|---|---|---|---|---|---|---|---|
| 24.05.2011 | 14.09.1980 | M | | 1747 | 1804 | For FBC, U/Es, TFTs, LFTs, Fasting Glucose & Fasting Cholesterol | | LH | |
| 25.05.2011 | 02.01.1952 | F | | 949 | 1002 | Script for Levothyroxine, Quinine Sulphate & Simvastatin given | | PAD | |
| 25.05.2011 | 03.07.1945 | F | | 1002 | 1006 | Medication Review Done | | ES | |
| 25.05.2011 | 31.01.1941 | F | | 1006 | 1020 | Medication Review Done | | JAE | |
| 25.05.2011 | 24.12.1972 | M | | 1020 | 1028 | Referred to ENT Surgeon regarding the maxillary sinus retention cysts noted on his MRI scan & as advised by the Neurologist | | SS | |
| 25.05.2011 | 31.01.1969 | F | S/Leave | 1030 | 1043 | Med. 3 04/10 given for Throat infection and Dizziness from 25.05.11 for 2 weeks | | JP | Script for Amoxycillin & Venlalic XL given. |
| 25.05.2011 | 22.05.1931 | F | | 1043 | 1051 | For USScan of the Abdomen (urgent) | | DK | |
| 25.05.2011 | 23.04.2007 | M | URTI | 1051 | 1057 | Sore throat | Amoxycillin | HB | |
| 25.05.2011 | 14.05.1923 | M | | 1057 | 1105 | Referred to Physiotherapist regarding (L) shoulder pain | | AM | |

Result of a query that lists all consultations from the 22nd to the end of May 2011 (ConsultationsSeenFrom22ndTillEndOfMay2011)

| SurgeryDate | DateOfBirth | Sex | Diagnosis | TimeIn | TimeOut | Complaints | Treatments | Initials | Notes |
|---|---|---|---|---|---|---|---|---|---|
| 25.05.2011 | 09.11.1967 | M | | 1105 | 1118 | Script for Codeine tablets given | | VEC | |
| 25.05.2011 | 07.06.1972 | M | | 1118 | 1122 | He will leave off steroid injection to his (L) shoulder as advised by the physiotherapist | | MJL | |
| 25.05.2011 | 27.02.1992 | M | | 1648 | 1658 | Referred to Physiotherapist regarding pain in the (R) hip region | | CPH | |
| 25.05.2011 | 11.09.1947 | M | | 1658 | 1708 | Script for Salicylic acid 26% solution given | | TSN | For FBC, U/Es & Fasting Glucose. |
| 25.05.2011 | 23.01.1947 | F | | 1708 | 1715 | For USScan of the abdomen (urgent) | | BW | |
| 25.05.2011 | 10.11.1976 | F | RTI | 1715 | 1723 | Chesty cough | Amoxycillin | DPS | |
| 25.05.2011 | 25.01.1955 | F | | 1723 | 1727 | Script for Co-phenotrope given | | CYR | |
| 25.05.2011 | 20.11.1936 | M | | 1727 | 1734 | Referred to General Surgeon regarding (R) direct inguinal hernia | | NN | |
| 25.05.2011 | 09.03.2006 | F | RTI | 1742 | 1748 | Chesty cough | Amoxycillin | IKR | |
| 25.05.2011 | 26.08.1982 | M | S/Leave | 1748 | 1754 | Med. 3 04/10 given for Stress from 25.05.11 for 12 months | | BLS | |

Result of a query that lists all consultations from the 22nd to the end of May 2011 (ConsultationsSeenFrom22ndTillEndOfMay2011)

| SurgeryDate | DateOfBirth | Sex | Diagnosis | TimeIn | TimeOut | Complaints | Treatments | Initials | Notes |
|---|---|---|---|---|---|---|---|---|---|
| 25.05.2011 | 24.12.1972 | F | | 1756 | 1801 | Referred to Dermatologist regarding mole on (R) side of her chest | | CC | |
| 26.05.2011 | 15.04.1951 | F | S/Leave | 945 | 955 | Med. 3 04/10 given for Pelvic floor repair from 19.05.11 for 3 months | | MM | |
| 26.05.2011 | 05.03.1972 | M | | 955 | 1055 | Script for Mirtazapine given | | WDJGW | |
| 26.05.2011 | 21.11.1948 | M | | 1005 | 1022 | Patient informed that he has Diabetes mellitus | | PCB | |
| 26.05.2011 | 10.01.2010 | F | | 1022 | 1032 | Script for Aveeno cream, Ibuprofen & Amoxycillin given | | SMH | |
| 26.05.2011 | 17.04.1923 | M | | 1032 | 1042 | Script for Temazepam given | | JWD | |
| 26.05.2011 | 09.04.1944 | F | | 1042 | 1053 | Medication Review Done | | JN | |
| 26.05.2011 | 07.02.1948 | M | | 1053 | 1059 | Infected insect bite | Flucloxacillin | GRC | |
| 26.05.2011 | 18.04.1978 | F | | 1059 | 1104 | Medication Review Done | | SL | |
| 26.05.2011 | 31.07.1961 | F | | 1645 | 1658 | Script for Norethisterone given | | CMW | For FBC, U/Es, B12, Folate, Ferritin & FSH. |
| 26.05.2011 | 21.05.1958 | F | | 1658 | 1703 | Script for Dixarit & Hydrocortisone/ Miconazole cream given | | SB | |

Result of a query that lists all consultations from the 22nd to the end of May 2011 (ConsultationsSeenFrom22ndTillEndOfMay2011)

| SurgeryDate | DateOfBirth | Sex | Diagnosis | TimeIn | TimeOut | Complaints | Treatments | Initials | Notes |
|---|---|---|---|---|---|---|---|---|---|
| 26.05.2011 | 23.04.1950 | F | | 1703 | 1707 | Script for Hydrocortisone/ Fusidic acid cream given | | PEH | |
| 26.05.2011 | 10.03.2004 | M | | 1707 | 1715 | Script for Salicylic acid 26% solution given | | CJCCB | Referred to Child Psychiatrist regarding his obstructive behaviour. |
| 26.05.2011 | 10.08.1963 | M | S/Leave | 1725 | 1733 | Med. 3 04/10 given for (R) Cataract operation for 2 months from 21.05.11 | | FN | Script for Carmellose 0.5% eye drops given. |
| 26.05.2011 | 03.12.1989 | F | | 1733 | 1741 | For USScan of the abdomen | | EDB | |
| 26.05.2011 | 11.08.2000 | M | | 1741 | 1747 | Cellulitis (L) ear lobe after piercing ear | Flucloxacillin | CALB | |
| 26.05.2011 | 14.11.1963 | F | S/Leave | 1753 | 1807 | Med. 3 04/10 given for Abdominal distension for one week from 25.05.11 | | SJK | Script for Omeprazole given. |
| 27.05.2011 | 09.10.1926 | M | | 931 | 941 | Referred to Nephrologist regarding recurrence of his nephrotic syndrome | | RAC | |
| 27.05.2011 | 24.03.1973 | M | S/Leave | 941 | 947 | Med. 3 04/10 given for Pain in the (R) foot for one week from 23.05.11 | | JCM | |

Result of a query that lists all consultations from the 22nd to the end of May 2011 (ConsultationsSeenFrom22ndTillEndOfMay2011)

| SurgeryDate | DateOfBirth | Sex | Diagnosis | TimeIn | TimeOut | Complaints | Treatments | Initials | Notes |
|---|---|---|---|---|---|---|---|---|---|
| 27.05.2011 | 10.03.1936 | M | URTI | 956 | 1005 | Sore throat | Amoxycillin | TCC | |
| 27.05.2011 | 18.02.1956 | F | | 1005 | 1013 | Referred to One stop Breast clinic regarding her ache at the back of her (L) breast | | CJF | |
| 27.05.2011 | 09.08.1927 | F | | 1013 | 1020 | Medication Review Done | | SW | |
| 27.05.2011 | 19.08.1939 | F | | 1020 | 1037 | Referred to One stop Haematuria clinic regarding her persistent microscopic haematuria | | JEN | Script for |
| 27.05.2011 | 05.06.2010 | M | | 1037 | 1043 | Referred to Paediatrician regarding his persistent chesty cough at night when he lies down | | EM | |
| 27.05.2011 | 27.07.1948 | M | | 1043 | 1054 | Script for Bendroflumethiazide & Lisinopril given | | BAG | |
| 27.05.2011 | 27.08.1935 | M | | 1054 | 1102 | Script for Sudocrem given | | AAS | His wife came to the Surgery. |

Result of a query that lists all consultations from the 22nd to the end of May 2012 (ConsultationsSeenFrom22ndTillEndOfMay2012)

| SurgeryDate | DateOfBirth | Sex | Diagnosis | TimeIn | TimeOut | Complaints | Treatments | Initials | Notes |
|---|---|---|---|---|---|---|---|---|---|
| 23.05.2012 | 23.01.1926 | F | | 945 | 953 | Script for Prochlorperazine given | | FGN | |
| 23.05.2012 | 16.03.1956 | F | | 956 | 1007 | To see the nurse for asthma check | | SPD | |
| 23.05.2012 | 25.12.1944 | M | | 1007 | 1020 | Referred to ENT Surgeon regarding the feeling of wanting to clear his throat all the time | | CDC | Referred to Dermatologist regarding the macular rash on the (R) fore-arm. |
| 23.05.2012 | 27.10.1960 | F | S/Leave | 1020 | 1029 | Med. 3 04/10 given for Back Pain from 22.05.12 for 3 months | | DLK | Referred to Physiotherapist regarding exacerbation of her ongoing back pain. Script for Co-dydramol & Oramorph given. |
| 23.05.2012 | 26.04.1944 | F | | 1029 | 1034 | Referred to Physiotherapist regarding her back pain | | AW | |
| 23.05.2012 | 04.08.1936 | M | | 1041 | 1047 | Script for Amoxycillin given | | ECM | |
| 23.05.2012 | 03.05.1944 | F | | 1047 | 1052 | Referred to Physiotherapist regarding her persistent (R) elbow pain | | JM | |
| 23.05.2012 | 04.11.1966 | F | | 1052 | 1057 | Script for Ferrous Fumarate given | | SJOB | |

Result of a query that lists all consultations from the 22nd to the end of May 2012 (ConsultationsSeenFrom22ndTillEndOfMay2012)

| SurgeryDate | DateOfBirth | Sex | Diagnosis | TimeIn | TimeOut | Complaints | Treatments | Initials | Notes |
|---|---|---|---|---|---|---|---|---|---|
| 23.05.2012 | 08.01.1972 | M | | 1100 | 1107 | To contact the Cardiologist regarding his missed appointment | | EM | |
| 23.05.2012 | 18.03.1967 | F | | 1635 | 1648 | Script for Transvasin Heat Rub cream given | | SO | |
| 23.05.2012 | 03.02.1957 | M | | 1648 | 1705 | BP 135/76 | | ER | |
| 23.05.2012 | 23.03.1967 | F | | 1705 | 1720 | Script for Fucidin H cream given | | TPW | |
| 23.05.2012 | 12.02.1996 | M | | 1720 | 1726 | Script for Fucidin H cream & Amoxycillin given | | JW | |
| 23.05.2012 | 05.10.1974 | M | | 1726 | 1735 | For KUB USScan | | SMG | |
| 23.05.2012 | 04.09.1967 | M | | 1735 | 1743 | to see the nurse in 6 months for repeat U/Es & serum cholesterol | | DPM | |
| 23.05.2012 | 31.05.1967 | M | RTI | 1743 | 1751 | Chesty cough | Ciprofloxacin | GKP | Penicillin & Erythromycin allergy. |
| 23.05.2012 | 10.12.1986 | F | RTI | 1751 | 1756 | Chesty cough | Amoxycillin | HEB | |
| 23.05.2012 | 18.04.1957 | F | | 1756 | 1810 | Script for Janumet given | | SK | |
| 24.05.2012 | 22.02.1944 | M | | 948 | 1001 | Script for Nortriptyline given | | AS | Referred to Orthopaedic Surgeon regarding his back pain & pain in the (L) leg. |

Result of a query that lists all consultations from the 22nd to the end of May 2012 (ConsultationsSeenFrom22ndTillEndOfMay2012)

| SurgeryDate | DateOfBirth | Sex | Diagnosis | TimeIn | TimeOut | Complaints | Treatments | Initials | Notes |
|---|---|---|---|---|---|---|---|---|---|
| 24.05.2012 | 18.01.1977 | F | | 1001 | 1006 | Med. 3 04/10 given for Depression from 22.05.12 for 3 months | | MP | |
| 24.05.2012 | 14.11.1959 | M | | 1006 | 1014 | Script for Salbutamol inhaler given | | PBD | For Chest X-Rays. |
| 24.05.2012 | 13.04.1942 | M | | 1014 | 1026 | Script for Furosemide given | | HJM | |
| 24.05.2012 | 15.12.1939 | M | | 1026 | 1040 | Script for Ferrous fumarate, Senna & Simvastatin given | | ERC | Referred to Dermatologist regarding possible BCC lesions on his neck & (L) thigh. |
| 24.05.2012 | 24.03.1977 | M | S/Leave | 1040 | 1045 | Med. 3 04/10 given for Depression from 21.05.12 for 1 week | | JCM | |
| 24.05.2012 | 07.03.1958 | M | | 1045 | 1051 | Referred to Physiotherapist regarding pain in his (R) shoulder & neck | | JDP | |
| 24.05.2012 | 27.03.1931 | F | | 1051 | 1059 | Script for Ferrous fumarate given | | MMA | |
| 24.05.2012 | 24.09.1930 | F | | 1110 | 1140 | For USScan of the abdomen | | JMC | |
| 24.05.2012 | 08.04.1945 | M | | 1642 | 1652 | Cryotherapy to warts on the (R) hand | | GTW | For X-Rays of the (R) hip & the (R) knee. |
| 24.05.2012 | 02.04.1987 | F | | 1652 | 1700 | For Pelvic USScan | | NTNW | |

**Result of a query that lists all consultations from the 22nd to the end of May 2012 (ConsultationsSeenFrom22ndTillEndOfMay2012)**

| SurgeryDate | DateOfBirth | Sex | Diagnosis | TimeIn | TimeOut | Complaints | Treatments | Initials | Notes |
|---|---|---|---|---|---|---|---|---|---|
| 24.05.2012 | 16.10.1996 | F | | 1700 | 1712 | Cryotherapy to wars on the (L) index finger | | YM | Script for Flucloxacillin given. |
| 24.05.2012 | 03.05.1996 | F | | 1712 | 1719 | Script for Duac gel & Flucloxacillin given | | EMH | |
| 24.05.2012 | 30.05.2007 | M | | 1719 | 1725 | Referred to Paediatrician regarding his speech impediment | | LFK | |
| 24.05.2012 | 13.10.1955 | F | S/Leave | 1782 | 1744 | Med. 3 04/10 given for (R) knee arthroscopy & debridement from 20.05.12 until 22.05.12 | | TK | Script for Xenical given. |
| 24.05.2012 | 02.12.1954 | M | | 1744 | 1809 | Script for Lansoprazole given | | OAK | |
| 24.05.2012 | 30.09.1961 | M | | 1810 | 1816 | Script for Canesten HC cream, Zineryt lotion & Flucloxacillin given | | IMB | |
| 24.05.2012 | 12.05.1990 | M | | 1816 | 1821 | Script for Amoxycillin, Budesonide nasal spray, Cetirizine tablets & Sodium cromoglicate eye drops given | | APS | |

Result of a query that lists all consultations from the 22nd to the end of May 2012 (ConsultationsSeenFrom22ndTillEndOfMay2012)

| SurgeryDate | DateOfBirth | Sex | Diagnosis | TimeIn | TimeOut | Complaints | Treatments | Initials | Notes |
|---|---|---|---|---|---|---|---|---|---|
| 24.05.2012 | 17.09.1977 | F | | 1821 | 1826 | Pregnancy test negative | | NJS | |
| 25.05.2012 | 09.09.2006 | M | | 947 | 956 | Script for Amoxycillin given | | JWCC | |
| 25.05.2012 | 27.07.1948 | M | | 956 | 1002 | Script for Co-codamol & Diprosalic ointment given | | BAG | |
| 25.05.2012 | 15.10.1969 | F | S/Leave | 1002 | 1018 | Med. 3 04/10 given for Fractured (L) ring finger from 25.05.12 for 2 weeks | | MAC | |
| 25.05.2012 | 13.01.1966 | M | | 1018 | 1026 | Script for Canesten HC cream given | | PJB | For FBC, U/Es, LFTs, serum cholesterol & fasting Glucose. |
| 25.05.2012 | 11.12.1944 | F | | 1026 | 1034 | For USScan of the abdomen | | GMW | |
| 25.05.2012 | 14.08.1935 | M | | 1036 | 1044 | Script for Amitripyline, Flucloxacillin & Metrogel given | | RAT | |
| 25.05.2012 | 22.02.2012 | M | | 1047 | 1056 | Script for Sunsense daily face cream given | | RNEL | |
| 25.05.2012 | 21.02.1961 | F | | 1056 | 1102 | Script for Trimethoprim given | | CHO | For Chest X-Rays. |
| 25.05.2012 | 02.06.1955 | F | | 1102 | 1111 | Script for Fluoxetine given | | JPS | |

Result of a query that lists all consultations from the 22nd to the end of May 2012 (ConsultationsSeenFrom22ndTillEndOfMay2012)

| SurgeryDate | DateOfBirth | Sex | Diagnosis | TimeIn | TimeOut | Complaints | Treatments | Initials | Notes |
|---|---|---|---|---|---|---|---|---|---|
| 28.05.2012 | 09.10.1926 | M | | 946 | 957 | Script for Prochlorperazine given | | RAC | |
| 28.05.2012 | 03.10.1941 | M | | 957 | 1005 | Script for Flucloxacillin given | | JJD | |
| 28.05.2012 | 01.03.1947 | M | | 1005 | 1010 | For X-Rays of the hips | | JRW | |
| 28.05.2012 | 13.04.1985 | F | | 1010 | 1025 | Script for Fluoxetine, Quetiapine & Zopiclone given | | CLA | For FBC, U/Es, fasting Glucose, Fasting lipids, B12, Folate, LFTs & Ferritin. |
| 28.05.2012 | 01.06.1947 | F | | 1025 | 1030 | Script for Lansoprazole given | | VP | |
| 28.05.2012 | 08.10.1961 | M | | 1030 | 1036 | For X-Rays of the (L) wrist with scaphoid views | | GRL | |
| 28.05.2012 | 27.05.1954 | F | | 1036 | 1045 | She will come back later for extension of her sick leave | | CAA | |
| 28.05.2012 | 16.09.1989 | F | | 1049 | 1057 | Script for Amoxycillin & Fucidin H cream given | | SLW | For Chest X-Rays. |
| 28.05.2012 | 18.02.1968 | F | | 1057 | 1107 | Script for Co-Amoxiclav & Olopatadine eye drops given | | DG | |
| 28.05.2012 | 31.01.1969 | F | | 1409 | 1427 | Script for Amoxycillin & Stemetil given | | JP | Home visit. |

Result of a query that lists all consultations from the 22nd to the end of May 2012 (ConsultationsSeenFrom22ndTillEndOfMay2012)

| SurgeryDate | DateOfBirth | Sex | Diagnosis | TimeIn | TimeOut | Complaints | Treatments | Initials | Notes |
|---|---|---|---|---|---|---|---|---|---|
| 28.05.2012 | 14.04.1946 | F | | 1640 | 1649 | Script for Fucidin H cream given | | VBB | |
| 28.05.2012 | 23.04.1923 | F | | 1649 | 1658 | Script for Furosemide & Temazepam given | | JD | |
| 28.05.2012 | 08.04.1942 | M | | 1658 | 1706 | Script for Ketoconazole shampoo & Loratadine given | | GFT | |
| 28.05.2012 | 20.03.1959 | F | | 1706 | 1720 | Script for Flucloxacillin & Naproxen given | | TS | |
| 28.05.2012 | 22.06.1955 | M | | 1722 | 1733 | Script for Canesten HC cream & Nizoral shampoo given | | MT | |
| 28.05.2012 | 29.06.1985 | M | | 1759 | 1814 | Referred to Dermatologist regarding the raised mole on his (R) fore-arm | | JLO | |
| 29.05.2012 | 06.05.1929 | F | | 954 | 1000 | Script for Curanail given | | JAE | |
| 29.05.2012 | 22.02.1963 | M | S/Leave | 1002 | 1013 | Med. 3 04/10 given for Back Pain from 07.05.12 for 3 weeks | | JBP | Referred to Physiotherapist regarding his back pain. |
| 29.05.2012 | 21.04.1949 | M | | 1013 | 1028 | Script for Co-codamol given | | RL | For USScan of the neck lump. |

300

## Result of a query that lists all consultations from the 22nd to the end of May 2012 (ConsultationsSeenFrom22ndTillEndOfMay2012)

| SurgeryDate | DateOfBirth | Sex | Diagnosis | TimeIn | TimeOut | Complaints | Treatments | Initials | Notes |
|---|---|---|---|---|---|---|---|---|---|
| 29.05.2012 | 26.08.1962 | F | | 1033 | 1056 | Script for Metformin given | | HD | For X-Rays of the (R) hand & (R) wrist with scaphoid views. |
| 29.05.2012 | 24.07.1956 | M | URTI | 1056 | 1100 | Sore throat | Amoxycillin | SS | |
| 29.05.2012 | 23.09.1936 | M | | 1100 | 1112 | Script for Co-codamol, Nystatin suspension, Omeprazole & Temazepam given | | TH | |
| 29.05.2012 | 29.06.1939 | M | | 1112 | 1120 | Script for Salbutamol inhaler & Amoxycillin given | | CRG | |
| 29.05.2012 | 13.02.1950 | M | | 1120 | 1132 | Script for Prochlorperazine given | | DCF | For FBC, U/Es, fasting Glucose, cholesterol, LFTs, PSA & MSU. |
| 29.05.2012 | 31.07.1923 | M | | 1641 | 1656 | Cryotherapy blasts applied to lesion on the scalp | | HO | |
| 29.05.2012 | 26.01.1991 | M | S/Leave | 1656 | 1704 | Med. 3 04/10 given for Drug Induced Psychosis from 23.05.12 for 3 months | | LM | |
| 29.05.2012 | 22.11.1992 | F | | 1723 | 1730 | Script for Cetirizine & Salbutamol inhaler given | | RKC | |

Result of a query that lists all consultations from the 22nd to the end of May 2012 (ConsultationsSeenFrom22ndTillEndOfMay2012)

| SurgeryDate | DateOfBirth | Sex | Diagnosis | TimeIn | TimeOut | Complaints | Treatments | Initials | Notes |
|---|---|---|---|---|---|---|---|---|---|
| 29.05.2012 | 17.05.2011 | M | URTI | 1740 | 1751 | Running nose & fever | Amoxycillin | SPS | |
| 29.05.2012 | 29.12.2000 | F | | 1804 | 1810 | Referred to Dermatologist regarding her severe eczema | | MMS | |
| 29.05.2012 | 23.01.1961 | F | | 1810 | 1822 | Fostering Medical Examination done | | JJH | |
| 30.05.2012 | 04.05.1963 | M | | 945 | 955 | For FBC, U/Es, Fasting lipids, LFTs, fasting cholesterol & TFTs | | DPF | |
| 30.05.2012 | 09.05.1973 | M | | 955 | 1004 | Referred to Spinal Surgeon as advised by the physiotherapist regarding his back pain | | MPC | Script for Dihydrocodeine given. |
| 30.05.2012 | 24.03.1973 | M | S/Leave | 1004 | 1016 | Med. 3 04/10 given for Pain in the (R) foot from 28.05.12 for 1 week | | JCM | Referred to Dermatologist regarding the mole on his back. |
| 30.05.2012 | 14.01.1974 | F | | 1016 | 1027 | Script for Cetirizine, Co-codamol & Norrtriptyline given | | LBA | |
| 30.05.2012 | 07.05.1938 | F | | 1027 | 1037 | Script for Amoxycillin & E45 cream given | | ILB | For Chest X-Rays. |

Result of a query that lists all consultations from the 22nd to the end of May 2012 (ConsultationsSeenFrom22ndTillEndOfMay2012)

| SurgeryDate | DateOfBirth | Sex | Diagnosis | TimeIn | TimeOut | Complaints | Treatments | Initials | Notes |
|---|---|---|---|---|---|---|---|---|---|
| 30.05.2012 | 20.07.1989 | F | | 1037 | 1043 | To see her new GP in Kent regarding her investigations of polycystic ovarian syndrome | | AP | |
| 30.05.2012 | 04.09.1952 | M | RTI | 1102 | 1108 | Chesty cough | Amoxycillin | DJB | |
| 30.05.2012 | 01.12.1933 | F | | 1320 | 1345 | Script for Trimethoprim given | | JM | Home visit. Penicillin allergy. |
| 30.05.2012 | 25.11.1943 | M | | 1645 | 1649 | For FBC, Fasting Glucose, serum cholesterol, LFTs & U/Es | | AES | |
| 30.05.2012 | 25.12.1946 | F | | 1659 | 1707 | For X-Rays of the (L) shoulder | | AS | |
| 30.05.2012 | 25.11.1949 | M | | 1707 | 1713 | To see the nurse in 6 months for repeat PSA | | GJD | |
| 30.05.2012 | 31.03.1956 | F | S/Leave | 1713 | 1719 | Med. 3 04/10 given for Chest Infection from 25.05.12 for 1 week | | SD | |
| 30.05.2012 | 20.11.1946 | M | | 1719 | 1730 | Medication Review Done | | LPH | |
| 30.05.2012 | 15.09.1939 | F | | 1737 | 1745 | Script for Flucloxacillin given | | EH | |
| 30.05.2012 | 10.01.2010 | F | | 1749 | 1756 | To continue with her OTC Piriton for her hay fever | | SMH | |

303

Result of a query that lists all consultations from the 22nd to the end of May 2012 (ConsultationsSeenFrom22ndTillEndOfMay2012)

| SurgeryDate | DateOfBirth | Sex | Diagnosis | TimeIn | TimeOut | Complaints | Treatments | Initials | Notes |
|---|---|---|---|---|---|---|---|---|---|
| 30.05.2012 | 02.03.1971 | F | | 1805 | 1815 | Script for Absorbent perforated plastic film faced dressings, Co-codamol, Flucloxacillin, Levemir Penfil & Novorapid Penfil Insulins given | | DLM | |
| 30.05.2012 | 25.03.2011 | M | | 1802 | 1826 | To use his own Calamine lotion & Calpol for his possible measles rash | | JAB | |

Result of a query that lists all consultations from the 22nd to the end of May 2013 (ConsultationsSeenFrom22ndTillEndOfMay2013)

| SurgeryDate | DateOfBirth | Sex | Diagnosis | TimeIn | TimeOut | Complaints | Treatments | Initials | Notes |
|---|---|---|---|---|---|---|---|---|---|
| 22.05.2013 | 27.10.1960 | F | S/Leave | 937 | 947 | Med. 3 04/10 given for Back Pain for 3 months from 22.05.13 | | DLK | Script for Cetraben cream, Co-dydramol & Oramorph given. |
| 22.05.2013 | 02.12.1954 | M | | 947 | 1009 | BP 127/92 | | OAK | |
| 22.05.2013 | 31.01.1933 | M | | 1009 | 1020 | Referred to Dermatologist regarding his scaly, itchy scalp | | MPB | Referred for Colonoscopy regarding his persistent diarrhoea. |
| 22.05.2013 | 26.08.1962 | F | RTI | 1020 | 1028 | Chesty cough | Amoxycillin | HD | |

Result of a query that lists all consultations from the 22nd to the end of May 2013 (ConsultationsSeenFrom22ndTillEndOfMay2013)

| SurgeryDate | DateOfBirth | Sex | Diagnosis | TimeIn | TimeOut | Complaints | Treatments | Initials | Notes |
|---|---|---|---|---|---|---|---|---|---|
| 22.05.2013 | 16.08.1983 | F | | 1028 | 1036 | Script for Balneum Plus bath oil & Fexofenadine was given | | CEC | |
| 22.05.2013 | 13.02.1950 | M | | 1036 | 1042 | He says when he saw the ENT Surgeon he was advised to stop the Serc & the Tamsulosin | | DCF | |
| 22.05.2013 | 31.07.1961 | F | | 1042 | 1055 | Script for Erythromycin given | | CMW | Referred to Breast Surgeon (2WW) regarding the (L) breast abscess in the same breast that she had cancer in 2 years ago. |
| 22.05.2013 | 08.11.1929 | M | | 1055 | 1107 | Referred to Occupational therapist regarding being fitted with a strong support for his (R) knee which keeps giving way | | FAD | |
| 22.05.2013 | 25.10.1966 | M | | 1107 | 1120 | Script for Omeprazole given | | WBG | |
| 22.05.2013 | 12.08.1993 | M | | 1644 | 1708 | I explained to the lady from family Mosaic that I am unable to sign the bus pass application form | | DTA | |

Result of a query that lists all consultations from the 22nd to the end of May 2013 (ConsultationsSeenFrom22ndTillEndOfMay2013)

| SurgeryDate | DateOfBirth | Sex | Diagnosis | TimeIn | TimeOut | Complaints | Treatments | Initials | Notes |
|---|---|---|---|---|---|---|---|---|---|
| 22.05.2013 | 07.10.1981 | M | S/Leave | 1708 | 1726 | Med. 3 04/10 given for Injury (R) ankle for 2 months from 09.04.13 | | JPB | |
| 22.05.2013 | 15.04.2003 | F | | 1726 | 1733 | Script for Flucloxacillin given | | LMC | |
| 22.05.2013 | 07.03.1999 | F | | 1733 | 1742 | Script for Acyclovir given | | SAW | |
| 22.05.2013 | 07.01.1998 | F | | 1742 | 1748 | Script for Mefenamic acid given | | ECAS | |
| 22.05.2013 | 17.07.1983 | F | | 1748 | 1802 | Referred to Dermatologist with view to having allergy testing | | DLR | Referred for Colonoscopy regarding her recurrent constipation. |
| 22.05.2013 | 03.07.1950 | F | | 1802 | 1810 | For X-Rays of the (R) hip | | YC | |
| 22.05.2013 | 24.03.1973 | M | S/Leave | 1810 | 1819 | Private Sick Leave given for Pain in the (R) foot for 1 week from 17.05.13 | | JCM | |
| 22.05.2013 | 25.04.1951 | F | | 1820 | 1830 | Script for Co-codamol given | | SM | For X-Rays of both feet. |
| 23.05.2013 | 08.05.1956 | F | | 942 | 949 | Script for Propranolol given | | SH | |
| 23.05.2013 | 23.11.1946 | M | | 949 | 956 | Script for Mometasone nasal spray given | | TSM | For X-Rays of the (R) hip. |

Result of a query that lists all consultations from the 22nd to the end of May 2013 (ConsultationsSeenFrom22ndTillEndOfMay2013)

| SurgeryDate | DateOfBirth | Sex | Diagnosis | TimeIn | TimeOut | Complaints | Treatments | Initials | Notes |
|---|---|---|---|---|---|---|---|---|---|
| 23.05.2013 | 18.04.1965 | M | | 956 | 1007 | Script for Citalopram given | | MGF | |
| 23.05.2013 | 23.11.1964 | M | | 1007 | 1014 | Script for Flucloxacillin given | | PAM | |
| 23.05.2013 | 15.01.1935 | F | | 1014 | 1022 | Script for Xanthan gum given | | JRS | |
| 23.05.2013 | 05.07.1931 | F | | 1022 | 1038 | Script for Flucloxacillin & Furosemide given | | AVD | |
| 23.05.2013 | 19.05.1944 | F | | 1051 | 1102 | Script for Hirudoid gel given | | AWB | |
| 23.05.2013 | 16.07.1969 | F | | 1102 | 1113 | For FBC, U/Es, CRP, Rheumatoid factor & Bone Profile | | NB | |
| 23.05.2013 | 06.07.1957 | F | | 1648 | 1658 | Script for Lansoprazole given | | WS | |
| 23.05.2013 | 17.05.1939 | M | | 1658 | 1705 | Script for Co-codamol & Transvasin Heat Rub cream given | | JTN | |
| 23.05.2013 | 07.02.1997 | M | | 1705 | 1710 | Medication Review Done | | JAW | |
| 23.05.2013 | 11.11.1981 | F | | 1710 | 1716 | Urine Pregnancy test is positive | | SC | |
| 23.05.2013 | 09.01.1962 | F | | 1716 | 1726 | Referred to Orthopaedic Surgeon regarding her scoliosis & back pain | | VVB | |

Result of a query that lists all consultations from the 22nd to the end of May 2013 (ConsultationsSeenFrom22ndTillEndOfMay2013)

| SurgeryDate | DateOfBirth | Sex | Diagnosis | TimeIn | TimeOut | Complaints | Treatments | Initials | Notes |
|---|---|---|---|---|---|---|---|---|---|
| 23.05.2013 | 09.06.1993 | F | | 1743 | 1756 | The antenatal booking form is completed with the patient, by asking her the questions directly | | AL | |
| 23.05.2013 | 08.10.1963 | M | | 1756 | 1803 | Script for Lisinopril given | | RBA | |
| 23.05.2013 | 11.06.1968 | F | | 1803 | 1809 | She is going on skydiving for charity on 25.06.13 for charity & has brought in a form to be signed | | TR | |
| 24.05.2013 | 01.09.1946 | M | | 935 | 952 | Medication Review Done | | PAH | |
| 24.05.2013 | 01.01.1953 | M | | 952 | 958 | Private script for Viagra given | | TPH | Script for Amoxycillin given. |
| 24.05.2013 | 26.02.1934 | F | | 1004 | 1013 | BP 126/88 | | DIM | |
| 24.05.2013 | 18.11.1982 | F | | 1013 | 1024 | For FBC, U/Es & TFTs | | VAB | |
| 24.05.2013 | 04.08.1936 | M | | 1024 | 1040 | Script for Lansoprazole given | | ECM | |
| 24.05.2013 | 28.08.1984 | M | S/Leave | 1045 | 1102 | Private Sick Leave given for Nose bleed for 1 week from 21.05.13 | | JTP | |
| 24.05.2013 | 11.05.1972 | M | S/Leave | 1102 | 1110 | Med. 3 04/10 given for Abdominal pain for 1 month from 24.05.13 | | JRG | |

Result of a query that lists all consultations from the 22nd to the end of May 2013 (ConsultationsSeenFrom22ndTillEndOfMay2013)

| SurgeryDate | DateOfBirth | Sex | Diagnosis | TimeIn | TimeOut | Complaints | Treatments | Initials | Notes |
|---|---|---|---|---|---|---|---|---|---|
| 24.05.2013 | 05.07.1981 | F | | 1112 | 1122 | Routine immediate post-natal check done | | THO | |
| 28.05.2013 | 16.10.2009 | F | | 945 | 952 | To continue with Lactulose twice daily | | LP | |
| 28.05.2013 | 18.05.1949 | M | | 952 | 1006 | For TFTs | | JJ | Script for Lisinopril given. |
| 28.05.2013 | 30.08.1945 | M | | 1006 | 1016 | Medication Review Done | | AJS | |
| 28.05.2013 | 19.08.1917 | F | | 1016 | 1028 | For MSU | | VL | |
| 28.05.2013 | 05.11.1924 | F | | 1028 | 1036 | For FBC, U/Es & TFTs | | BM | |
| 28.05.2013 | 20.02.1939 | F | | 1036 | 1048 | Script for Beconase Aqueous nasal spray given | | MJP | |
| 28.05.2013 | 20.01.1986 | F | | 1048 | 1056 | She is having 3 yearly regular smear | | JES | |
| 28.05.2013 | 02.01.1955 | M | | 1056 | 1104 | Medication Review Done | | TRE | |
| 28.05.2013 | 05.06.1924 | M | | 1300 | 1325 | Script for Furosemide & Ferrous Fumarate given | | DAC | For FBC & U/Es. Home visit. |
| 28.05.2013 | 27.01.1934 | F | | 1649 | 1704 | Script for Amlodipine given | | JWC | |
| 28.05.2013 | 04.10.1947 | F | | 1704 | 1713 | Script for Amorolfine 5% medicated nail lacquer given | | PVD | |

Result of a query that lists all consultations from the 22nd to the end of May 2013 (ConsultationsSeenFrom22ndTillEndOfMay2013)

| SurgeryDate | DateOfBirth | Sex | Diagnosis | TimeIn | TimeOut | Complaints | Treatments | Initials | Notes |
|---|---|---|---|---|---|---|---|---|---|
| 28.05.2013 | 24.03.1973 | M | S/Leave | 1713 | 1720 | Med. 3 04/10 given for Pain in the (R) foot from 24.05.13 to 03.06.13 | | JCM | |
| 28.05.2013 | 31.05.1967 | M | | 1720 | 1731 | Script for Cefalexin given | | GKP | For X-Rays of both Tibia. |
| 28.05.2013 | 22.10.2009 | F | | 1731 | 1736 | Script for Erythromycin & Otosporin ear drops given | | CMGM | |
| 28.05.2013 | 08.09.1981 | M | | 1736 | 1741 | Script for Amoxycillin & Codeine tablets given | | SK | |
| 28.05.2013 | 31.03.1956 | F | | 1756 | 1806 | Referred to Dermatologist (urgent) regarding recurrent ulcer on the 2nd (L) toe | | SD | |
| 28.05.2013 | 24.09.1976 | M | | 1806 | 1814 | Referred for Gastroscopy regarding his indigestion | | DIB | Script for Omeprazole given. |
| 28.05.2013 | 28.11.2012 | F | RTI | 1814 | 1820 | Chesty cough | Amoxycillin | ARM | |
| 29.05.2013 | 13.05.1992 | F | | 949 | 1004 | Referred to Ophthalmologist regarding her recurrent (L) iritis | | AVB | Referred to Dermatologist regarding possible Lichen planus on her ankles & wrists. |

310

Result of a query that lists all consultations from the 22nd to the end of May 2013 (ConsultationsSeenFrom22ndTillEndOfMay2013)

| SurgeryDate | DateOfBirth | Sex | Diagnosis | TimeIn | TimeOut | Complaints | Treatments | Initials | Notes |
|---|---|---|---|---|---|---|---|---|---|
| 29.05.2013 | 04.11.1966 | F | | 1004 | 1008 | Advised to take the iron tablets three times daily | | SJOB | |
| 29.05.2013 | 28.03.1970 | F | | 1008 | 1019 | Referred to Orthopaedic Surgeon regarding pain in her (R) ankle | | LJ | |
| 29.05.2013 | 23.01.1947 | F | | 1019 | 1028 | She will bring in a copy of her MSU result from Wellesley hospital which we have not yet got | | BW | |
| 29.05.2013 | 04.07.1929 | M | | 1033 | 1041 | Referred for Gastroscopy regarding his abdominal pain, persistent anaemia & weight loss | | RMC | |
| 29.05.2013 | 17.09.1965 | F | URTI | 1041 | 1045 | Sore throat | Amoxycillin | PAE | |
| 29.05.2013 | 16.01.1986 | M | S/Leave | 1045 | 1051 | Med. 3 04/10 given for Infection in the (R) testicle for 2 weeks from 27.05.13 | | ANI | |
| 29.05.2013 | 20.07.1956 | M | | 1054 | 1122 | Referred to Chest Physician regarding his wheezing & shortness of breath | | MDJ | Script for Campral EC given. |
| 29.05.2013 | 27.03.1940 | F | | 1126 | 1152 | Script for Cetraben emollient cream, GelTears 0.2% & Salivix pastilles given | | MAD | |

## Result of a query that lists all consultations from the 22nd to the end of May 2013 (ConsultationsSeenFrom22ndTillEndOfMay2013)

| SurgeryDate | DateOfBirth | Sex | Diagnosis | TimeIn | TimeOut | Complaints | Treatments | Initials | Notes |
|---|---|---|---|---|---|---|---|---|---|
| 29.05.2013 | 15.10.1969 | F | | 1647 | 1657 | For USScan of the upper abdomen | | MAC | |
| 29.05.2013 | 17.10.1998 | M | | 1703 | 1710 | For X-Rays of the (R) foot | | KRC | Script for Ibuprofen given. |
| 29.05.2013 | 05.11.1946 | M | | 1710 | 1718 | Script for Doxazosin given | | BDD | |
| 29.05.2013 | 14.08.1935 | M | | 1718 | 1727 | Referred to ENT Surgeon regarding | | RAT | |
| 29.05.2013 | 11.05.1959 | F | | 1734 | 1742 | Script for Erythromycin given | | LJE | |
| 29.05.2013 | 09.02.1969 | F | | 1751 | 1758 | Script for Ferrous Fumarate given | | OLF | |
| 29.05.2013 | 29.09.2006 | M | | 1758 | 1805 | Referred to ENT Surgeon regarding deafness & possible foreign body in the (R) ear canal | | ODO | |
| 30.05.2013 | 10.04.1969 | F | | 945 | 1000 | Script for Propranolol given | | LAJ | |
| 30.05.2013 | 02.07.1943 | M | | 1000 | 1011 | Referred to ENT Surgeon regarding swallowing problems & blockage feeling in his throat | | WRW | |
| 30.05.2013 | 17.05.1935 | F | | 1011 | 1019 | Advised to see the nurse in 6 months for repeat FBC, LFTs, TFTs & serum cholesterol | | CSS | |

Result of a query that lists all consultations from the 22nd to the end of May 2013 (ConsultationsSeenFrom22ndTillEndOfMay2013)

| SurgeryDate | DateOfBirth | Sex | Diagnosis | TimeIn | TimeOut | Complaints | Treatments | Initials | Notes |
|---|---|---|---|---|---|---|---|---|---|
| 30.05.2013 | 13.04.1985 | F | | 1019 | 1026 | Script for Amoxycillin & Prochlorperazine given | | CLA | |
| 30.05.2013 | 09.08.1987 | F | | 1026 | 1036 | Script for Fucidin H cream given | | RJM | For Urine Pregnancy test. |
| 30.05.2013 | 15.07.1956 | M | S/Leave | 1034 | 1042 | Med. 3 04/10 given for Depression for 2 weeks from 30.05.13 | | DHC | |
| 30.05.2013 | 13.05.1992 | F | | 1047 | 1058 | Referred to Ophthalmologist regarding her (L) iritis | | ZLB | For TFTs. |
| 30.05.2013 | 15.11.1969 | M | | 1058 | 1108 | Referred to Podiatrist regarding his (R) big toe nail which is growing thick rather than growing long | | DWK | Referred to Physiotherapist regarding his back pain since being involved in accident whilst riding his motor-bike. |
| 30.05.2013 | 14.04.1946 | F | | 1108 | 1113 | Script for Amoxycillin & Otosporin ear drops given | | VBB | |
| 30.05.2013 | 03.07.1957 | F | | 1645 | 1656 | Referred to Ophthalmologist regarding her Thyroid eye disease from her Grave's disease | | EGL | |
| 30.05.2013 | 08.07.1998 | F | | 1656 | 1702 | Script for Amoxycillin given | | COSP | |
| 30.05.2013 | 27.05.2008 | F | RTI | 1702 | 1707 | Chesty cough | Amoxycillin | HCJN | |

Result of a query that lists all consultations from the 22nd to the end of May 2013 (ConsultationsSeenFrom22ndTillEndOfMay2013)

| SurgeryDate | DateOfBirth | Sex | Diagnosis | TimeIn | TimeOut | Complaints | Treatments | Initials | Notes |
|---|---|---|---|---|---|---|---|---|---|
| 30.05.2013 | 16.08.1989 | F | | 1707 | 1714 | For MSU | | SLW | |
| 30.05.2013 | 11.12.2008 | M | URTI | 1714 | 1719 | Ear ache | Amoxycillin | MBB | |
| 30.05.2013 | 18.05.1975 | F | | 1719 | 1725 | For X-Rays of the (L) elbow | | EGHG | |

Result of a query that lists all consultations from the 22nd to the end of May 2014 (ConsultationsSeenFrom22ndTillEndOfMay2014)

| SurgeryDate | DateOfBirth | Sex | Diagnosis | TimeIn | TimeOut | Complaints | Treatments | Initials | Notes |
|---|---|---|---|---|---|---|---|---|---|
| 22.05.2014 | 05.08.1994 | F | | 943 | 950 | Script for Duac Once Daily gel given | | GLJ | |
| 22.05.2014 | 13.02.1950 | M | | 950 | 1003 | BP 120/79 | | DCF | |
| 22.05.2014 | 16.03.1963 | F | S/Leave | 1013 | 1019 | Med. 3 04/10 given for Depression for 3 months from 15.05.14 | | TJC | |
| 22.05.2014 | 09.10.1926 | M | | 1019 | 1031 | To see me in 3 to 4 months for repeat HbA1c | | RAC | |
| 22.05.2014 | 04.07.1961 | F | | 1031 | 1044 | BP 90/67 | | JB | |
| 22.05.2014 | 27.03.1935 | M | | 1044 | 1100 | Referred to Orthopaedic Surgeon regarding his frozen (R) shoulder as advised by the Radiologist | | RH | For FBC, HbA1c, LFTs, Cholesterol, U/Es & Urine microalbumin screen. |

Result of a query that lists all consultations from the 22nd to the end of May 2014 (ConsultationsSeenFrom22ndTillEndOfMay2014)

| SurgeryDate | DateOfBirth | Sex | Diagnosis | TimeIn | TimeOut | Complaints | Treatments | Initials | Notes |
|---|---|---|---|---|---|---|---|---|---|
| 22.05.2014 | 26.06.1946 | M | | 1100 | 1107 | X-Rays of the finger did not show any bony injury but showed degenerative changes of the pip joint of her (L) middle finger | | PGB | |
| 22.05.2014 | 21.12.1945 | F | | 1107 | 1113 | Script for Atorvastatin given | | JAL | |
| 22.05.2014 | 23.01.1968 | F | | 1113 | 1120 | Script for Doxycycline & Sofradex ear drops given | | KS | |
| 22.05.2014 | 08.08.1953 | M | | 1651 | 1701 | Script for Candesartan given | | BP | |
| 22.05.2014 | 14.07.1965 | M | | 1701 | 1720 | Referred to Orthopaedic Surgeon regarding pain in both knees worse on the (L) side | | SM | For FBC, U/Es, Fasting Glucose, TFTs, Fasting Lipids & LFTs. |
| 22.05.2014 | 05.07.1970 | F | | 1720 | 1727 | Script for Doxycycline & Otomize ear spray given | | SLS | |
| 22.05.2014 | 09.06.1993 | F | | 1727 | 1737 | Referred to Plastic Surgeon regarding her unequal sized breasts which she is very self-conscious about | | AL | |
| 22.05.2014 | 02.01.1988 | M | URTI | 1737 | 1743 | Sore throat | Co-Amoxiclav | AHK | |

315

Result of a query that lists all consultations from the 22nd to the end of May 2014 (ConsultationsSeenFrom22ndTillEndOfMay2014)

| SurgeryDate | DateOfBirth | Sex | Diagnosis | TimeIn | TimeOut | Complaints | Treatments | Initials | Notes |
|---|---|---|---|---|---|---|---|---|---|
| 22.05.2014 | 05.03.1943 | M | | 1743 | 1753 | Script for Calcitriol ointment & Doxycycline given | | HTB | Private script for Sildenafil given. |
| 22.05.2014 | 08.11.1988 | F | | 1753 | 1801 | Script for Cetirizine, Qvar 50 & Ventolin inhalers given | | JAP | Referred to Psychiatrist (Dr. Mirg) as she DNA'd her last appointment. |
| 22.05.2014 | 16.08.1943 | M | | 1801 | 1812 | For B12, Folate, Ferritin & repeat MSU | | MJG | |
| 23.05.2014 | 22.08.1963 | M | | 944 | 953 | Script for Codeine tablets, Co-Amoxiclav & Prednisolone given | | GWM | |
| 23.05.2014 | 02.09.1941 | F | | 953 | 1006 | Script for Nifedipine given | | MS | |
| 23.05.2014 | 23.02.1951 | F | RTI | 1009 | 1019 | Chesty cough | Doxycycline | JPN | |
| 23.05.2014 | 13.08.1923 | F | | 1021 | 1040 | Referred to Neurologist (urgent) regarding swallowing & speech problems | | TRC | For Chest X-Rays. |
| 23.05.2014 | 14.12.1944 | M | | 1040 | 1051 | Script for Forxiga given | | NH | |
| 23.05.2014 | 01.12.1934 | F | | 1051 | 1102 | For Clotting screen | | LFM | |
| 23.05.2014 | 15.11.1933 | M | | 1102 | 1108 | Script for Co-codamol & Naproxen given | | TJJ | |
| 23.05.2014 | 18.02.1968 | F | | 1108 | 1122 | Script for Tapentadol m/r & Naproxen given | | PAC | |

Result of a query that lists all consultations from the 22nd to the end of May 2014 (ConsultationsSeenFrom22ndTillEndOfMay2014)

| SurgeryDate | DateOfBirth | Sex | Diagnosis | TimeIn | TimeOut | Complaints | Treatments | Initials | Notes |
|---|---|---|---|---|---|---|---|---|---|
| 27.05.2014 | 05.03.1950 | M | | 944 | 1004 | Referred to Orthopaedic Surgeon regarding his ankle & (R) | | TMJC | |
| 27.05.2014 | 15.12.1939 | M | | 1004 | 1011 | Script for Doxycycline & Sofradex ear drops given | | ERC | |
| 27.05.2014 | 04.08.1936 | M | | 1011 | 1020 | Referred to Neurologist for investigation regarding him developing Parkinson's disease as requested by the Community Podiatrist | | ECM | |
| 27.05.2014 | 25.11.1945 | F | | 1020 | 1027 | Script for Codeine Linctus, Doxycycline, Prednisolone & Ventolin evohaler given | | CLH | |
| 27.05.2014 | 06.12.1940 | F | | 1027 | 1035 | BP 143/83 | | MC | |
| 27.05.2014 | 03.04.1987 | F | S/Leave | 1035 | 1050 | Med. 3 04/10 given for UTI for 1 week from 26.05.14 | | LJP | For repeat MSU. |
| 27.05.2014 | 31.05.1967 | M | | 1050 | 1100 | Script for Doxycycline given | | GKP | |

317

Result of a query that lists all consultations from the 22nd to the end of May 2014 (ConsultationsSeenFrom22ndTillEndOfMay2014)

| SurgeryDate | DateOfBirth | Sex | Diagnosis | TimeIn | TimeOut | Complaints | Treatments | Initials | Notes |
|---|---|---|---|---|---|---|---|---|---|
| 27.05.2014 | 18.05.1952 | F | | 1107 | 1114 | To see the nurse in a couple of months for for TFTs & serum cholesterol | | JN | |
| 27.05.2014 | 18.03.1967 | F | | 1648 | 1701 | Script for Canesten HC cream & Metronidazole tablets given | | SO | |
| 27.05.2014 | 07.10.1981 | M | | 1701 | 1716 | Script for Nizoral 2% shampoo given | | JPB | |
| 27.05.2014 | 18.01.1950 | F | | 1716 | 1723 | Advised to keep to her usual dose of Levothyroxine | | JS | |
| 27.05.2014 | 05.07.1931 | F | | 1727 | 1747 | For B12, Folate & Ferritin | | AVD | |
| 27.05.2014 | 11.08.1983 | F | | 1747 | 1756 | For FBC, Ferritin, Folate, B12, Fasting Glucose, Fasting Lipids, TFTs, HbA1c & U/Es | | RJN | |
| 27.05.2014 | 09.10.1974 | F | | 1756 | 1806 | Script for Ferrous Fumarate & Co-Amoxiclav given | | MJF | For U/Es, TFTs & Fasting Glucose. |
| 27.05.2014 | 11.07.1962 | M | | 1806 | 1816 | Script for Amlodipine, Doxazosin & Bendroflumethiazide given | | JEG | |

Result of a query that lists all consultations from the 22nd to the end of May 2014 (ConsultationsSeenFrom22ndTillEndOfMay2014)

| SurgeryDate | DateOfBirth | Sex | Diagnosis | TimeIn | TimeOut | Complaints | Treatments | Initials | Notes |
|---|---|---|---|---|---|---|---|---|---|
| 27.05.2014 | 11.03.1986 | M | | 1816 | 1824 | To try OTC Imodium & Dioralyte for his diarrhoea in the first instance | | LTB | |
| 28.05.2014 | 12.10.1948 | F | | 943 | 953 | Script for Co-codamol & Atorvastatin given | | SFC | |
| 28.05.2014 | 27.09.1984 | M | | 953 | 1010 | Referred to ENT Surgeon (Mr. Warwick-Brown) as he DNA'd his last appointment | | DGC | Script for Occlusal 26% solution given. For U/Es & FBC. |
| 28.05.2014 | 21.11.1948 | M | | 1010 | 1025 | Script for Allopurinol, Ibuprofen & Omeprazole given | | PCB | For FBC, serum Testosterone, HbA1c, Cholesterol, U/Es, Urine microalbuminuria screen, LFTs & Uric acid. |
| 28.05.2014 | 18.03.1979 | F | | 1025 | 1035 | Script for Citalopram given | | MJH | |
| 28.05.2014 | 06.11.1968 | M | | 1035 | 1047 | For USScan of his testicles (urgent) | | ARP | |
| 28.05.2014 | 08.12.1962 | F | | 1047 | 1104 | Script for Doxycycline given | | BJM | |
| 28.05.2014 | 20.02.1930 | M | | 1104 | 1116 | Referred to Memory Clinic regarding his short-term memory loss | | AL | Referred to Gastroenterologist regarding his persistent diarrhoea. |

Result of a query that lists all consultations from the 22nd to the end of May 2014 (ConsultationsSeenFrom22ndTillEndOfMay2014)

| SurgeryDate | DateOfBirth | Sex | Diagnosis | TimeIn | TimeOut | Complaints | Treatments | Initials | Notes |
|---|---|---|---|---|---|---|---|---|---|
| 28.05.2014 | 06.11.1981 | F | | 1116 | 1124 | For Urine Pregnancy test in one week, form given to the patient | | CL | |
| 28.05.2014 | 20.10.2010 | M | | 1646 | 1654 | Script for Erythromycin, Clenil Modulite & Prednisolone given | | JH | |
| 28.05.2014 | 06.08.1921 | F | | 1654 | 1701 | Script for Co-codamol given | | EE | Daughter came to Surgery. |
| 28.05.2014 | 09.08.1939 | M | | 1701 | 1710 | For FBC, U/Es & serum Uric acid | | JL | |
| 28.05.2014 | 12.09.1986 | F | | 1713 | 1725 | Script for Clotrimazole pessary given | | OK | for serum Ferritin, Folate & B12. |
| 28.05.2014 | 20.05.1987 | F | | 1725 | 1734 | Script for Propranolol given | | DADS | |
| 28.05.2014 | 21.03.1973 | M | | 1734 | 1743 | Script for Pregabalin & Tegretol Retard given | | DRK | |
| 28.05.2014 | 07.08.1971 | F | | 1743 | 1752 | Referred to Physiotherapist regarding her persistent back pain | | LPH | |
| 28.05.2014 | 03.11.1971 | F | | 1752 | 1803 | Script for Diazepam tablets & Premarin given | | KDM | |
| 28.05.2014 | 16.07.1969 | F | | 1803 | 1813 | Script for Co-Amoxiclav & Otomize ear spray given | | NB | |

Result of a query that lists all consultations from the 22nd to the end of May 2014 (ConsultationsSeenFrom22ndTillEndOfMay2014)

| SurgeryDate | DateOfBirth | Sex | Diagnosis | TimeIn | TimeOut | Complaints | Treatments | Initials | Notes |
|---|---|---|---|---|---|---|---|---|---|
| 29.05.2014 | 19.01.1954 | F | | 946 | 952 | To come back later for the extension of her sick leave | | DGD | |
| 29.05.2014 | 18.01.1977 | F | | 952 | 1009 | Referred to Psychiatrist regarding feeling low & depressed | | MP | |
| 29.05.2014 | 02.12.1995 | F | | 1009 | 1020 | Script for Cerelle given | | JAM | For FBC, U/Es, Fasting Glucose & TFTs. |
| 29.05.2014 | 08.03.1920 | M | | 1053 | 1103 | Referred to Dermatologist (urgent) regarding his recurrent red patch area on his penis | | CB | Script for Trimovate cream given. |
| 29.05.2014 | 01.06.1989 | F | URTI | 1103 | 1110 | Sore throat | Amoxycillin | SRN | |
| 29.05.2014 | 19.06.1943 | M | | 1235 | 1250 | Script for Codeine tablets, Codeine Linctus & Clarithromycin given | | BFS | Home visit. |
| 29.05.2014 | 17.07.1983 | F | | 1646 | 1652 | Script for Citalopram given | | DLR | |
| 29.05.2014 | 15.03.1984 | F | | 1652 | 1701 | Referred to Counsellor regarding feeling low & depressed following the death of her nan | | SLL | |
| 29.05.2014 | 06.01.1955 | M | | 1701 | 1706 | Private script for Sildenafil given | | MAS | |

Result of a query that lists all consultations from the 22nd to the end of May 2014 (ConsultationsSeenFrom22ndTillEndOfMay2014)

| SurgeryDate | DateOfBirth | Sex | Diagnosis | TimeIn | TimeOut | Complaints | Treatments | Initials | Notes |
|---|---|---|---|---|---|---|---|---|---|
| 29.05.2014 | 01.01.1951 | F | | 1706 | 1718 | Script for Trimethoprim given | | CR | for MSU, FBC, U/Es, TFTs, Ferritin, Folate & B12. |
| 29.05.2014 | 17.10.1953 | F | | 1741 | 1804 | For HbA1c in 3 months, form given to the patient | | MS | |
| 29.05.2014 | 22.05.1966 | F | | 1804 | 1813 | Referred to Oral Surgeon regarding likely benign (L) parotid gland | | KP | |
| 29.05.2014 | 01.07.1997 | F | URTI | 1813 | 1819 | Sore throat | Amoxycillin | MJB | |
| 30.05.2014 | 09.05.1964 | F | | 949 | 1004 | For X-Rays of the (L) wrist with scaphoid views, 5th (L) metatarsal & (L) ankle | | CAC | |
| 30.05.2014 | 23.10.1941 | M | | 1004 | 1012 | Script for Lansoprazole given | | RJH | |
| 30.05.2014 | 10.10.1992 | F | | 1012 | 1034 | Script for Rigevidon given | | AEH | |
| 30.05.2014 | 06.02.1944 | M | | 1034 | 1040 | Script for Gabapentin given | | AMC | |
| 30.05.2014 | 14.08.1935 | M | | 1040 | 1058 | Script for Gliclazide given | | RAT | |
| 30.05.2014 | 19.06.1944 | F | | 1058 | 1107 | Script for Doxycycline given | | PJL | |
| 30.05.2014 | 06.06.1961 | M | | 1107 | 1114 | Script for Citalopram given | | LG | |

Result of a query that lists all consultations from the 22nd to the end of May 2014 (ConsultationsSeenFrom22ndTillEndOfMay2014)

| SurgeryDate | DateOfBirth | Sex | Diagnosis | TimeIn | TimeOut | Complaints | Treatments | Initials | Notes |
|---|---|---|---|---|---|---|---|---|---|
| 30.05.2014 | 20.08.1939 | F | | 1114 | 1126 | Script for Itraconazole given | | SLT | |
| 30.05.2014 | 25.08.1949 | F | RTI | 1225 | 1231 | Chesty cough | Doxycycline | JP | |

Result of a query that lists all consultations from the 22nd to the end of May 2015 (ConsultationsSeenFrom22ndTillEndOfMay2015)

| SurgeryDate | DateOfBirth | Sex | Diagnosis | TimeIn | TimeOut | Complaints | Treatments | Initials | Notes |
|---|---|---|---|---|---|---|---|---|---|
| 22.05.2015 | 04.04.1953 | M | | 942 | 952 | Script for Tramadol & 1% Hydrocortisone cream given | | GC | |
| 22.05.2015 | 05.03.1950 | M | | 952 | 1005 | Script for Indapamide given | | TMJC | Referred to Community Diabetic specialist nurses regarding his high HbA1c results. |
| 22.05.2015 | 11.10.1954 | M | | 1005 | 1018 | He will come back later for his sick leave preferably with a copy of his latest one | | PWC | |
| 22.05.2015 | 11.11.1934 | M | | 1018 | 1027 | Script for Codeine tablets given | | VRB | |
| 22.05.2015 | 21.08.1934 | F | | 1027 | 1035 | Script for Gliclazide given | | IEW | |
| 22.05.2015 | 26.03.1965 | F | | 1035 | 1042 | She will come back later for the extension of her sick leave | | CP | |

Result of a query that lists all consultations from the 22nd to the end of May 2015 (ConsultationsSeenFrom22ndTillEndOfMay2015)

| SurgeryDate | DateOfBirth | Sex | Diagnosis | TimeIn | TimeOut | Complaints | Treatments | Initials | Notes |
|---|---|---|---|---|---|---|---|---|---|
| 22.05.2015 | 03.11.1994 | F | | 1042 | 1055 | Script for Pregaday tablets given | | SMB | |
| 22.05.2015 | 01.01.1983 | F | | 1055 | 1110 | Routine 6 weeks post-natal check done | | LB | |
| 26.05.2015 | 13.03.1932 | M | | 945 | 959 | Referred to Urologist (2ww) regarding his painless haematuria | | BJC | |
| 26.05.2015 | 04.09.1970 | M | | 959 | 1007 | For FBC, U/Es, TFTs, Fasting Glucose, Bone profile, Fasting Lipids & LFTs | | PSG | |
| 26.05.2015 | 08.01.1942 | F | | 1007 | 1014 | Script for | | SM | |
| 26.05.2015 | 13.05.1992 | F | | 1014 | 1023 | For FBC, U/Es, TFTs, Ferritin, Folate & B12 | | ZLB | |
| 26.05.2015 | 21.06.1961 | F | | 1023 | 1030 | Medications Review Done | | CHO | |
| 26.05.2015 | 09.03.1947 | F | | 1030 | 1036 | Her MSU is normal | | PAN | |
| 26.05.2015 | 16.10.1996 | F | | 1036 | 1044 | To use OTC Sodium bicarbonate ear drops | | YM | |
| 26.05.2015 | 28.07.1943 | F | | 1051 | 1059 | Script for Amorolfine 5% medicated nail lacquer given | | BS | Penicillin allergy. |
| 26.05.2015 | 22.03.1931 | F | | 1059 | 1117 | Script for Qvar inhaler given | | HH | For Chest X-Rays. |
| 26.05.2015 | 11.07.1956 | F | | 1644 | 1653 | For FBC, U/Es & serum Ferritin | | SAC | |
| 26.05.2015 | 16.05.1964 | M | | 1653 | 1700 | Medications Review Done | | GDC | |

Result of a query that lists all consultations from the 22nd to the end of May 2015 (ConsultationsSeenFrom22ndTillEndOfMay2015)

| SurgeryDate | DateOfBirth | Sex | Diagnosis | TimeIn | TimeOut | Complaints | Treatments | Initials | Notes |
|---|---|---|---|---|---|---|---|---|---|
| 26.05.2015 | 02.02.2009 | M | | 1705 | 1714 | Referred to Paediatrician regarding his leg pains & peeling of the tips of the toes & fingers | | OCM | |
| 26.05.2015 | 12.01.1970 | F | | 1720 | 1740 | He will come back later for extension of his sick leave | | AL | |
| 26.05.2015 | 31.12.1953 | F | | 1740 | 1747 | Script for Codeine Linctus given | | JWH | |
| 26.05.2015 | 18.03.1979 | F | | 1747 | 1752 | For Urine Pregnancy test | | MJH | |
| 26.05.2015 | 15.06.1986 | F | | 1752 | 1801 | Referred to Breast Surgeon (One stop Breast clinic) regarding lump in the (R) breast | | LP | Script for Cerelle given. |
| 26.05.2015 | 06.08.1941 | M | | 1801 | 1815 | Referred to ENT Surgeon regarding his persistent cough | | AJM | |
| 27.05.2015 | 22.03.1933 | F | | 1003 | 1009 | The Managing Neck and Back Pain booklet has been given to the patient | | LLW | |
| 27.05.2015 | 28.09.1998 | M | | 1010 | 1017 | Script for Balneum Plus bath oil, Cetirizine & Cetraben cream given | | LJS | |

Result of a query that lists all consultations from the 22nd to the end of May 2015 (ConsultationsSeenFrom22ndTillEndOfMay2015)

| SurgeryDate | DateOfBirth | Sex | Diagnosis | TimeIn | TimeOut | Complaints | Treatments | Initials | Notes |
|---|---|---|---|---|---|---|---|---|---|
| 27.05.2015 | 04.04.1953 | M | S/Leave | 1017 | 1029 | Med. 3 04/10 given for (L) ankle revision for 2 months from 25.05.15 | | GC | |
| 27.05.2015 | 25.05.1970 | F | S/Leave | 1041 | 1056 | Med. 3 04/10 given for Stress & Anxiety for 3 months from 28.04.15 | | KB | Script for Tramadol given. |
| 27.05.2015 | 05.12.1956 | M | | 1056 | 1103 | For MSU, FBC, U/Es & PSA | | DTB | |
| 27.05.2015 | 04.05.1956 | M | | 1646 | 1704 | For USScan of the abdomen | | JAP | |
| 27.05.2015 | 18.05.1952 | F | | 1704 | 1711 | Script for Ranitidine given | | CAE | |
| 27.05.2015 | 01.01.1951 | F | | 1711 | 1720 | Referred to Gastroenterologist regarding her persistent low serum Ferritin | | CR | |
| 27.05.2015 | 19.03.1952 | M | S/Leave | 1720 | 1739 | Private Sick Leave given for Shingles for 1 week from 25.05.15 | | RJB | Script for Acyclovir tablets given. For FBC, U/Es, HbA1c, Cholesterol, LFTs, TFTs & Urine microalbumin screen. |
| 27.05.2015 | 04.11.1977 | F | | 1739 | 1745 | Script for Amoxycillin given | | KOH | |

Result of a query that lists all consultations from the 22nd to the end of May 2015 (ConsultationsSeenFrom22ndTillEndOfMay2015)

| SurgeryDate | DateOfBirth | Sex | Diagnosis | TimeIn | TimeOut | Complaints | Treatments | Initials | Notes |
|---|---|---|---|---|---|---|---|---|---|
| 27.05.2015 | 08.01.1972 | M | | 1745 | 1755 | Referred to Pain Management Specialist as he missed his appointment to be seen in the clinic on 18.05.15 | | EM | |
| 28.05.2015 | 12.05.1935 | F | | 943 | 952 | Script for Prednisolone & Ventolin Evohaler given | | SJN | |
| 28.05.2015 | 02.11.1938 | M | | 952 | 1000 | To use the Fucidin H cream for the forehead rash which has now cleared for further 2 weeks | | MSH | |
| 28.05.2015 | 26.12.1932 | F | | 1011 | 1022 | Referred to Breast Surgeon (2ww) regarding bloody discharge from the (R) nipple | | JB | |
| 28.05.2015 | 25.04.1935 | M | | 1022 | 1036 | Referred to Incontinence clinic regarding getting pants for his double incontinence rather than pads | | KGB | Script for Bisoprolol & Furosemide given. |
| 28.05.2015 | 04.07.1959 | F | | 1036 | 1047 | BP 113/87 | | SAB | |
| 28.05.2015 | 13.11.1952 | F | | 1047 | 1054 | Script for Otomize ear spray given | | LH | |

Result of a query that lists all consultations from the 22nd to the end of May 2015 (ConsultationsSeenFrom22ndTillEndOfMay2015)

| SurgeryDate | DateOfBirth | Sex | Diagnosis | TimeIn | TimeOut | Complaints | Treatments | Initials | Notes |
|---|---|---|---|---|---|---|---|---|---|
| 28.05.2015 | 31.12.1969 | F | | 1054 | 1102 | Referred to Counsellor regarding depression & being unable to cope | | BV | |
| 28.05.2015 | 06.10.1933 | M | | 1102 | 1110 | Script for Nasacort Allergy nasal spray given | | RJK | |
| 28.05.2015 | 09.10.1926 | M | | 1110 | 1120 | Script for Amitriptyline given | | RAC | |
| 28.05.2015 | 25.03.2005 | F | URTI | 1120 | 1130 | Sore throat | Amoxycillin | HJT | |
| 28.05.2015 | 04.04.1938 | M | | 1644 | 1701 | Script for Amoxycillin given | | DB | |
| 28.05.2015 | 08.10.1940 | F | | 1701 | 1714 | Script for Trifluoperazine oral solution given | | MRH | |
| 28.05.2015 | 23.06.1962 | M | S/Leave | 1714 | 1727 | Med. 3 04/10 given for Back Pain for 3 months from 28.05.15 | | RJE | |
| 28.05.2015 | 07.12.2011 | M | | 1732 | 1742 | Parents are to mention to the Paediatrician regarding pain in the (R) ankle when he is seen in the Paediatric clinic | | NDM | |
| 28.05.2015 | 18.04.1978 | F | | 1742 | 1748 | To continue with the Aldomet & to see me a few days before they are due to finish for review | | SL | |

Result of a query that lists all consultations from the 22nd to the end of May 2015 (ConsultationsSeenFrom22ndTillEndOfMay2015)

| SurgeryDate | DateOfBirth | Sex | Diagnosis | TimeIn | TimeOut | Complaints | Treatments | Initials | Notes |
|---|---|---|---|---|---|---|---|---|---|
| 28.05.2015 | 25.06.2001 | M | | 1748 | 1758 | Referred to Paediatrician regarding his behavioural problems | | JJP | |
| 28.05.2015 | 22.07.1961 | M | | 1758 | 1808 | Script for Sumatriptan given | | PWL | |
| 29.05.2015 | 08.10.1956 | M | | 945 | 959 | Script for Codeine tablets, Diazepam & Naproxen given | | GPS | |
| 29.05.2015 | 29.02.1944 | F | | 959 | 1004 | Her MSU was essentially normal | | CFC | |
| 29.05.2015 | 06.08.1921 | F | | 1004 | 1009 | Referred to District Nurses regarding dressing of the (L) lower leg wound | | EE | Her daughter came in on her behalf. |
| 29.05.2015 | 07.06.1971 | M | | 1009 | 1020 | To see the nurse in 3 months for repeat blood test for LFTs & Cholesterol | | DAE | Penicillin allergy. |
| 29.05.2015 | 04.11.1966 | F | | 1020 | 1030 | Referred to Podiatrist regarding pain & tenderness in the (L) heel | | SJOB | Script for Amoxycillin given. For MSU. |
| 29.05.2015 | 04.04.1992 | F | | 1030 | 1040 | Script for Zelleta given | | SAG | |
| 29.05.2015 | 22.03.1986 | F | | 1040 | 1047 | For Urine Pregnancy test | | KAR | |
| 29.05.2015 | 29.11.1946 | F | | 1047 | 1056 | Script for Doxycycline given | | PW | |

Result of a query that lists all consultations from the 22nd to the end of May 2015 (ConsultationsSeenFrom22ndTillEndOfMay2015)

| SurgeryDate | DateOfBirth | Sex | Diagnosis | TimeIn | TimeOut | Complaints | Treatments | Initials | Notes |
|---|---|---|---|---|---|---|---|---|---|
| 29.05.2015 | 08.11.1966 | F | | 1056 | 1103 | Script for Ferrous Sulphate given | | AJK | |
| 29.05.2015 | 22.05.2015 | M | | 1103 | 1113 | Script for Nystan oral suspension & Chloramphenicol eye drops given | | OM | |
| 29.05.2015 | 24.08.2012 | M | | 1113 | 1118 | Script for Amoxycillin & Paracetamol given | | FSDPH | |

# RESULTS OF QUERIES THAT LIST ALL CONSULTATIONS FROM THE 22$^{ND}$ TO THE END OF JUNE 1997 TO JUNE 2015

Result of a query that lists all consultations from the 22nd to the end of June 1997 (ConsultationsSeenFrom22ndTillEndOfJun1997)

| SurgeryDate | DateOfBirth | Sex | Diagnosis | TimeIn | TimeOut | Complaints | Treatments | NumbersID | Notes |
|---|---|---|---|---|---|---|---|---|---|
| 23.06.97 | 26.05.13 | F | RTI | 1225 | 1245 | Cough | Erymax | Temp | Home visit. Penicillin allergy. Also has chest pain, Rx. GTN spray. |
| 26.06.97 | 29.10.49 | F | Pain | 1026 | 1031 | Pain (R) side | Co-dydramol | NP | Transvasin cream also prescribed. |
| 27.06.97 | 03.01.49 | M | Lump | 931 | 935 | Subcutaneous tiny lumps on chest & thigh | To observe | NP | |
| 27.06.97 | 28.04.73 | F | | 1640 | 1654 | See notes | | Temp | Script for Human Insulatard, Human Actrapid, Canesten cream & Pregaday. |
| 30.01.97 | 19.02.72 | M | Pain | 945 | 954 | Pain (R) arm | Co-dydramol & Transvasin cream | 1424 | For physiotherapy. |
| 24.06.97 | 13.05.14 | M | RTI | 1205 | 1230 | Cough | Ciprofloxacin | 1466 | Bendrofluazide & Aspirin. Home visit. |
| 30.01.97 | 23.01.30 | M | | 1015 | 1020 | Constipated | Senna tablets & Lactulose | 1495 | |
| 23.06.97 | 23.08.25 | F | | 1657 | 1704 | Blurred vision (R) eye | To see Optician | 1613 | |
| 24.06.97 | 24.12.50 | F | | 1707 | 1711 | (R) ear pain | Amoxycillin | 1638 | |
| 23.06.97 | 23.06.53 | M | S/Leave | 1741 | 1743 | Alcoholism & depression | | 1681 | |
| 30.01.97 | 20.05.38 | F | RTI | 1005 | 1009 | Cough | Ciprofloxacin | 1869 | |
| 26.06.97 | 03.07.27 | F | Pain | 1639 | 1644 | Back pain | Co-dydramol | 1920 | |

Result of a query that lists all consultations from the 22nd to the end of June 1997 (ConsultationsSeenFrom22ndTillEndOfJun1997)

| SurgeryDate | DateOfBirth | Sex | Diagnosis | TimeIn | TimeOut | Complaints | Treatments | NumbersID | Notes |
|---|---|---|---|---|---|---|---|---|---|
| 25.06.97 | 01.09.54 | F | Rash | 952 | 959 | Dry, itchy & scaly rash on leg | To Dermatologist (BUPA) | 2025 | Inadequate bladder & bowel function since she had forceps delivery 4 years ago, referred to Gynaecologist (BUPA). |
| 28.06.97 | 23.09.68 | M | URTI | 1036 | 1040 | Sore throat | Penicillin V | 2136 | |
| 30.01.97 | 25.04.62 | M | URTI | 1000 | 1004 | Sore throat | Erymax | 2142 | |
| 30.01.97 | 06.08.80 | F | URTI | 1840 | 1848 | Sore throat | Augmentin & Junifen | 2298 | |
| 25.06.97 | 01.03.84 | F | URTI | 923 | 926 | Sore throat | Amoxycillin | 2349 | |
| 27.06.97 | 08.05.86 | F | UTI | 1849 | 1855 | Dysuria & haematuria | Amoxycillin | 2350 | |
| 27.06.97 | 11.05.59 | F | URTI | 1806 | 1813 | Sore throat | Erythromycin | 2351 | |
| 24.06.97 | 03.12.35 | M | Hypertension | 930 | 942 | BP 180/110 | Atenolol | 2353 | For FBC, U/Es, Cholesterol & Glucose. |
| 24.06.97 | 09.07.41 | F | Revisit | 1712 | 1721 | Back pain worse | X-Ray Lumbosacral spine | 2393 | For Physiotherapy. |
| 24.06.97 | 19.06.37 | M | Revisit | 1722 | 1732 | Persistent cough | For CXR | 2394 | Also has back pain, for Physiotherapy. Simple Linctus also prescribed. |
| 30.01.97 | 23.01.26 | F | | 927 | 939 | Piles & bleeding pr. | For FBC, ESR & faecal occult blood | 2479 | |

## Result of a query that lists all consultations from the 22nd to the end of June 1997 (ConsultationsSeenFrom22ndTillEndOfJun1997)

| SurgeryDate | DateOfBirth | Sex | Diagnosis | TimeIn | TimeOut | Complaints | Treatments | NumbersID | Notes |
|---|---|---|---|---|---|---|---|---|---|
| 27.06.97 | 03.09.88 | F | Conjunctivitis | 1750 | 1755 | Stye (L) upper eye lid | Chloramphenicol eye ointment | 2565 | Penicillin allergy. |
| 24.06.97 | 24.10.48 | M | S/Leave | 907 | 919 | Low back ache | | 2706 | |
| 27.06.97 | 05.04.57 | M | S/Leave | 1718 | 1723 | Pain (L) shoulder - Private | | 277 | For X-Ray (L) shoulder. |
| 24.06.97 | 27.06.59 | F | | 1803 | 1829 | Seen by Gynaecologist | | 2869 | She was told that she has endometriosis, to go & have a chat with her own GP. |
| 30.01.97 | 21.09.19 | M | Pain | 1010 | 1014 | Back pain | Co-dydramol & Senna tablets | 2917 | |
| 23.06.97 | 08.12.62 | F | Pain | 1807 | 1813 | Pain & swelling (R) ankle | To Orthopaedic Surgeon at Basildon hospital | 294 | |
| 27.06.97 | 25.07.38 | F | | 1116 | 1116 | DNA | | 2964 | |
| 23.06.97 | 15.06.53 | M | URTI | 1722 | 1726 | Sinusitis | Amoxycillin | 2974 | |
| 23.06.97 | 24.04.90 | F | Rash | 1733 | 1740 | Reddish rash on fore-arms | Calamine lotion & Paracetamol | 2989 | |
| 28.06.97 | 25.02.86 | F | URTI | 1102 | 1112 | Sore throat | Augmentin-Duo | 3035 | |
| 30.01.97 | 15.02.32 | F | Pain | 1646 | 1703 | Pain (L) shoulder | For X-Ray | 3043 | Injection Depo-Medrone with Lidocaine given. |
| 23.06.97 | 04.10.83 | M | Revisit | 1640 | 1645 | Acne worse | To Dermatologist | 3046 | |
| 25.06.97 | 22.02.91 | M | | 913 | 919 | Dysuria on & off | For MSU | 3196 | |
| 23.06.97 | 24.08.91 | M | Rash | 1814 | 1817 | Warts on back, (R) palm & (R) sole | Salactol | 3306 | Referred to Dermatologist. |

Result of a query that lists all consultations from the 22nd to the end of June 1997 (ConsultationsSeenFrom22ndTillEndOfJun1997)

| SurgeryDate | DateOfBirth | Sex | Diagnosis | TimeIn | TimeOut | Complaints | Treatments | NumbersID | Notes |
|---|---|---|---|---|---|---|---|---|---|
| 27.06.97 | 26.03.58 | F | URTI | 1711 | 1717 | Infected rhinorrhoea | Amoxycillin | 335 | |
| 28.06.97 | 04.01.58 | F | RTI | 1054 | 1057 | Cough | Amoxycillin | 3420 | |
| 25.06.97 | 23.12.56 | M | URTI | 1031 | 1036 | Discharge (L) ear | Co-Amoxiclav & Otosporin | 3435 | Recurrent boil (L) nostril over past 2 yrs., referred to ENT Surgeon. |
| 26.06.97 | 02.03.48 | M | Pain | 1747 | 1800 | Abdominal pain | Buscopan | 3473 | |
| 26.06.97 | 05.04.87 | M | Pain | 1743 | 1745 | Injury (R) thumb | To A/E | 349 | |
| 27.06.97 | 04.02.90 | F | RTI | 1734 | 1738 | Cough | Amoxycillin | 3527 | |
| 30.01.97 | 25.09.70 | F | URTI | 1850 | 1854 | Sore throat | Penicillin V | 3533 | |
| 23.06.97 | 19.05.92 | F | URTI | 1005 | 1009 | Sore throat | Amoxycillin & Paracetamol | 3581 | |
| 26.06.97 | 06.03.64 | F | | 1713 | 1718 | Verruca (R) big toe | Salactol | 3582 | To see Chiropodist. |
| 30.01.97 | 10.08.68 | F | S/Leave | 917 | 926 | Abdominal pain | | 3629 | Script for Geston injection. |
| 24.06.97 | 13.05.92 | F | | 1748 | 1752 | D&V | Dioralyte | 3630 | |
| 24.06.97 | 13.05.92 | F | | 1744 | 1747 | D&V | Dioralyte | 3631 | |
| 23.06.97 | 23.04.37 | F | | 1705 | 1708 | WCC 15.6 x 10^9/L | For rpt. FBC in 2/52 | 3708 | |
| 27.06.97 | 23.04.37 | F | URTI | 1814 | 1828 | Sore throat | Suprax | 3708 | Paracetamol soluble script also given. Recurrent sore throat, referred to ENT Surgeon. |
| 28.06.97 | 02.11.20 | F | Depression | 1017 | 1035 | Panic attacks | To CPN | 3789 | Patient is to increase dose of Amitriptyline. |

335

Result of a query that lists all consultations from the 22nd to the end of June 1997 (ConsultationsSeenFrom22ndTillEndOfJun1997)

| SurgeryDate | DateOfBirth | Sex | Diagnosis | TimeIn | TimeOut | Complaints | Treatments | NumbersID | Notes |
|---|---|---|---|---|---|---|---|---|---|
| 26.06.97 | 07.06.40 | M | | 954 | 1004 | Sore & raw looking groin areas | Flucloxacillin & Fucidin H cream | 38 | |
| 23.06.97 | 19.03.15 | F | | 908 | 918 | Nicorandil script | | 3888 | Ikorel studies - 3rd visit. |
| 30.01.97 | 19.03.15 | F | RTI | 1704 | 1707 | Cough | Amoxycillin | 3888 | |
| 24.06.97 | 10.02.69 | M | | 1753 | 1756 | Tender cyst (L) groin | Flucloxacillin | 3894 | |
| 30.01.97 | 23.06.90 | M | Pain | 1729 | 1737 | Pain lower back | Diclofenac & Co-dydramol | 4081 | |
| 23.06.97 | 27.10.58 | F | | 1744 | 1753 | NHS script for Gonal F & Suprecur (fertility drugs) | | 4160 | Also has hay fever, Rx. Loratadine. |
| 23.06.97 | 26.02.36 | F | RTI | 1210 | 1225 | Cough | Amoxycillin | 4240 | Home visit. |
| 24.06.97 | 09.01.91 | M | URTI | 1830 | 1833 | Sore throat | Amoxycillin & Paracetamol | 4258 | |
| 24.06.97 | 11.12.62 | M | | 1646 | 1651 | Diarrhoea | Loperamide | 4315 | |
| 24.06.97 | 11.01.64 | F | URTI | 1757 | 1802 | Sore throat | Amoxycillin | 4320 | |
| 28.06.97 | 16.02.94 | F | URTI | 1058 | 1101 | Infected rhinorrhoea | Amoxycillin | 4339 | |
| 24.06.97 | 11.11.30 | M | S/Leave | 956 | 1002 | Back strain | | 4410 | Co-dydramol script also given. |
| 26.06.97 | 26.11.75 | M | S/Leave | 1039 | 1043 | Back strain | | 4410 | |
| 23.06.97 | 22.03.18 | F | | 923 | 935 | Script for Hirudoid cream & Paracetamol | | 4411 | |
| 27.06.97 | 18.11.91 | M | RTI | 919 | 921 | Cough | Amoxycillin | 4475 | |
| 27.06.97 | 08.04.93 | M | RTI | 922 | 926 | Cough | Amoxycillin & Paracetamol | 4476 | |
| 27.06.97 | 28.05.88 | M | RTI | 915 | 918 | Cough | Amoxycillin | 4477 | |
| 27.06.97 | 06.11.68 | F | RTI | 927 | 930 | Cough | Erymax | 4479 | Penicillin allergy. |

## Result of a query that lists all consultations from the 22nd to the end of June 1997 (ConsultationsSeenFrom22ndTillEndOfJun1997)

| SurgeryDate | DateOfBirth | Sex | Diagnosis | TimeIn | TimeOut | Complaints | Treatments | NumbersID | Notes |
|---|---|---|---|---|---|---|---|---|---|
| 26.06.97 | 29.09.32 | F | Pain | 1654 | 1700 | (R) shoulder pain | Co-dydramol & Transvasin cream | 4487 | |
| 23.06.97 | 15.02.27 | F | | 953 | 1004 | Co-Amilozide script | | 4495 | |
| 26.06.97 | 03.04.69 | F | Pain | 1645 | 1653 | Abdominal pain | Buscopan | 4508 | For MSU. |
| 27.06.97 | 01.07.65 | M | | 1739 | 1749 | Wants appointment to see Orthopaedic Surgeon brought forward | Done | 4593 | |
| 24.06.97 | 29.05.94 | F | URTI | 1120 | 1128 | Sore throat | Amoxycillin | 4598 | |
| 26.06.97 | 24.03.90 | F | RTI | 1701 | 1704 | Cough | Amoxycillin | 4680 | |
| 24.06.97 | 21.10.91 | F | RTI | 920 | 929 | Cough | Amoxycillin | 4739 | Incontinent of urine. For MSU. Referred to Paediatrician. |
| 24.06.97 | 16.03.95 | F | Rash | 1639 | 1644 | ?Insect bites on legs | Use own Calamine lotion | 4773 | |
| 23.06.97 | 09.05.72 | F | | 1650 | 1656 | Abscess on lower abdomen | Erymax | 4789 | Fucidin cream also prescribed. |
| 23.06.97 | 21.03.92 | F | RTI | 1646 | 1649 | Cough | Amoxycillin | 4794 | |
| 25.06.97 | 14.02.76 | F | | 906 | 912 | Microgynon script | | 4868 | |
| 30.01.97 | 14.02.76 | F | URTI | 1708 | 1711 | Sore throat | Penicillin V | 4868 | |
| 30.01.97 | 12.01.84 | M | RTI | 1826 | 1830 | Cough | Amoxycillin | 4878 | |
| 30.01.97 | 07.08.86 | F | URTI | 1831 | 1839 | Sore throat | Augmentin-Duo & Paracetamol | 4881 | |
| 25.06.97 | 30.05.68 | F | URTI | 1009 | 1017 | Sore throat | Augmentin | 4898 | On Logynon. FP1001 (GMS4) form signed. |

Result of a query that lists all consultations from the 22nd to the end of June 1997 (ConsultationsSeenFrom22ndTillEndOfJun1997)

| SurgeryDate | DateOfBirth | Sex | Diagnosis | TimeIn | TimeOut | Complaints | Treatments | NumbersID | Notes |
|---|---|---|---|---|---|---|---|---|---|
| 23.06.97 | 21.10.38 | F | | 1709 | 1713 | Infection (R) fore-arm | Amoxycillin & Flucloxacillin | 4918 | On Cyclosporin-type drug. |
| 30.01.97 | 11.07.33 | M | Pain | 1748 | 1756 | Fleeting joint pains | To Rheumatologist | 4968 | |
| 30.01.97 | 07.02.31 | F | | 906 | 916 | Script for Dramamine & Loperamide | | 5036 | |
| 27.06.97 | 26.06.88 | M | | 1724 | 1727 | Impetigo | Fucidin cream & Flucloxacillin | 5073 | |
| 23.06.97 | 20.11.70 | F | | 1150 | 1200 | Routine P/Natal visit | | 5109 | Home visit. |
| 26.06.97 | 11.01.57 | F | Rash | 1723 | 1728 | Non-itchy dry rash on face | Aqueous cream | 5113 | |
| 26.06.97 | 02.05.85 | F | URTI | 1729 | 1733 | Ear infection | Amoxycillin | 5114 | |
| 23.06.97 | 13.12.27 | F | URTI | 1010 | 1017 | Sore throat | Amoxycillin | 5118 | Furuncle on bridge of nose, Rx. Fucidin cream. |
| 24.06.97 | 17.09.75 | F | Rash | 1657 | 1706 | Sore rashes on legs | Flucloxacillin & Fucidin cream | 5148 | |
| 27.06.97 | 05.10.59 | F | | 1019 | 1025 | Cervical glands enlarged, tired | For FBC, TFT's & Glandular fever screen | 5197 | |
| 25.06.97 | 06.06.78 | F | | 1037 | 1037 | DNA | | 5232 | |
| 30.01.97 | 11.11.59 | F | S/Leave | 1757 | 1806 | Painful haemorrhoids | | 5252 | Scheriproct suppositories also given. |
| 28.06.97 | 01.06.93 | M | URTI | 1041 | 1052 | Sore throat | Augmentin-Duo | 5318 | |
| 23.06.97 | 18.07.79 | M | | 919 | 922 | Known depressed patient | To CPN | 5417 | Wants to be referred to CPN. |

**Result of a query that lists all consultations from the 22<sup>nd</sup> to the end of June 1997 (ConsultationsSeenFrom22ndTillEndOfJun1997)**

| SurgeryDate | DateOfBirth | Sex | Diagnosis | TimeIn | TimeOut | Complaints | Treatments | NumbersID | Notes |
|---|---|---|---|---|---|---|---|---|---|
| 27.06.97 | 03.08.48 | M | S/Leave | 905 | 914 | Depression | | 5418 | Lustral script also given. |
| 30.01.97 | 14.11.89 | M | Rash | 1029 | 1039 | Itchy rash on arms & legs | Clarityn & Calamine lotion | 5429 | |
| 27.06.97 | 18.11.96 | F | URTI | 1632 | 1637 | Has red (L) ear | Amoxycillin | 5442 | |
| 30.01.97 | 13.12.96 | M | RTI | 955 | 959 | Cough | Amoxycillin | 5461 | |
| 28.06.97 | 21.01.23 | F | | 1003 | 1017 | Fever & unwell | Amoxycillin | 5465 | She also has vaginal irritation, Rx. Daktarin cream. |
| 25.06.97 | 21.03.51 | F | RTI | 1018 | 1030 | Cough | Amoxycillin | 5479 | She also complained of hay fever, Rx. Zirtek. |
| 30.01.97 | 07.07.76 | F | Pain | 1718 | 1728 | Pain (L) shoulder | For X-Ray | 5480 | Co-dydramol script also given. |
| 30.01.97 | 20.01.97 | F | Conjunctivitis | 1819 | 1825 | Sticky (L) eye | Chloramphenicol eye drops | 5496 | |
| 26.06.97 | 17.01.65 | F | | 940 | 952 | Difficulty passing urine | For MSU | 5511 | She also feels bloated, Rx. Bendrofluazide. |
| 28.06.97 | 20.02.28 | F | | 1119 | 1139 | Haematemesis | To Medics on call, Southend Hosp. | 5517 | She had laparotomy for Duodenal ulcer 29 years ago. |
| 30.01.97 | 27.01.80 | F | URTI | 1712 | 1717 | Sore throat | Co-Amoxiclav | 5530 | Loestrin 20 script also given. |
| 27.06.97 | 15.05.88 | M | URTI | 1031 | 1035 | Tonsillitis | Penicillin V | 5533 | |
| 27.06.97 | 28.10.95 | F | URTI | 1031 | 1035 | Sore throat | Amoxycillin | 5536 | |

Result of a query that lists all consultations from the 22nd to the end of June 1997 (ConsultationsSeenFrom22ndTillEndOfJun1997)

| SurgeryDate | DateOfBirth | Sex | Diagnosis | TimeIn | TimeOut | Complaints | Treatments | NumbersID | Notes |
|---|---|---|---|---|---|---|---|---|---|
| 23.06.97 | 04.06.68 | M | Revisit | 936 | 954 | Rash on body getting worse | To Dermatology clinic | 5564 | |
| 30.01.97 | 07.07.59 | M | Hypertension | 1634 | 1645 | BP 150/100 | Bendrofluazide | 5584 | For U/Es & FBC. |
| 27.06.97 | 03.10.35 | F | | 1655 | 1659 | Tooth ache | Amoxycillin & Co-dydramol | 5606 | |
| 26.06.97 | 26.08.49 | F | S/Leave | 1006 | 1025 | Thrombosis (R) leg | | 610 | Script for Hirudoid cream & Frusemide also given. |
| 30.01.97 | 21.01.30 | M | RTI | 1807 | 1812 | Cough | Augmentin | 733 | |
| 24.06.97 | 05.05.49 | M | | 1834 | 1844 | Wax in ears | Cerumol ear drops | 910 | For ear syringing. Fell & banged his elbow. To use own Paracetamol. |
| 24.06.97 | 28.01.80 | F | | 1733 | 1743 | Unwell | Amoxycillin | 912 | For FBC & Glandular fever screen. |
| 25.06.97 | 14.02.44 | M | ?Otitis Ext. | 944 | 951 | Deafness (L) ear | Otosporin ear drops | 984 | He also has a spot on his nose which is getting darker & bigger, referred to Dermatologist (BUPA). |

Result of a query that lists all consultations from the 22nd to the end of June 1998 (ConsultationsSeenFrom22ndTillEndOfJun1998)

| SurgeryDate | DateOfBirth | Sex | Diagnosis | TimeIn | TimeOut | Complaints | Treatments | NumbersID | Notes |
|---|---|---|---|---|---|---|---|---|---|
| 23.06.98 | 26.06.32 | F | Revisit | 957 | 1006 | (L) foot still painful | For X-Ray (L) foot | 3265 | New patient check done. |
| 22.06.98 | 20.11.46 | M | | 1008 | 1020 | Prozac script | | 1011 | Referred to Psychiatrist. New patient check done. |
| 22.06.98 | 23.09.54 | M | | 936 | 944 | Prozac script | | 1017 | New patient check done. Tetanus toxoid given. |
| 25.06.98 | 21.12.73 | M | Pain | 1001 | 1011 | Back pain | Diclofenac enteric coated & Co-dydramol | 1085 | New patient check done. |
| 26.06.98 | 20.07.56 | M | | 1644 | 1649 | New patient check done. | | 1126 | |
| 29.06.98 | 08.02.39 | F | | 1748 | 1755 | Prolapse underneath | To see P/Nurse | 113 | New patient check done. |
| 30.06.98 | 26.07.47 | M | Pain | 1738 | 1746 | Pain (L) groin | Co-dydramol | 1143 | New patient check done. |
| 30.06.98 | 29.03.46 | F | Rash | 1732 | 1738 | Rash on face is worse | Referred to Dermatologist | 1146 | New patient check done. |
| 24.06.98 | 16.08.44 | M | Lump | 1640 | 1645 | Infected facial lump | Flucloxacillin | 1304 | New patient check done. Referred to Surgeon. |
| 29.06.98 | 26.06.34 | M | | 935 | 945 | LFTs slightly elevated | | 1334 | New patient check done. |
| 26.06.98 | 08.04.83 | M | URTI | 1838 | 1847 | Vomiting & fever | Maxolon, Augmentin-Duo, Ibuprofen & Paracetamol | 134 | New patient check done. |

Result of a query that lists all consultations from the 22nd to the end of June 1998 (ConsultationsSeenFrom22ndTillEndOfJun1998)

| SurgeryDate | DateOfBirth | Sex | Diagnosis | TimeIn | TimeOut | Complaints | Treatments | NumbersID | Notes |
|---|---|---|---|---|---|---|---|---|---|
| 23.06.98 | 15.01.20 | F | | 1057 | 1105 | Script for Zopiclone & Multivitamins | | 1432 | New patient check done. |
| 23.06.98 | 29.07.47 | F | Pain | 1739 | 1745 | Pain (R) foot | Referred to Orthopaedic Surgeon - BUPA | 1455 | New patient check done. |
| 24.06.98 | 17.09.16 | F | | 920 | 927 | Legs feel spastic | Referred back to Neuro-Surgeon | 1531 | New patient check done. |
| 23.06.98 | 17.01.26 | F | UTI | 1030 | 1035 | Dysuria | Trimethoprim | 1537 | New patient check done. Penicillin allergy. |
| 30.06.98 | 04.03.13 | F | | 1405 | 1415 | Giddy | To observe | 1541 | New patient check done. Home visit. |
| 27.06.98 | 16.09.80 | F | | 1035 | 1050 | Initially requested tablets to delay her period whilst she is on holidays, later declined | | 1572 | New patient check done. |
| 30.06.98 | 21.03.12 | F | | 1006 | 1017 | Wax in ears | Cerumol ear drops | 1582 | New patient check done. For syringing. |
| 29.06.98 | 20.08.66 | F | Rash | 1032 | 1035 | Acne on face | Tetracycline | 1602 | New patient check done. |
| 24.06.98 | 06.04.37 | F | | 1042 | 1049 | (L) sided facial swelling & (L) ear ache | Sofradex ear drops & Amoxycillin | 1604 | New patient check done. |
| 27.06.98 | 06.04.37 | F | Revisit | 1001 | 1012 | Shingles | Famciclovir & Co-dydramol | 1604 | |
| 25.06.98 | 17.10.40 | M | | 917 | 925 | Headaches & dizziness | For FBC & ESR | 1652 | New patient check done. |

Result of a query that lists all consultations from the 22nd to the end of June 1998 (ConsultationsSeenFrom22ndTillEndOfJun1998)

| SurgeryDate | DateOfBirth | Sex | Diagnosis | TimeIn | TimeOut | Complaints | Treatments | NumbersID | Notes |
|---|---|---|---|---|---|---|---|---|---|
| 25.06.98 | 24.03.31 | F |  | 1025 | 1040 | Loss of weight | For CXR, FBC & TFTs | 1750 | New patient check done. Seroxat, Co-Proxamol & Nitrazepam script. |
| 23.06.98 | 30.10.35 | M | URTI | 1824 | 1828 | Sore throat | Amoxycillin | 1790 | New patient check done. |
| 26.06.98 | 01.03.23 | M |  | 1820 | 1826 | Sub-conjunctival haemorrhage | Chloramphenicol eye drops | 1823 | New patient check done. |
| 29.06.98 | 20.06.38 | M | RTI | 1820 | 1827 | Cough | Ciprofloxacin | 1855 | New patient check done. Penicillin allergy. |
| 29.06.98 | 04.01.62 | F |  | 1055 | 1100 | Dizziness & unwell | Prochlorperazine & Amoxycillin | 1884 |  |
| 24.06.98 | 03.09.80 | F |  | 1740 | 1746 | Fuci-bet ointment, Balneum Plus bath oil, Klaricid & Cetirizine script given |  | 1901 | New patient check done. |
| 26.06.98 | 09.10.21 | M | URTI | 1720 | 1725 | Infected rhinorrhoea | Amoxycillin | 1998 | New patient check done. |
| 30.06.98 | 04.04.36 | F | RTI | 935 | 944 | Cough | Ciprofloxacin | 1999 | New patient check done. |
| 26.06.98 | 11.03.68 | F |  | 939 | 945 | Cilest script given |  | 2 | New patient check done. |
| 26.06.98 | 21.11.54 | M | RTI | 1004 | 1013 | Cough | Amoxycillin | 2018 | New patient check done. Tetanus toxoid booster. |
| 25.06.98 | 22.09.83 | F | Pain | 1709 | 1717 | Headaches & neck ache | Ibuprofen | 2026 | New patient check done. |

343

Result of a query that lists all consultations from the 22nd to the end of June 1998 (ConsultationsSeenFrom22ndTillEndOfJun1998)

| SurgeryDate | DateOfBirth | Sex | Diagnosis | TimeIn | TimeOut | Complaints | Treatments | NumbersID | Notes |
|---|---|---|---|---|---|---|---|---|---|
| 22.06.98 | 08.04.48 | M | Lump | 1125 | 1143 | Swollen (L) scrotum | Referred to Urology Dr. on call | 2062 | Lyclear Dermal cream script also given. |
| 25.06.98 | 23.11.60 | M | Pain | 1826 | 1831 | Pain (R) elbow | X-Ray (R) elbow | 2064 | New patient check done. He also banged his elbow. |
| 30.06.98 | 06.06.69 | M | | 1825 | 1831 | (R) eye sight is worse | Referred to Ophthalmologist | 2065 | New patient check done. |
| 26.06.98 | 14.10.38 | F | | 1014 | 1040 | To use own Zoton | | 2081 | New patient check done. |
| 23.06.98 | 02.03.18 | F | Conjunctivitis | 932 | 940 | Sticky eyes | Chloramphenicol eye drops | 2134 | New patient check done. Tetanus toxoid booster. |
| 25.06.98 | 02.03.18 | F | Revisit | 1717 | 1725 | (R) eye sticky & swollen, but better | | 2134 | |
| 22.06.98 | 25.04.62 | M | | 1848 | 1855 | Hay fever | Salbutamol inhaler & Loratadine | 2142 | New patient check done. |
| 23.06.98 | 07.10.20 | M | | 1714 | 1725 | Side effects from Zoton | Referred to Care of the elderly consultant | 2263 | New patient check done. |
| 29.06.98 | 07.09.27 | F | | 1024 | 1032 | Generalised pruritus | Referred to Dermatologist | 2276 | New patient check done. Loratadine not helping. |

344

Result of a query that lists all consultations from the 22nd to the end of June 1998 (ConsultationsSeenFrom22ndTillEndOfJun1998)

| SurgeryDate | DateOfBirth | Sex | Diagnosis | TimeIn | TimeOut | Complaints | Treatments | NumbersID | Notes |
|---|---|---|---|---|---|---|---|---|---|
| 22.06.98 | 17.02.22 | F | | 1310 | 1326 | Abrasions & wounds on legs & arm | Flucloxacillin | 2285 | She fell one day ago. She also has sub-conjunctival haemorrhage, Rx. Chloramphenicol eye drops. Home visit. |
| 29.06.98 | 29.10.19 | F | RTI | 1648 | 1658 | Cough | Amoxycillin & Salbutamol inhaler | 2321 | New patient check done. |
| 24.06.98 | 10.10.64 | F | | 950 | 954 | Vaginal thrush is better | | 2355 | New patient check done. |
| 22.06.98 | 19.11.51 | M | | 1855 | 1903 | Pain & swelling (L) chest & neck | Co-Amoxiclav | 237 | New patient check done. |
| 24.06.98 | 18.12.26 | F | URTI | 1026 | 1032 | Infected rhinorrhoea | Amoxycillin, Co-dydramol & Pavacol-D | 238 | New patient check done. |
| 29.06.98 | 02.12.48 | M | Hypertension | 1804 | 1815 | 180/130 | Enalapril & Atenolol | 2380 | New patient check done. |
| 29.06.98 | 03.03.77 | M | RTI | 1815 | 1820 | Cough & chest pain | Amoxycillin & Co-dydramol | 2380 | New patient check done. |
| 29.06.98 | 07.11.57 | F | Pain | 1710 | 1722 | NNeck pain & unwell | Co-dydramol & Amoxycillin | 2382 | New patient check done. FP1001 (GMS4) Form signed. |

Result of a query that lists all consultations from the 22nd to the end of June 1998 (ConsultationsSeenFrom22ndTillEndOfJun1998)

| SurgeryDate | DateOfBirth | Sex | Diagnosis | TimeIn | TimeOut | Complaints | Treatments | NumbersID | Notes |
|---|---|---|---|---|---|---|---|---|---|
| 24.06.98 | 06.11.20 | M |  | 1000 | 1010 | Bilateral ankle oedema | Frusemide | 2423 | New patient check done. He also has generalised pruritus, referred to Dermatologist (BUPA). |
| 22.06.98 | 01.10.20 | M |  | 951 | 1000 | Itchy blistery rash | Flucloxacillin & Cetirizine | 2463 | New patient check done. Tetanus toxoid given. |
| 30.06.98 | 14.10.80 | F | URTI | 1040 | 1045 | Sinusitis | Amoxicillin, Buccastem & Chloramphenicol eye drops | 256 | New patient check done. |
| 30.06.98 | 30.10.60 | F | Pain | 1812 | 1819 | (L) foot painful | Referred to Physiotherapy | 2572 | New patient check done. |
| 25.06.98 | 05.11.65 | M |  | 1806 | 1813 | Fever & tiredness | Amoxycillin & Co-dydramol | 2663 | New patient check done. |
| 30.06.98 | 17.11.89 | M | RTI | 1045 | 1049 | Cough | Amoxicillin | 2707 | New patient check done. |
| 23.06.98 | 05.09.73 | M | S/Leave | 1752 | 1901 | Injury (R) hand |  | 2779 | New patient check done. Salbutamol inhaler. |
| 25.06.98 | 04.06.66 | F |  | 915 | 917 | Feels tired | For FBC | 2781 | New patient check done. |
| 26.06.98 | 14.06.90 | F | URTI | 1714 | 1720 | Bilateral ear ache | Augmentin-Duo | 2823 | New patient check done. |
| 29.06.98 | 21.09.83 | M | URTI | 1702 | 1710 | Sore throat | Amoxycillin | 2843 | New patient check done. |

Result of a query that lists all consultations from the 22nd to the end of June 1998 (ConsultationsSeenFrom22ndTillEndOfJun1998)

| SurgeryDate | DateOfBirth | Sex | Diagnosis | TimeIn | TimeOut | Complaints | Treatments | NumbersID | Notes |
|---|---|---|---|---|---|---|---|---|---|
| 25.06.98 | 14.09.80 | M | RTI | 1738 | 1745 | Irritating cough | Amoxycillin | 2845 | New patient check done. He also has warts on his finger & toes, Rx. Cuplex gel. Referred to Dermatologist. |
| 22.06.98 | 18.02.86 | M | | 1750 | 1754 | New patient check done | | 286 | |
| 25.06.98 | 22.07.87 | F | | 1631 | 1637 | Persistent tickly cough over the past 6 months | Referred to Paediatrician | 293 | |
| 23.06.98 | 01.08.48 | F | Pain | 1649 | 1658 | Abdominal pain | Amoxycillin | 3009 | New patient check done. |
| 25.06.98 | 25.02.86 | F | Pain | 1745 | 1751 | Pain (L) ankle | Ibuprofen & Tubigrip | 3035 | New patient check done. |
| 23.06.98 | 06.10.34 | F | RTI | 1321 | 1335 | Cough | Amoxycillin | 312 | Home visit. She also has abdominal pain, Rx. Buscopan. |
| 26.06.98 | 30.04.85 | M | | 1706 | 1714 | Wants to have wound dressed | To see P/Nurse | 318 | |
| 22.06.98 | 22.02.91 | M | | 925 | 935 | Constipation | Glycerine suppositories | 3196 | CHS checked. Paracetamol script. On Lactulose. |
| 29.06.98 | 16.03.25 | M | | 1632 | 1637 | Dothiepin script given | | 3245 | New patient check done. |
| 23.06.98 | 16.06.66 | F | Rash | 948 | 957 | Itchy blisters on face | Fucidin cream & Flucloxacillin | 3265 | New patient check done. |

Result of a query that lists all consultations from the 22nd to the end of June 1998 (ConsultationsSeenFrom22ndTillEndOfJun1998).

| SurgeryDate | DateOfBirth | Sex | Diagnosis | TimeIn | TimeOut | Complaints | Treatments | NumbersID | Notes |
|---|---|---|---|---|---|---|---|---|---|
| 23.06.98 | 20.08.31 | F | | 1726 | 1735 | Eyes stinging | Livostin | 3266 | New patient check done. |
| 30.06.98 | 21.03.93 | M | RTI | 1049 | 1054 | Cough | Amoxicillin | 3294 | New patient check done. |
| 23.06.98 | 15.02.68 | M | S/Leave | 1706 | 1710 | Pain (R) hand | | 3308 | New patient check done. |
| 22.06.98 | 06.09.84 | M | Lump | 1720 | 1726 | Tender lump (R) breast | Flucloxacillin | 3340 | New patient check done |
| 29.06.98 | 14.08.35 | M | | 945 | 955 | New patient check done. | | 3353 | New patient check done. |
| 24.06.98 | 19.03.19 | M | | 1010 | 1016 | Dizziness | Prochlorperazine | 3392 | New patient check done. He also has pain in both legs, Rx. Diclofenac enteric coated. |
| 24.06.98 | 30.07.64 | F | | 933 | 944 | Diarrhoea & nausea | Referred to Gastro-enterologist | 3414 | New patient check done. Feels full after eating small meal. |
| 26.06.98 | 01.09.78 | F | | 945 | 954 | Burst condom | Schering PC4 | 3458 | New patient check done. FP1001 (GMS4) Form signed. |
| 24.06.98 | 16.08.27 | F | | 1728 | 1740 | Glucose 9.8 mmol/L | For fasting Glucose | 3477 | New patient check done. |
| 23.06.98 | 03.09.66 | M | S/Leave | 1640 | 1649 | Depression | | 3486 | New patient check done. |
| 25.06.98 | 19.06.43 | M | | 1012 | 1019 | Co-Amilofruse script given | | 3487 | New patient check done. |

**Result of a query that lists all consultations from the 22nd to the end of June 1998 (ConsultationsSeenFrom22ndTillEndOfJun1998)**

| SurgeryDate | DateOfBirth | Sex | Diagnosis | TimeIn | TimeOut | Complaints | Treatments | NumbersID | Notes |
|---|---|---|---|---|---|---|---|---|---|
| 29.06.98 | 11.04.21 | F | | 1255 | 1310 | Bruises (L) toes | Observe | 3495 | New patient check done. Tetanus toxoid booster. Home visit. She fell few days ago. |
| 24.06.98 | 03.12.44 | F | Pain | 1750 | 1808 | Back pain | Co-dydramol | 3509 | New patient check done. Fucidin-H ointment also prescribed. For CXR in view of loss of weight. |
| 26.06.98 | 26.07.25 | F | | 954 | 1004 | Canesten cream script given | | 3525 | New patient check done. Tetanus toxoid booster. |
| 27.06.98 | 09.12.33 | F | | 1012 | 1024 | Recurrent diarrhoea | Spasmonal | 3583 | New patient check done. |
| 30.06.98 | 05.04.73 | F | | 1645 | 1655 | Late period | For Pregnancy test | 3627 | New patient check done. |
| 29.06.98 | 05.12.39 | M | | 1004 | 1012 | Ciprofloxacin script given | | 3646 | New patient check done. |
| 30.06.98 | 27.02.54 | F | RTI | 1746 | 1754 | Cough | Amoxycillin | 370 | New patient check done. |
| 23.06.98 | 23.05.27 | M | | 905 | 917 | Awaiting appointment to see Rheumatologist | | 3716 | New patient check done. |
| 23.06.98 | 16.08.27 | F | Rash | 920 | 931 | Discoid eczema on palms | Fucidin cream & Flucloxacillin | 3717 | New patient check done. |
| 23.06.98 | 08.11.31 | F | URTI | 1831 | 1835 | Sore throat | Amoxycillin & Pavacol-D | 372 | New patient check done. |

Result of a query that lists all consultations from the 22nd to the end of June 1998 (ConsultationsSeenFrom22ndTillEndOfJun1998)

| SurgeryDate | DateOfBirth | Sex | Diagnosis | TimeIn | TimeOut | Complaints | Treatments | NumbersID | Notes |
|---|---|---|---|---|---|---|---|---|---|
| 22.06.98 | 08.09.92 | F | Revisit | 1000 | 1007 | Still chesty | To see P/Nurse re: asthma check | 3734 | |
| 24.06.98 | 08.09.92 | F | | 912 | 920 | Mum wonders if she has whooping cough | | 3734 | |
| 29.06.98 | 01.10.23 | F | Pain | 907 | 914 | Pain (L) leg | Diclofenac enteric coated | 3750 | New patient check done. |
| 30.06.98 | 03.12.88 | M | URTI | 1034 | 1040 | Sore throat & headache | Amoxycillin & Ibuprofen | 3785 | New patient check done. |
| 29.06.98 | 07.06.40 | M | | 927 | 935 | Amitriptyline script given | | 38 | New patient check done. |
| 23.06.98 | 29.09.37 | F | URTI | 1036 | 1045 | Discharge from (L) ear | Amoxycillin & Sofradex ear drops | 3835 | New patient check done. |
| 23.06.98 | 27.03.67 | M | | 1735 | 1739 | Hay fever | Telfast | 3862 | New patient check done. |
| 25.06.98 | 21.05.71 | F | | 1051 | 1055 | Hay fever | Loratadine & Rapitil eye drops | 39 | New patient check done. |
| 24.06.98 | 07.04.50 | M | Rash | 1808 | 1818 | Reddish rash on face | Doxycycline | 3914 | New patient check done. He also has pedal oedema, Rx. Bendrofluazide. |
| 22.06.98 | 16.10.56 | F | Revisit | 1738 | 1750 | Back ache still | Tylex | 3929 | New patient check done |
| 24.06.98 | 16.10.59 | F | | 1032 | 1037 | Tylex caused her to be sick | | 3929 | |
| 23.06.98 | 01.10.41 | F | S/Leave | 941 | 948 | Ruptured Baker's cyst. Acute renal failure. Med 5 | | 3944 | |

Result of a query that lists all consultations from the 22nd to the end of June 1998 (ConsultationsSeenFrom22ndTillEndOfJun1998)

| SurgeryDate | DateOfBirth | Sex | Diagnosis | TimeIn | TimeOut | Complaints | Treatments | NumbersID | Notes |
|---|---|---|---|---|---|---|---|---|---|
| 26.06.98 | 04.04.44 | F | UTI | 906 | 917 | Dysuria | Trimethoprim | 3968 | New patient check done. For MSU. |
| 25.06.98 | 07.10.68 | F | URTI | 1637 | 1641 | Sore throat | Amoxycillin | 3969 | New patient check done. FP1001 (GMS4) Form signed. |
| 25.06.98 | 01.08.47 | F | | 1758 | 1806 | Rocaltrol script | | 398 | New patient check done. |
| 26.06.98 | 06.02.44 | M | | 1810 | 1820 | Amitriptyline script | | 401 | He also has facial mole, referred to Dermatologist. New patient check done. |
| 23.06.98 | 02.07.91 | M | Pain | 1745 | 1752 | Pain (R) leg | Referred to Paediatrician | 4035 | New patient check done. |
| 25.06.98 | 02.11.39 | F | URTI | 1730 | 1735 | Sore throat | Penicillin V | 4065 | New patient check done. |
| 30.06.98 | 09.04.62 | M | Lump | 1831 | 1840 | ?(R) Inguinal hernia | Referred to Surgeon - BUPA | 4086 | New patient check done. |
| 30.06.98 | 21.01.29 | F | URTI | 1658 | 1705 | Sinusitis | Amoxycillin | 4116 | New patient check done. Tetanus toxoid booster. |
| 22.06.98 | 29.11.62 | M | S/Leave | 1056 | 1115 | Dizzy spells | | 4135 | New patient check done |
| 26.06.98 | 02.06.75 | M | | 1833 | 1838 | Gets sinus problems | Referred to ENT Surgeon - BUPA | 4213 | New patient check done. |
| 22.06.98 | 29.08.73 | F | | 1644 | 1707 | Irregular, painful periods | Referred to Gynaecologist - Basildon | 4262 | New patient check done. Tetanus toxoid given. |

**Result of a query that lists all consultations from the 22nd to the end of June 1998 (ConsultationsSeenFrom22ndTillEndOfJun1998)**

| SurgeryDate | DateOfBirth | Sex | Diagnosis | TimeIn | TimeOut | Complaints | Treatments | NumbersID | Notes |
|---|---|---|---|---|---|---|---|---|---|
| 22.06.98 | 04.09.90 | M | Revisit | 1714 | 1720 | Still coughing | Klaricid | 4278 | New patient check done. Codeine linctus also prescribed. |
| 29.06.98 | 23.06.72 | F | | 900 | 907 | Dianette script given | | 4336 | New patient check done. |
| 30.06.98 | 07.11.58 | F | Pain | 1017 | 1025 | Pain in jaws | Referred to Maxillo-facial Surgeon | 4374 | New patient check done. For syringing. Script for Dothiepin & Salbutamol. |
| 23.06.98 | 22.03.31 | F | | 917 | 920 | Hb 11.4 g/dl | For B12, Folate & Ferritin | 4393 | New patient check done. |
| 23.06.98 | 22.03.18 | F | | 1340 | 1355 | Swollen (L) ankle | Klaricid & Frusemide | 4411 | Home visit. |
| 25.06.98 | 24.05.94 | M | | 958 | 1001 | 2.5 yr. old check | | 4469 | |
| 23.06.98 | 23.06.94 | M | Revisit | 1045 | 1049 | Still drinking a lot, lethargic | Referred to Paediatrician | 4494 | |
| 26.06.98 | 24.10.82 | M | Pain | 1749 | 1801 | Pain lower back | Ibuprofen & Paracetamol | 4560 | New patient check done. |
| 26.06.98 | 29.05.94 | F | URTI | 926 | 931 | (L) ear ache | Augmentin-Duo | 4598 | |
| 24.06.98 | 02.05.86 | M | S/Leave | 1656 | 1701 | Chest infection - Private | | 4603 | New patient check done. He was also given script for Amoxycillin. |
| 24.06.98 | 04.06.61 | F | URTI | 1650 | 1656 | Infected rhinorrhoea | | 4605 | New patient check done. |

352

Result of a query that lists all consultations from the 22nd to the end of June 1998 (ConsultationsSeenFrom22ndTillEndOfJun1998)

| SurgeryDate | DateOfBirth | Sex | Diagnosis | TimeIn | TimeOut | Complaints | Treatments | NumbersID | Notes |
|---|---|---|---|---|---|---|---|---|---|
| 24.06.98 | 01.12.24 | F | URTI | 927 | 933 | Catarrh in throat | Amoxycillin | 4628 | New patient check done. |
| 25.06.98 | 18.11.79 | M | | 925 | 935 | Constipation | Co-danthramer | 4635 | New patient check done. |
| 29.06.98 | 29.04.56 | M | Revisit | 1755 | 1804 | Carpal tunnel syndrome (L) wrist | Frusemide | 466 | New patient check done. Referred to Orthopaedic Surgeon. |
| 27.06.98 | 16.11.94 | M | | 1058 | 1105 | Needs to see speech therapist | Advised to see H/Visitor | 4665 | |
| 24.06.98 | 02.07.43 | M | | 1037 | 1041 | Infected swelling (L) side of cheek | Co-Amoxiclav | 4667 | New patient check done. |
| 22.06.98 | 26.04.36 | M | | 1047 | 1056 | Chest pain, ?angina | Referred to Cardiologist | 4675 | New patient check done |
| 23.06.98 | 07.01.81 | F | URTI | 1820 | 1824 | Sore throat | Amoxycillin | 4686 | New patient check done. |
| 24.06.98 | 07.08.42 | F | RTI | 1706 | 1711 | Cough | Co-Amoxiclav | 4695 | New patient check done. |
| 23.06.98 | 16.08.74 | M | | 1828 | 1831 | Hay fever | Loratadine | 471 | New patient check done. |
| 23.06.98 | 10.08.72 | F | Pain | 1659 | 1706 | Pain (L) wrist | Co-dydramol | 4714 | New patient check done. |
| 22.06.98 | 05.06.71 | F | Rash | 1819 | 1829 | Itchy red rash on neck | Piriton | 4717 | New patient check done. Five and a half months pregnant. |
| 24.06.98 | 16.03.95 | F | | 944 | 950 | Recurrent tonsillitis | Referred to ENT Surgeon | 4733 | New patient check done. |

Result of a query that lists all consultations from the 22nd to the end of June 1998 (ConsultationsSeenFrom22ndTillEndOfJun1998)

| SurgeryDate | DateOfBirth | Sex | Diagnosis | TimeIn | TimeOut | Complaints | Treatments | NumbersID | Notes |
|---|---|---|---|---|---|---|---|---|---|
| 23.06.98 | 01.03.95 | M | | 1110 | 1115 | Bruised fore-skin | Augmentin-Duo | 4742 | New patient check done. |
| 30.06.98 | 02.09.21 | F | | 1025 | 1031 | Goes deaf | Cerumol ear drops | 478 | New patient check done. For syringing. She also has dizziness, for FBC. |
| 25.06.98 | 28.03.31 | F | | 1040 | 1050 | Low Hb & Ferritin quite low | Ferrous Sulphate | 4781 | Referred to Endocrinologist. |
| 22.06.98 | 22.04.62 | F | | 909 | 924 | To continue Propranolol | | 4831 | New patient check done. Tetanus toxoid given. |
| 30.06.98 | 22.04.62 | F | | 1705 | 1720 | Propranolol script given | | 4831 | |
| 22.06.98 | 17.03.67 | M | | 1726 | 1736 | Frusemide script | | 4854 | New patient check done |
| 29.06.98 | 17.03.67 | M | S/Leave | 1733 | 1738 | Tenosynovitis (R) wrist | | 4854 | |
| 23.06.98 | 18.06.32 | M | RTI | 1415 | 1427 | Cough | Ciprofloxacin & Salbutamol | 4874 | Home visit. |
| 30.06.98 | 12.01.84 | M | URTI | 1054 | 1059 | Sore throat | Co-Amoxiclav | 4878 | New patient check done. |
| 30.06.98 | 07.08.86 | F | URTI | 1059 | 1103 | Sore throat | Augmentin-Duo & Paracetamol | 4881 | New patient check done. |
| 25.06.98 | 28.10.91 | M | | 944 | 952 | Sore throat | Dimotane & Simple Linctus | 4896 | |
| 22.06.98 | 24.09.66 | F | S/Leave | 1845 | 1848 | Back pain | | 4907 | |

## Result of a query that lists all consultations from the 22nd to the end of June 1998 (ConsultationsSeenFrom22ndTillEndOfJun1998)

| SurgeryDate | DateOfBirth | Sex | Diagnosis | TimeIn | TimeOut | Complaints | Treatments | NumbersID | Notes |
|---|---|---|---|---|---|---|---|---|---|
| 26.06.98 | 26.06.98 | F | UTI | 1634 | 1644 | Dysuria | Trimethoprim | 491 | Rapitil eye drops & Telfast script also given. |
| 24.06.98 | 18.09.92 | F | Revisit | 1635 | 1640 | Infected wart (R) thumb | Suprax & Cuplex gel | 4956 | New patient check done. |
| 23.06.98 | 11.07.33 | M | | 1801 | 1808 | Flaky scalp | Nizoral shampoo | 4968 | New patient check done. Synalar-N script given. |
| 25.06.98 | 05.10.95 | F | | 952 | 958 | Crusty nostrils | Naseptin cream | 5053 | 2.5 yr. old check |
| 24.06.98 | 08.09.89 | M | | 1701 | 1706 | Sore throat | Erythromycin | 5069 | New patient check done. Penicillin allergy. |
| 25.06.98 | 18.09.55 | F | | 1651 | 1705 | Ear lobes splitting | Referred to ENT Surgeon | 5071 | New patient check done. She also has (R) bunion, referred to Orthopaedic Surgeon. |
| 30.06.98 | 30.04.62 | M | | 1800 | 1810 | Wax in both ears | Cerumol ear drops | 5076 | New patient check done. |
| 24.06.98 | 20.11.70 | F | RTI | 954 | 1000 | Cough | Amoxycillin | 5109 | New patient check done. |
| 22.06.98 | 11.06.80 | M | URTI | 1029 | 1039 | Sore throat | Penicillin V | 5115 | New patient check done. He also has warts on his fingers, Rx. Cuplex. |
| 27.06.98 | 13.12.27 | F | Rash | 1050 | 1055 | Scabies | Lyclear Dermal cream & Loratadine | 5118 | New patient check done. |

Result of a query that lists all consultations from the 22nd to the end of June 1998 (ConsultationsSeenFrom22ndTillEndOfJun1998)

| SurgeryDate | DateOfBirth | Sex | Diagnosis | TimeIn | TimeOut | Complaints | Treatments | NumbersID | Notes |
|---|---|---|---|---|---|---|---|---|---|
| 26.06.98 | 19.10.78 | M | | 919 | 926 | Unwell | Amoxycillin | 5134 | New patient check done. |
| 30.06.98 | 23.05.78 | F | | 1727 | 1732 | Palpitations | For FBC & TFTs | 5204 | New patient check done. |
| 26.06.98 | 20.04.55 | F | | 1740 | 1749 | Infected insect bite (L) lower eye lid | Flucloxacillin | 5253 | Loratadine also prescribed. She also has panic attacks, Rx. Seroxat. |
| 29.06.98 | 08.12.78 | F | | 915 | 920 | Cilest script | | 5293 | New patient check done. FP1001 (GMS4) Form signed. |
| 29.06.98 | 28.06.46 | F | | 1743 | 1748 | Kapake script given | | 5361 | New patient check done. |
| 26.06.98 | 03.05.72 | F | | 931 | 939 | Vaginal thrush | Diflucan | 5373 | New patient check done. Moles on (L) breast & neck, referred to Dermatologist. |
| 25.06.98 | 23.02.85 | F | | 1735 | 1738 | Sepsis (L) big toe | Flucloxacillin | 543 | New patient check done. |
| 30.06.98 | 20.02.28 | F | | 958 | 1006 | Script for Colofac, Fosamax & Kapake | | 5517 | |
| 26.06.98 | 30.11.85 | M | Rash | 857 | 906 | Facial acne | Zineryt lotion | 5562 | |
| 29.06.98 | 27.03.85 | F | | 1729 | 1733 | Paronychia (R) thumb | Flucloxacillin | 5586 | |
| 22.06.98 | 03.10.35 | F | UTI | 1755 | 1807 | Dysuria | Trimethoprim | 5606 | |
| 27.06.98 | 01.07.97 | F | Rash | 1055 | 1058 | Nappy rash | Timodine cream | 5656 | |
| 24.06.98 | 27.10.56 | M | | 906 | 912 | Co-Proxamol & Multivitamin script | | 5698 | |

356

## Result of a query that lists all consultations from the 22nd to the end of June 1998 (ConsultationsSeenFrom22ndTillEndOfJun1998)

| SurgeryDate | DateOfBirth | Sex | Diagnosis | TimeIn | TimeOut | Complaints | Treatments | NumbersID | Notes |
|---|---|---|---|---|---|---|---|---|---|
| 26.06.98 | 21.08.97 | M | URTI | 1801 | 1810 | Infected rhinorrhoea | Amoxycillin | 5724 | |
| 23.06.98 | 24.04.35 | F | RTI | 1049 | 1056 | Cough | Co-Amoxiclav | 5770 | For nebulizer. |
| 22.06.98 | 16.09.40 | F | | 1039 | 1047 | Fainted yesterday | For FBC, U/Es, TFTs, Glucose & Cholesterol | 5866 | |
| 29.06.98 | 08.08.24 | F | | 1035 | 1040 | Wants to know about hepatitis | | 5868 | Husband came to Surgery. |
| 24.06.98 | 19.04.84 | F | URTI | 1017 | 1021 | Sore throat | | 5884 | |
| 24.06.98 | 15.07.87 | M | URTI | 1022 | 1026 | Sore throat | | 5887 | |
| 25.06.98 | 08.10.97 | M | RTI | 910 | 915 | Cough | Amoxycillin & Paracetamol | 5906 | |
| 30.06.98 | 15.03.74 | F | | 927 | 935 | Worms | Vermox | 5927 | |
| 29.06.98 | 14.08.56 | M | Pain | 955 | 1003 | Back pain | Diclofenac enteric coated & Co-dydramol | 5936 | |
| 26.06.98 | 02.02.98 | F | RTI | 1649 | 1658 | Cough | Amoxycillin | 5967 | |
| 25.06.98 | 01.02.98 | M | | 1814 | 1820 | Fever & infected rhinorrhoea | Amoxycillin & Paracetamol | 5973 | |
| 30.06.98 | 01.02.98 | M | | 1754 | 1800 | Diarrhoea | Electrolade & Sudocrem | 5973 | |
| 26.06.98 | 01.01.53 | M | Conjunctivitis | 1659 | 1706 | Red & painful (R) eye | Fucithalmic eye drops | 5975 | |
| 30.06.98 | 03.01.33 | F | UTI | 1031 | 1034 | Dysuria | Trimethoprim | 5976 | |
| 23.06.98 | 29.08.43 | M | | 1024 | 1030 | Gets dizzy on Cardura | To stop | 5999 | |
| 23.06.98 | 24.05.29 | M | | 1808 | 1820 | Son wants his dad's heart checking | Referred to Physician - BUPA | 6 | New patient check done. |
| 23.06.98 | 13.10.45 | F | | 1015 | 1024 | Bendrofluazide script | | 6000 | |

357

Result of a query that lists all consultations from the 22nd to the end of June 1998 (ConsultationsSeenFrom22ndTillEndOfJun1998)

| SurgeryDate | DateOfBirth | Sex | Diagnosis | TimeIn | TimeOut | Complaints | Treatments | NumbersID | Notes |
|---|---|---|---|---|---|---|---|---|---|
| 25.06.98 | 05.12.20 | M | Hypertension | 1055 | 1102 | BP 170/120 | Atenolol | 6015 | |
| 27.06.98 | 14.05.71 | M | RTI | 958 | 1001 | Cough | Amoxycillin | 6017 | |
| 25.06.98 | 20.10.96 | M | Rash | 1019 | 1025 | Eczema | Fucidin-H ointment | 6022 | |
| 22.06.98 | 12.04.98 | M | RTI | 1829 | 1845 | Cough & vomiting | Amoxycillin, Maxolon & Paracetamol | 6034 | |
| 29.06.98 | 19.05.55 | F | | 920 | 927 | Amitriptyline script given | | 6071 | |
| 22.06.98 | 03.05.98 | M | Conjunctivitis | 1020 | 1028 | Sticky eyes | Chloramphenicol eye drops | 6072 | |
| 24.06.98 | 03.05.98 | M | Revisit | 1746 | 1759 | Still coughing | Simple Linctus & Amoxycillin | 6072 | |
| 29.06.98 | 03.05.98 | M | | 1738 | 1743 | Paracetamol script given | | 6072 | He is on Amoxycillin & Paracetamol already. |
| 30.06.98 | 27.01.45 | M | Pain | 1819 | 1825 | Back pain | Diclofenac enteric coated & Kapake | 6086 | |
| 29.06.98 | 23.05.98 | M | | 1040 | 1054 | Unwell & refusing feeds | Referred to Paediatric Dr. on call, SGH | 6088 | |
| 27.06.98 | 20.09.28 | F | RTI | 1024 | 1030 | Cough | Amoxycillin | 663 | |
| 29.06.98 | 30.06.42 | M | | 1656 | 1702 | New patient check done. | | 672 | New patient check done. |
| 23.06.98 | 19.10.24 | F | | 1403 | 1412 | Vomiting | Maxolon | 677 | Home visit. |
| 22.06.98 | 26.01.53 | F | RTI | 1808 | 1814 | Cough | Ciprofloxacin | 686 | |

## Result of a query that lists all consultations from the 22nd to the end of June 1998 (ConsultationsSeenFrom22ndTillEndOfJun1998)

| SurgeryDate | DateOfBirth | Sex | Diagnosis | TimeIn | TimeOut | Complaints | Treatments | NumbersID | Notes |
|---|---|---|---|---|---|---|---|---|---|
| 30.06.98 | 12.02.08 | F |  | 1425 | 1435 | Sepsis (L) big toe | Flucloxacillin | 73 | New patient check done. Home visit. |
| 23.06.98 | 02.11.54 | F | Lump | 1710 | 1714 | Lump (R) breast | To examine with Practice Nurse | 780 |  |
| 29.06.98 | 18.10.74 | F |  | 1012 | 1023 | PER VAGINA bleeding & burst condom | For pregnancy test | 784 | New patient check done. |
| 30.06.98 | 04.09.85 | F |  | 1720 | 1727 | Hyperventilation attacks |  | 811 | New patient check done. |
| 30.06.98 | 05.09.53 | F | Pain | 903 | 917 | Abdominal pain | Co-Amoxiclav & Buscopan | 844 | New patient check done. Tetanus toxoid booster. |
| 30.06.98 | 18.02.62 | F | Rash | 917 | 927 | Rosacea | Tetracycline | 857 | New patient check done. |
| 22.06.98 | 09.06.54 | F | S/Leave | 1707 | 1714 | Sub-total thyroidectomy |  | 927 | New patient check done. Frusemide script also given. |
| 25.06.98 | 05.03.75 | F |  | 935 | 944 | Late period | For Pregnancy test | 934 | New patient check done. FP1001 (GMS4) Form signed. |
| 22.06.98 | 26.06.45 | F |  | 1814 | 1819 | Wants to know how to use the antibiotics prescribed |  | 939 |  |
| 24.06.98 | 15.04.43 | M | Rash | 1712 | 1720 | Rash on legs | 1% OH Cortisone cream | 946 | He also has wax in both ears, Rx. Cerumol ear drops. |
| 22.06.98 | 20.10.25 | F |  | 946 | 951 | Deafness (R) ear, wax | Continue Cerumol ear drops | 952 | For ear syringing. |

### Result of a query that lists all consultations from the 22nd to the end of June 1998 (ConsultationsSeenFrom22ndTillEndOfJun1998)

| SurgeryDate | DateOfBirth | Sex | Diagnosis | TimeIn | TimeOut | Complaints | Treatments | NumbersID | Notes |
|---|---|---|---|---|---|---|---|---|---|
| 22.06.98 | 04.07.59 | F | | 1628 | 1643 | Chest pain | Referred to Cardiologist | 96 | New patient check done. Tetanus toxoid given. |
| 30.06.98 | 25.05.50 | M | | 944 | 958 | Inferior wall myocardial infarction | | 968 | New patient check done. He also has chest infection, Rx. Amoxycillin. |
| 23.06.98 | 30.10.84 | F | URTI | 1007 | 1015 | Sore throat | Amoxycillin | 980 | New patient check done. |
| 22.06.98 | 01.04.70 | F | Rash | 1119 | 1125 | Scabies | Lyclear Dermal cream | Temp | |
| 24.06.98 | 02.09.26 | F | | 1631 | 1635 | Script for Transderm Nitro patch, Aspirin & Diltiazem | | Temp | |
| 25.06.98 | 26.08.71 | F | | 1726 | 1730 | Amoxycillin script | | Temp | |

### Result of a query that lists all consultations from the 22nd to the end of June 1999 (ConsultationsSeenFrom22ndTillEndOfJun1999)

| SurgeryDate | DateOfBirth | Sex | Diagnosis | TimeIn | TimeOut | Complaints | Treatments | NumbersID | Notes |
|---|---|---|---|---|---|---|---|---|---|
| 22.06.99 | 07.06.74 | F | URTI | 1804 | 1814 | (L) ear ace | Amoxycillin | NP | Script for Microgynon-30 was also given. |
| 23.06.99 | 27.09.47 | F | | 1052 | 1100 | Inj. Clopixol given im | | Temp | |
| 23.06.99 | 16.01.41 | F | | 1100 | 1104 | Dysuria | For MSU | Temp | |

Result of a query that lists all consultations from the 22nd to the end of June 1999 (ConsultationsSeenFrom22ndTillEndOfJun1999)

| SurgeryDate | DateOfBirth | Sex | Diagnosis | TimeIn | TimeOut | Complaints | Treatments | NumbersID | Notes |
|---|---|---|---|---|---|---|---|---|---|
| 23.06.99 | 13.06.99 | M | Conjunctivitis | 1658 | 1708 | Sticky (R) eye | Chloramphenicol eye drops | NP | Script for Cicatrin, Aqueous cream & Nystatin oral suspension |
| 24.06.99 | 16.11.74 | F | | 1110 | 1119 | Injury (R) big toe | Erythromycin | Temp | |
| 29.06.99 | 17.05.77 | F | URTI | 1021 | 1027 | Sore throat | Amoxycillin | Temp | |
| 30.06.99 | 27.11.50 | F | Depression | 1644 | 1652 | Weepy & unable to cope | | Temp | |
| 29.06.99 | 03.08.35 | M | Pain | 1714 | 1728 | (L) hip pain & (L) testicle | For MSU & X-Ray (L) hip | 1071 | New Patient check done. |
| 30.06.99 | 27.10.29 | F | | 955 | 1010 | Red & itchy lower legs | Erythromycin, Fucidin-H cream & Support stockings | 1129 | Penicillin allergy. |
| 30.06.99 | 25.07.25 | M | | 1254 | 1315 | General condition poor & pressure sores have broken down | Zinc effervescent, Vit. C Tabs, Ciprofloxacin & Kapake | 1135 | Home visit. |
| 28.06.99 | 15.05.81 | F | URTI | 1802 | 1807 | Sore throat | Amoxycillin | 1136 | |
| 24.06.99 | 18.05.49 | M | Pain | 1814 | 1819 | Pain (R) big toe | Ibuprofen | 1160 | |
| 23.06.99 | 26.01.74 | M | RTI | 1714 | 1719 | Cough | Ciprofloxacin | 1248 | He also has hay fever, Rx. Nasonex nasal spray. |
| 29.06.99 | 27.08.70 | M | | 1712 | 1714 | Script for Xyloproct given | | 1262 | |
| 25.06.99 | 26.11.35 | M | | 1910 | 1930 | Diarrhoea & infected (R) knee | Ciprofloxacin & Loperamide | 1276 | Home visit. He had a (R) operation about 10 days ago. |

Result of a query that lists all consultations from the 22nd to the end of June 1999 (ConsultationsSeenFrom22ndTillEndOfJun1999)

| SurgeryDate | DateOfBirth | Sex | Diagnosis | TimeIn | TimeOut | Complaints | Treatments | NumbersID | Notes |
|---|---|---|---|---|---|---|---|---|---|
| 29.06.99 | 15.07.36 | F | S/Leave | 906 | 916 | Back problems - private | | 1309 | She also has catarrh in her throat, Rx. Amoxycillin. |
| 30.06.99 | 08.01.42 | F | | 1756 | 1804 | Her solicitor wants steroid inj; to be given to her (R) shoulder | I declined | 1435 | |
| 30.06.99 | 21.07.32 | M | Revisit | 901 | 908 | Dizziness & bitter taste in the mouth much better | | 1439 | |
| 25.06.99 | 12.05.63 | F | | 914 | 918 | Hay fever | Loratadine | 1506 | Script for Betnovate cream given. |
| 28.06.99 | 12.05.63 | F | | 1724 | 1727 | Skin infection around the eyes | Flucloxacillin | 1506 | |
| 30.06.99 | 12.05.63 | F | Revisit | 1044 | 1052 | Blistery rash around (L) eye & sore | Acyclovir eye ointment | 1506 | |
| 25.06.99 | 15.03.25 | F | | 902 | 908 | Hb 11.3 g/dl | Ferrous Sulphate | 1585 | |
| 24.06.99 | 24.12.50 | F | | 1721 | 1734 | (L) ear ache | Amoxycillin | 1638 | New Patient check done. She also has headaches, Rx. Clotam Rapid. Her thyroid gland seems enlarged. She is also T.A.T.T. For FBC, TFTs, LH & FSH. |
| 24.06.99 | 23.07.23 | M | | 1709 | 1715 | USScan: Large hydrocele around (L) testicle | | 175 | |

362

Result of a query that lists all consultations from the 22nd to the end of June 1999 (ConsultationsSeenFrom22ndTillEndOfJun1999)

| SurgeryDate | DateOfBirth | Sex | Diagnosis | TimeIn | TimeOut | Complaints | Treatments | NumbersID | Notes |
|---|---|---|---|---|---|---|---|---|---|
| 25.06.99 | 01.01.51 | F |  | 1058 | 1104 | Recurrent neck pain | Referred to Orthopaedic Surgeon | 1769 |  |
| 24.06.99 | 12.11.31 | F | Revisit | 949 | 1003 | USScan: ?bowel mass | Referred to Surgeon (urgent) | 184 |  |
| 30.06.99 | 19.01.40 | F | Pain | 1020 | 1030 | Pain (L) leg | Co-Proxamol & Ibuprofen | 1850 |  |
| 25.06.99 | 16.09.49 | M |  | 1813 | 1824 | Cholesterol 7.8 mmols/L | Diet sheet given | 1893 | Script for Atenolol was given. |
| 29.06.99 | 23.07.69 | M |  | 1728 | 1734 | Furunculosis (R) axilla | Flucloxacillin & Fucidin cream | 1989 |  |
| 22.06.99 | 04.04.36 | F |  | 1005 | 1024 | Script for Adalat LA 60 given |  | 1999 |  |
| 29.06.99 | 17.08.61 | F |  | 1640 | 1652 | Fishy vaginal discharge |  | 2095 |  |
| 24.06.99 | 23.12.29 | F |  | 1130 | 1138 | ?Allergic rash to Tetracycline | Hydroxyzine | 2104 |  |
| 23.06.99 | 21.06.59 | F | URTI | 1033 | 1037 | Sore throat | Amoxycillin | 2174 |  |
| 23.06.99 | 22.03.33 | F | Pain | 1643 | 1647 | Neck ache | Co-dydramol & Movelat cream | 2179 |  |
| 23.06.99 | 08.01.24 | F |  | 1041 | 1052 | Script for Ferrous Sulphate given |  | 2269 |  |
| 22.06.99 | 23.08.37 | F |  | 909 | 914 | Persistent chesty cough | For CXR | 2304 |  |
| 28.06.99 | 23.04.50 | F |  | 1703 | 1724 | Burst condom | Schering PC4 | 236 |  |
| 23.06.99 | 02.12.48 | M |  | 1027 | 1033 | Tingling both hands |  | 2380 |  |

Result of a query that lists all consultations from the 22nd to the end of June 1999 (ConsultationsSeenFrom22ndTillEndOfJun1999)

| SurgeryDate | DateOfBirth | Sex | Diagnosis | TimeIn | TimeOut | Complaints | Treatments | NumbersID | Notes |
|---|---|---|---|---|---|---|---|---|---|
| 24.06.99 | 02.12.48 | M | | 1028 | 1037 | Abnormal U/Es | For repeat U/Es & Creatinine clearance test | 2380 | He is also on Lipitor, for LFTs. |
| 28.06.99 | 08.02.21 | F | | 1031 | 1038 | Script for Adalat LA 30 given | | 2500 | |
| 28.06.99 | 27.01.65 | M | Pain | 1807 | 1813 | Epigastric pain | Omeprazole | 2504 | New Patient check done. |
| 23.06.99 | 09.01.38 | F | URTI | 1759 | 1802 | Sinuses tender | Amoxycillin | 2508 | |
| 24.06.99 | 22.09.39 | F | | 1647 | 1653 | Script for Co-dydramol & Ibuprofen given | | 2510 | |
| 28.06.99 | 29.06.59 | M | | 1756 | 1800 | Verruca (R) foot | Cuplex gel | 2533 | He also has painful (L) shoulder, Rx. Diclofenac enteric coated. |
| 23.06.99 | 04.04.38 | M | | 1802 | 1810 | Inj. Depo-Medrone with Lidocaine was given to (L) shoulder | | 262 | |
| 29.06.99 | 13.05.95 | M | | 1652 | 1702 | Diarrhoea & abdominal pain | Loperamide, Merbentyl & Ibuprofen | 2820 | |
| 28.06.99 | 14.06.90 | F | | 1744 | 1749 | Verrucae (R) foot | Cuplex gel | 2823 | |
| 22.06.99 | 04.06.84 | M | Lump | 1640 | 1646 | Lump (L) breast | Flucloxacillin | 288 | New Patient check done. |
| 22.06.99 | 05.07.52 | F | Lump | 1701 | 1711 | Lump (L) thigh | referred to Surgeon | 2894 | Script for Co-Proxamol was also given. |

Result of a query that lists all consultations from the 22nd to the end of June 1999 (ConsultationsSeenFrom22ndTillEndOfJun1999)

| SurgeryDate | DateOfBirth | Sex | Diagnosis | TimeIn | TimeOut | Complaints | Treatments | NumbersID | Notes |
|---|---|---|---|---|---|---|---|---|---|
| 23.06.99 | 30.01.46 | F | | 1021 | 1027 | Advised to take Dixarit 50 mcg bd instead of 25 mcg which she now takes | | 290 | Septrin allergy. |
| 30.06.99 | 05.11.19 | M | | 1652 | 1704 | The Orange badge was apparently refused | | 291 | His wife came to the Surgery. |
| 24.06.99 | 17.02.58 | M | | 903 | 906 | Appointment to see the Gastro-enterologist to be expedited | | 3 | |
| 22.06.99 | 31.01.38 | M | Pain | 953 | 1001 | Pain (L) shoulder | Co-Proxamol | 3001 | T.A.T.T., for FBC & TFTs. |
| 23.06.99 | 01.08.48 | F | | 1810 | 1813 | Script for Doxazosin was given | | 3009 | |
| 25.06.99 | 10.08.68 | F | Pain | 1030 | 1035 | Neck pain | Diclofenac enteric coated & Zopa fwan foam | 3033 | RTA fee of £21.30 paid. |
| 30.06.99 | 29.01.56 | F | Rash | 1010 | 1020 | Mole on neck & (R) arm | Referred to Dermatologist | 3034 | She also has irritable bowel syndrome, Rx. Spasmonal. She also has headaches, Rx. Clotam Rapid. |
| 29.06.99 | 07.07.83 | F | | 1754 | 1759 | She wants to know about commencing the contraceptive pill | | 3085 | |

Result of a query that lists all consultations from the 22nd to the end of June 1999 (ConsultationsSeenFrom22ndTillEndOfJun1999)

| SurgeryDate | DateOfBirth | Sex | Diagnosis | TimeIn | TimeOut | Complaints | Treatments | NumbersID | Notes |
|---|---|---|---|---|---|---|---|---|---|
| 24.06.99 | 15.03.87 | M | RTI | 915 | 920 | Cough | Amoxycillin | 3143 | He also has fever, Rx. Telfast. The Loratadine is not helping. |
| 24.06.99 | 09.08.61 | M | | 945 | 949 | Advised to continue Omeprazole | | 3217 | |
| 30.06.99 | 15.04.53 | M | Pain | 1709 | 1717 | Pain (L) big toe & in (L) shoulder | Diclofenac enteric coated | 3228 | For Uric Acid & X-Ray (L) shoulder. |
| 30.06.99 | 10.12.74 | F | Revisit | 932 | 936 | Still getting lump feeling at the back of the throat | Referred to ENT Surgeon | 3315 | |
| 25.06.99 | 11.06.56 | F | | 1742 | 1749 | Small hiatus hernia on Endoscopy | Ranitidine | 3371 | |
| 25.06.99 | 20.07.61 | M | URTI | 1723 | 1727 | Sore throat | Amoxycillin | 3412 | |
| 22.06.99 | 02.03.48 | M | Pain | 1057 | 1106 | Pain (L) loin | Colpermin | 3437 | For MSU. |
| 22.06.99 | 04.11.91 | M | Conjunctivitis | 1725 | 1733 | Eyes are sticky | Fucithalmic eye drops | 3445 | Script for Sotalol & Warfarin was also given. |
| 25.06.99 | 15.11.88 | M | | 1644 | 1647 | Hay fever | Loratadine | 3466 | |
| 25.06.99 | 07.10.91 | F | | 1641 | 1644 | Hay fever | Loratadine | 3469 | Script for Simple Linctus Paediatric. |
| 22.06.99 | 15.07.56 | M | RTI | 905 | 909 | Cough | Amoxycillin | 352 | She also has hay fever, Rx. Loratadine |
| 24.06.99 | 07.11.54 | F | | 1807 | 1814 | Bloated feeling in abdomen & constipated | Colpermin & Lactulose | 3520 | She also has hot flushes & no periods for 1 year, for LH & FSH. |

Result of a query that lists all consultations from the 22nd to the end of June 1999 (ConsultationsSeenFrom22ndTillEndOfJun1999)

| SurgeryDate | DateOfBirth | Sex | Diagnosis | TimeIn | TimeOut | Complaints | Treatments | NumbersID | Notes |
|---|---|---|---|---|---|---|---|---|---|
| 25.06.99 | 25.02.75 | M | RTI | 1002 | 1006 | Cough | Co-Amoxiclav | 3535 | |
| 22.06.99 | 09.12.23 | F | Pain | 1024 | 1030 | (R) lower abdominal pain | For USScan abdomen | 3583 | Tetracycline Allergy. |
| 29.06.99 | 09.12.33 | F | | 921 | 933 | Worried about PER VAGINA discharge | | 3583 | |
| 30.06.99 | 23.08.87 | M | Pain | 1750 | 1756 | Pain (R) knee | Referred to Orthopaedic Surgeon | 3680 | |
| 29.06.99 | 09.06.53 | M | Rash | 949 | 1001 | Broken infected skin both groins | Fucidin-H cream | 3695 | Script for Lansoprazole was also given. |
| 28.06.99 | 29.08.34 | F | Pain | 1813 | 1831 | Chest pain | GTN spray & Adalat LA 30 | 3729 | New Patient check done. |
| 28.06.99 | 01.10.23 | F | | 928 | 935 | Script for Adalat LA 20 given | | 3750 | |
| 22.06.99 | 24.09.41 | F | S/Leave | 1711 | 1718 | COPD, Depression & Insomnia - Med 4 | | 3760 | |
| 29.06.99 | 16.11.87 | F | URTI | 944 | 949 | Sore throat | Amoxycillin | 3770 | |
| 23.06.99 | 16.02.67 | F | UTI | 1037 | 1041 | Dysuria | Trimethoprim | 3814 | FP1001 (GMS4) form signed. |
| 24.06.99 | 29.09.37 | F | Revisit | 1023 | 1028 | Pain (R) upper arm persists | For X-Ray of (R) Humerus | 3835 | |
| 23.06.99 | 29.12.51 | M | | 1708 | 1714 | Advised to complete a self-Certificate | | 3874 | |
| 25.06.99 | 16.10.59 | F | | 930 | 941 | LFTs, TFTs, Folate & B12 were all normal | | 3929 | |

Result of a query that lists all consultations from the 22nd to the end of June 1999 (ConsultationsSeenFrom22ndTillEndOfJun1999)

| SurgeryDate | DateOfBirth | Sex | Diagnosis | TimeIn | TimeOut | Complaints | Treatments | NumbersID | Notes |
|---|---|---|---|---|---|---|---|---|---|
| 30.06.99 | 11.01.91 | F | Pain | 1704 | 1709 | Injury (L) ankle | Referred to Orthopaedic Surgeon | 3945 | |
| 28.06.99 | 18.06.93 | F | RTI | 1051 | 1057 | Cough | Amoxycillin | 4038 | She also has hay fever, Rx. Loratadine. |
| 22.06.99 | 09.03.93 | M | Lump | 1741 | 1749 | Lump (L) knee | Ibuprofen | 4047 | New Patient check done. Referred to Orthopaedic Surgeon. |
| 28.06.99 | 09.03.93 | M | | 1644 | 1651 | X-Ray (L) knee: foreign body (?glass) just inferior to the Patella | | 4047 | |
| 30.06.99 | 07.10.33 | M | | 936 | 941 | Script for Haloperidol & Procyclidine given | | 4055 | |
| 22.06.99 | 10.04.58 | F | Pain | 1753 | 1804 | Chest pain | GTN spray | 4129 | |
| 23.06.99 | 20.11.38 | M | Pain | 950 | 1010 | Back pain | Kapake & Diclofenac enteric coated | 4187 | He is also incontinent of urine at night, Rx. Desmospray. He also has gross pedal oedema, referred to Physician. |
| 30.06.99 | 18.09.93 | F | RTI | 1728 | 1732 | Cough | Amoxycillin | 4188 | |
| 23.06.99 | 29.07.54 | F | Pain | 1108 | 1113 | Back pain | Tramadol | 4197 | Referred to Orthopaedic Surgeon. |

368

Result of a query that lists all consultations from the 22nd to the end of June 1999 (ConsultationsSeenFrom22ndTillEndOfJun1999)

| SurgeryDate | DateOfBirth | Sex | Diagnosis | TimeIn | TimeOut | Complaints | Treatments | NumbersID | Notes |
|---|---|---|---|---|---|---|---|---|---|
| 24.06.99 | 06.07.92 | M | URTI | 936 | 938 | Sore throat | Amoxycillin | 4231 | |
| 23.06.99 | 10.03.36 | M | Pain | 1638 | 16436 | Pain (R) calf | Referred to Orthopaedic Surgeon | 425 | |
| 29.06.99 | 30.10.69 | F | | 1027 | 1036 | Paronychia (L) Ring finger | Flucloxacillin | 4275 | |
| 23.06.99 | 25.12.16 | M | | 1725 | 1744 | Awaiting letter from Orthopaedic Surgeon before referring him to Nephrologist | | 4286 | |
| 24.06.99 | 25.12.16 | M | | 1003 | 1023 | Awaiting letter from Orthopaedic Surgeon. His daughters came to Surgery | | 4286 | |
| 24.06.99 | 24.06.28 | M | | 906 | 915 | Cholesterol 7.4 mmols/L | Diet sheet given | 4312 | |
| 30.06.99 | 07.02.94 | M | Pain | 1717 | 1728 | Recurrent headaches & nasally | Amoxycillin, Ibuprofen & Flixonase nasal spray | 4318 | |
| 28.06.99 | 21.01.45 | M | | 945 | 1001 | Infected abrasions on (L) knee | Flucloxacillin & Fucidin ointment | 4329 | Tetanus toxoid booster given. |
| 23.06.99 | 03.12.60 | M | Conjunctivitis | 1744 | 1749 | Sticky eyes | Chloramphenicol eye drops | 4335 | |
| 30.06.99 | 09.03.63 | F | | 1642 | 1644 | Vaginal thrush | Fluconazole | 4368 | |
| 22.06.99 | 16.05.93 | F | | 1045 | 1057 | She saw her mum being molested & attacked by her husband | Referred to Child Psychiatrist | 4397 | |

Result of a query that lists all consultations from the 22nd to the end of June 1999 (ConsultationsSeenFrom22ndTillEndOfJun1999)

| SurgeryDate | DateOfBirth | Sex | Diagnosis | TimeIn | TimeOut | Complaints | Treatments | NumbersID | Notes |
|---|---|---|---|---|---|---|---|---|---|
| 30.06.99 | 06.08.44 | M | RTI | 1807 | 1810 | Cough | Amoxycillin | 440 | |
| 23.06.99 | 10.04.45 | F | | 902 | 917 | She will contact Kent Elms surgery regarding foot surgery | | 4413 | |
| 29.06.99 | 22.07.47 | F | RTI | 1014 | 1021 | Cough | Amoxycillin | 443 | |
| 28.06.99 | 24.03.35 | F | RTI | 1700 | 1703 | Cough | Amoxycillin | 4466 | |
| 25.06.99 | 31.12.22 | M | RTI | 1808 | 1813 | Chesty cough & wheezy | Ciprofloxacin, Prednisolone & Combivent inhaler | 4470 | |
| 22.06.99 | 08.01.87 | F | Rash | 1718 | 1722 | Itchy red rash between toes | Terbinafine cream | 45 | |
| 28.06.99 | 24.12.91 | M | | 1657 | 1700 | Hay fever | Loratadine | 4526 | |
| 25.06.99 | 19.06.27 | F | | 1749 | 1808 | Fractured (L) Humerus | Ibuprofen & Co-dydramol | 4527 | |
| 25.06.99 | 22.04.59 | F | | 1727 | 1737 | Itchy & sore breasts | Efamast & Hydroxyzine | 463 | |
| 25.06.99 | 21.05.35 | M | S/Leave | 918 | 930 | Cancer of Oesophagus | | 4788 | Script for Chloramphenicol eye drops, Metoclopramide syrup & Lansoprazole was also given. |
| 22.06.99 | 03.01.14 | F | | 1035 | 10345 | Panic attacks & difficulty breathing | Diazepam & Singulaire | 4877 | |
| 23.06.99 | 09.04.55 | F | Lump | 937 | 950 | Lump (R) breast | Referred to breast Surgeon | 491 | |

**Result of a query that lists all consultations from the 22nd to the end of June 1999 (ConsultationsSeenFrom22ndTillEndOfJun1999)**

| SurgeryDate | DateOfBirth | Sex | Diagnosis | TimeIn | TimeOut | Complaints | Treatments | NumbersID | Notes |
|---|---|---|---|---|---|---|---|---|---|
| 29.06.99 | 19.06.85 | F | | 1759 | 1805 | Involved in accident on the fair ground | Advised to go to A/E | 494 | |
| 22.06.99 | 11.03.61 | M | Pain | 900 | 905 | Injury to both Achilles tendon | For Physiotherapy | 4954 | |
| 23.06.99 | 12.09.05 | M | | 1134 | 1145 | The consultant Physician would like some of her medications discontinued: Betahistine, Spasmonal & Digoxin. Her son came to Surgery. | | 4980 | |
| 24.06.99 | 30.03.17 | M | | 1037 | 1047 | 1st & 2nd (R) toes purplish | Referred to Vascular Surgeon | 5005 | He also has a mole on his (R) temple, referred to Dermatologist. Pseudomonas aeruginosa was cultured on toes wound, Rx. Ciprofloxacin. |
| 28.06.99 | 29.09.95 | M | | 1102 | 1107 | Cheeks are red, sore & itchy | Flucloxacillin & Loratadine | 5022 | His eczema is also quite bad, Rx. Unguentum Merck cream. |
| 28.06.99 | 08.09.89 | M | RTI | 1727 | 1732 | Cough | Erythromycin | 5069 | Penicillin allergy. |
| 28.06.99 | 01.10.56 | M | Pain | 1732 | 1739 | Ongoing back pain | For Physiotherapy | 5070 | |

371

Result of a query that lists all consultations from the 22nd to the end of June 1999 (ConsultationsSeenFrom22ndTillEndOfJun1999)

| SurgeryDate | DateOfBirth | Sex | Diagnosis | TimeIn | TimeOut | Complaints | Treatments | NumbersID | Notes |
|---|---|---|---|---|---|---|---|---|---|
| 30.06.99 | 11.08.38 | M | Pain | 1848 | 1857 | Severe abdominal pain | Referred to Surgeon | 5093 | Home visit. |
| 28.06.99 | 31.10.20 | F |  | 1041 | 1051 | Infection along (R) varicose veins | Flucloxacillin & Lasonil cream | 5160 | She also has itchy & sore (L) eye, Rx. Fucithalmic eye drops. |
| 23.06.99 | 18.02.43 | M | Pain | 1753 | 1759 | Epigastric pain | Omeprazole | 519 | Script for Lactulose was also given. For FBC |
| 23.06.99 | 06.06.78 | F |  | 1719 | 1725 | USScan: Viable intra-uterine pregnancy |  | 5232 |  |
| 22.06.99 | 26.10.60 | F |  | 914 | 917 | Smelly vaginal discharge | To see P/Nurse for HVS | 5319 |  |
| 24.06.99 | 11.11.69 | F | Rash | 1715 | 1725 | Itchy rash, ?Viral | Loratadine & Calamine lotion | 5363 |  |
| 25.06.99 | 10.11.57 | F | Pain | 1035 | 1050 | Abdominal pain | For MSU & USScan | 5385 |  |
| 22.06.99 | 25.06.62 | M | RTI | 1722 | 1725 | Cough | Amoxycillin | 5393 |  |
| 25.06.99 | 29.12.37 | F | RTI | 1824 | 1827 | Cough | Co-Amoxiclav | 5395 |  |
| 23.06.99 | 27.07.96 | M |  | 1813 | 1817 | Mouth quite sore | Erythromycin | 5407 |  |
| 24.06.99 | 07.02.53 | M | Revisit | 1759 | 1807 | USScan of the Gall bladder - normal |  | 5425 | The pain persists & bread gets stuck on swallowing, referred to Gastro-enterologist. Script for Co-dydramol was also given. |
| 25.06.99 | 04.04.54 | M | S/Leave | 1705 | 1723 | RTA - Multiple trauma - Med 5 |  | 544 |  |

Result of a query that lists all consultations from the 22nd to the end of June 1999 (ConsultationsSeenFrom22ndTillEndOfJun1999)

| SurgeryDate | DateOfBirth | Sex | Diagnosis | TimeIn | TimeOut | Complaints | Treatments | NumbersID | Notes |
|---|---|---|---|---|---|---|---|---|---|
| 30.06.99 | 08.05.76 | M | | 1732 | 1736 | Recurrent (R) thigh furunculosis | Flucloxacillin | 5454 | For Glucose. |
| 22.06.99 | 20.02.25 | M | RTI | 934 | 937 | Cough | Amoxycillin | 5468 | |
| 29.06.99 | 03.11.67 | F | | 933 | 939 | Late period | For Pregnancy test | 5537 | |
| 28.06.99 | 02.12.93 | M | URTI | 1632 | 1636 | Sore throat | Erythromycin | 5569 | Penicillin allergy. |
| 22.06.99 | 28.09.21 | F | Rash | 937 | 953 | Stinging rash both legs | Zacin cream | 5597 | |
| 29.06.99 | 17.04.23 | M | | 1005 | 1008 | X-Ray both knees - normal | | 560 | |
| 29.06.99 | 30.03.84 | F | Pain | 1036 | 1041 | Abdominal pain | For MSU | 5608 | |
| 23.06.99 | 06.05.97 | M | URTI | 1017 | 1021 | Sore throat | Erythromycin | 5645 | Penicillin allergy. |
| 29.06.99 | 04.12.09 | F | RTI | 1200 | 1215 | Cough | Clarithromycin | 5721 | Home visit. |
| 28.06.99 | 07.08.96 | F | RTI | 1038 | 1041 | Cough | Amoxycillin | 5784 | |
| 25.06.99 | 03.02.68 | M | | 1737 | 1742 | Hay fever | Rhinocort Aqua nasal spray & Telfast | 5805 | |
| 23.06.99 | 30.10.97 | M | Rash | 1010 | 1017 | Eczema on legs & arms | Fucidin-H ointment | 5847 | |
| 28.06.99 | 15.01.48 | F | | 901 | 908 | She would like to stop smoking | | 5859 | |
| 22.06.99 | 16.02.37 | F | Pain | 917 | 923 | Chest pain | GTN spray | 5875 | Script for Co-Proxamol was also given. |
| 29.06.99 | 20.07.63 | F | | 1734 | 1744 | Body pains | Tylex | 5892 | |

373

## Result of a query that lists all consultations from the 22nd to the end of June 1999 (ConsultationsSeenFrom22ndTillEndOfJun1999)

| SurgeryDate | DateOfBirth | Sex | Diagnosis | TimeIn | TimeOut | Complaints | Treatments | NumbersID | Notes |
|---|---|---|---|---|---|---|---|---|---|
| 29.06.99 | 03.05.36 | F | | 1744 | 1750 | Constipated | Lactulose & Co-Danthramer | 5892 | Script for Bendrofluazide was also given. She is also tired all the time, & she is on Thyroxine. For FBC & TFTs. |
| 28.06.99 | 23.01.89 | M | Pain | 914 | 922 | Pain & swollen (R) ankle | Flucloxacillin | 5894 | For X-Ray (R) ankle. |
| 25.06.99 | 26.09.64 | M | | 1632 | 1641 | Pain (R) groin | Ibuprofen | 5918 | |
| 29.06.99 | 22.12.97 | F | | 1001 | 1005 | Fever & miserable | Amoxycillin | 5919 | |
| 24.06.99 | 25.12.63 | F | | 1047 | 1100 | Script for Dianette & Telfast given | | 5934 | |
| 28.06.99 | 23.03.26 | M | | 1001 | 1013 | Wax in the ears | Cerumol ear drops | 5954 | |
| 24.06.99 | 02.02.98 | F | | 1653 | 1656 | Impetigo affecting nostril | Flucloxacillin & Naseptin cream | 5967 | |
| 30.06.99 | 17.12.31 | M | RTI | 929 | 932 | Cough | Amoxycillin | 5978 | |
| 29.06.99 | 20.02.98 | F | RTI | 1041 | 1046 | Cough | Amoxycillin & Paracetamol | 5985 | |
| 28.06.99 | 24.05.29 | M | | 1013 | 1031 | Son came to Surgery regarding his dad's long-term in-dwelling urethral catheter | | 6 | |
| 24.06.99 | 20.08.59 | M | S/Leave | 1734 | 1741 | (L) wrist pain - private | | 6029 | |
| 30.06.99 | 13.01.28 | F | | 1040 | 1044 | Kapake script given | | 6045 | |
| 24.06.99 | 17.04.30 | M | | 938 | 945 | Script for Movelat cream was given | | 6059 | |

Result of a query that lists all consultations from the 22nd to the end of June 1999 (ConsultationsSeenFrom22ndTillEndOfJun1999)

| SurgeryDate | DateOfBirth | Sex | Diagnosis | TimeIn | TimeOut | Complaints | Treatments | NumbersID | Notes |
|---|---|---|---|---|---|---|---|---|---|
| 28.06.99 | 03.11.60 | F | | 908 | 914 | Script for Co-Proxamol & Evorel-25 patch given | | 6062 | |
| 23.06.99 | 06.03.97 | F | | 917 | 929 | Banged her head 2 days ago | For skull X-Ray | 6090 | She also has fever, Rx. Amoxycillin & Ibuprofen. |
| 22.06.99 | 05.06.60 | M | RTI | 1749 | 1753 | Cough | Amoxycillin | 6123 | He also has pain in his (L) shoulder, Rx. Ibuprofen. He also has hay fever, Rx. Loratadine. |
| 28.06.99 | 05.06.60 | M | Revisit | 1651 | 1657 | Still wheezy | Co-Amoxiclav | 6123 | He gets recurrent injury to his (L) shoulder, for Physiotherapy. |
| 29.06.99 | 10.03.30 | F | Revisit | 916 | 921 | Script for Omeprazole given | | 6166 | She still gets indigestion, referred to Gastro-enterologist. |
| 25.06.99 | 13.05.82 | F | URTI | 1026 | 1030 | Sore throat | Co-Amoxiclav | 6210 | Her (L) eye is also sticky, Rx. Fucithalmic eye drops. |
| 29.06.99 | 30.10.45 | F | | 1708 | 1712 | Hay fever | Loratadine | 6213 | |
| 25.06.99 | 03.05.36 | M | | 941 | 952 | Patient is not aware of missing hospital appointment | | 6236 | |
| 28.06.99 | 25.02.80 | F | Rash | 922 | 928 | Itchy feet | Fucidin-H cream & Loratadine | 6255 | |

Result of a query that lists all consultations from the 22nd to the end of June 1999 (ConsultationsSeenFrom22ndTillEndOfJun1999)

| SurgeryDate | DateOfBirth | Sex | Diagnosis | TimeIn | TimeOut | Complaints | Treatments | NumbersID | Notes |
|---|---|---|---|---|---|---|---|---|---|
| 22.06.99 | 07.07.27 | M | | 1656 | 1701 | Light-headed two days ago | For FBC, Cholesterol & Glucose | 6287 | |
| 24.06.99 | 04.07.71 | F | | 1635 | 1639 | Hay fever | Telfast | 6291 | Clarityn was not helping. |
| 23.06.99 | 10.02.42 | M | Pain | 929 | 934 | (L) kidney pain & night sweats | Co-Amoxiclav | 6310 | |
| 25.06.99 | 06.01.69 | F | | 952 | 959 | (R) mastitis | Co-Amoxiclav | 6316 | She had a baby 2 weeks ago. |
| 30.06.99 | 30.07.75 | F | | 1804 | 1807 | (L) big toe nail is lifting up, not sore | Advised to see a Chiropodist | 6323 | |
| 30.06.99 | 08.12.68 | M | | 1810 | 1814 | Constipated | Lactulose & Co-Danthramer | 6324 | |
| 29.06.99 | 24.01.99 | M | | 1008 | 1014 | Script for Normal Saline nasal drops given | | 6336 | |
| 25.06.99 | 14.09.72 | F | | 1006 | 1026 | Cat scratch (R) upper eye lid | Erythromycin | 6337 | Penicillin allergy. 1st dose of a course of Tetanus vaccination given. |
| 23.06.99 | 28.03.45 | M | Revisit | 934 | 937 | He still has boils on the nose | Tetracycline | 6357 | |
| 29.06.99 | 02.10.27 | M | | 939 | 944 | Constipated | Lactulose & Co-danthramer | 6360 | |
| 25.06.99 | 23.05.48 | F | S/Leave | 1628 | 1632 | Loss of memory | | 6361 | |
| 30.06.99 | 15.03.89 | F | URTI | 908 | 920 | Sore throat | Amoxycillin | 6378 | |
| 30.06.99 | 12.06.60 | F | | 920 | 929 | Watery eyes | Fucithalmic eye drops | 6380 | |
| 29.06.99 | 16.01.93 | M | | 1702 | 1708 | Dysuria | For MSU | 6391 | |

## Result of a query that lists all consultations from the 22nd to the end of June 1999 (ConsultationsSeenFrom22ndTillEndOfJun1999)

| SurgeryDate | DateOfBirth | Sex | Diagnosis | TimeIn | TimeOut | Complaints | Treatments | NumbersID | Notes |
|---|---|---|---|---|---|---|---|---|---|
| 24.06.99 | 15.12.98 | M | | 1754 | 1759 | (L) leg swollen with abrasion & itchy | Flucloxacillin & Calamine lotion | 6394 | |
| 23.06.99 | 24.03.60 | M | | 1749 | 1753 | Hay fever | Flixonase & Loratadine | 640 | |
| 29.06.99 | 28.12.72 | M | | 1805 | 1815 | He wants to stop taking drugs | Advised to contact the Roche Unit | 6410 | |
| 25.06.99 | 08.12.98 | M | URTI | 1649 | 1658 | Infected rhinorrhoea | Amoxycillin | 6434 | |
| 22.06.99 | 20.09.28 | F | Conjunctivitis | 1646 | 1656 | Blepharitis (L) eye | Chloramphenicol eye ointment | 663 | |
| 24.06.99 | 16.02.71 | M | | 1741 | 1754 | Family history of heart disease | For cholesterol | 715 | New Patient check done. Tetanus toxoid Booster given. |
| 29.06.99 | 12.02.08 | F | Rash | 1230 | 1240 | Raw & sore rash on lower abdomen | Flucloxacillin & Fucidin cream | 73 | Home visit. Script for Lactulose was also given. |
| 24.06.99 | 04.09.85 | F | | 1707 | 1709 | Verrucae both feet | Cuplex gel | 811 | |
| 22.06.99 | 13.09.18 | M | | 1001 | 1005 | CXR normal | | 841 | |
| 22.06.99 | 05.07.50 | M | Pain | 1030 | 1035 | Injury lower abdomen | Ibuprofen | 877 | |
| 28.06.99 | 15.03.75 | F | | 1636 | 1644 | Bleeding piles | Scheriproct suppositories & Scheriproct ointment | 934 | She also has sore throat & heartburn, Rx. Amoxycillin & Omeprazole. |
| 30.06.99 | 03.03.29 | M | | 1736 | 1750 | Script for Co-Proxamol given | | 979 | He is also quite pale, for FBC. |
| 29.06.99 | 08.12.62 | F | | 1046 | 1049 | Itching in the vagina | Fluconazole | 981 | |
| 25.06.99 | 01.06.32 | M | RTI | 1658 | 1705 | Cough | Amoxycillin | 997 | |

Result of a query that lists all consultations from the 22$^{nd}$ to the end of June 2000 (ConsultationsSeenFrom22ndTillEndOfJun2000)

| SurgeryDate | DateOfBirth | Sex | Diagnosis | TimeIn | TimeOut | Complaints | Treatments | NumbersID | Notes |
|---|---|---|---|---|---|---|---|---|---|
| 27.06.2000 | 24.02.1942 | M | | 1007 | 1009 | Advised to see P/Nurse for asthma check | | 1031 | |
| 22.06.2000 | 08.02.1939 | F | Pain | 1013 | 1021 | Pain in the back of neck & Sore throat | Amoxycillin & Movelat cream | 113 | Unwell, for FBC. |
| 27.06.2000 | 18.05.1949 | M | S/Leave | 947 | 952 | Pain (R) foot | | 1160 | |
| 22.06.2000 | 13.03.1954 | F | | 955 | 1013 | Script for Minocin MR, Rosex cream, Nizoral shampoo & ROC 25 given | | 1172 | |
| 27.06.2000 | 19.06.1959 | M | RTI | 1022 | 1026 | Cough | Amoxycillin | 1191 | |
| 29.06.2000 | 24.10.1929 | F | Pain | 1656 | 1702 | Pain (R) elbow | Co-dydramol | 1255 | |
| 29.06.2000 | 12.09.1962 | F | RTI | 1750 | 1758 | Cough | Amoxycillin & Simple Linctus | 1411 | |
| 29.06.2000 | 24.09.1984 | M | RTI | 1801 | 1806 | Cough | Amoxycillin & Simple Linctus | 1412 | Verruca of (R) foot, referred to Dermatologist. |
| 27.06.2000 | 21.09.1924 | F | Pain | 1250 | 1310 | Multiple joint pains | Referred to MAU, SGH - tomorrow | 1419 | Home visit. |
| 29.06.2000 | 20.10.1938 | F | | 1108 | 1115 | Advised to stop St. John's Wort unless it is absolutely necessary to continue | | 1583 | |
| 26.06.2000 | 12.07.1983 | F | | 943 | 953 | She passed out at work | For FBC, fasting Glucose & U/Es | 160 | |
| 29.06.2000 | 02.10.1943 | M | Rash | 1741 | 1744 | Birth mark on (R) thigh is bigger & aches | Referred to Dermatologist (Basildon hospital) | 1852 | |

378

Result of a query that lists all consultations from the 22nd to the end of June 2000 (ConsultationsSeenFrom22ndTillEndOfJun2000)

| SurgeryDate | DateOfBirth | Sex | Diagnosis | TimeIn | TimeOut | Complaints | Treatments | NumbersID | Notes |
|---|---|---|---|---|---|---|---|---|---|
| 23.06.2000 | 16.09.1949 | M | | 1754 | 1801 | Script for Adalat LA 60 given | | 1893 | |
| 29.06.2000 | 23.09.1951 | F | | 1806 | 1812 | Infection of the (R) lower gum | Amoxycillin | 1969 | |
| 26.06.2000 | 19.09.1984 | F | | 1818 | 1825 | Hay fever | Loratadine | 1978 | Collapse, ?cause. For FBC & fasting Glucose. |
| 29.06.2000 | 20.05.1980 | M | S/Leave | 1736 | 1741 | Abdominal pain - Private | | 2085 | Script for Buscopan given. |
| 28.06.2000 | 06.01.1931 | M | Revisit | 1744 | 1758 | He still has bilateral pitting ankle oedema | Inj. Frusemide & Bumetanide | 2208 | Itchy mole on (L) chest, referred to Dermatologist (Basildon). |
| 27.06.2000 | 01.03.1947 | M | | 1700 | 1712 | Wheezes a lot | Amoxycillin & Salbutamol inhaler | 2215 | For CXR, U/Es & fasting Cholesterol. Skin tags in axillae, referred to Dermatologist. |
| 26.06.2000 | 14.08.1927 | M | | 1010 | 1023 | Urine is bloody & cloudy | For MSU & PSA | 2289 | |
| 22.06.2000 | 25.01.1931 | M | | 1804 | 1814 | Script for Omeprazole given | | 2307 | Unwell & T.A.T.T., for FBC & TFTs. |
| 23.06.2000 | 06.11.1920 | M | | 907 | 922 | X-Ray Lumbar spine: The bones are rather poorly | Calcichew D3 | 2423 | Septrin & Cefadroxil allergy. |
| 28.06.2000 | 07.11.1984 | F | URTI | 119 | 1124 | Sore throat & neck pain | Amoxycillin & Paracetamol | 2438 | |

379

## Result of a query that lists all consultations from the 22nd to the end of June 2000 (ConsultationsSeenFrom22ndTillEndOfJun2000)

| SurgeryDate | DateOfBirth | Sex | Diagnosis | TimeIn | TimeOut | Complaints | Treatments | NumbersID | Notes |
|---|---|---|---|---|---|---|---|---|---|
| 29.06.2000 | 01.10.1920 | M | | 940 | 957 | Letter to whom it may concern that he is fit to travel to Canada | | 2463 | |
| 23.06.2000 | 22.09.1939 | F | | 1644 | 1658 | Script for Enalapril & Aspirin given | | 2510 | |
| 27.06.2000 | 16.09.1927 | M | | 1843 | 1855 | Vomiting & dizziness | Buccastem, Amoxycillin & Electrolade | 2558 | Home visit. |
| 22.06.2000 | 08.02.1951 | M | | 1706 | 1715 | Script for Amitriptyline given | | 2593 | |
| 23.06.2000 | 24.06.1932 | F | | 1009 | 1016 | Septic insect bite on both legs | Flucloxacillin & Fucidin-H cream | 2629 | Tetanus Toxoid Booster given. |
| 28.06.2000 | 02.03.1971 | F | URTI | 1701 | 1705 | Infected rhinorrhoea | Amoxycillin | 2787 | |
| 26.06.2000 | 11.04.1920 | F | | 1716 | 1730 | Infected (L) leg wound | Flucloxacillin | 2891 | New Patient check done. D/Nurse to dress wound. |
| 29.06.2000 | 27.09.1937 | F | | 1056 | 1101 | Whitlow (R) big toe | Flucloxacillin | 2893 | |
| 23.06.2000 | 24.09.1970 | F | S/Leave | 922 | 926 | Abdominal pain | | 2935 | Script for Tylex given. |
| 29.06.2000 | 27.10.1961 | F | UTI | 1717 | 1724 | Dysuria | Trimethoprim | 2973 | For MSU. |
| 29.06.2000 | 01.08.1948 | F | | 901 | 908 | Snoring | Referred to Snoring clinic (BUPA) | 3009 | |
| 27.06.2000 | 15.02.1932 | F | | 1215 | 1245 | Fell, head injury | Referred to A/E Dr., SGH | 3043 | Home visit. |
| 22.06.2000 | 06.04.1968 | M | | 1724 | 1727 | Advised to continue Kapake | | 3088 | |

380

Result of a query that lists all consultations from the 22nd to the end of June 2000 (ConsultationsSeenFrom22ndTillEndOfJun2000)

| SurgeryDate | DateOfBirth | Sex | Diagnosis | TimeIn | TimeOut | Complaints | Treatments | NumbersID | Notes |
|---|---|---|---|---|---|---|---|---|---|
| 26.06.2000 | 03.02.1951 | M | Lump | 1745 | 1752 | (L) testicle is larger & sore | Co-Amoxiclav | 3089 | For USScan of testicles. |
| 27.06.2000 | 15.03.1987 | M | RTI | 1758 | 1802 | Cough at night & headaches | Amoxycillin & Co-dydramol | 3143 | |
| 22.06.2000 | 12.07.1967 | M | | 1715 | 1724 | Chesty cough & hay fever | Amoxycillin & Loratadine | 3153 | |
| 23.06.2000 | 13.08.1979 | M | Rash | 1005 | 1009 | Skin of the feet & palms are peeling off | Fuci-bet cream | 320 | |
| 29.06.2000 | 13.08.1979 | M | Revisit | 1030 | 1033 | Skins of palms & feet are still peeling but not worse | See in 3/52 | 320 | |
| 23.06.2000 | 25.10.1968 | F | | 1032 | 1046 | Her mother-in-law & husband beat her up | Co-dydramol | 3214 | She feels sick, Rx. Metoclopramide. Health Visitor advised her to come to Surgery. |
| 28.06.2000 | 20.11.1965 | M | Otitis Externa | 1037 | 1044 | Throbbing (R) ear pain | Flucloxacillin & Otomize ear spray | 3254 | Stye in the (L) eye, Rx. Chloramphenicol eye ointment. Referred to ENT Surgeon for recurrent Otitis externa. For fasting Glucose. |
| 26.06.2000 | 22.05.1991 | M | Rash | 1637 | 1642 | Itchy rash on (R) leg | Calamine lotion | 3257 | Mole on (R) side of neck, referred to Dermatologist. |

## Result of a query that lists all consultations from the 22ⁿᵈ to the end of June 2000 (ConsultationsSeenFrom22ndTillEndOfJun2000)

| SurgeryDate | DateOfBirth | Sex | Diagnosis | TimeIn | TimeOut | Complaints | Treatments | NumbersID | Notes |
|---|---|---|---|---|---|---|---|---|---|
| 28.06.2000 | 15.12.1939 | M | URTI | 1732 | 1737 | (R) ear is sore | Gentamicin-HC ear drops | 3277 | |
| 23.06.2000 | 26.03.1958 | F | | 952 | 1000 | For repeat TFTs in 3 months | | 335 | Tetanus Toxoid Booster given. |
| 23.06.2000 | 19.07.1952 | M | Revisit | 1751 | 1754 | He still has a lump on the (L) anterior chest wall | Referred to Surgeon (BUPA) | 3430 | |
| 28.06.2000 | 22.09.1960 | F | | 1003 | 1037 | Infected cold sores on lower lips & mouth ulcers and body pains | Co-codamol dispersible, Flucloxacillin & Metronidazole | 3499 | |
| 23.06.2000 | 22.07.1982 | F | | 926 | 942 | Script for Loestrin 20 given | | 3504 | Penicillin allergy. |
| 26.06.2000 | 07.05.1961 | F | Depression | 1735 | 1741 | Her husband has walked out & she can't cope | Citalopram | 3653 | |
| 27.06.2000 | 31.07.1935 | M | | 917 | 928 | (R) ear ache | Erythromycin | 3709 | Penicillin allergy. |
| 28.06.2000 | 13.02.1987 | M | | 1640 | 1647 | He is very hard to handle in school | Referred to child Psychiatrist | 3931 | |
| 22.06.2000 | 04.09.1985 | M | | 1646 | 1652 | Advised go wait for at least 6 weeks after fractured Clavicle before commencing car racing again | | 3959 | |
| 26.06.2000 | 16.12.1949 | M | Conjunctivitis | 1757 | 1807 | Blood shot (R) eye | Chloramphenicol eye ointment | 3960 | Penicillin allergy. Script for Lansoprazole given. |

Result of a query that lists all consultations from the 22nd to the end of June 2000 (ConsultationsSeenFrom22ndTillEndOfJun2000)

| SurgeryDate | DateOfBirth | Sex | Diagnosis | TimeIn | TimeOut | Complaints | Treatments | NumbersID | Notes |
|---|---|---|---|---|---|---|---|---|---|
| 23.06.2000 | 01.08.1947 | F | Pain | 1808 | 1817 | Pain (R) loin | Diclofenac enteric coated & Co-Proxamol | 398 | Constipation, Rx. Senna tablets & Lactulose. Redness & tender head of 5$^{th}$ (L) Meta-tarsal bone, for X-Ray (L) foot. |
| 26.06.2000 | 03..1.1915 | M | | 931 | 943 | Script for Detrunorm given | | 3981 | For PSA. |
| 29.06.2000 | 09.03.1993 | F | | 1033 | 1056 | Allergic asthma attack | Bricanyl & Pulmicort turbohaler | 4048 | Nebulizer. |
| 23.06.2000 | 07.10.1933 | M | | 1000 | 1005 | Script for Haloperidol & Procyclidine given | | 4055 | |
| 27.06.2000 | 29.11.1962 | M | Pain | 1002 | 1007 | Low back pain - Med. 5 | | 4135 | |
| 23.06.2000 | 26.07.1924 | M | Pain | 1725 | 1734 | Pain in both legs & pedal oedema | Bumetanide & Co-dydramol | 4270 | Constipation, Rx. Lactulose. |
| 28.06.2000 | 26.07.1924 | M | | 1737 | 1744 | Weight loss | See in 3 months for repeat weighing | 4270 | |
| 28.06.2000 | 25.05.1968 | F | Pain | 1654 | 1701 | Neck pain following RTA | Ibuprofen & Co-dydramol | 429 | Septrin, Penicillin & Erythromycin allergy. To pay £21.30 BMA RTA fee. |
| 28.06.2000 | 07.03.1958 | M | URTI | 1815 | 1820 | Sore throat & cough | Amoxycillin & Codeine Linctus | 4321 | |

383

Result of a query that lists all consultations from the 22nd to the end of June 2000 (ConsultationsSeenFrom22ndTillEndOfJun2000)

| SurgeryDate | DateOfBirth | Sex | Diagnosis | TimeIn | TimeOut | Complaints | Treatments | NumbersID | Notes |
|---|---|---|---|---|---|---|---|---|---|
| 27.06.2000 | 19.09.1922 | F | RTI | 1736 | 1748 | Cough | Amoxycillin | 4371 | For CXR & FBC. Aspirin allergy. |
| 29.06.2000 | 08.09.1992 | M | | 1744 | 1750 | Hay fever | Loratadine | 4387 | Script for Pulmicort & Bricanyl turbohalers given. |
| 22.06.2000 | 18.03.1983 | F | | 1652 | 1659 | Nausea & vomiting | Metoclopramide | 4428 | She is unable to face people & food. Insomnia. Referred to CPN. |
| 28.06.2000 | 25.04.1935 | M | | 1705 | 1713 | Dizziness & fever | Prochlorperazine & Amoxycillin | 4438 | T.A.T.T., for FBC & TFTs. |
| 26.06.2000 | 24.03.1935 | F | Revisit | 1730 | 1735 | (L) toe still sore & swollen | Flucloxacillin | 4466 | |
| 27.06.2000 | 28.06.1994 | F | URTI | 1632 | 1637 | Sore throat | Amoxycillin & Paracetamol | 4502 | |
| 23.06.2000 | 13.02.1961 | F | RTI | 1721 | 1725 | Cough | Amoxycillin | 4522 | |
| 27.06.2000 | 24.12.1991 | M | | 1748 | 1758 | Script for Flixonase nasal spray given | | 4526 | |
| 23.06.2000 | 21.06.1945 | M | S/Leave | 902 | 907 | Low back pain | Diclofenac enteric coated & Kapake | 4566 | |
| 26.06.2000 | 10.09.1994 | M | Revisit | 1752 | 1757 | Rash on leg & scalp has been recurrent | Referred to Dermatologist | 4587 | |
| 28.06.2000 | 07.06.1966 | F | URTI | 1647 | 1654 | Sore throat | Penicillin V | 46 | |
| 23.06.2000 | 25.03.1925 | F | | 1640 | 1644 | Script for Atenolol given | | 4625 | Script for Fluconazole given. |
| 22.06.2000 | 22.04.1959 | F | | 1744 | 1747 | She wants her period delayed | Norethisterone | 463 | |

Result of a query that lists all consultations from the 22nd to the end of June 2000 (ConsultationsSeenFrom22ndTillEndOfJun2000)

| SurgeryDate | DateOfBirth | Sex | Diagnosis | TimeIn | TimeOut | Complaints | Treatments | NumbersID | Notes |
|---|---|---|---|---|---|---|---|---|---|
| 22.06.2000 | 22.11.1983 | F | | 1747 | 1751 | She wants her period delayed | Norethisterone | 464 | |
| 29.06.2000 | 06.04.1978 | F | RTI | 913 | 922 | Cough | Ciprofloxacin | 4647 | Penicillin allergy. |
| 27.06.2000 | 16.11.1962 | F | URTI | 1009 | 1022 | Sore throat | Penicillin V | 4655 | |
| 27.06.2000 | 27.07.1995 | F | RTI | 1650 | 1656 | Cough | Amoxycillin | 4964 | Script for Diprobase cream & Aveeno bath oil given. |
| 28.06.2000 | 10.06.1920 | F | Revisit | 902 | 914 | She still gets pain in the buttocks & in (L) leg | Referred to Vascular Surgeon | 4969 | Script for Movelat cream given. |
| 29.06.2000 | 12.02.1996 | M | RTI | 908 | 913 | Cough | Augmentin-Duo | 5156 | |
| 28.06.2000 | 09.05.1927 | M | | 941 | 1003 | Red spot in (L) ear | Otomize ear spray | 5162 | Pitting ankle oedema, Rx. Frusemide. Script for Movelat cream given. |
| 27.06.2000 | 06.06.1978 | F | Pain | 933 | 947 | Migraine & (R) upper abdominal pain | Paramax & Buscopan | 5232 | Diet sheet given. For USScan of the upper abdomen. Penicillin allergy. |
| 28.06.2000 | 11.05.1996 | M | RTI | 932 | 936 | Cough | Amoxycillin | 5254 | |
| 23.06.2000 | 04.04.1996 | M | | 942 | 946 | Infected eczema | Augmentin-Duo | 5282 | |
| 27.06.2000 | 04.07.1986 | F | Pain | 1637 | 1643 | Pain (R) knee | Ibuprofen | 5386 | New Patient check. |
| 27.06.2000 | 16.10.1996 | F | URTI | 1643 | 1650 | Infected rhinorrhoea & fever | Amoxycillin & Ibuprofen | 5409 | |
| 27.06.2000 | 29.03.1984 | F | | 1727 | 1736 | Burst condom | Schering PC4 | 5411 | |

Result of a query that lists all consultations from the 22nd to the end of June 2000 (ConsultationsSeenFrom22ndTillEndOfJun2000)

| SurgeryDate | DateOfBirth | Sex | Diagnosis | TimeIn | TimeOut | Complaints | Treatments | NumbersID | Notes |
|---|---|---|---|---|---|---|---|---|---|
| 22.06.2000 | 24.02.1918 | M | | 1026 | 1048 | Nightmares from war problems | Dosulepin (Dothiepin) | 5490 | |
| 26.06.2000 | 06.01.1978 | M | | 919 | 922 | Hay fever | Fexofenadine | 555 | |
| 29.06.2000 | 06.03.1910 | F | Pain | 922 | 936 | Abdominal pain & constipation | Senna, Lactulose & Buscopan | 5550 | |
| 26.06.2000 | 06.07.1942 | F | | 922 | 931 | Dizziness & ear ache | EarCalm, Amoxicillin & Prochlorperazine | 556 | |
| 29.06.2000 | 03.04.1997 | M | RTI | 957 | 1002 | Cough | Erythromycin & Simple Linctus | 5566 | Penicillin allergy. |
| 26.06.2000 | 17.08.1947 | F | | 1642 | 1651 | Abdominal distension | Colofac MR & Colpermin | 56 | For USScan of the abdomen. |
| 29.06.2000 | 17.08.1947 | F | Pain | 1019 | 1030 | Clicking & painful (R) temporo-mandibular joint | Diclofenac enteric coated & Co-dydramol | 56 | |
| 23.06.2000 | 27.12.1959 | F | URTI | 1027 | 1032 | Sore throat | Ceporex | 5609 | Penicillin allergy. |
| 29.06.2000 | 07.06.1997 | F | | 936 | 940 | Persistent constipation | Referred to Paediatrician | 5623 | |
| 29.06.2000 | 27.12.1941 | F | | 1225 | 1245 | Vomiting & abdominal pain | Referred to Surgical Dr. on call, SGH | 5790 | Home visit |
| 22.06.2000 | 17.01.1956 | F | Revisit | 911 | 921 | Still unable to fully extend the (R) Index finger | Referred to Orthopaedic Surgeon (BUPA) | 5796 | Aspirin allergy. |
| 29.06.2000 | 09.10.1997 | F | RTI | 1758 | 1801 | Cough | Amoxicillin & Simple Linctus | 5871 | |
| 29.06.2000 | 27.01.1940 | F | S/Leave | 1702 | 1707 | Chest infection - Private | | 588 | Cough, Rx. Amoxycillin. |

Result of a query that lists all consultations from the 22nd to the end of June 2000 (ConsultationsSeenFrom22ndTillEndOfJun2000)

| SurgeryDate | DateOfBirth | Sex | Diagnosis | TimeIn | TimeOut | Complaints | Treatments | NumbersID | Notes |
|---|---|---|---|---|---|---|---|---|---|
| 28.06.2000 | 25.12.1963 | F | Rash | 1103 | 1107 | Itchy & sore red rash under the chin | Fucidin-H cream | 5934 | Persistent itchy & flaky scalp with hair loss, referred to Dermatologist. |
| 28.06.2000 | 20.04.1984 | M | URTI | 1059 | 1103 | Infected rhinorrhoea | Penicillin V & Paracetamol | 5937 | |
| 22.06.2000 | 12.06.1969 | M | | 903 | 911 | Mole on neck is quite sore & bleeding | Flucloxacillin & Fucidin cream | 6021 | |
| 26.06.2000 | 21.05.1981 | F | | 1712 | 1716 | I advised her to contact Gynaecological clinic regarding missed appointment | | 6076 | |
| 26.06.2000 | 23.05.1998 | M | URTI | 1651 | 1700 | Infected rhinorrhoea | Amoxycillin | 6088 | Injury (L) side of face, for X-Ray (L) Maxilla. |
| 22.06.2000 | 06.03.1997 | F | | 1021 | 1026 | Cough | Simple Linctus | 6090 | |
| 23.06.2000 | 20.04.1933 | M | | 946 | 952 | Advised to increase the Tramadol dose from 50 mg qds to 100mg qds | | 6110 | |
| 28.06.2000 | 01.07.1998 | M | Conjunctivitis | 936 | 941 | Sticky eyes | Chloramphenicol eye drops | 6120 | Cough, Rx. Amoxycillin. |
| 28.06.2000 | 23.09.1948 | M | Revisit | 1635 | 1640 | He still gets pain in the knee | Referred to Physiotherapy | 6143 | |
| 23.06.2000 | 22.07.1917 | F | | 1734 | 1751 | To expedite appointment to see Orthopaedic Surgeon | | 6182 | Penicillin & Vallergan allergy. |
| 28.06.2000 | 30.11.1975 | F | | 1044 | 1054 | Bloated abdomen | She will observe | 6272 | |

Result of a query that lists all consultations from the 22nd to the end of June 2000 (ConsultationsSeenFrom22ndTillEndOfJun2000)

| SurgeryDate | DateOfBirth | Sex | Diagnosis | TimeIn | TimeOut | Complaints | Treatments | NumbersID | Notes |
|---|---|---|---|---|---|---|---|---|---|
| 22.06.2000 | 03.03.1994 | F | URTI | 1754 | 1757 | Sore throat | Amoxycillin | 6297 | |
| 22.06.2000 | 04.02.1972 | F | | 1757 | 1804 | She wants her period delayed | Norethisterone | 6311 | |
| 26.06.2000 | 06.01.1969 | F | Rash | 1023 | 1027 | Mole on (R) anterior abdominal wall | Referred to Dermatologist | 6316 | |
| 23.06.2000 | 12.04.1952 | M | Pain | 1717 | 1721 | Back pain | Ibuprofen & Co-Proxamol | 6322 | Plaster allergy. |
| 26.06.2000 | 14.04.1946 | F | | 1700 | 1712 | Heavy bleeding vaginally whilst on holidays | For USScan of the Pelvis & FBC | 6333 | |
| 23.06.2000 | 28.03.1945 | M | Pain | 1021 | 1027 | Pain in (R) knee | Co-dydramol | 6357 | For X-Ray (R) knee. |
| 27.06.2000 | 17.12.1946 | M | | 1712 | 1716 | Itchy moles on chest arm | Referred to Dermatologist | 6425 | |
| 27.06.2000 | 08.11.1963 | F | | 1716 | 1727 | Headaches & pain down (L) side once only & patch of hair loss on that side | To observe | 6432 | |
| 22.06.2000 | 08.12.1998 | M | URTI | 1751 | 1754 | Infected rhinorrhoea | Amoxycillin | 6434 | |
| 27.06.2000 | 04.07.1976 | M | | 1026 | 1040 | Irritable bowel syndrome | Colofac MR | 6448 | |
| 28.06.2000 | 31.03.1967 | F | | 1713 | 1732 | She doesn't want to see a Private Neurologist for her epilepsy | Referred to Neurologist | 6462 | |
| 28.06.2000 | 21.05.1960 | M | Pain | 1806 | 1811 | Low back pain | Ibuprofen & Co-dydramol | 6493 | |

Result of a query that lists all consultations from the 22nd to the end of June 2000 (ConsultationsSeenFrom22ndTillEndOfJun2000)

| SurgeryDate | DateOfBirth | Sex | Diagnosis | TimeIn | TimeOut | Complaints | Treatments | NumbersID | Notes |
|---|---|---|---|---|---|---|---|---|---|
| 28.06.2000 | 08.11.1993 | F | | 1758 | 1806 | Sore throat & Diarrhoea | Paracetamol, Loperamide, Electrolade & Merbentyl | 6519 | |
| 23.06.2000 | 27.07.1999 | M | URTI | 1016 | 1021 | Pulling (R) ear & fever | Amoxycillin | 6534 | |
| 26.06.2000 | 27.07.1999 | M | Rash | 1027 | 1031 | Viral rash on body | To observe | 6534 | |
| 27.06.2000 | 11.02.1963 | F | Pain | 1802 | 1806 | Migraine headaches | Imigran | 6552 | T.A.T.T., for FBC &TFTs. |
| 22.06.2000 | 16.04.1942 | F | | 1727 | 1731 | Persistent chesty cough | For CXR | 6594 | |
| 22.06.2000 | 19.09.1925 | F | Lump | 921 | 926 | Lump (R) palm | Referred to Orthopaedic Surgeon | 665 | |
| 22.06.2000 | 30.08.1998 | F | | 1048 | 1052 | Script for Simple Linctus & Lactulose given | | 6660 | |
| 26.06.2000 | 08.10.1940 | F | | 900 | 913 | Cholesterol 6.3 mmols/L | Simvastatin | 6705 | For LFTs. |
| 27.06.2000 | 25.08.1990 | M | URTI | 958 | 933 | Infected rhinorrhoea | Augmentin-Duo | 6718 | |
| 27.06.2000 | 17.02.1957 | F | | 900 | 906 | She wants Mat. B1 form | Advised to come back for this | 6724 | |
| 28.06.2000 | 26.02.1951 | F | Hypertension | 914 | 922 | BP 190/100 | Adalat LA 30 | 6769 | |
| 29.06.2000 | 07.12.1966 | M | Revisit | 1002 | 1009 | Red rash in the flexures has persisted | Penicillin V, Flucloxacillin & Fucidin-H cream | 6787 | For FBC & fasting Glucose. |

## Result of a query that lists all consultations from the 22nd to the end of June 2000 (ConsultationsSeenFrom22ndTillEndOfJun2000)

| SurgeryDate | DateOfBirth | Sex | Diagnosis | TimeIn | TimeOut | Complaints | Treatments | NumbersID | Notes |
|---|---|---|---|---|---|---|---|---|---|
| 29.06.2000 | 27.10.1952 | F | | 1643 | 1650 | Streamy eyes | She will come back when her notes are back here as she has just joined the Surgery | 6797 | |
| 28.06.2000 | 14.12.1974 | M | | 1054 | 1059 | Script for Salbutamol Diskhaler given | | 6800 | |
| 28.06.2000 | 01.03.1994 | M | URTI | 1811 | 1815 | Fever & neck pain | Amoxycillin | 6810 | |
| 28.06.2000 | 06.06.1970 | M | | 1107 | 1119 | His sore throat is a lot better | | 6813 | |
| 23.06.2000 | 24.12.1945 | F | S/Leave | 1801 | 1818 | Anterior Colporrhaphy | | 771 | On Tibolone, for LFTs. |
| 23.06.2000 | 14.02.1976 | M | RTI | 1817 | 1821 | Cough | Amoxycillin | 778 | |
| 22.06.2000 | 08.10.1981 | F | | 1659 | 1706 | Late period | For Pregnancy test | 779 | |
| 29.06.2000 | 08.10.1981 | F | | 1724 | 1736 | Pregnancy test positive | | 779 | For TOP. |
| 23.06.2000 | 18.10.1974 | F | UTI | 1635 | 1640 | Dysuria | Amoxycillin | 784 | For MSU. Erythromycin allergy. |
| 29.06.2000 | 14.10.1982 | F | URTI | 1650 | 1656 | Sore throat | Penicillin V & Paracetamol | 795 | |
| 23.06.2000 | 19.10.1975 | F | | 1658 | 1717 | She will come back for sick leave | | 819 | |

## Result of a query that lists all consultations from the 22nd to the end of June 2000 (ConsultationsSeenFrom22ndTillEndOfJun2000)

| SurgeryDate | DateOfBirth | Sex | Diagnosis | TimeIn | TimeOut | Complaints | Treatments | NumbersID | Notes |
|---|---|---|---|---|---|---|---|---|---|
| 27.06.2000 | 14.08.1960 | M | Pain | 952 | 1002 | Pain (L) chest | GTN spray & Co-dydramol | 881 | Script for Lansoprazole given. (R) ear ache, Rx. Otosporin ear drops. Penicillin, Erythromycin & Tetracycline allergy. |
| 29.06.2000 | 03.03.1929 | F | Pain | 1707 | 1717 | Pain (L) foot | For X-Ray (L) foot | 979 | |
| 26.06.2000 | 31.12.1930 | F | | 953 | 1010 | She will contact the Pain Management Clinic | | 989 | |
| 22.06.2000 | 06.06.1970 | M | URTI | 1731 | 1734 | Sore throat | Penicillin V | Temp | |
| 23.06.2000 | 31.07.1976 | F | | 1046 | 1054 | Script for Diazepam & Temazepam given | | Temp | Patient is a drug addict. |
| 26.06.2000 | 01.03.1935 | M | | 1807 | 1818 | Script for Kapake & Oxazepam given | | Temp | |

## Result of a query that lists all consultations from the 22nd to the end of June 2001 (ConsultationsSeenFrom22ndTillEndOfJun2001)

| SurgeryDate | DateOfBirth | Sex | Diagnosis | TimeIn | TimeOut | Complaints | Treatments | NumbersID | Notes |
|---|---|---|---|---|---|---|---|---|---|
| 26.06.2001 | 28.09.1980 | M | | 1811 | 1817 | Septic (L) facial wounds | Flucloxacillin & Fucidin cream | 1012 | Hay fever, Rx. Cetirizine. |
| 22.06.2001 | 24.07.1948 | F | | 1731 | 1735 | She would need the Norethisterone to postpone her periods | | 1067 | |

391

Result of a query that lists all consultations from the 22nd to the end of June 2001 (ConsultationsSeenFrom22ndTillEndOfJun2001)

| SurgeryDate | DateOfBirth | Sex | Diagnosis | TimeIn | TimeOut | Complaints | Treatments | NumbersID | Notes |
|---|---|---|---|---|---|---|---|---|---|
| 29.06.2001 | 08.02.1939 | F | | 954 | 1000 | Dysuria & frequency of urine | For MSU | 113 | Trimethoprim allergy. |
| 22.06.2001 | 18.05.1949 | M | S/Leave | 1655 | 1659 | Injury (R) shoulder | | 1160 | |
| 26.06.2001 | 29.12.1930 | F | | 945 | 952 | CXR: (R) apical fibrosis | | 1188 | Penicillin allergy. |
| 26.06.2001 | 03.10.1969 | F | | 1042 | 1048 | For MSU in two weeks | | 1206 | Trimethoprim allergy. |
| 28.06.2001 | 03.10.1969 | F | S/Leave | 930 | 936 | Urinary tract infection | | 1206 | Trimethoprim allergy. |
| 26.06.2001 | 05.02.1946 | F | Revisit | 1038 | 1042 | Still coughing & weak | Erythromycin & Multivitamins | 1268 | |
| 26.06.2001 | 23.10.1929 | F | | 952 | 1002 | Script for Simvastatin given | | 1279 | Penicillin allergy. For LFTs. |
| 26.06.2001 | 07.12.1982 | F | | 1640 | 1650 | Burst Condom | Schering PC4 | 1323 | |
| 22.06.2001 | 06.08.1941 | M | Pain | 1748 | 1755 | Pain (R) side of chest | For Chest X-Ray | 1425 | |
| 22.06.2001 | 15.01.1926 | F | | 919 | 934 | Dizziness | Betahistine | 1432 | Septic wound on (L) arm, Rx. Flucloxacillin & Fucidin cream. Script for Multivitamins given. For FBC. |
| 29.06.2001 | 15.06.1987 | M | Pain | 928 | 936 | Back pain | Ibuprofen & Paracetamol | 1447 | Persistent verruca (L) foot, referred to Dermatologist (Basildon hospital). |
| 29.06.2001 | 28.07.1936 | M | | 939 | 949 | Private prescription for Viagra given | | 1508 | |

Result of a query that lists all consultations from the 22nd to the end of June 2001 (ConsultationsSeenFrom22ndTillEndOfJun2001)

| SurgeryDate | DateOfBirth | Sex | Diagnosis | TimeIn | TimeOut | Complaints | Treatments | NumbersID | Notes |
|---|---|---|---|---|---|---|---|---|---|
| 25.06.2001 | 08.05.1966 | M | Lump | 1644 | 1652 | Lump on penile shaft | Referred to Urologist (BUPA) | 1745 | |
| 27.06.2001 | 28.07.1960 | F | | 930 | 937 | Advised not to wear her contact lenses for a couple of weeks after scratching her (R) eye | | 189 | |
| 22.06.2001 | 19.08.1926 | F | | 1659 | 1711 | For repeat FBC in 3 months | | 1907 | |
| 29.06.2001 | 19.08.1926 | F | | 1631 | 1636 | Isotard XL 60 discontinued | | 1907 | |
| 29.06.2001 | 07.08.1985 | M | RTI | 1736 | 1741 | Cough | Amoxycillin | 191 | |
| 28.06.2001 | 22.09.1981 | M | Rash | 1739 | 1742 | Facial acne rash | Zineryt lotion | 2165 | |
| 22.06.2001 | 11.06.1968 | F | | 943 | 950 | Queensway clinic is unable to insert IUCD, advised to come back after her period | | 2261 | |
| 29.06.2001 | 17.12.1931 | F | | 1652 | 1657 | Pedal oedema | Frusemide | 2409 | |
| 29.06.2001 | 16.06.1915 | M | | 1034 | 1042 | PSA normal, Awaiting CXR result | | 245 | |
| 27.06.2001 | 20.06.1950 | M | Pain | 1801 | 1812 | Pain in (L) big toe, ?Gout | Co-dydramol & Diclofenac enteric coated | 2475 | For Uric Acid in 4 weeks. |
| 26.06.2001 | 07.09.1980 | F | Revisit | 919 | 929 | Fungal infection (R) middle toe is worse | Terbinafine tablets & Terbinafine cream | 2577 | For LFTs, FBC & Fasting Glucose. |
| 25.06.2001 | 07.05.1978 | F | URTI | 1758 | 1811 | Sore throat | Amoxycillin | 2684 | For Pregnancy test. |

## Result of a query that lists all consultations from the 22nd to the end of June 2001 (ConsultationsSeenFrom22ndTillEndOfJun2001)

| SurgeryDate | DateOfBirth | Sex | Diagnosis | TimeIn | TimeOut | Complaints | Treatments | NumbersID | Notes |
|---|---|---|---|---|---|---|---|---|---|
| 28.06.2001 | 22.12.1989 | M | Rash | 1659 | 1706 | Itchy rash both feet | Daktacort | 2725 | |
| 29.06.2001 | 23.02.1945 | M | RTI | 909 | 913 | Cough | Erythromycin | 2750 | |
| 27.06.2001 | 05.07.1952 | F | Hypertension | 1812 | 1821 | BP 150/100 | Ramipril & Adalat LA 30 | 2894 | |
| 27.06.2001 | 01.06.1969 | F | Pain | 1702 | 1707 | Pins & needles both hands & pain, ?Carpal tunnel syndrome | Referred to Plastic Surgeon | 2903 | |
| 29.06.2001 | 05.05.1953 | F | URTI | 949 | 954 | Pain at the back of the throat | Amoxycillin | 3000 | |
| 28.06.2001 | 26.06.1946 | M | S/Leave | 912 | 922 | Depression | | 3025 | |
| 25.06.2001 | 20.03.1959 | F | Rash | 948 | 956 | Itchy & sore moles on the neck | Referred to Dermatologist (Basildon hospital) | 3166 | Septrin & Ceporex allergy. |
| 25.06.2001 | 27.04.1976 | M | S/Leave | 1015 | 1018 | Back pain | | 3184 | |
| 25.06.2001 | 16.03.1925 | M | | 939 | 943 | Diarrhoea | Lomotil | 3245 | |
| 27.06.2001 | 08.10.1969 | F | Pain | 1740 | 1750 | Low back pain | Co-dydramol & Diclofenac enteric coated | 3270 | For MSU. |
| 25.06.2001 | 31.07.1959 | F | | 1002 | 1015 | Recurrent vaginal thrush | Clotrimazole pessary | 3327 | For Fasting Glucose. |
| 28.06.2001 | 20.05.1938 | F | | 922 | 930 | Blood shot (R) eye | Chloramphenicol eye drops | 336 | |
| 26.06.2001 | 18.07.1978 | F | | 1200 | 1212 | Routine P/Natal visit | | 337 | Home visit. |
| 28.06.2001 | 11.06.1956 | F | Rash | 1635 | 1642 | ?Shingles rash L2/L3 | Famciclovir | 3371 | |
| 25.06.2001 | 19.03.1919 | M | | 1050 | 1057 | Painful (R) ribs following fall | Advised to use own Co-dydramol | 3392 | |

394

Result of a query that lists all consultations from the 22nd to the end of June 2001 (ConsultationsSeenFrom22ndTillEndOfJun2001)

| SurgeryDate | DateOfBirth | Sex | Diagnosis | TimeIn | TimeOut | Complaints | Treatments | NumbersID | Notes |
|---|---|---|---|---|---|---|---|---|---|
| 25.06.2001 | 01.09.1978 | F | | 915 | 925 | Script for Noriday given | | 3458 | FP1001 (GMS4) form signed. |
| 29.06.2001 | 28.10.1960 | M | URTI | 1753 | 1758 | Lump on the back of the throat | Amoxycillin | 3501 | |
| 22.06.2001 | 27.02.1992 | M | Pain | 1726 | 1731 | Injury (R) ankle | Ibuprofen & Paracetamol | 3589 | Penicillin allergy. |
| 28.06.2001 | 14.06.1957 | F | Hypertension | 1650 | 1659 | BP 170/100 | Celiprolol | 3661 | |
| 27.06.2001 | 17.02.1992 | F | URTI | 1735 | 1740 | Sore throat & fever | Erythromycin, Paracetamol & Ibuprofen | 3669 | Penicillin allergy. |
| 27.06.2001 | 12.08.1974 | F | Conjunctivitis | 1726 | 1732 | Yellow discharge both eyes | Chloramphenicol eye ointment | 3693 | |
| 27.06.2001 | 07.06.1940 | M | | 1750 | 1801 | Patient was informed that his Kapake will be changed to Dihydrocodeine | | 38 | |
| 27.06.2001 | 25.01.1983 | F | | 905 | 911 | Septic (R)IGTN | Flucloxacillin | 3930 | |
| 27.06.2001 | 16.06.1966 | F | URTI | 1824 | 1830 | Sore throat & ear ache | Erythromycin, Sofradex ear drops & Diclofenac enteric coated | 3944 | |
| 25.06.2001 | 10.06.1970 | F | | 1709 | 1714 | Hay fever | Fexofenadine | 4104 | Penicillin allergy. |
| 22.06.2001 | 21.01.1929 | F | Revisit | 1648 | 1655 | Pain (R) hip & (R) knee is still present | Referred to Orthopaedic Surgeon | 4116 | Moles on arm, Referred to Dermatologist (Basildon hospital). Zantac allergy. |

## Result of a query that lists all consultations from the 22nd to the end of June 2001 (ConsultationsSeenFrom22ndTillEndOfJun2001)

| SurgeryDate | DateOfBirth | Sex | Diagnosis | TimeIn | TimeOut | Complaints | Treatments | NumbersID | Notes |
|---|---|---|---|---|---|---|---|---|---|
| 28.06.2001 | 04.11.1947 | F | | 1028 | 1036 | Advised to change to period-free HRT when she is 34 years old | | 4165 | Penicillin & Klaricid allergy. |
| 27.06.2001 | 03.06.1974 | F | S/Leave | 1637 | 1646 | Intra Uterine growth Retardation | | 4219 | Script for Pregaday given. |
| 26.06.2001 | 24.06.1970 | F | URTI | 915 | 919 | Thick greenish running nose | Erythromycin | 4295 | |
| 27.06.2001 | 24.12.1989 | F | URTI | 1646 | 1650 | Sore throat | Amoxycillin | 4328 | |
| 29.06.2001 | 12.04.1927 | M | | 936 | 939 | Septic scrotal wound | Flucloxacillin | 4394 | |
| 25.06.2001 | 31.07.1972 | F | Depression | 925 | 939 | She is afraid that her boyfriend is cheating in her & can't cope | Citalopram | 4398 | |
| 22.06.2001 | 03.10.1926 | M | | 915 | 919 | Script for Lansoprazole given | | 4399 | |
| 28.06.2001 | 28.11.1925 | F | | 1006 | 1028 | Pain in legs & heavy | Co-dydramol & Naftidrofuryl | 4400 | (R) eye is blurred, referred to Ophthalmologist. |
| 25.06.2001 | 28.07.1977 | M | URTI | 1714 | 1721 | Sore throat, fever & diarrhoea | Erythromycin & Ibuprofen | 4637 | |
| 27.06.2001 | 03.07.1967 | F | URTI | 1036 | 1048 | (L) ear ache | Sofradex ear drops & Amoxycillin | 4657 | |
| 25.06.2001 | 27.04.1962 | F | URTI | 1652 | 1658 | ?Boil in the (L) ear | Flucloxacillin & sofradex ear drops | 4724 | |
| 28.06.2001 | 19.05.1989 | M | | 901 | 912 | Dizziness & fainting attacks after & during exercise | Referred to Paediatrician | 4895 | For FBC, TFTs & Fasting Glucose. |

396

Result of a query that lists all consultations from the 22nd to the end of June 2001 (ConsultationsSeenFrom22ndTillEndOfJun2001)

| SurgeryDate | DateOfBirth | Sex | Diagnosis | TimeIn | TimeOut | Complaints | Treatments | NumbersID | Notes |
|---|---|---|---|---|---|---|---|---|---|
| 22.06.2001 | 03.08.1993 | F | | 934 | 940 | Hay fever | Loratadine | 4914 | Wart on (L) palm, Rx. Cuplex gel. |
| 22.06.2001 | 16.10.1963 | F | | 940 | 943 | Hay fever | Loratadine | 4916 | |
| 22.06.2001 | 10.06.1921 | M | | 950 | 954 | I explained to him that Celebrex & Bendrofluazide will not clash | | 4972 | |
| 28.06.2001 | 24.09.1995 | F | RTI | 1709 | 1712 | Cough | Amoxycillin | 5040 | |
| 26.06.2001 | 26.08.1913 | F | | 1650 | 1700 | Eyes are red & hot | Referred to eye Surgeon | 5046 | |
| 22.06.2001 | 28.11.1991 | M | URTI | 1817 | 1827 | Sore throat | Amoxycillin & Paracetamol | 5079 | |
| 26.06.2001 | 06.06.1978 | F | Depression | 1020 | 1038 | Unable to cope & insomnia | Citalopram | 5232 | Penicillin allergy. |
| 25.06.2001 | 24.10.1989 | F | Pain | 902 | 908 | Injury (R) thumb | Ibuprofen suspension | 5236 | |
| 29.06.2001 | 04.04.1996 | M | Pain | 1710 | 1716 | Nose injury & epistaxis | For X-Ray of nose | 5282 | |
| 22.06.2001 | 10.05.1958 | M | S/Leave | 954 | 1026 | Tiredness & chest pain - Med. 5 | | 5377 | |
| 28.06.2001 | 24.06.1937 | M | Revisit | 1758 | 1804 | Pruritus ani persists | Mebendazole | 5437 | |
| 28.06.2001 | 15.11.1944 | F | | 1742 | 1758 | Script for Simvastatin given | | 5438 | |
| 25.06.2001 | 13.12.1996 | M | | 1041 | 1045 | Cough | Dimotane Plus | 5461 | |
| 26.06.2001 | 08.01.1973 | F | | 1009 | 1020 | For Fasting Cholesterol | | 5592 | |

Result of a query that lists all consultations from the 22nd to the end of June 2001 (ConsultationsSeenFrom22ndTillEndOfJun2001)

| SurgeryDate | DateOfBirth | Sex | Diagnosis | TimeIn | TimeOut | Complaints | Treatments | NumbersID | Notes |
|---|---|---|---|---|---|---|---|---|---|
| 29.06.2001 | 19.12.1978 | F | URTI | 1758 | 1803 | (L) Otitis ext. | Flucloxacillin & Sofradex ear drops | 5626 | |
| 22.06.2001 | 06.05.1997 | M | | 1028 | 1033 | Hay fever | Cetirizine | 5645 | Penicillin allergy. |
| 27.06.2001 | 05.12.1938 | M | Pain | 1125 | 1133 | Pain (R) knee & swelling | Flucloxacillin, Co-dydramol & Diclofenac enteric coated | 5651 | |
| 22.06.2001 | 31.01.1941 | F | | 908 | 915 | Script for Estraderm MX patches given | | 5867 | |
| 22.06.2001 | 06.01.1935 | M | | 1719 | 1726 | Advised to contact the smoking cessation clinic | | 5872 | |
| 28.06.2001 | 21.11.1997 | M | RTI | 1706 | 1709 | Cough | Amoxycillin | 5898 | |
| 26.06.2001 | 21.08.1946 | F | | 929 | 936 | Stabbing pain in (R) breast | Advised to use own Co-Proxamol | 5902 | |
| 29.06.2001 | 14.08.1956 | M | | 1702 | 1710 | Excessive salivation since tooth extraction | Metronidazole | 5936 | |
| 26.06.2001 | 29.09.1975 | F | | 1745 | 1756 | Diarrhoea & headaches | Advised to use own Dioralyte & Paracetamol | 5970 | Penicillin allergy. 16 weeks gestation. |
| 25.06.2001 | 06.01.1987 | F | | 1658 | 1709 | ?Chicken pox rash | Paracetamol & Calamine lotion | 5981 | |
| 27.06.2001 | 30.01.1931 | F | Rash | 920 | 930 | Bilateral ankle swelling & red sore areas on the legs | Frusemide & Flucloxacillin | 600 | |

398

Result of a query that lists all consultations from the 22nd to the end of June 2001 (ConsultationsSeenFrom22ndTillEndOfJun2001)

| SurgeryDate | DateOfBirth | Sex | Diagnosis | TimeIn | TimeOut | Complaints | Treatments | NumbersID | Notes |
|---|---|---|---|---|---|---|---|---|---|
| 25.06.2001 | 02.08.1970 | F | | 1018 | 1041 | Script for Triamcinolone Inj. & Ventolin inhaler given | | 6019 | |
| 27.06.2001 | 28.05.1944 | M | | 1018 | 1036 | Hay fever | Loratadine | 609 | |
| 27.06.2001 | 19.09.1937 | M | | 1821 | 1824 | U/Es & Cholesterol normal | | 6104 | |
| 22.06.2001 | 25.04.1984 | M | | 1026 | 1028 | Hay fever | Fexofenadine | 6116 | Penicillin allergy. |
| 22.06.2001 | 28.09.1939 | F | Revisit | 1809 | 1817 | Sore throat & feeling of lump in the throat | Referred to ENT Surgeon | 6176 | |
| 29.06.2001 | 19.1.1964 | F | Pain | 901 | 909 | Pain & throbbing (R) thigh | Naftidrofuryl | 6196 | Indigestion, Rx. Lansoprazole. |
| 28.06.2001 | 19.12.1974 | M | | 1730 | 1739 | Palpable & tender (L) femoral glands | Flucloxacillin | 6319 | For FBC & X-Ray (L) big toe. |
| 27.06.2001 | 23.05.1948 | F | | 1650 | 1655 | Nausea | Metoclopramide | 6361 | Script for Aspirin dispersible given. |
| 28.06.2001 | 29.09.1949 | F | | 1804 | 1811 | Heavy periods with clots | Norethisterone | 6365 | |
| 28.06.2001 | 02.07.1987 | M | Rash | 1036 | 1047 | (L) T3 shingles rash | Famciclovir, Ibuprofen & Calamine lotion | 6388 | |
| 22.06.2001 | 17.06.1941 | F | | 1755 | 1809 | Hay fever | Beclomethasone nasal spray & fexofenadine | 6435 | Script for Atenolol & Cuplex gel given. Penicillin allergy. |
| 28.06.2001 | 08.11.1993 | F | Revisit | 1712 | 1716 | Chesty cough again | Erythromycin | 6519 | |
| 28.06.2001 | 26.02.1934 | F | Rash | 1002 | 1006 | Mole on (L) thigh | Referred to Dermatologist (Basildon hospital) | 6536 | |

**Result of a query that lists all consultations from the 22nd to the end of June 2001 (ConsultationsSeenFrom22ndTillEndOfJun2001)**

| SurgeryDate | DateOfBirth | Sex | Diagnosis | TimeIn | TimeOut | Complaints | Treatments | NumbersID | Notes |
|---|---|---|---|---|---|---|---|---|---|
| 22.06.2001 | 01.09.1999 | M | | 1639 | 1648 | Injury (L) face, tender & swollen | For X-Ray (L) facial bones | 6564 | |
| 27.06.2001 | 09.04.1944 | F | | 1655 | 1702 | Script for Lansoprazole given | | 6592 | |
| 25.06.2001 | 29.11.1963 | F | | 1721 | 1735 | Indigestion Pain | Lansoprazole | 6631 | FP1001 (GMS4) form signed. |
| 27.06.2001 | 24.02.1969 | F | | 956 | 1003 | Mouth ulcers | Metronidazole | 6700 | |
| 26.06.2001 | 25.02.1988 | F | | 1817 | 1820 | Hay fever | Loratadine | 6701 | |
| 29.06.2001 | 25.08.1990 | M | URTI | 1731 | 1734 | (R) ear ache | Amoxycillin | 6718 | |
| 26.06.2001 | 16.07.1969 | F | Revisit | 1730 | 1733 | Feeling of a lump in the throat despite taking 2 courses of antibiotics | Referred to ENT Surgeon (Basildon hospital) | 6747 | |
| 26.06.2001 | 13.06.1945 | M | | 1002 | 1009 | Sore & tender lump under (R) foot | For X-Ray (R) foot | 6767 | History of inoperable (R) lung carcinoma. |
| 29.06.2001 | 01.10.1949 | M | | 1636 | 1640 | Face is swollen following insect bite | Flucloxacillin & Loratadine | 6795 | |
| 25.06.2001 | 20.10.1998 | F | | 1744 | 1748 | Hay fever | Chlorpheniramine | 6919 | |
| 25.06.2001 | 30.01.1949 | F | | 1811 | 1820 | Weepy | Benfleet Open Door suggested | 6932 | |
| 28.06.2001 | 11.09.2000 | M | Rash | 1059 | 1109 | ?Chicken Pox | Paracetamol & Calamine lotion | 6934 | |
| 28.06.2001 | 17.09.1966 | F | | 959 | 1002 | Script for Fexofenadine given | | 6939 | |
| 22.06.2001 | 16.05.1964 | M | | 1711 | 1719 | Swollen & painful (R) knee | Flucloxacillin & for X-Ray (R) knee | 6940 | |

Result of a query that lists all consultations from the 22nd to the end of June 2001 (ConsultationsSeenFrom22ndTillEndOfJun2001)

| SurgeryDate | DateOfBirth | Sex | Diagnosis | TimeIn | TimeOut | Complaints | Treatments | NumbersID | Notes |
|---|---|---|---|---|---|---|---|---|---|
| 29.06.2001 | 25.06.1990 | F | Pain | 1657 | 1702 | Injury (L) ring finger, tender | For X-Ray (L) ring finger | 6951 | |
| 25.06.2001 | 05.01.1960 | F | Pain | 1735 | 1744 | Back pain & pain in (L) leg | Dihydrocodeine | 6958 | |
| 26.06.2001 | 04.03.1946 | F | Pain | 1718 | 1723 | Pain & swelling both wrists | Dihydrocodeine | 6983 | For RA Latex test. |
| 26.06.2001 | 24.01.1924 | M | | 1714 | 1718 | Uric Acid normal | | 6985 | |
| 25.06.2001 | 01.04.1937 | M | S/Leave | 956 | 1002 | (R) knee joint replacement - Med. 5 | | 6987 | Brittle nails, referred to Dermatologist (Basildon hospital). |
| 26.06.2001 | 19.12.1939 | F | | 936 | 945 | Her sister has osteoporosis, hence she needs a test for this | | 6998 | |
| 29.06.2001 | 19.12.1939 | F | Revisit | 1640 | 1652 | For DEXA scan | | 6998 | |
| 25.06.2001 | 17.03.1968 | F | | 1748 | 1758 | Late period | For pregnancy test | 7008 | |
| 27.06.2001 | 08.10.1997 | F | RTI | 1732 | 1735 | Cough | Amoxycillin | 7018 | |
| 28.06.2001 | 07.07.1980 | M | | 1053 | 1059 | Script for Quetiapine given | | 7057 | |
| 28.06.2001 | 07.07.1980 | M | Revisit | 1811 | 1818 | Quetiapine makes him float | Advised to stop it | 7057 | |
| 29.06.2001 | 02.06.2001 | F | | 1722 | 1731 | Constipation | Lactulose | 7121 | |
| 27.06.2001 | 22.08.1928 | F | | 911 | 920 | Awaiting official letter from Optician before referral to Ophthalmologist for her cataract | | 7122 | |

Result of a query that lists all consultations from the 22nd to the end of June 2001 (ConsultationsSeenFrom22ndTillEndOfJun2001)

| SurgeryDate | DateOfBirth | Sex | Diagnosis | TimeIn | TimeOut | Complaints | Treatments | NumbersID | Notes |
|---|---|---|---|---|---|---|---|---|---|
| 26.06.2001 | 03.03.1938 | F | RTI | 1705 | 1714 | Cough | Amoxycillin | 783 | |
| 26.06.2001 | 18.10.1974 | F | | 1723 | 1730 | Legs feel heavy with pins & needles | For Fasting Glucose | 784 | Erythromycin allergy. |
| 28.06.2001 | 10.09.1919 | F | | 1047 | 1055 | Script for Prednisolone enteric coated & Lansoprazole given | | 823 | |
| 27.06.2001 | 05.07.1950 | M | Lump | 1707 | 1716 | Lump on (L) sclera | Referred to eye Surgeon (BUPA) | 877 | |
| 28.06.2001 | 05.10.1974 | M | Revisit | 949 | 959 | (R) shoulder is painful again | Referred to Rheumatologist | 918 | |
| 22.06.2001 | 20.10.1925 | F | Revisit | 1033 | 1041 | X-Ray: (R) knee - mild osteo-arthritis. X-Ray Lumbar: mild to moderate spondylosis affecting L2/3 | Referred to Physiotherapist | 952 | Penicillin & Aspirin allergy. |
| 26.06.2001 | 15.03.1975 | F | | 903 | 915 | Pregnancy test positive | | 954 | |
| 27.06.2001 | 10.06.2001 | F | | 1003 | 1010 | Oral thrush | Nystatin oral suspension | NP | |
| 26.06.2001 | 12.05.1945 | M | | 1700 | 1705 | Septic wounds on arm | Flucloxacillin | Temp | For FBC & Fasting Glucose. |
| 26.06.2001 | 31.01.1958 | M | Depression | 1756 | 1811 | Depressed & insomnia | Citalopram | Temp | |
| 27.06.2001 | 09.06.1924 | F | | 937 | 956 | Script for Lansoprazole given | | Temp | |

402

Result of a query that lists all consultations from the 22nd to the end of June 2003 (ConsultationsSeenFrom22ndTillEndOfJun2003)

| SurgeryDate | DateOfBirth | Sex | Diagnosis | TimeIn | TimeOut | Complaints | Treatments | NumbersID | Notes |
|---|---|---|---|---|---|---|---|---|---|
| 24.06.2003 | 20.04.1947 | F | S/Leave | 934 | 940 | Depression | | 11 | Penicillin allergy. |
| 27.06.2003 | 08.02.1939 | F | URTI | 1013 | 1024 | Sore throat | Erythromycin & Otomize ear spray | 113 | Dizziness, Rx. Prochlorperazine. Trimethoprim allergy. |
| 25.06.2003 | 15.06.1974 | F | Rash | 1727 | 1734 | Moles on face & back | Referred to Dermatologist | 1219 | Script for Fluoxetine given. Dalacin allergy. |
| 25.06.2003 | 06.07.1948 | M | Rash | 1746 | 1749 | Mole on fore-head | Referred to Dermatologist | 1356 | |
| 24.06.2003 | 26.10.1943 | F | Revisit | 919 | 923 | (L) leg cellulitis is a lot better but still quite solid | Penicillin V | 1365 | |
| 23.06.2003 | 08.10.1940 | M | | 927 | 932 | Script for Nicotine '20' patch given | | 1396 | |
| 23.06.2003 | 28.07.1939 | F | | 921 | 927 | Script for Nicotine '20' patch given | | 1398 | |
| 27.06.2003 | 17.10.1967 | F | RTI | 1747 | 1756 | Chesty cough | Cefalexin | 1646 | Metronidazole, Penicillin, Vancomycin & Erythromycin allergy. |
| 27.06.2003 | 30.09.1933 | M | | 938 | 943 | Giddy spells on & off | For FBC & Fasting Glucose | 1758 | |
| 24.06.2003 | 02.09.1941 | F | Revisit | 926 | 934 | (R) elbow is still painful | Amitriptyline | 1797 | |

403

Result of a query that lists all consultations from the 22nd to the end of June 2003 (ConsultationsSeenFrom22ndTillEndOfJun2003)

| SurgeryDate | DateOfBirth | Sex | Diagnosis | TimeIn | TimeOut | Complaints | Treatments | NumbersID | Notes |
|---|---|---|---|---|---|---|---|---|---|
| 25.06.2003 | 27.05.2003 | M | | 1734 | 1738 | Bunged up | Normal Saline nasal drops | 1802 | Script for Infacol given. |
| 26.06.2003 | 20.05.1938 | F | Rash | 951 | 955 | Itchy rash on heels | Clotrimazole 1% + 1% Hydrocortisone cream | 1869 | |
| 24.06.2003 | 25.09.1987 | F | URTI | 1033 | 1037 | Sore throat & ear ache | Penicillin V | 1968 | |
| 23.06.2003 | 10.08.1931 | M | | 1009 | 1020 | Diabetic Clinic | | 2182 | |
| 24.06.2003 | 31.07.1921 | M | Rash | 1024 | 1033 | Lesion on (R) heel is quite painful & looks like a wound | Flucloxacillin & Fusidic Acid cream | 2275 | Referred to Dermatologist. |
| 27.06.2003 | 22.08.1980 | F | | 905 | 911 | Hay fever & itchy eyes | Fexofenadine & Sodium Cromoglicate eye drops | 2303 | FP1001 (GMS4) form signed. |
| 24.06.2003 | 22.03.1936 | F | | 948 | 955 | Script for Metformin given | | 2348 | |
| 23.06.2003 | 16.03.1927 | F | | 1020 | 1037 | Diabetic Clinic | | 2415 | For CXR. |
| 24.06.2003 | 23.01.1926 | F | | 940 | 948 | Script for Alendronate & Proctosedyl ointment given | | 2479 | |
| 24.06.2003 | 04.04.1938 | M | | 1706 | 1717 | CXR - normal | | 262 | |
| 24.06.2003 | 17.12.1924 | M | | 1810 | 1825 | Injection Depo-Medrone with Lidocaine given to (R) knee | | 2635 | |

## Result of a query that lists all consultations from the 22nd to the end of June 2003 (ConsultationsSeenFrom22ndTillEndOfJun2003)

| SurgeryDate | DateOfBirth | Sex | Diagnosis | TimeIn | TimeOut | Complaints | Treatments | NumbersID | Notes |
|---|---|---|---|---|---|---|---|---|---|
| 25.06.2003 | 20.05.1921 | F | | 930 | 955 | Persistent pressure sore on the (R) heel | Referred to Dermatologist | 2809 | The Parking Badge Scheme for Disabled People Medical Practitioner form completed. |
| 27.06.2003 | 15.02.1932 | F | Revisit | 1005 | 1013 | Still unable to speak properly | Referred to ENT Surgeon | 3043 | |
| 26.06.2003 | 18.03.1978 | M | | 921 | 928 | Script for Acrivastine given | | 3115 | |
| 24.06.2003 | 13.11.1953 | M | S/Leave | 1637 | 1643 | Multiple joint pains - Med. 5 | | 3119 | |
| 23.06.2003 | 22.05.1983 | F | | 1728 | 1736 | She would like to have IUCD fitted | | 3142 | FP1001 (GMS4) form signed. |
| 23.06.2003 | 15.03.1987 | F | RTI | 1633 | 1638 | Chesty cough | Amoxycillin & Salbutamol inhaler | 3143 | |
| 25.06.2003 | 06.03.1991 | M | Rash | 912 | 921 | Multiple rash on the buttocks, face & arms | Flucloxacillin & Fusidic Acid cream | 3158 | Referred to Dermatologist. |
| 23.06.2003 | 04.07.1929 | M | Pain | 937 | 945 | Pain (L) elbow | Injection MethylPrednisolone 40mg, Lidocaine 10mg/ml. 1ml | 322 | Scaly rash on (R) wrist, Rx. Clotrimazole 1% + 1% Hydrocortisone cream. Penicillin allergy. |

Result of a query that lists all consultations from the 22nd to the end of June 2003 (ConsultationsSeenFrom22ndTillEndOfJun2003)

| SurgeryDate | DateOfBirth | Sex | Diagnosis | TimeIn | TimeOut | Complaints | Treatments | NumbersID | Notes |
|---|---|---|---|---|---|---|---|---|---|
| 27.06.2003 | 04.07.1929 | M | | 1815 | 1827 | Injection Depo-Medrone with Lidocaine given to (L) elbow | | 322 | Penicillin allergy. |
| 24.06.2003 | 15.04.1953 | M | S/Leave | 1717 | 1733 | Stress - Private | | 3228 | Script for Amitriptyline given. |
| 25.06.2003 | 12.08.1932 | M | Hypertension | 1749 | 1756 | BP 195/84 | Atenolol | 3344 | Script for Bendrofluazide & Coracten XL. Impotence, Rx. Viagra (Private script). |
| 26.06.2003 | 18.07.1978 | F | Pain | 928 | 932 | Joint pains | For Rheumatoid Factor & ESR | 337 | |
| 24.06.2003 | 23.05.1927 | M | | 904 | 919 | Fear of flying | Diazepam | 3716 | Penicillin allergy. |
| 24.06.2003 | 07.07.1961 | F | S/Leave | 923 | 926 | Whiplash injury | | 3768 | |
| 23.06.2003 | 31.01.1959 | M | S/Leave | 1736 | 1741 | Pain & tender (L) elbow | | 3795 | |
| 27.06.2003 | 07.06.1940 | M | | 1725 | 1735 | Mild bilateral pedal oedema since starting Amlodipine | | 38 | |
| 24.06.2003 | 16.07.1967 | F | | 955 | 1003 | Vaginal thrush | Fluconazole | 3993 | For Fasting Glucose & FBC. |
| 25.06.2003 | 21.01.1929 | F | | 1110 | 1117 | Serum Ferritin 16ng/L | Ferrous Sulphate | 4116 | Zantac allergy. |

Result of a query that lists all consultations from the 22nd to the end of June 2003 (ConsultationsSeenFrom22ndTillEndOfJun2003)

| SurgeryDate | DateOfBirth | Sex | Diagnosis | TimeIn | TimeOut | Complaints | Treatments | NumbersID | Notes |
|---|---|---|---|---|---|---|---|---|---|
| 25.06.2003 | 21.02.1916 | F | | 1808 | 1819 | Injection Depo-Medrone with Lidocaine given to (L) knee | | 4178 | Penicillin allergy. |
| 23.06.2003 | 02.02.1994 | M | Rash | 1741 | 1749 | Sun burn on the back of the neck & itchy rash on body | Loratadine syrup & Fusidic Acid cream | 4319 | |
| 25.06.2003 | 24.01.1957 | M | Pain | 1128 | 1138 | Pain (L) leg following injury | Diclofenac enteric coated & Co-codamol | 4354 | For X-Ray. |
| 27.06.2003 | 22.05.1966 | F | | 957 | 1005 | She wants her period postponed whilst on holidays | Norethisterone | 4391 | |
| 25.06.2003 | 10.03.1936 | F | | 1103 | 1110 | Breasts feel normal on examination | | 4442 | |
| 25.06.2003 | 03.04.1969 | F | URTI | 925 | 930 | Bilateral ear ache | Erythromycin & Otomize ear spray | 4508 | Penicillin allergy. |
| 23.06.2003 | 09.10.1926 | F | Revisit | 1041 | 1052 | Still has bilateral pedal oedema | For Echocardiography | 4567 | Penicillin allergy. |
| 24.06.2003 | 13.03.1932 | M | RTI | 1048 | 1102 | Chesty cough | Amoxycillin | 4699 | Injection Zoladex given. |
| 24.06.2003 | 16.09.1988 | F | Lump | 1757 | 1803 | Tender lump on the front of the (R) ankle & (R) lower leg | Referred to Orthopaedic Surgeon (Basildon Hospital) | 4712 | |
| 24.06.2003 | 10.03.1960 | F | | 1751 | 1757 | To try OTC Vit. B Co for her (L) thumb that moves by itself - not trigger thumb | | 4713 | |

Result of a query that lists all consultations from the 22nd to the end of June 2003 (ConsultationsSeenFrom22ndTillEndOfJun2003)

| SurgeryDate | DateOfBirth | Sex | Diagnosis | TimeIn | TimeOut | Complaints | Treatments | NumbersID | Notes |
|---|---|---|---|---|---|---|---|---|---|
| 25.06.2003 | 23.04.1921 | F | Revisit | 904 | 912 | Still coughing | Erythromycin | 5108 | For CXR & for MSU. |
| 23.06.2003 | 02.05.1985 | F | URTI | 910 | 914 | Sore throat | Amoxycillin | 5114 | |
| 26.06.2003 | 11.06.1980 | M | | 1009 | 1014 | To go to GUM clinic regarding warts on penis | | 5115 | |
| 25.06.2003 | 26.05.1976 | M | | 1014 | 1024 | He is requesting a form to be completed as he is joining the Police Force | | 512 | |
| 23.06.2003 | 14.10.1928 | M | Rash | 1150 | 1200 | Penile & groin rash | Clotrimazole 1% + 1% Hydrocortisone cream | 539 | Home visit. |
| 27.06.2003 | 13.12.1996 | M | Rash | 1645 | 1650 | Verruca under (L) big toe area | Occlusal | 5461 | |
| 26.06.2003 | 27.03.1985 | F | | 906 | 921 | Script for Doxycycline given | | 5586 | FP1001 (GMS4) form signed. |
| 23.06.2003 | 17.04.1923 | M | | 951 | 957 | (L) testicular pain has improved with Paracetamol | | 560 | |
| 23.06.2003 | 06.04.1955 | F | | 1655 | 1705 | To take Dihydrocodeine often for her (R) knee pain | | 579 | |
| 27.06.2003 | 15.10.1962 | F | URTI | 1024 | 1030 | Bilateral ear ache | Otomize ear spray | 5883 | |
| 25.06.2003 | 19.04.1985 | F | URTI | 921 | 925 | Sore throat | Amoxycillin | 5885 | FP1001 (GMS4) form signed. |

408

Result of a query that lists all consultations from the 22nd to the end of June 2003 (ConsultationsSeenFrom22ndTillEndOfJun2003)

| SurgeryDate | DateOfBirth | Sex | Diagnosis | TimeIn | TimeOut | Complaints | Treatments | NumbersID | Notes |
|---|---|---|---|---|---|---|---|---|---|
| 23.06.2003 | 12.02.1938 | M | Revisit | 1800 | 1812 | Cellulitis area is still sore but improving | Flucloxacillin, Penicillin V & Etoricoxib | 5997 | For X-Ray (L) Tibia. For FBC, Fasting Glucose & ESR. |
| 25.06.2003 | 05.12.1920 | M | Revisit | 1024 | 1056 | Still has pain in the (R) lower gum | Referred to Oral Surgeon (BUPA) | 6015 | Script for Senna given. |
| 27.06.2003 | 14.05.1971 | M | Hypertension | 943 | 957 | BP 160/112 | Atenolol & Bendrofluazide | 6017 | For FBC, Lipids, HBA1c, U/Es & Fasting Glucose. |
| 26.06.2003 | 19.01.1964 | F |  | 1006 | 1009 | Varicose veins on legs | Referred to Vascular Surgeon (BUPA) | 6196 |  |
| 27.06.2003 | 10.01.1973 | F | UTI | 1030 | 1034 | Dysuria & frequency of micturition | Amoxycillin | 6309 | For MSU. |
| 27.06.2003 | 01.01.1924 | M |  | 927 | 938 | Letter to whom it may concern regarding his medications |  | 6353 |  |
| 27.06.2003 | 31.07.1997 | F |  | 1716 | 1722 | Wound on the (L) heel after stepping on glass | Flucloxacillin & Fusidic Acid cream | 6409 | For X-Ray. |
| 27.06.2003 | 06.12.1962 | M | URTI | 1709 | 1716 | Sore throat | Amoxycillin | 6415 |  |
| 27.06.2003 | 17.09.1965 | F | URTI | 918 | 927 | Sore throat | Amoxycillin | 6518 | FP1001 (GMS4) form signed. |
| 23.06.2003 | 27.07.1999 | M | URTI | 1650 | 1655 | Sore throat | Amoxycillin | 6534 | Script for Loratadine syrup given. |

## Result of a query that lists all consultations from the 22nd to the end of June 2003 (ConsultationsSeenFrom22ndTillEndOfJun2003)

| SurgeryDate | DateOfBirth | Sex | Diagnosis | TimeIn | TimeOut | Complaints | Treatments | NumbersID | Notes |
|---|---|---|---|---|---|---|---|---|---|
| 25.06.2003 | 11.12.1968 | F | | 1700 | 1709 | Sores breaking up on her body | Flucloxacillin & Fusidic Acid cream | 6579 | Insomnia, Rx. Temazepam. |
| 26.06.2003 | 20.11.1945 | M | Rash | 1014 | 1019 | Rash on limbs | Referred to Dermatologist | 6617 | Penicillin allergy. |
| 25.06.2003 | 14.10.1997 | F | RTI | 1744 | 1746 | Cough | Amoxycillin | 6626 | |
| 23.06.2003 | 20.02.1953 | F | Revisit | 1643 | 1650 | Still coughing & chest pain | Salbutamol easi-breathe inhaler, GTN & Amoxycillin | 6633 | |
| 26.06.2003 | 08.05.1939 | F | | 959 | 1006 | Pallor | For FBC | 6643 | |
| 24.06.2003 | 22.02.1963 | M | S/Leave | 1733 | 1744 | Injury (R) knee - Private | | 6739 | Script for Dihydrocodeine given. |
| 25.06.2003 | 21.03.2000 | F | Rash | 1722 | 1727 | Multiple red rash on face & arm | Calamine lotion | 6788 | |
| 24.06.2003 | 12.04.1932 | F | | 1003 | 1024 | Script for Co-codamol given | | 6825 | For FBC, Ferritin & Folate. |
| 24.06.2003 | 10.03.1951 | F | | 1648 | 1706 | Script for Simvastatin given | | 683 | |
| 26.06.2003 | 01.01.1962 | M | URTI | 955 | 959 | Sore throat | Amoxycillin | 6879 | |
| 26.06.2003 | 06.12.1983 | F | Depression | 1019 | 1039 | Weepy after TOP | Referred to Practice Counsellor | 6893 | |
| 27.06.2003 | 25.09.1960 | M | Pain | 1807 | 1810 | He fell on his (L) knee, painful | For X-Ray | 6898 | |
| 24.06.2003 | 11.01.1964 | F | URTI | 1803 | 1810 | Sore throat | Amoxycillin | 6976 | |

410

Result of a query that lists all consultations from the 22nd to the end of June 2003 (ConsultationsSeenFrom22ndTillEndOfJun2003)

| SurgeryDate | DateOfBirth | Sex | Diagnosis | TimeIn | TimeOut | Complaints | Treatments | NumbersID | Notes |
|---|---|---|---|---|---|---|---|---|---|
| 25.06.2003 | 03.03.1934 | M | Pain | 1117 | 1128 | Cramps at back of leg | Quinine Bisulphate | 6984 | |
| 25.06.2003 | 31.10.2000 | M | RTI | 1740 | 1744 | Cough | Amoxycillin | 6986 | |
| 25.06.2003 | 13.07.1946 | F | Conjunctivitis | 1804 | 1808 | Grit in (L) eye | Chloramphenicol eye ointment | 7188 | |
| 24.06.2003 | 29.06.1949 | M | | 1643 | 1648 | Diarrhoea | Ciprofloxacin | 7196 | |
| 27.06.2003 | 04.09.2001 | F | Rash | 914 | 918 | Skin blemishes, dry & itchy | Fusidic Acid 2% + 1% Hydrocortisone cream | 7204 | |
| 25.06.2003 | 15.03.1922 | F | URTI | 1056 | 1103 | Sore throat & ear ache | Amoxycillin & Otomize ear spray | 7229 | |
| 25.06.2003 | 14.02.1952 | M | Revisit | 1709 | 1722 | Still coughing & chest pain | Erythromycin & GTN spray | 7298 | Referred to Cardiologist. |
| 23.06.2003 | 26.04.1944 | F | S/Leave | 905 | 910 | (R) Shoulder pain | | 7376 | |
| 25.06.2003 | 13.02.2002 | F | RTI | 1738 | 1740 | Cough | Amoxycillin & Paracetamol | 7392 | |
| 27.06.2003 | 25.02.2002 | F | RTI | 1810 | 1815 | Chesty cough | Amoxycillin & Paracetamol | 7402 | |
| 23.06.2003 | 29.04.2002 | M | RTI | 1723 | 1728 | Chesty cough | Amoxycillin | 7452 | |
| 25.06.2003 | 06.03.1957 | F | Pain | 955 | 1000 | Aches & pains both legs | Referred to Rheumatologist | 7478 | |
| 23.06.2003 | 20.06.2002 | M | | 1001 | 1009 | Pyrexial & not eating | Erythromycin | 7480 | |
| 26.06.2003 | 05.03.1954 | F | Pain | 1055 | 1105 | Epigastric & Posterior chest pain | Esomeprazole & Dihydrocodeine | 7492 | For FBC, TFTs, CXR & U/Es. |
| 23.06.2003 | 03.05.1944 | F | | 1705 | 1714 | Fed up of her voice getting hoarse | Referred to ENT Surgeon | 7499 | Aching in (R) chest, for CXR. |

Result of a query that lists all consultations from the 22nd to the end of June 2003 (ConsultationsSeenFrom22ndTillEndOfJun2003)

| SurgeryDate | DateOfBirth | Sex | Diagnosis | TimeIn | TimeOut | Complaints | Treatments | NumbersID | Notes |
|---|---|---|---|---|---|---|---|---|---|
| 25.06.2003 | 23.07.1931 | F | | 1643 | 1700 | For FBC, ESR, U/Es, LFTs, TFTs, Fasting Glucose & Fasting Cholesterol | | 7575 | |
| 27.06.2003 | 07.03.1968 | F | | 1650 | 1657 | Vaginal thrush | Fluconazole | 7577 | Script for Paramax given. T.A.T.T., for FBC & TFTs. |
| 26.06.2003 | 26.07.1960 | F | | 1039 | 1045 | ?Peri-menopausal | For LH & FSH | 7591 | |
| 25.06.2003 | 08.10.1938 | M | | 1009 | 1014 | Script for Beconase nasal spray given | | 7606 | |
| 27.06.2003 | 18.11.1999 | M | URTI | 1722 | 1725 | (R) ear ache | Amoxycillin | 7619 | |
| 24.06.2003 | 05.12.2002 | M | | 1744 | 1751 | Script for Normal Saline nasal drops | | 7637 | |
| 24.06.2003 | 06.05.1960 | F | Pain | 1037 | 1048 | Pain in neck & (R) elbow after her husband tried to take her bag off her | Co-codamol & Ibuprofen | 7691 | |
| 26.06.2003 | 26.09.1937 | M | | 1045 | 1055 | Injection Depo-Medrone with Lidocaine given to (L) heel | | 7693 | |
| 24.06.2003 | 20.02.2003 | F | | 1632 | 1637 | To give own Calpol | | 7721 | |
| 23.06.2003 | 31.05.1930 | F | Pain | 1714 | 1723 | Pain & swelling (L) knee | For X-Ray | 7730 | |
| 23.06.2003 | 05.12.1934 | F | Pain | 945 | 951 | Pain in the knees | Dihydrocodeine | 7757 | |

## Result of a query that lists all consultations from the 22nd to the end of June 2003 (ConsultationsSeenFrom22ndTillEndOfJun2003)

| SurgeryDate | DateOfBirth | Sex | Diagnosis | TimeIn | TimeOut | Complaints | Treatments | NumbersID | Notes |
|---|---|---|---|---|---|---|---|---|---|
| 27.06.2003 | 17.02.1949 | M | S/Leave | 1034 | 1043 | Non-ST elevation Myocardial Infarction - Med. 3 & Private | | 7758 | |
| 26.06.2003 | 28.03.1947 | F | | 932 | 951 | Awaiting all her Medical Records | | 7760 | |
| 25.06.2003 | 23.12.1946 | M | | 1000 | 1009 | Script for Gliclazide, Diclofenac enteric coated & Rabeprazole given | | 7761 | |
| 23.06.2003 | 02.02.1949 | F | | 914 | 921 | Dizzy spells & nausea | Prochlorperazine | 7771 | |
| 27.06.2003 | 02.02.1949 | F | S/Leave | 911 | 914 | Dizziness | | 7771 | |
| 27.06.2003 | 17.05.1947 | M | | 1635 | 1645 | Script for Co-codamol & Mometasone given | | 7772 | |
| 25.06.2003 | 11.11.1909 | F | | 1756 | 1804 | For home visit tomorrow | | 7824 | Her son came to Surgery. |
| 27.06.2003 | 11.11.1909 | M | | 1756 | 1807 | I explained to her son that she is due to be seen at home by the Psychogeriatrician | | 7824 | |
| 27.06.2003 | 16.07.1983 | F | | 1735 | 1747 | Script for Venlafaxine XL given | | 967 | |

413

Result of a query that lists all consultations from the 22nd to the end of June 2004 (ConsultationsSeenFrom22ndTillEndOfJun2004)

| SurgeryDate | DateOfBirth | Sex | Diagnosis | TimeIn | TimeOut | Complaints | Treatments | NumbersID | Notes |
|---|---|---|---|---|---|---|---|---|---|
| 25.06.2004 | 05.01.1971 | F | | 1659 | 1711 | Pregnancy test positive | | 1003 | |
| 28.06.2004 | 31.12.1953 | F | Hypertension | 908 | 916 | BP 178/112 | Atenolol | 1075 | |
| 22.06.2004 | 30.07.1952 | F | | 1047 | 1055 | Referred to Neurologist as advised by the Chiropractor | | 1170 | |
| 25.06.2004 | 24.10.1929 | F | | 1020 | 1027 | Bleeding pr | For rectal examination with P/Nurse | 1255 | |
| 24.06.2004 | 03.05.1951 | F | | 905 | 915 | Script for Conjugated oestrogens equine with Medroxyprogesterone (continuous combined) 300mcg + 1.5mg given | | 162 | Cefaclor allergy. |
| 25.06.2004 | 08.11.1981 | M | | 1742 | 1750 | Enlarged inguinal nodes | For FBC | 1699 | |
| 25.06.2004 | 03.07.1927 | F | | 1652 | 1659 | To stop the Bendrofluazide for one month as she has possible side effects from them | | 1929 | Penicillin allergy. |
| 25.06.2004 | 06.07.1957 | F | S/Leave | 1730 | 1742 | Low back pain | | 1954 | |
| 25.06.2004 | 11.07.1950 | M | | 1721 | 1728 | Build-up of wax in the ears | Sodium bicarbonate ear drops | 1971 | |

Result of a query that lists all consultations from the 22nd to the end of June 2004 (ConsultationsSeenFrom22ndTillEndOfJun2004)

| SurgeryDate | DateOfBirth | Sex | Diagnosis | TimeIn | TimeOut | Complaints | Treatments | NumbersID | Notes |
|---|---|---|---|---|---|---|---|---|---|
| 23.06.2004 | 10.08.1931 | M | | 923 | 931 | Script for Co-codamol & Erodolac given | | 2182 | Aspirin allergy. |
| 25.06.2004 | 14.08.1927 | M | | 1002 | 1012 | Hair loss | For FBC, TFTs, LFTs, Cholesterol & U/Es | 2289 | |
| 22.06.2004 | 22.03.1936 | F | | 912 | 927 | Script for Doxazosin & Bendrofluazide given | | 2348 | |
| 23.06.2004 | 23.04.1950 | F | | 1745 | 1756 | Script for Conjugated Oestrogens equine with Medroxyprogesterone (continuous combined) 300mcgs + 1.5mg given | | 2369 | |
| 28.06.2004 | 28.03.1970 | F | | 1032 | 1039 | Script for Fluconazole given | | 2375 | |
| 23.06.2004 | 16.03.1927 | F | | 931 | 954 | Script for Atenolol & Doxazosin given | | 2415 | |
| 25.06.2004 | 07.03.1968 | F | | 922 | 927 | For B12, Folate & Ferritin | | 2421 | |
| 28.06.2004 | 27.11.1987 | M | S/Leave | 1025 | 1032 | Diarrhoea - Private | | 2427 | |
| 22.06.2004 | 30.05.1955 | F | | 932 | 949 | Black spot in (L) groin, sore | Flucloxacillin | 2608 | |
| 29.06.2004 | 04.04.1938 | M | | 1737 | 1746 | Script for Omeprazole & Private script for Viagra given | | 262 | |

415

## Result of a query that lists all consultations from the 22nd to the end of June 2004 (ConsultationsSeenFrom22ndTillEndOfJun2004)

| SurgeryDate | DateOfBirth | Sex | Diagnosis | TimeIn | TimeOut | Complaints | Treatments | NumbersID | Notes |
|---|---|---|---|---|---|---|---|---|---|
| 23.06.2004 | 19.03.1925 | F | | 914 | 923 | Script for Metformin given | | 2634 | |
| 28.06.2004 | 06.01.1943 | F | | 928 | 940 | Script for Doxazosin & Frusemide given | | 2642 | |
| 29.06.2004 | 16.01.1971 | M | | 1752 | 1757 | Boil on (R) thigh | Flucloxacillin & Fusidic Acid cream | 2674 | For FBC & Fasting Glucose. |
| 25.06.2004 | 24.03.1973 | M | S/Leave | 947 | 952 | Injury (R) toe - Med. 5 | | 2784 | |
| 23.06.2004 | 08.04.1990 | M | URTI | 1716 | 1720 | Sore throat | Amoxycillin | 2789 | Cefaclor allergy. |
| 23.06.2004 | 10.09.1936 | M | | 1004 | 1019 | Script for Allopurinol given | | 284 | |
| 23.06.2004 | 31.05.1968 | M | Rash | 1733 | 1736 | Mole on (R) shoulder | Referred to Dermatologist (BUPA) | 2920 | |
| 25.06.2004 | 27.10.1961 | F | Pain | 1034 | 1046 | Neck pain | Co-codamol & Diclofenac e/c | 2973 | For Cervical X-Ray. |
| 22.06.2004 | 07.07.1962 | M | | 1755 | 1807 | T.A.T.T. | For FBC, TFTs, Fasting Glucose & Fasting Cholesterol | 3240 | |
| 29.06.2004 | 26.03.1958 | F | | 1801 | 1805 | Septic insect bite on the (R) leg | Flucloxacillin | 33 | |
| 23.06.2004 | 23.03.1967 | F | URTI | 1736 | 1741 | Sore throat | Amoxycillin | 3529 | Septrin allergy. |
| 29.06.2004 | 08.04.1945 | M | | 1012 | 1022 | Low serum Ferritin | Ferrous Sulphate | 3574 | |
| 29.06.2004 | 12.08.1944 | M | S/Leave | 1733 | 1737 | Pain in (R) heel | Referred to Orthopaedic Surgeon (Basildon Hospital) | 364 | Script for Flucloxacillin given. |

416

Result of a query that lists all consultations from the 22nd to the end of June 2004 (ConsultationsSeenFrom22ndTillEndOfJun2004)

| SurgeryDate | DateOfBirth | Sex | Diagnosis | TimeIn | TimeOut | Complaints | Treatments | NumbersID | Notes |
|---|---|---|---|---|---|---|---|---|---|
| 28.06.2004 | 26.04.1942 | F | | 1004 | 1025 | Script for Metformin & Simvastatin given | | 3697 | |
| 22.06.2004 | 06.02.1944 | M | | 1810 | 1818 | As Amitriptyline was initiated privately, not given | | 401 | |
| 24.06.2004 | 07.04.1964 | F | | 1031 | 1036 | HVS - vaginal candidiasis | Fluconazole | 4101 | |
| 22.06.2004 | 21.02.1916 | F | Conjunctivitis | 1712 | 1722 | Painful & watery eyes | Chloramphenicol eye drops | 4178 | Penicillin allergy. |
| 25.06.2004 | 30.10.1969 | F | | 1757 | 1805 | For MSU | | 4275 | |
| 29.06.2004 | 27.08.1990 | F | Pain | 1034 | 1042 | Injury (L) ankle | For X-Ray | 4303 | |
| 25.06.2004 | 16.04.1993 | F | | 1646 | 1652 | Script for Salbutamol inhaler given | | 4327 | |
| 28.06.2004 | 26.01.1935 | M | | 1636 | 1648 | He had cystoscopy 8 days ago | | 4505 | |
| 24.06.2004 | 21.09.1923 | M | | 915 | 928 | Script for Doxazosin & Co-codamol given | | 4692 | |
| 25.06.2004 | 13.03.1932 | M | | 1105 | 1115 | Injection Zoladex given | | 4699 | |
| 29.06.2004 | 24.06.1964 | M | | 1757 | 1801 | (L) ankle is red & sore | Flucloxacillin | 4769 | |
| 23.06.2004 | 25.09.1922 | F | | 1405 | 1428 | Swollen legs | Frusemide & Aqueous cream | 484 | |
| 24.06.2004 | 02.04.1967 | F | | 958 | 1006 | Script for Atenolol given | | 4894 | Penicillin allergy. |
| 22.06.2004 | 27.11.1992 | F | URTI | 1740 | 1743 | (R) ear ache | Amoxycillin | 4913 | |

Result of a query that lists all consultations from the 22nd to the end of June 2004 (ConsultationsSeenFrom22ndTillEndOfJun2004)

| SurgeryDate | DateOfBirth | Sex | Diagnosis | TimeIn | TimeOut | Complaints | Treatments | NumbersID | Notes |
|---|---|---|---|---|---|---|---|---|---|
| 28.06.2004 | 28.04.1947 | M | | 940 | 949 | Advised to see the Optician regarding the 2 black shadows in his (R) eye | | 502 | |
| 29.06.2004 | 17.05.1986 | F | | 1042 | 1051 | To see P/Nurse for HVS & Chlamydial swab | | 5135 | |
| 23.06.2004 | 12.02.1996 | M | URTI | 1741 | 1745 | Sore throat | Amoxycillin | 5165 | Plaster allergy. |
| 28.06.2004 | 27.02.1945 | M | | 1047 | 1054 | Diarrhoea & abdominal pain | Loperamide & Hyoscine butylbromide | 5302 | Stool for C&S. |
| 29.06.2004 | 31.01.1964 | F | | 1642 | 1654 | She will go home & think about her gall bladder stones | | 5334 | |
| 28.06.2004 | 30.03.1985 | M | | 1632 | 1636 | Advised to go to A/E regarding the injury to his (L) elbow | | 534 | Penicillin allergy. |
| 29.06.2004 | 11.11.1969 | F | | 1350 | 1400 | Routine P/Natal visit | | 5363 | Home visit. |
| 25.06.2004 | 22.06.1973 | F | Pain | 1027 | 1034 | Abdominal pain | Hyoscine butylbromide | 5488 | |
| 29.06.2004 | 03.02.1920 | M | | 1022 | 1034 | He is happy to continue with prn Dihydrocodeine for his back pain | | 5557 | |
| 22.06.2004 | 10.05.1980 | F | | 1747 | 1755 | Script for Propranolol given | | 557 | |
| 22.06.2004 | 13.06.1997 | F | | 1743 | 1747 | Hay fever | Loratadine syrup | 5632 | |

Result of a query that lists all consultations from the 22nd to the end of June 2004 (ConsultationsSeenFrom22ndTillEndOfJun2004)

| SurgeryDate | DateOfBirth | Sex | Diagnosis | TimeIn | TimeOut | Complaints | Treatments | NumbersID | Notes |
|---|---|---|---|---|---|---|---|---|---|
| 25.06.2004 | 17.07.1997 | M | Conjunctivitis | 902 | 904 | Sticky, sore & red (R) eye | Chloramphenicol eye drops | 5673 | |
| 29.06.2004 | 13.12.1948 | F | | 953 | 958 | Septic insect bite on (R) arm | Flucloxacillin | 6033 | |
| 28.06.2004 | 30.06.1998 | M | Rash | 1807 | 1810 | Small reddish warts above the (R) eye | Fusidic Acid cream | 6159 | |
| 22.06.2004 | 06.11.1998 | M | URTI | 1704 | 1712 | Discharging (R) ear | Amoxycillin | 6301 | Referred to ENT Surgeon. |
| 29.06.2004 | 08.05.1974 | M | URTI | 950 | 953 | Fever & sore throat | Amoxycillin | 6352 | Script for Co-codamol given. |
| 25.06.2004 | 06.12.1962 | M | | 927 | 947 | Script for Amoxycillin given | | 6415 | |
| 29.06.2004 | 06.12.1962 | M | | 1654 | 1723 | Feels panicky about his forthcoming cardiology test | Propranolol | 6415 | Referred to P/Counsellor. |
| 29.06.2004 | 06.06.1959 | M | Pain | 936 | 950 | Abdominal pain | Amoxycillin & Buscopan | 6461 | Private script for Viagra given. |
| 28.06.2004 | 14.11.1916 | F | | 1358 | 1405 | Paronychia (R) middle finger | Flucloxacillin & Fusidic Acid cream | 6591 | Home visit. |
| 28.06.2004 | 02.03.1948 | F | | 1759 | 1807 | Unable to hear properly | Dexamethasone with neomycin ear spray | 6631 | Penicillin allergy. |
| 28.06.2004 | 25.06.1953 | M | Hypertension | 1810 | 1819 | BP 141/103 | Bendrofluazide | 6632 | |
| 23.06.2004 | 26.03.1965 | F | | 1029 | 1036 | T.A.T.T. | For FBC, TFTs, U/Es, LFTs, Cholesterol & Fasting Glucose | 6656 | |

Result of a query that lists all consultations from the 22nd to the end of June 2004 (ConsultationsSeenFrom22ndTillEndOfJun2004)

| SurgeryDate | DateOfBirth | Sex | Diagnosis | TimeIn | TimeOut | Complaints | Treatments | NumbersID | Notes |
|---|---|---|---|---|---|---|---|---|---|
| 24.06.2004 | 24.04.1966 | M | UTI | 1040 | 1049 | Dysuria | Amoxycillin | 669 | For MSU. |
| 25.06.2004 | 22.02.1963 | M | | 908 | 922 | I told him that I could not request for AIDs test for his private IVF treatment | | 6739 | |
| 29.06.2004 | 19.10.1924 | F | RTI | 1310 | 1320 | Cough & congested | Erythromycin | 677 | Home visit. Penicillin allergy. |
| 23.06.2004 | 21.02.1928 | F | | 1642 | 1650 | Night cramps | Quinine Sulphate | 6770 | |
| 22.06.2004 | 03.09.1952 | F | | 1652 | 1704 | (R) upper abdominal pain | For USScan of the upper abdomen | 6790 | |
| 23.06.2004 | 15.07.1971 | F | | 902 | 914 | Script for Norethisterone given | | 6808 | She has a strong family history of ovarian cancer, referred to Gynaecologist (Basildon Hospital). |
| 28.06.2004 | 16.01.1998 | F | | 1039 | 1047 | Script for extrafine particle inhaler given | | 6809 | |
| 22.06.2004 | 23.11.1946 | M | | 1024 | 1028 | For repeat FBC & Cholesterol in 1 year | | 6822 | |
| 25.06.2004 | 16.05.1964 | M | | 1016 | 1020 | Sprain to the (R) thigh | To use own Co-codamol | 6940 | |
| 22.06.2004 | 08.09.1978 | M | | 1036 | 1047 | Vomiting & hyperventilating | Advised to go to A/E | 6950 | |
| 25.06.2004 | 16.05.1997 | F | RTI | 1754 | 1757 | Chesty cough | Amoxycillin | 7006 | |

Result of a query that lists all consultations from the 22nd to the end of June 2004 (ConsultationsSeenFrom22ndTillEndOfJun2004)

| SurgeryDate | DateOfBirth | Sex | Diagnosis | TimeIn | TimeOut | Complaints | Treatments | NumbersID | Notes |
|---|---|---|---|---|---|---|---|---|---|
| 24.06.2004 | 27.05.1991 | M | | 1049 | 1054 | To take own Calpol/ Nurofen for his chest pain after it was banged at school | | 7084 | |
| 22.06.2004 | 09.02.1980 | F | | 1009 | 1016 | Recurrent diarrhoea | Loperamide | 7148 | Stool for C&S. Penicillin allergy. |
| 24.06.2004 | 04.01.2000 | M | | 1036 | 1040 | Septic wound on lip | Amoxycillin | 7156 | |
| 24.06.2004 | 05.11.1971 | M | RTI | 955 | 958 | Chesty cough | Amoxycillin | 7195 | |
| 22.06.2004 | 13.09.1946 | F | | 1636 | 1642 | (R) Carpal tunnel syndrome | Referred to Orthopaedic Surgeon (Basildon Hospital) | 7222 | |
| 23.06.2004 | 27.01.1934 | F | | 1720 | 1733 | She has a blur in her (R) eye | Referred to Ophthalmologist | 7252 | |
| 22.06.2004 | 15.08.1949 | F | | 1722 | 1740 | She will stop the HRT as she has been on it for more than 10 years | | 7325 | |
| 28.06.2004 | 04.11.1924 | F | | 919 | 924 | She will leave off the Ibuprofen | | 7363 | |
| 29.06.2004 | 04.11.1924 | F | | 1746 | 1752 | I explained to her that Opticrom eye drops contains Sodium Cromoglycate, which she currently takes | | 7363 | |
| 25.06.2004 | 25.02.2002 | F | URTI | 1750 | 1754 | Infected rhinorrhoea & sticky eyes | Amoxycillin & Chloramphenicol eye drops | 7402 | |

Result of a query that lists all consultations from the 22nd to the end of June 2004 (ConsultationsSeenFrom22ndTillEndOfJun2004)

| SurgeryDate | DateOfBirth | Sex | Diagnosis | TimeIn | TimeOut | Complaints | Treatments | NumbersID | Notes |
|---|---|---|---|---|---|---|---|---|---|
| 22.06.2004 | 12.06.1934 | M |  | 1642 | 1649 | To take OTC Co-codamol for his painful (L) knee |  | 7415 |  |
| 24.06.2004 | 12.06.1934 | M | Pain | 949 | 955 | Pain (L) knee | Dihydrocodeine | 7415 |  |
| 28.06.2004 | 03.07.1950 | F |  | 1720 | 1727 | Infection up her (R) nostril | Erythromycin & Mupirocin nasal cream | 7468 |  |
| 22.06.2004 | 15.01.1935 | F |  | 1016 | 1024 | For MSU |  | 7511 |  |
| 29.06.2004 | 28.03.1960 | F |  | 923 | 931 | Smelly discharge from navel |  | 7518 | Script for Fluoxetine given. |
| 22.06.2004 | 20.02.1953 | F |  | 927 | 932 | CXR shows mild COAD | Flucloxacillin | 7559 |  |
| 23.06.2004 | 07.02.1997 | M |  | 1650 | 1656 | To apply own Calamine lotion for probable Chicken Pox rash |  | 7570 |  |
| 29.06.2004 | 07.10.2002 | F | Revisit | 931 | 936 | Recurrent rash on body | Referred to Dermatologist (Basildon Hospital) | 7593 |  |
| 29.06.2004 | 21.10.1962 | M |  | 1726 | 1733 | For MSU, Fasting Glucose & PSA |  | 7594 |  |
| 25.06.2004 | 30.11.1945 | F |  | 1711 | 1718 | Pain in (R) eye | Chloramphenicol eye ointment | 7595 |  |
| 29.06.2004 | 22.06.1974 | F |  | 910 | 914 | Hay fever | Fexofenadine | 7596 |  |
| 28.06.2004 | 01.11.1936 | M | Rash | 1727 | 1734 | Lesion on the (R) anterior chest wall | Referred to Dermatologist (Basildon Hospital) | 7608 | Script for Inj. MethylPrednisolone with lignocaine given. |

422

## Result of a query that lists all consultations from the 22nd to the end of June 2004 (ConsultationsSeenFrom22ndTillEndOfJun2004)

| SurgeryDate | DateOfBirth | Sex | Diagnosis | TimeIn | TimeOut | Complaints | Treatments | NumbersID | Notes |
|---|---|---|---|---|---|---|---|---|---|
| 23.06.2004 | 06.04.1938 | M | | 1044 | 1053 | (R) eye is sticky with swollen lower eye lid | Flucloxacillin & Chloramphenicol eye ointment | 7626 | |
| 23.06.2004 | 04.07.1938 | M | | 1053 | 1145 | HGV Medical Examination Done | | 7631 | |
| 24.06.2004 | 04.07.1938 | F | | 1018 | 1031 | Script for Dihydrocodeine given | | 7647 | For MSU. |
| 28.06.2004 | 20.09.2000 | F | Pain | 924 | 928 | Headaches & vomiting | Referred to Paediatrician | 7657 | |
| 22.06.2004 | 26.04.1943 | M | Pain | 905 | 912 | (R) hip pain | Co-codamol | 7697 | Penicillin allergy. |
| 23.06.2004 | 26.04.1943 | M | S/Leave | 1637 | 1642 | Pain in (R) hip - Private | | 7697 | |
| 29.06.2004 | 24.10.1946 | F | Revisit | 920 | 923 | Still has pain in (L) foot | Referred to Podiatrist | 7704 | |
| 28.06.2004 | 07.01.1944 | M | Depression | 956 | 1004 | Stress at home | Fluoxetine | 7714 | |
| 23.06.2004 | 07.11.1968 | F | | 954 | 1004 | Sore throat | Amoxycillin | 7739 | Script for Clotrimazole given |
| 23.06.2004 | 23.12.1946 | M | Revisit | 1656 | 1711 | Still coughing | Erythromycin | 7761 | |
| 28.06.2004 | 04.04.1920 | M | | 1734 | 1747 | Script for Penicillin V, Fusidic Acid cream & Co-codamol given | | 7766 | |
| 28.06.2004 | 08.04.1942 | M | | 1707 | 1711 | Wax in the ears | Sodium bicarbonate ear drops | 7774 | Tetanus allergy. |

Result of a query that lists all consultations from the 22nd to the end of June 2004 (ConsultationsSeenFrom22ndTillEndOfJun2004)

| SurgeryDate | DateOfBirth | Sex | Diagnosis | TimeIn | TimeOut | Complaints | Treatments | NumbersID | Notes |
|---|---|---|---|---|---|---|---|---|---|
| 22.06.2004 | 18.05.1963 | M | | 949 | 1004 | Script for Venlafaxine, Diazepam, Disulfiram, Sodium Valproate & Zopiclone given | | 7803 | |
| 25.06.2004 | 08.12.1938 | F | | 1718 | 1721 | Injury to (L) little toe | For X-Ray | 7811 | |
| 29.06.2004 | 18.10.1974 | F | | 1335 | 1340 | Patient not at home | | 784 | Home visit. |
| 24.06.2004 | 19.10.1938 | M | | 928 | 936 | To continue with Meloxicam for the arthritis in his neck | | 7847 | |
| 25.06.2004 | 15.03.1946 | M | | 952 | 1002 | Script for Simvastatin given | | 7916 | |
| 22.06.2004 | 22.01.1991 | M | Lump | 1807 | 1810 | Slightly tender (L) breast tissue | Flucloxacillin | 7923 | |
| 24.06.2004 | 28.08.1946 | F | | 1006 | 1018 | Script for Co-codamol & Hydrocortisone 17-Buryrate 0.1% given | | 799 | |
| 29.06.2004 | 10.09.1919 | F | | 1633 | 1642 | Script for Prednisolone given | | 823 | |
| 22.06.2004 | 17.11.1975 | M | Revisit | 901 | 905 | He is still seeing shadows in front of the eyes | Referred to Ophthalmologist | 826 | |
| 25.06.2004 | 28.09.1958 | M | S/Leave | 1642 | 1646 | Pain (L) elbow | | 905 | |
| 22.06.2004 | 03.10.2003 | M | | 1004 | 1009 | To observe the area in front of (R) ear lobe which is red following removal of skin tag | | NP (BA) | |

424

Result of a query that lists all consultations from the 22nd to the end of June 2004 (ConsultationsSeenFrom22ndTillEndOfJun2004)

| SurgeryDate | DateOfBirth | Sex | Diagnosis | TimeIn | TimeOut | Complaints | Treatments | NumbersID | Notes |
|---|---|---|---|---|---|---|---|---|---|
| 29.06.2004 | 03.10.2003 | M | | 1007 | 1012 | Pussy head on wound next to the (R) ear | Flucloxacillin | NP (BA) | |
| 28.06.2004 | 21.05.1930 | F | | 1711 | 1720 | Letter sent to Ophthalmologist regarding her (L) ectropion | | NP (DD) | Penicillin allergy. |
| 24.06.2004 | 06.09.1927 | F | | 936 | 949 | Bilateral pedal oedema | Frusemide & Bumetanide | NP (DL) | |
| 25.06.2004 | 23.02.1982 | M | Rash | 1639 | 1642 | Red scabs on bridge of the nose | Mupirocin cream | NP (GO) | |
| 28.06.2004 | 31.10.1986 | F | Rash | 900 | 905 | Roundish rash on the (L) upper arm | Clotrimazole 1% + 1% Hydrocortisone cream | NP (JJ) | |
| 28.06.2004 | 06.02.1946 | F | | 949 | 956 | Script for Propranolol given | | NP (KT) | |
| 23.06.2004 | 30.06.1981 | M | Depression | 1711 | 1716 | Separated from her children & quite low | Fluoxetine | NP (LW) | |
| 23.06.2004 | 15.04.1956 | M | | 1029 | 1036 | Serum B12 is low | Referred to Haematologist | NP (MO) | |
| 28.06.2004 | 15.04.1956 | M | | 1648 | 1707 | Script for Amoxycillin & Lisinopril given | | NP (MO) | |
| 25.06.2004 | 23.12.1976 | F | URTI | 1012 | 1016 | Sore throat | Amoxycillin | NP (NB) | |
| 23.06.2004 | 08.11.2002 | M | RTI | 1036 | 1044 | Sticky eyes & cough | Amoxycillin & Chloramphenicol eye drops | NP (OJ) | |
| 29.06.2004 | 25.01.1939 | F | | 914 | 920 | For Dexascan | | NP (PC) | Penicillin allergy. |

425

Result of a query that lists all consultations from the 22nd to the end of June 2004 (ConsultationsSeenFrom22ndTillEndOfJun2004)

| SurgeryDate | DateOfBirth | Sex | Diagnosis | TimeIn | TimeOut | Complaints | Treatments | NumbersID | Notes |
|---|---|---|---|---|---|---|---|---|---|
| 22.06.2004 | 08.10.2003 | M | Revisit | 1818 | 1821 | One of the rash on his body seems a little infected | Flucloxacillin | NP (RA) | |
| 29.06.2004 | 15.05.1980 | F | | 1805 | 1811 | Letter to whom it may concern regarding her (R) knee | | NP (SP) | Erythromycin allergy. |
| 22.06.2004 | 07.02.1972 | F | | 1028 | 1036 | To see P/Nurse for HVS | | NP (SR) | |
| 29.06.2004 | 01.06.1967 | F | Rash | 1723 | 1726 | Raised red spot on the (L) lower leg | Referred to Dermatologist (Basildon Hospital) | NP (SW) | |
| 22.06.2004 | 17.05.2004 | M | | 1649 | 1652 | To apply own Sudocrem for his facial rash | | NP (TB) | |

Result of a query that lists all consultations from the 22nd to the end of June 2005 (ConsultationsSeenFrom22ndTillEndOfJun2005)

| SurgeryDate | DateOfBirth | Sex | Diagnosis | TimeIn | TimeOut | Complaints | Treatments | NumbersID | Notes |
|---|---|---|---|---|---|---|---|---|---|
| 28.06.2005 | 15.06.1974 | F | | 1813 | 1816 | Script for Propranolol given | | 1219 | |
| 23.06.2005 | 26.01.1974 | M | | 1707 | 1712 | Hay fever | Desloratadine | 1248 | |
| 22.06.2005 | 25.03.1944 | M | Rash | 1713 | 1719 | Bright red, weepy rash on chest & legs | Flucloxacillin | 125 | |
| 28.06.2005 | 24.10.1929 | F | | 1029 | 1044 | For repeat FBC | | 1255 | |

Result of a query that lists all consultations from the 22nd to the end of June 2005 (ConsultationsSeenFrom22ndTillEndOfJun2005)

| SurgeryDate | DateOfBirth | Sex | Diagnosis | TimeIn | TimeOut | Complaints | Treatments | NumbersID | Notes |
|---|---|---|---|---|---|---|---|---|---|
| 29.06.2005 | 26.06.1981 | F | | 1013 | 1018 | To take OTC co-codamol for her neck pain | | 1574 | |
| 28.06.2005 | 27.06.1944 | M | | 1652 | 1702 | Script for Phenobarbitone given | | 1673 | |
| 23.06.2005 | 30.05.1916 | M | | 938 | 943 | Referred to Audiology clinic for hearing aid assessment | | 1712 | |
| 22.06.2005 | 11.10.1938 | F | UTI | 1727 | 1732 | Frequency of micturition | Amoxycillin | 1832 | For MSU. |
| 22.06.2005 | 02.10.1943 | M | | 1751 | 1758 | To contact the DVT clinic regarding his painful & swollen (L) calf | | 1852 | |
| 23.06.2005 | 19.08.1926 | F | | 1712 | 1715 | Script for Ezetimibe given | | 1907 | |
| 29.06.2005 | 31.08.1982 | F | Rash | 919 | 929 | Itchy rash on hands & feet | Fusidic Acid 2% + 1% Hydrocortisone cream | 1924 | |
| 24.06.2005 | 29.11.1929 | F | | 1752 | 1803 | (L) Carpal tunnel syndrome | Referred to Orthopaedic Surgeon (Basildon Hospital) | 193 | |
| 27.06.2005 | 21.03.1988 | F | | 1738 | 1744 | Pregnancy test negative | | 1951 | |
| 24.06.2005 | 02.03.1918 | F | | 1005 | 1014 | To continue with Atenolol for now | | 2134 | Chloramphenicol allergy. |

Result of a query that lists all consultations from the 22nd to the end of June 2005 (ConsultationsSeenFrom22ndTillEndOfJun2005)

| SurgeryDate | DateOfBirth | Sex | Diagnosis | TimeIn | TimeOut | Complaints | Treatments | NumbersID | Notes |
|---|---|---|---|---|---|---|---|---|---|
| 27.06.2005 | 10.08.1931 | M | | 1041 | 1046 | Diet controlled Diabetic | | 2182 | Aspirin allergy. |
| 29.06.2005 | 18.09.1980 | F | Pain | 1719 | 1727 | Back pain over (L) shoulder | Referred to Orthopaedic Surgeon (BUPA) | 2193 | |
| 22.06.2005 | 31.03.1913 | M | | 1649 | 1656 | Script for Co-codamol given | | 228 | Daughter came to Surgery. |
| 24.06.2005 | 14.08.1927 | M | | 1807 | 1818 | Dizziness | Prochlorperazine | 2289 | |
| 24.06.2005 | 08.06.1958 | F | S/Leave | 931 | 946 | Fractured 3rd (L) toe | | 2385 | |
| 29.06.2005 | 02.11.1977 | F | | 929 | 935 | Late Period | For Pregnancy test | 2487 | |
| 28.06.2005 | 13.11.1970 | F | Rash | 1802 | 1806 | Moles on legs | Referred to Dermatologist (Basildon Hospital) | 2578 | |
| 22.06.2005 | 15.08.1953 | F | | 1656 | 1701 | For Physiotherapy | | 2625 | |
| 24.06.2005 | 07.05.1978 | F | | 925 | 931 | To attend Family Planning Clinic | | 2684 | |
| 29.06.2005 | 25.05.1976 | F | | 1704 | 1719 | Script for Fluoxetine & Propranolol given | | 2797 | |
| 27.06.2005 | 06.04.1924 | F | | 1026 | 1041 | Deafness in the (L) ear | Referred to ENT Surgeon | 2909 | Diabetic Clinic check. Penicillin allergy. |
| 28.06.2005 | 15.03.1946 | F | | 1732 | 1753 | Script for Script for Acarbose given | | 2975 | |

Result of a query that lists all consultations from the 22$^{nd}$ to the end of June 2005 (ConsultationsSeenFrom22ndTillEndOfJun2005)

| SurgeryDate | DateOfBirth | Sex | Diagnosis | TimeIn | TimeOut | Complaints | Treatments | NumbersID | Notes |
|---|---|---|---|---|---|---|---|---|---|
| 23.06.2005 | 25.12.1946 | F | | 1655 | 1701 | Script for Conjugated oestrogens equine with Medroxyprogesterone (continuous combined) 300mcg + 1.5mg | | 3197 | |
| 24.06.2005 | 16.03.1925 | M | | 1036 | 1044 | Blood Pressure normal | | 3245 | |
| 24.06.2005 | 16.03.1950 | M | S/Leave | 1742 | 1752 | Stress - Med. 5 | | 3317 | |
| 22.06.2005 | 12.08.1932 | M | | 1641 | 1649 | Script for Sodium bicarbonate ear drops given | | 3344 | |
| 27.06.2005 | 06.06.1947 | M | Pain | 915 | 923 | Deep pain in the ears | Referred to ENT Surgeon | 3588 | |
| 23.06.2005 | 04.11.1966 | F | Rash | 1753 | 1757 | Mole on (R) shoulder | Referred to Dermatologist (BUPA) | 3632 | Trimethoprim allergy. |
| 23.06.2005 | 23.05.1943 | M | | 1012 | 1028 | PSA - 59.5 mcg/L, elevated | Referred to Urologist (urgent) | 3684 | Script for Simvastatin given. |
| 27.06.2005 | 16.08.1927 | F | | 1020 | 1026 | To try own Co-codamol | | 3717 | |
| 24.06.2005 | 26.01.1991 | M | S/Leave | 946 | 957 | Sore throat - Private | | 3724 | Script for Erythromycin allergy. Penicillin allergy. |
| 22.06.2005 | 07.07.1961 | F | | 905 | 911 | Script for Erythromycin given | | 3768 | |
| 29.06.2005 | 21.05.1971 | F | | 940 | 945 | Vaginal thrush | Clotrimazole pessary | 39 | |

Result of a query that lists all consultations from the 22nd to the end of June 2005 (ConsultationsSeenFrom22ndTillEndOfJun2005)

| SurgeryDate | DateOfBirth | Sex | Diagnosis | TimeIn | TimeOut | Complaints | Treatments | NumbersID | Notes |
|---|---|---|---|---|---|---|---|---|---|
| 23.06.2005 | 29.01.1956 | M | S/Leave | 943 | 946 | Depression | | 3935 | |
| 24.06.2005 | 18.01.1968 | M | | 1730 | 1738 | Referred to Ophthalmologist regarding possible ocular hypertension | | 3992 | Penicillin allergy. |
| 24.06.2005 | 11.06.1962 | F | | 919 | 925 | Script for Citalopram given | | 4023 | |
| 28.06.2005 | 22.05.1991 | M | Pain | 1759 | 1802 | Back Pain | Referred to Orthopaedic Surgeon (Basildon Hospital) | 4093 | |
| 29.06.2005 | 04.09.1952 | M | | 1033 | 1050 | Script for Atorvastatin given | | 4128 | |
| 29.06.2005 | 18.03.1987 | F | Rash | 1747 | 1755 | Itchy rash on body & legs | Fexofenadine | 4132 | |
| 24.06.2005 | 30.10.1947 | M | S/Leave | 1803 | 1807 | Waldenstrom's macroglobulinemia | | 431 | Scoline allergy. |
| 23.06.2005 | 20.05.1992 | F | URTI | 1718 | 1722 | Sore throat | Amoxycillin | 4396 | |
| 28.06.2005 | 31.12.1922 | M | | 944 | 1005 | Script for Cisclosonide inhaler, Miconazole 2% + 1% Hydrocortisone cream & Temazepam given | | 4470 | |
| 22.06.2005 | 30.05.1953 | F | Revisit | 1000 | 1003 | Rash on (L) fore-arm is still present | Referred to Dermatologist (Basildon Hospital) | 4618 | |
| 28.06.2005 | 25.03.1952 | F | Pain | 1022 | 1029 | Injury (R) foot | For X-Ray | 4625 | |

Result of a query that lists all consultations from the 22nd to the end of June 2005 (ConsultationsSeenFrom22ndTillEndOfJun2005)

| SurgeryDate | DateOfBirth | Sex | Diagnosis | TimeIn | TimeOut | Complaints | Treatments | NumbersID | Notes |
|---|---|---|---|---|---|---|---|---|---|
| 23.06.2005 | 01.03.1961 | F | | 1648 | 1655 | Mouth ulcers | Amoxycillin | 4880 | |
| 22.06.2005 | 10.06.1921 | M | Pain | 1320 | 1330 | Pain & redness both legs | Flucloxacillin & Frusemide | 4972 | Home visit. |
| 29.06.2005 | 09.02.1965 | F | Revisit | 904 | 909 | Still has dizzy spells | Referred to ENT Surgeon | 5077 | |
| 22.06.2005 | 09.04.1926 | M | | 1020 | 1028 | Script for Omeprazole given | | 5248 | |
| 27.06.2005 | 24.04.1935 | F | Pain | 1646 | 1650 | Painful knees | | 5770 | |
| 22.06.2005 | 17.01.1986 | F | | 1044 | 1106 | For Physiotherapy | for X-Ray | 5796 | Aspirin allergy. |
| 27.06.2005 | 03.01.1941 | M | | 923 | 937 | Copy of Glenworth financial Medical Certificate Claim form altered appropriately | | 587 | Wife came to Surgery. |
| 24.06.2005 | 13.04.1942 | M | | 1636 | 1642 | For repeat TFTs in 4 to 6 months | | 5876 | |
| 23.06.2005 | 07.05.1974 | M | S/Leave | 1737 | 1746 | Headaches. Diarrhoea & vomiting - Private | | 5951 | |
| 29.06.2005 | 07.05.1974 | M | S/Leave | 909 | 913 | Headaches. Diarrhoea & Vomiting | | 5951 | |
| 22.06.2005 | 06.01.1987 | F | | 1758 | 1801 | Script for Bupropion m/r given | | 5981 | |
| 22.06.2005 | 30.01.1931 | F | | 1701 | 1713 | She will be moving Surgery soon (change of her address) | | 600 | |
| 27.06.2005 | 28.09.1939 | F | Lump | 1641 | 1646 | Lump on (R) chest wall | Referred to Surgeon | 6176 | |

Result of a query that lists all consultations from the 22nd to the end of June 2005 (ConsultationsSeenFrom22ndTillEndOfJun2005)

| SurgeryDate | DateOfBirth | Sex | Diagnosis | TimeIn | TimeOut | Complaints | Treatments | NumbersID | Notes |
|---|---|---|---|---|---|---|---|---|---|
| 23.06.2005 | 14.01.1934 | F |  | 926 | 932 | Script for Co-codamol & Etodolac given |  | 6234 |  |
| 22.06.2005 | 11.09.1978 | M | URTI | 1740 | 1744 | (L) ear is sore with leakage | Erythromycin | 6244 | Penicillin allergy. |
| 24.06.2005 | 10.01.1973 | F |  | 1014 | 1021 | Script for Citalopram given |  | 6305 |  |
| 24.06.2005 | 24.11.1985 | M |  | 1738 | 1742 | To attend ROCHE unit regarding smoking cannabis |  | 6576 |  |
| 28.06.2005 | 02.11.1984 | F | RTI | 937 | 944 | Chesty cough | Amoxycillin | 6604 |  |
| 23.06.2005 | 08.10.1940 | F |  | 901 | 907 | She will observe her painful (L) knee for now |  | 6705 | Penicillin & desloratadine allergy. |
| 29.06.2005 | 20.03.1952 | F |  | 1800 | 1803 | Flare-up of diverticulitis | Amoxycillin | 6741 | Erythromycin allergy. Husband came to Surgery. |
| 29.06.2005 | 13.02.1950 | M | URTI | 1803 | 1807 | Sore throat | Amoxycillin | 6765 |  |
| 23.06.2005 | 23.11.1946 | M |  | 1004 | 1012 | Script for Atorvastatin given |  | 6822 |  |
| 22.06.2005 | 16.09.1936 | M |  | 920 | 924 | Private script for Viagra given |  | 693 |  |
| 28.06.2005 | 25.02.1949 | M |  | 1721 | 1732 | Lloyds TSB Insurance Medical Claim form completed |  | 6956 |  |
| 22.06.2005 | 18.04.1965 | M | URTI | 1719 | 1723 | (L) ear ache & discharge | Amoxycillin | 7014 | Aspirin allergy. |

## Result of a query that lists all consultations from the 22nd to the end of June 2005 (ConsultationsSeenFrom22ndTillEndOfJun2005)

| SurgeryDate | DateOfBirth | Sex | Diagnosis | TimeIn | TimeOut | Complaints | Treatments | NumbersID | Notes |
|---|---|---|---|---|---|---|---|---|---|
| 29.06.2005 | 18.04.1965 | M | Revisit | 1755 | 1800 | (L) ear is still weeping | Erythromycin & Dexamethasone with neomycin ear spray | 7014 | |
| 23.06.2005 | 01.01.1968 | F | | 1638 | 1644 | Vaginal hysterectomy | | 7021 | |
| 27.06.2005 | 23.12.1929 | F | Lump | 944 | 950 | Something coming down vaginally | Referred to Gynaecologist (Basildon Hospital) | 7078 | |
| 28.06.2005 | 14.08.1984 | M | S/Leave | 931 | 937 | Diarrhoea - Private | | 708 | |
| 24.06.2005 | 11.04.1974 | F | | 902 | 919 | To lose 2.5kg in one month | | 7083 | |
| 23.06.2005 | 14.02.2001 | F | URTI | 1644 | 1648 | Sore throat | Amoxycillin | 7140 | |
| 27.06.2005 | 24.06.2001 | M | RTI | 1719 | 1722 | Cough | Amoxycillin | 7155 | |
| 27.06.2005 | 05.11.1971 | M | RTI | 1753 | 1759 | Chesty cough & wheezy | Amoxycillin & Salbutamol inhaler | 7159 | |
| 28.06.2005 | 04.01.1932 | F | | 912 | 931 | Script for Bendrofluazide & Simvastatin given | | 7247 | |
| 23.06.2005 | 02.02.1968 | F | | 1042 | 1048 | Swollen lower lip & split in mouth following cold sore | Tetracycline | 7269 | Penicillin allergy. |
| 29.06.2005 | 24.06.1969 | M | | 1727 | 1732 | Penile thrush | Fluconazole | 7273 | |
| 22.06.2005 | 18.05.1936 | M | | 924 | 931 | Script for Sodium bicarbonate ear drops given | | 7356 | |

Result of a query that lists all consultations from the 22nd to the end of June 2005 (ConsultationsSeenFrom22ndTillEndOfJun2005)

| SurgeryDate | DateOfBirth | Sex | Diagnosis | TimeIn | TimeOut | Complaints | Treatments | NumbersID | Notes |
|---|---|---|---|---|---|---|---|---|---|
| 22.06.2005 | 27.03.1931 | F | Revisit | 946 | 950 | Still has pain in the (L) leg | Referred to Orthopaedic Surgeon (Basildon Hospital) | 7356 | |
| 28.06.2005 | 20.10.1935 | F | | 1055 | 1115 | Due to go on Sulfasalazine 1g bd soon | | 7444 | |
| 29.06.2005 | 27.09.1969 | F | | 1050 | 1058 | Script for Microgynon 30 given | | 7495 | |
| 24.06.2005 | 27.04.1925 | M | | 957 | 1005 | Patient informed that the nephrologist advised that he should not go on ACE inhibitors or "Sartans" | | 751 | |
| 27.06.2005 | 06.04.1930 | M | | 1656 | 1707 | For MSU, PSA & FBC | | 7512 | |
| 22.06.2005 | 27.08.1935 | M | Pain | 1031 | 1044 | (R) calf tenderness | Referred to DVT Clinic, SGH | 7514 | Flu vaccine allergy. |
| 28.06.2005 | 20.02.1953 | F | S/Leave | 902 | 906 | Sprained (R) ankle | | 7559 | |
| 22.06.2005 | 27.10.1966 | M | | 1744 | 1751 | He will come back for Private sick leave | | 7571 | |
| 23.06.2005 | 27.10.1966 | M | S/Leave | 1746 | 1750 | Stress - Private | | 7571 | |
| 23.06.2005 | 06.04.1938 | M | | 1028 | 1037 | Pain in (L) big toe has gone | | 7624 | Diclofenac allergy. |
| 28.06.2005 | 22.08.1952 | F | | 1044 | 1055 | To see Nurse for HVS & Chlamydial swab | | 7626 | |
| 28.06.2005 | 18.10.1966 | F | | 1005 | 1015 | Script for Amoxycillin with Clarithromycin & Lansoprazole given | | 7634 | |

Result of a query that lists all consultations from the 22nd to the end of June 2005 (ConsultationsSeenFrom22ndTillEndOfJun2005)

| SurgeryDate | DateOfBirth | Sex | Diagnosis | TimeIn | TimeOut | Complaints | Treatments | NumbersID | Notes |
|---|---|---|---|---|---|---|---|---|---|
| 28.06.2005 | 26.09.1937 | M | Pain | 1636 | 1643 | Pain (L) shoulder | Diclofenac e/c & Omeprazole | 7693 | |
| 27.06.2005 | 09.10.1966 | F | | 937 | 944 | For Fasting Glucose | | 7710 | |
| 29.06.2005 | 01.06.1947 | F | Pain | 1642 | 1646 | Pain both groins | For X-Ray of hips & pelvis | 7754 | |
| 23.06.2005 | 15.04.2003 | F | URTI | 1757 | 1803 | Recurrent discharge from (R) ear with ache | Amoxycillin | 7769 | Referred to ENT Surgeon. |
| 28.06.2005 | 04.03.1952 | M | | 1715 | 1721 | Script for Simvastatin given | | 7830 | |
| 23.06.2005 | 13.01.1997 | F | | 1722 | 1726 | To see Practice Nurse for Peak flow measurement | | 7834 | Penicillin allergy. |
| 29.06.2005 | 03.10.1958 | F | Revisit | 1646 | 153 | Pain in (R) foot is still bad | Referred to Physiotherapy | 7891 | Penicillin allergy. |
| 23.06.2005 | 27.05.2000 | M | | 1037 | 1042 | Fell into a garden pond | Flucloxacillin | 7921 | |
| 28.06.2005 | 18.05.1935 | M | Pain | 1702 | 1715 | Pain (L) knee | For X-Ray | 83 | For PSA. |
| 22.06.2005 | 21.07.1963 | F | S/Leave | 1028 | 1031 | Tired all the time & Depression - Med. 5 | | 835 | |
| 23.06.2005 | 05.10.1974 | M | | 1731 | 1735 | Hay fever | Desloratadine | 918 | |
| 29.06.2005 | 08.12.1962 | F | | 1732 | 1747 | Multiple small intramural fibroids noten on USScan | Referred to Gynaecologist (Basildon Hospital) | 981 | Penicillin allergy. |
| 27.06.2005 | 06.04.1937 | M | | 1650 | 1656 | Script for Prochlorperazine given | | 988 | |

Result of a query that lists all consultations from the 22nd to the end of June 2005 (ConsultationsSeenFrom22ndTillEndOfJun2005)

| SurgeryDate | DateOfBirth | Sex | Diagnosis | TimeIn | TimeOut | Complaints | Treatments | NumbersID | Notes |
|---|---|---|---|---|---|---|---|---|---|
| 29.06.2005 | 12.05.1936 | M | Pain | 945 | 954 | Pain (R) hip | For X-Ray | NP (AM) | |
| 22.06.2005 | 26.06.1954 | M | S/Leave | 917 | 920 | Back Pain | | NP (CDP) | |
| 27.06.2005 | 08.04.2005 | M | RTI | 1707 | 1714 | Chesty cough | Amoxycillin | NP (CE) | |
| 24.06.2005 | 12.10.1946 | F | Rash | 1021 | 1036 | Septic rash on (L) leg | Flucloxacillin | NP (CS) | Septrin allergy. |
| 28.06.2005 | 02.02.1939 | M | UTI | 1806 | 1813 | Dysuria | Amoxycillin | NP (DH) | Script for Atorvastatin given. For MSU. |
| 29.06.2005 | 22.11.1981 | M | | 1004 | 1013 | Hay fever | Fexofenadine | NP (DP) | |
| 23.06.2005 | 02.06.1931 | M | | 1726 | 1729 | Bruised discoloured area on back | To observe | NP (EE) | |
| 27.06.2005 | 08.12.1930 | M | RTI | 950 | 1005 | Chesty cough | Amoxycillin | NP (FR) | Script for Atorvastatin given. |
| 28.06.2005 | 14.04.1970 | M | | 1643 | 1652 | Heart missing a beat | To come in with a record of this in 3 months | NP (GB) | Penicillin allergy. |
| 29.06.2005 | 02.09.1961 | F | | 954 | 959 | Nails are brittle & discoloured | Referred to Dermatologist (Basildon Hospital) | NP (IK) | |
| 22.06.2005 | 03.04.1920 | F | Pain | 1305 | 1320 | Burning pain in the (L) leg | Flucloxacillin & Paracetamol | NP (JA) | Home visit. |
| 27.06.2005 | 25.07.1939 | F | | 905 | 915 | Script for Simvastatin given | | NP (JB) | |
| 24.06.2005 | 23.04.1923 | F | UTI | 1719 | 1725 | Dysuria | Amoxycillin | NP (JD) | For MSU. |
| 22.06.2005 | 12.07.1948 | F | S/Leave | 1723 | 1727 | Removal of brain tumour | | NP (JE) | |

Result of a query that lists all consultations from the 22nd to the end of June 2005 (ConsultationsSeenFrom22ndTillEndOfJun2005)

| SurgeryDate | DateOfBirth | Sex | Diagnosis | TimeIn | TimeOut | Complaints | Treatments | NumbersID | Notes |
|---|---|---|---|---|---|---|---|---|---|
| 22.06.2005 | 18.07.1929 | F | Rash | 911 | 917 | Eczema rash on palms | Referred to Dermatologist (Basildon Hospital) | NP (JG) | |
| 29.06.2005 | 21.02.1951 | M | Rash | 959 | 1004 | Tender & itchy rash on face | Fusidic Acid 2% + 1% Hydrocortisone cream | NP (JH) | |
| 23.06.2005 | 12.03.1954 | M | Lump | 907 | 917 | Lump (L) testicle | For USScan of testicles (BUPA) | NP (JL) | |
| 23.06.2005 | 09.01.1987 | F | Rash | 917 | 921 | Warts on (L) arm & fingers | Referred to Dermatologist (Basildon Hospital) | NP (JW) | |
| 24.06.2005 | 22.07.1974 | F | S/Leave | 1652 | 1700 | Sore throat - Med. 5 | | NP (KR) | Script for Salbutamol inhaler given. Penicillin allergy. |
| 22.06.2005 | 02.02.1949 | F | | 1635 | 1641 | Script for Bupropion m/r given | | NP (LL) | |
| 24.06.2005 | 13.01.1993 | M | | 1716 | 1719 | Hay fever | Loratadine | NP (LP) | |
| 28.06.2005 | 23.05.1952 | F | Conjunctivitis | 1015 | 1022 | Sticky eyes | Chloramphenicol eye drops | NP (MEH) | |
| 29.06.2005 | 20.11.1948 | F | Pain | 1633 | 1642 | Joints pains | Diclofenac e/c | NP (MS) | |
| 22.06.2005 | 19.06.1983 | F | Revisit | 1016 | 1020 | Advised to go to A/E regarding pain in her (L) breast | | NP (NS) | |

437

Result of a query that lists all consultations from the 22nd to the end of June 2005 (ConsultationsSeenFrom22ndTillEndOfJun2005)

| SurgeryDate | DateOfBirth | Sex | Diagnosis | TimeIn | TimeOut | Complaints | Treatments | NumbersID | Notes |
|---|---|---|---|---|---|---|---|---|---|
| 24.06.2005 | 04.11.1924 | F | | 1700 | 1716 | Script for Bendrofluazide given | | NP (OR) | Script for Omeprazole given. |
| 27.06.2005 | 07.12.1947 | M | Rash | 1005 | 1009 | Skin tags & mole on (L) shoulder & back | Referred to Dermatologist (Basildon Hospital) | NP (PB) | |
| 28.06.2005 | 30.05.1991 | M | Pain | 1753 | 1759 | Methylphenidate m/r given | | NP (RA) | |
| 27.06.2005 | 16.03.1955 | F | | 1009 | 1020 | Blood tests & USScan of abdomen all normal | | NP (SJL) | |
| 27.06.2005 | 17.05.2004 | M | | 1714 | 1719 | He probably has a viral rash | | NP (TB) | |
| 24.06.2005 | 15.07.1936 | F | | 1642 | 1652 | Loss of weight & diarrhoea | Referred to Gastro-enterologist (Basildon Hospital) | NP (TL) | |
| 27.06.2005 | 30.01.1949 | M | | 1744 | 1753 | Septic blister on dorsum of (L) foot | Flucloxacillin | NP (WD) | |
| 23.06.2005 | 13.02.1985 | F | | 950 | 1000 | To get OTC Co-codamol for her headaches | | Temp | |
| 23.06.2005 | 26.11.1965 | M | | 1701 | 1707 | Script for Co-codamol, Diclofenac m/r, Lansoprazole & Temazepam given | | Temp | |

438

Result of a query that lists all consultations from the 22nd to the end of June 2006 (ConsultationsSeenFrom22ndTillEndOfJun2006)

| SurgeryDate | DateOfBirth | Sex | Diagnosis | TimeIn | TimeOut | Complaints | Treatments | Initials | Notes |
|---|---|---|---|---|---|---|---|---|---|
| 22.06.2006 | 24.04.1935 | F | | 942 | 1000 | Referred to P/ Counsellor regarding rows with her family | | DAS | |
| 22.06.2006 | 20.08.1966 | F | | 1000 | 1010 | Script for MethylPrednisolone with Lidocaine given | | LDD | |
| 22.06.2006 | 28.05.1985 | F | | 1010 | 1020 | Referred to ENT Surgeon regarding her (L) ear lobe lump | | JLH | Script for Cetirizine given. |
| 22.06.2006 | 01.06.1907 | F | | 1020 | 1028 | Daughter will inform her mum of urine test result | | WT | |
| 22.06.2006 | 17.10.1953 | F | | 1034 | 1054 | Physical Activity Referral form completed | | MS | |
| 22.06.2006 | 14.12.1954 | F | | 1054 | 1102 | Script for Norgestrel & Conjugate oestrogens given | | SAH | |
| 22.06.2006 | 12.10.1946 | F | | 1102 | 1118 | Script for Clobetasol given | | CPS | |
| 22.06.2006 | 06.10.1952 | M | S/Leave | 1118 | 1127 | Possible broken ribs | | CJG | |
| 22.06.2006 | 18.01.1968 | M | | 1137 | 1150 | Referred to Rheumatologist regarding multiple joints pain | | IGN | |
| 22.06.2006 | 28.09.1921 | F | Pain | 1300 | 1310 | Headaches | Co-codamol & Etodolac capsules | RG | Home visit. |

Result of a query that lists all consultations from the 22nd to the end of June 2006 (ConsultationsSeenFrom22ndTillEndOfJun2006)

| SurgeryDate | DateOfBirth | Sex | Diagnosis | TimeIn | TimeOut | Complaints | Treatments | Initials | Notes |
|---|---|---|---|---|---|---|---|---|---|
| 22.06.2006 | 13.16.1932 | M | | 1317 | 1327 | Diarrhoea | Loperamide & Electrolade | AP | Home visit. |
| 22.06.2006 | 06.05.1932 | F | | 1410 | 1425 | Script for Amoxycillin, Citalopram & Prochlorperazine given | | RT | Home visit. |
| 22.06.2006 | 21.02.1916 | F | | 1657 | 1708 | Script for Pentoxifyline & Quinine Sulphate given | | EFH | |
| 22.06.2006 | 09.07.1969 | M | | 1708 | 1715 | Script for Fexofenadine & Fusidic acid cream given | | DBJD | |
| 22.06.2006 | 18.06.1993 | F | | 1715 | 1725 | Script for Beclomethasone inhaler & Loratadine given | | LT | |
| 22.06.2006 | 04.10.1968 | F | S/Leave | 1721 | 1734 | Heavy Bleeding | | AC | |
| 22.06.2006 | 25.05.1939 | F | | 1734 | 1745 | Script for Rosiglitazone with Metformin given | | DET | |
| 22.06.2006 | 07.07.1962 | M | RTI | 1745 | 1750 | Chesty cough | Erythromycin | CB | |
| 22.06.2006 | 09.02.1965 | F | | 1750 | 1756 | For MSU | | JAJ | |
| 22.06.2006 | 26.10.1959 | F | | 1756 | 1803 | Referred to ENT Surgeon regarding deafness in her (L) ear | | JAE | |

Result of a query that lists all consultations from the 22nd to the end of June 2006 (ConsultationsSeenFrom22ndTillEndOfJun2006)

| SurgeryDate | DateOfBirth | Sex | Diagnosis | TimeIn | TimeOut | Complaints | Treatments | Initials | Notes |
|---|---|---|---|---|---|---|---|---|---|
| 22.06.2006 | 29.12.1920 | M | | 1803 | 1817 | For Ferritin, B12 & Folate | | WN | |
| 22.06.2006 | 19.05.1935 | F | RTI | 1817 | 1823 | Chesty cough | Amoxycillin | SMK | |
| 22.06.2006 | 23.04.1950 | F | | 1823 | 1833 | Sore on upper lip | Amoxycillin | PEH | |
| 23.06.2006 | 11.08.2000 | M | | 943 | 950 | Reviewed post tonsillectomy | | CALB | |
| 23.06.2006 | 18.10.1920 | F | | 950 | 1006 | Script for Co-codamol & MethylPrednisolone with Lidocaine injection given | | QK | |
| 23.06.2006 | 23.07.1923 | M | | 1006 | 1024 | Script for Ferrous Sulphate & Lisinopril given | | KWB | |
| 23.06.2006 | 06.08.1921 | F | | 1024 | 1039 | Script for Alendronic acid & Calcium Carbonate with cholecalciferol given | | EE | |
| 23.06.2006 | 29.08.1924 | M | | 1039 | 1052 | eGFR compatible with stage 4 CKD | Referred to Nephrologist | VRH | |
| 23.06.2006 | 06.04.1955 | F | | 1052 | 1101 | Referred to Orthopaedic Surgeon regarding knees pain | | JD | |
| 23.06.2006 | 05.06.1930 | F | RTI | 1101 | 1107 | Chesty cough | Amoxycillin & Prednisolone e/c | JMF | |
| 23.06.2006 | 31.10.1915 | F | | 1107 | 1130 | To start Doxazosin again | | MEC | |

441

Result of a query that lists all consultations from the 22nd to the end of June 2006 (ConsultationsSeenFrom22ndTillEndOfJun2006)

| SurgeryDate | DateOfBirth | Sex | Diagnosis | TimeIn | TimeOut | Complaints | Treatments | Initials | Notes |
|---|---|---|---|---|---|---|---|---|---|
| 23.06.2006 | 02.02.1930 | M | | 1130 | 1140 | Script for Dihydrocodeine given | | KRC | |
| 23.06.2006 | 10.09.1999 | F | | 1140 | 1150 | To get earlier appointment with Paediatrician | | EHMK | |
| 23.06.2006 | 11.12.1988 | F | | 1150 | 1200 | Script for Microgynon 30 given | | VJR | |
| 23.06.2006 | 03.09.1980 | F | | 1200 | 1208 | Chesty cough | Ciprofloxacin | KCS | Penicillin allergy. |
| 23.06.2006 | 09.10.1924 | F | | 1648 | 1658 | Script for Amoxycillin, Prednisolone e/c & Salbutamol inhaler given | | VOM | |
| 23.06.2006 | 12.10.1946 | F | | 1658 | 1703 | Septic insect bit (L) ankle | Flucloxacillin | CPC | |
| 23.06.2006 | 25.09.1987 | F | | 1703 | 1708 | Septic insect bit (L) ankle | Flucloxacillin | AS | |
| 23.06.2006 | 03.08.1972 | M | | 1708 | 1717 | Script for Gaviscon Advance given | | Temp (PN) | |
| 23.06.2006 | 24.03.1973 | M | S/Leave | 1717 | 1728 | Eczema flare-up - Med. 5 | | JCM | |
| 23.06.2006 | 10.08.1931 | M | | 1722 | 1728 | For repeat FBC in 3 months | | REW | |
| 23.06.2006 | 28.04.1957 | M | | 1728 | 1736 | Awaiting hospital letter | | RAS | |
| 23.06.2006 | 04.10.1962 | M | | 1736 | 1745 | Script for Cefalexin & Furosemide given | | JAS | |

442

Result of a query that lists all consultations from the 22nd to the end of June 2006 (ConsultationsSeenFrom22ndTillEndOfJun2006)

| SurgeryDate | DateOfBirth | Sex | Diagnosis | TimeIn | TimeOut | Complaints | Treatments | Initials | Notes |
|---|---|---|---|---|---|---|---|---|---|
| 23.06.2006 | 11.08.1952 | F | | 1745 | 1753 | For urgent USScan of pelvis & for MSU | | MK | |
| 23.06.2006 | 20.03.1952 | F | | 1753 | 1759 | Script for Amoxycillin & Furosemide given | | LJF | |
| 23.06.2006 | 13.02.1950 | M | | 1759 | 1811 | Referred to Urologist regarding Prostatic problems | | DCF | |
| 23.06.2006 | 17.03.1967 | F | | 1811 | 1822 | Script for Macrogol compound npf oral powder 13.8g given | | SOOSP | |
| 23.06.2006 | 15.07.2002 | F | | 1822 | 1828 | Script for Amoxycillin given | | CGD | For MSU. |
| 23.06.2006 | 30.01.1999 | F | | 1828 | 1834 | Lip ulcer | Amoxycillin | ALCW | |
| 23.06.2006 | 18.06.1993 | F | | 1834 | 1842 | Script for Beclomethasone inhaler given | | LT | |
| 26.06.2006 | 08.09.1964 | F | | 951 | 1002 | She may need removal of the Mirena IUS | | DMB | |
| 26.06.2006 | 20.11.1945 | M | | 1002 | 1009 | Referred to Dermatologist regarding rash | | CJM | |
| 26.06.2006 | 24.11.1933 | F | | 1009 | 1021 | Script for Omeprazole & Ibuprofen given | | PAB | |
| 26.06.2006 | 10.08.1952 | F | S/Leave | 1021 | 1029 | (L) Cataract Operation - MED. 5 | | SAG | |
| 26.06.2006 | 23.03.1926 | M | | 1029 | 1041 | Referred to Counsellor regarding being unable to cope | | JWH | |

443

Result of a query that lists all consultations from the 22nd to the end of June 2006 (ConsultationsSeenFrom22ndTillEndOfJun2006)

| SurgeryDate | DateOfBirth | Sex | Diagnosis | TimeIn | TimeOut | Complaints | Treatments | Initials | Notes |
|---|---|---|---|---|---|---|---|---|---|
| 26.06.2006 | 06.08.1930 | F | | 1041 | 1055 | To see nurse for BP check in one month | | LP | |
| 26.06.2006 | 26.10.1943 | F | | 1105 | 1119 | Script for Mupirocin cream given | | APM | For MSU. |
| 26.06.2006 | 02.03.1948 | M | | 1100 | 1105 | Referred to Orthopaedic Surgeon (BUPA) regarding (R) carpal tunnel syndrome | | SAM | |
| 26.06.2006 | 26.01.1959 | F | | 1105 | 1119 | Script for Trimethoprim given | | JHH | |
| 26.06.2006 | 28.09.1921 | F | | 1119 | 1131 | For Home visit | | REG | Niece came to Surgery. |
| 26.06.2006 | 09.06.1981 | M | | 1131 | 1138 | Sore gum | Amoxycillin | KS | |
| 26.06.2006 | 06.01.1943 | F | | 1138 | 1142 | She does not want any more follow-up in hospital regarding her double vision | | PC | |
| 26.06.2006 | 28.09.1973 | F | | 1142 | 1150 | Phlebitis (R) leg | Flucloxacillin | DMS | |
| 26.06.2006 | 28.09.1921 | F | | 1405 | 1455 | Social Service Respite care being arranged | | REG | Home visit. |
| 26.06.2006 | 13.11.1952 | F | | 1646 | 1654 | Referred to Orthopaedic Surgeon regarding Coccyx Pain | | LH | |
| 26.06.2006 | 17.04.1966 | M | | 1654 | 1704 | Hay fever | Cetirizine | JRB | |
| 26.06.2006 | 04.01.2000 | M | | 1704 | 1710 | Sore throat & ear ache | Amoxycillin & Paracetamol | ALKP | |

444

## Result of a query that lists all consultations from the 22nd to the end of June 2006 (ConsultationsSeenFrom22ndTillEndOfJun2006)

| SurgeryDate | DateOfBirth | Sex | Diagnosis | TimeIn | TimeOut | Complaints | Treatments | Initials | Notes |
|---|---|---|---|---|---|---|---|---|---|
| 26.06.2006 | 11.01.1986 | F | | 1710 | 1717 | Script for Flucloxacillin given | | SJW | |
| 26.06.2006 | 13.09.1948 | F | | 1717 | 1727 | Script for Diclofenac e/c & Dihydrocodeine given | | LP | Referred to Podiatrist regarding (R) foot pain. |
| 26.06.2006 | 02.12.1992 | M | | 1727 | 1734 | Script for Tetracycline topical solution given | | TJN | |
| 26.06.2006 | 28.04.1981 | F | Rash | 1734 | 1737 | Facial rash | Fusidic acid with hydrocortisone cream | NKL | |
| 26.06.2006 | 14.10.1969 | F | | 1737 | 1746 | Script for Norgestrel and Conjugated Oestrogens (equine) given | | LB | |
| 26.06.2006 | 27.09.1967 | F | S/Leave | 1746 | 1754 | Chest infection | | JTR | |
| 26.06.2006 | 02.05.1992 | M | | 1754 | 1800 | Referred to Orthopaedic Surgeon (BUPA) regarding his (L)IGT nail | | LIC | |
| 26.06.2006 | 23.02.1979 | F | | 1800 | 1806 | Script for Paroxetine given | | CLC | |
| 26.06.2006 | 03.03.1984 | M | | 1806 | 1814 | Script for Salicylic acid topical solution 26% given | | PWK | |
| 26.06.2006 | 31.01.1938 | F | RTI | 1817 | 1825 | Chesty cough | Amoxycillin | JMS | |
| 26.06.2006 | 26.05.1986 | M | URTI | 1825 | 1831 | (L) ear ache | Amoxycillin | BF | |
| 26.06.2006 | 18.11.1979 | M | | 1831 | 1841 | Script for Acyclovir tablets & Amoxycillin given | | JAS | |

Result of a query that lists all consultations from the 22nd to the end of June 2006 (ConsultationsSeenFrom22ndTillEndOfJun2006)

| SurgeryDate | DateOfBirth | Sex | Diagnosis | TimeIn | TimeOut | Complaints | Treatments | Initials | Notes |
|---|---|---|---|---|---|---|---|---|---|
| 27.06.2006 | 21.08.1946 | F | | 945 | 956 | Referred to Vascular Surgeon regarding aching varicose veins | | JK | |
| 27.06.2006 | 15.04.1927 | M | | 956 | 1008 | Referred to Dermatologist regarding moles & referred to Haematologist regarding persistent high WCC | | JB | |
| 27.06.2006 | 15.03.1934 | F | | 1008 | 1015 | BP 158/89 | | PJB | |
| 27.06.2006 | 07.03.1999 | F | | 1015 | 1025 | Script for Flucloxacillin & Metoclopramide given | | SAW | |
| 27.06.2006 | 04.05.1937 | F | | 1025 | 1035 | Script for Furosemide & Spironolactone given | | DMB | |
| 27.06.2006 | 03.02.1966 | F | | 1035 | 1040 | Script for Loratadine given | | LJR | |
| 27.06.2006 | 21.09.1999 | M | | 1040 | 1044 | He is okay with his medications | | VB | |
| 27.06.2006 | 08.03.1961 | M | S/Leave | 1044 | 1100 | Pain in the (R) elbow - Private | | RAB | |
| 27.06.2006 | 01.02.1988 | M | URTI | 1100 | 1105 | Sore throat | Amoxycillin | DJL | |
| 27.06.2006 | 26.05.1936 | M | | 1105 | 1113 | Script for Dihydrocodeine given | | TC | |
| 27.06.2006 | 07.10.1933 | M | | 1113 | 1124 | Script for Co-codamol, Etodolac & Olanzapine given | | FDF | |

446

## Result of a query that lists all consultations from the 22nd to the end of June 2006 (ConsultationsSeenFrom22ndTillEndOfJun2006)

| SurgeryDate | DateOfBirth | Sex | Diagnosis | TimeIn | TimeOut | Complaints | Treatments | Initials | Notes |
|---|---|---|---|---|---|---|---|---|---|
| 27.06.2006 | 27.03.1931 | F | | 1124 | 1132 | She developed itchy rash to Doxazosin | | MMA | |
| 27.06.2006 | 17.09.1998 | F | URTI | 1132 | 1139 | Sore throat | Erythromycin | SW | |
| 27.06.2006 | 24.04.2003 | M | | 1139 | 1147 | Unwell & pyrexial | Amoxycillin & Paracetamol | JPS | |
| 27.06.2006 | 10.09.1919 | F | Rash | 1147 | 1154 | Itchy rash on arms & legs | Loratadine & Calamine lotion | ALG | |
| 27.06.2006 | 10.06.1921 | M | | 1350 | 1415 | Chest infection, collapsed | To SGH, Medical Dr. on call | TH | Home visit. |
| 27.06.2006 | 11.09.1914 | F | | 1430 | 1440 | Patient not bothered by rash on arm | | PB | Home visit. |
| 27.06.2006 | 12.05.1936 | M | | 1645 | 1700 | For repeat MSU | | AM | |
| 27.06.2006 | 18.06.1993 | F | RTI | 1708 | 1712 | Chesty cough | Amoxycillin | LT | |
| 27.06.2006 | 06.12.1945 | M | S/Leave | 1712 | 1716 | Weakness in (L) hand | | BS | |
| 27.06.2006 | 04.11.1934 | M | | 1716 | 1720 | For USScan of the abdomen | | TEE | |
| 27.06.2006 | 09.06.1934 | M | | 1720 | 1728 | Script for Dihydrocodeine & Lansoprazole given | | MKC | |
| 27.06.2006 | 27.05.1993 | M | | 1728 | 1735 | To take the antibiotics prescribed by the dentist | | LRF | |
| 27.06.2006 | 14.05.1927 | F | | 1745 | 1754 | Bilateral pedal oedema | Bumetanide | 43070 | |
| 27.06.2006 | 24.07.1981 | F | | 1754 | 1802 | Facial spots | Erythromycin | CLN | |
| 27.06.2006 | 11.08.1980 | F | | 1802 | 1810 | For X-Ray (L) wrist | | MD | |

447

Result of a query that lists all consultations from the 22nd to the end of June 2006 (ConsultationsSeenFrom22ndTillEndOfJun2006)

| SurgeryDate | DateOfBirth | Sex | Diagnosis | TimeIn | TimeOut | Complaints | Treatments | Initials | Notes |
|---|---|---|---|---|---|---|---|---|---|
| 27.06.2006 | 29.09.1932 | F | | 1830 | 1845 | Script for Dihydrocodeine given | | SD | Referred to Orthopaedic Surgeon. Home visit. |
| 27.06.2006 | 13.11.1932 | M | | 1850 | 1900 | Script for Ciprofloxacin & Lomotil given | | AP | Home visit. |
| 28.06.2006 | 31.03.1956 | F | RTI | 938 | 945 | Wheezy & chesty cough | Amoxycillin, Prednisolone e/c & Peak flow meter | SD | |
| 28.06.2006 | 25.05.1973 | F | | 945 | 954 | Referred to General Surgeon regarding lump in her neck | | TJ | |
| 28.06.2006 | 04.07.1961 | F | | 954 | 1004 | Referred to Gynaecologist as her abdominal pain & per vagina bleeding are worse | | JB | |
| 28.06.2006 | 19.06.1927 | F | | 1004 | 1014 | Script for Fusidic acid with hydrocortisone cream & Loratadine given | | GEG | |
| 28.06.2006 | 25.08.1936 | M | | 1022 | 1034 | Script for Amoxycillin & Furosemide given | | CAJ | |
| 28.06.2006 | 01.04.1920 | F | | 1034 | 1044 | Anxious & panicky | Citalopram | HEW | |
| 28.06.2006 | 12.11.1950 | M | Pain | 1044 | 1051 | Back Pain | Dihydrocodeine | MJP | |
| 28.06.2006 | 31.08.1964 | M | | 1051 | 1055 | For MSU | | CJW | |

Result of a query that lists all consultations from the 22nd to the end of June 2006 (ConsultationsSeenFrom22ndTillEndOfJun2006)

| SurgeryDate | DateOfBirth | Sex | Diagnosis | TimeIn | TimeOut | Complaints | Treatments | Initials | Notes |
|---|---|---|---|---|---|---|---|---|---|
| 28.06.2006 | 03.01.1958 | F | | 1055 | 1101 | Script for Amoxycillin & Dexamethasone with given | | SABD | |
| 28.06.2006 | 14.12.1954 | F | | 1101 | 1115 | Script for Oestradiol & (Oestradiol with Levonorgestrel) given | | SAH | |
| 28.06.2006 | 11.01.1964 | F | | 1115 | 1124 | Script for Clotrimazole pessary given | | TJR | |
| 28.06.2006 | 13.12.1986 | F | | 1124 | 1136 | Script for Ferrous Sulphate given | | SAP | |
| 28.06.2006 | 02.06.1955 | F | RTI | 1136 | 1143 | Chesty cough | Erythromycin | JPS | Penicillin allergy. |
| 28.06.2006 | 17.10.1928 | M | | 1250 | 1300 | Script for Etodolac capsule given | | CW | |
| 28.06.2006 | 01.12.1933 | F | | 1643 | 1652 | Script for Co-codamol given | | JM | |
| 28.06.2006 | 19.01.1954 | F | | 1652 | 1658 | Reassured regarding lump on the (L) leg | | DD | |
| 28.06.2006 | 31.07.1956 | M | | 1702 | 1712 | Script for Furosemide given | | RUGH | |
| 28.06.2006 | 21.02.1916 | F | | 1712 | 1718 | Script for Loperamide given | | FEH | |
| 28.06.2006 | 04.01.1950 | F | | 1726 | 1737 | Dizziness | Prochlorperazine | JC | |
| 28.06.2006 | 14.08.1946 | M | Lump | 1743 | 1750 | Lumps (R) chest | Referred to General Surgeon | RBG | |
| 28.06.2006 | 17.09.1986 | F | Rash | 1751 | 1756 | Itchy rash on (L) leg | Loratadine & Fusidic with hydrocortisone cream | AK | |

Result of a query that lists all consultations from the 22nd to the end of June 2006 (ConsultationsSeenFrom22ndTillEndOfJun2006)

| SurgeryDate | DateOfBirth | Sex | Diagnosis | TimeIn | TimeOut | Complaints | Treatments | Initials | Notes |
|---|---|---|---|---|---|---|---|---|---|
| 28.06.2006 | 06.10.1981 | F |  | 1804 | 1815 | To see nurse for HVS & Chlamydial swab |  | WK |  |
| 28.06.2006 | 26.09.1957 | F |  | 1815 | 1830 | Script for Citalopram & Flucloxacillin given |  | KLD |  |
| 28.06.2006 | 06.08.1928 | F |  | 1840 | 1855 | To continue with her medications for now |  | GH | Home visit. |
| 29.06.2006 | 09.04.1944 | F |  | 940 | 954 | She will prefer not to take Methotrexate |  | JN |  |
| 29.06.2006 | 26.01.1953 | M |  | 954 | 1002 | Another USScan for abdomen card issued |  | BN |  |
| 29.06.2006 | 06.10.1952 | M | S/Leave | 1002 | 1007 | Possible broken ribs |  | CJG |  |
| 29.06.2006 | 23.12.1942 | F |  | 1025 | 1037 | She does not want her Diabetes medication altered |  | JASP |  |
| 29.06.2006 | 05.11.1941 | M |  | 1037 | 1045 | Private script for Viagra given |  | WB | Script for Diclofenac e/c given. |
| 29.06.2006 | 09.04.1926 | M |  | 1045 | 1107 | Referred to Gastro-enterologist regarding persistent low Hb |  | TS |  |
| 29.06.2006 | 21.05.1936 | M |  | 1107 | 1120 | Script for Chloramphenicol eye drops, Flucloxacillin & Loratadine given |  | CET |  |
| 29.06.2006 | 18.04.1978 | F | S/Leave | 11020 | 1129 | Stressed out, headaches & back pain in pregnancy |  | SL |  |

Result of a query that lists all consultations from the 22nd to the end of June 2006 (ConsultationsSeenFrom22ndTillEndOfJun2006)

| SurgeryDate | DateOfBirth | Sex | Diagnosis | TimeIn | TimeOut | Complaints | Treatments | Initials | Notes |
|---|---|---|---|---|---|---|---|---|---|
| 29.06.2006 | 25.09.1984 | M | | 1129 | 1137 | Patient will contact Dermatologist | | JW | |
| 29.06.2006 | 20.08.1966 | F | | 1137 | 1154 | Injection Depo-Medrone with Lidocaine given to the (R) shoulder | | LDD | |
| 29.06.2006 | 03.03.1994 | M | Pain | 1154 | 1204 | Pain (L) knee | Paracetamol & Ibuprofen | CGAP | |
| 29.06.2006 | 23.07.1969 | M | | 1645 | 1655 | Script for Selenium shampoo given | | JIS | |
| 29.06.2006 | 22.01.1932 | M | | 1655 | 1717 | Already on Lisinopril | | JBW | |
| 29.06.2006 | 22.04.2005 | M | Rash | 1717 | 1723 | Nappy rash | Timodine cream | DG | |
| 29.06.2006 | 12.11.1950 | M | | 1723 | 1730 | Script for Diclofenac e/c given | | MJP | |
| 29.06.2006 | 18.11.1979 | M | | 1730 | 1740 | For review in one week | | JAS | |
| 29.06.2006 | 05.10.1974 | M | | 1740 | 1754 | Script for Loratadine & Salbutamol inhaler given | | SMG | |
| 29.06.2006 | 08.11.1993 | F | URTI | 1754 | 1759 | Sore throat | Amoxycillin | MKE | |
| 29.06.2006 | 14.10.1969 | F | | 1759 | 1805 | Script for Estradiol & (Estradiol with Levonorgestrel) given | | LB | |
| 29.06.2006 | 15.05.1989 | F | | 1805 | 1812 | For Pregnancy test | | LEAP | |
| 29.06.2006 | 08.07.1976 | M | | 1818 | 1825 | Septic skin infection on chin | Flucloxacillin | IRP | |

451

Result of a query that lists all consultations from the 22nd to the end of June 2008 (ConsultationsSeenFrom22ndTillEndOfJun2008)

| SurgeryDate | DateOfBirth | Sex | Diagnosis | TimeIn | TimeOut | Complaints | Treatments | Initials | Notes |
|---|---|---|---|---|---|---|---|---|---|
| 23.06.2008 | 29.05.1967 | M | | 942 | 950 | For Lumbar Spine X-Rays | | CCS | |
| 23.06.2008 | 14.12.1944 | F | | 950 | 958 | Script for Beclomethasone aqueous nasal spray given | | PEF | |
| 23.06.2008 | 07.06.1955 | F | | 1006 | 1015 | Referred to Podiatrist regarding bilateral bunions | | JM | |
| 23.06.2008 | 26.09.1937 | M | | 1015 | 1032 | Referred to Dermatologist regarding lesion on the dorsum of the (L) hand | | DJD | |
| 23.06.2008 | 09.10.2003 | M | RTI | 1040 | 1049 | Chesty cough | Amoxycillin | WJ | |
| 23.06.2008 | 30.03.1923 | M | | 1049 | 1053 | He is still anaemic but his Hb is improving | | PGH | |
| 23.06.2008 | 24.12.1929 | F | | 1053 | 1057 | Medication Review Done | | ECH | Penicillin allergy. |
| 23.06.2008 | 07.07.1936 | F | | 1059 | 1110 | Script for Simvastatin given | | DR | |
| 23.06.2008 | 11.05.1962 | F | | 1110 | 1118 | Script for Diclofenac c/c & Co-codamol given | | JAB | |
| 23.06.2008 | 25.09.1987 | F | | 1118 | 1122 | Septic insect bite on the (L) leg | Flucloxacillin | AS | |

Result of a query that lists all consultations from the 22nd to the end of June 2008 (ConsultationsSeenFrom22ndTillEndOfJun2008)

| SurgeryDate | DateOfBirth | Sex | Diagnosis | TimeIn | TimeOut | Complaints | Treatments | Initials | Notes |
|---|---|---|---|---|---|---|---|---|---|
| 23.06.2008 | 03.02.2008 | F | | 1125 | 1138 | Script for Oral rehydration salts with rice powder given | | EEH | Stool for C&S. |
| 23.06.2008 | 06.04.1937 | M | | 1448 | 1500 | Script for Balneum Plus Bath oil, Telfast & Fucidin H cream given | | GWH | Home visit. |
| 23.06.2008 | 06.10.1933 | M | | 1646 | 1654 | Script for Simvastatin given | | RJK | |
| 23.06.2008 | 26.08.1913 | F | | 1654 | 1703 | Medication Review Done | | AEC | Her Daughter came to the Surgery. |
| 23.06.2008 | 28.01.1943 | F | | 1721 | 1726 | Script for Simvastatin given | | BH | |
| 23.06.2008 | 03.06.1937 | M | | 1726 | 1736 | Script for Omeprazole given | | AMH | Referred to Orthopaedic Surgeon regarding his bilateral Dupuytren's contracture. |
| 23.06.2008 | 09.01.1949 | M | | 1742 | 1750 | Referred to Oral Surgeon regarding burning sensation of the whole tongue | | DFH | |
| 23.06.2008 | 18.06.1981 | M | | 1750 | 1718 | Script for Trimethoprim given | | SCJ | For MSU. |
| 23.06.2008 | 16.06.2003 | F | | 1758 | 1804 | Script for Diprobase cream, Fusidic acid with Hydrocortisone cream & Soya with Lauromacrogols given | | FLR | |

453

Result of a query that lists all consultations from the 22$^{nd}$ to the end of June 2008 (ConsultationsSeenFrom22ndTillEndOfJun2008)

| SurgeryDate | DateOfBirth | Sex | Diagnosis | TimeIn | TimeOut | Complaints | Treatments | Initials | Notes |
|---|---|---|---|---|---|---|---|---|---|
| 23.06.2008 | 06.02.1968 | F | | 1809 | 1817 | Script for Citalopram given | | TH | For MSU. |
| 24.06.2008 | 08.11.1931 | F | | 946 | 955 | Script for Lisinopril given | | JC | |
| 24.06.2008 | 06.12.1947 | M | | 955 | 1005 | Medication Review Done | | BSK | |
| 24.06.2008 | 23.01.1926 | F | RTI | 1012 | 1019 | Chesty cough | Amoxycillin | FGN | |
| 24.06.2008 | 13.03.1932 | M | | 1019 | 1035 | Medication Review Done | | RJW | |
| 24.06.2008 | 09.05.1937 | F | | 1035 | 1050 | Medication Review Done | | KMN | |
| 24.06.2008 | 05.06.1930 | F | RTI | 1050 | 1059 | Chesty cough | Amoxycillin | JMF | Script for Elasticated C tubular bandage 6.75cm given. |
| 24.06.2008 | 02.10.1945 | F | | 1059 | 1103 | Script for Simvastatin given | | BT | |
| 24.06.2008 | 18.07.1965 | F | | 1103 | 1110 | Script for Acrivastine & Norethisterone given | | LSC | |
| 24.06.2008 | 18.06.1951 | M | | 1110 | 1120 | Script for Trimethoprim & Lisinopril given | | AL | |
| 24.06.2008 | 10.06.2005 | M | | 1120 | 1128 | Script for Maxolon Paediatric & Amoxycillin given | | SSD | |
| 24.06.2008 | 05.06.1960 | M | RTI | 1128 | 1132 | Chesty cough | Amoxycillin | GWP | |

454

Result of a query that lists all consultations from the 22nd to the end of June 2008 (ConsultationsSeenFrom22ndTillEndOfJun2008)

| SurgeryDate | DateOfBirth | Sex | Diagnosis | TimeIn | TimeOut | Complaints | Treatments | Initials | Notes |
|---|---|---|---|---|---|---|---|---|---|
| 24.06.2008 | 03.02.2008 | F | | 1132 | 1137 | To apply own Calamine lotion to the rash | | EEH | |
| 24.06.2008 | 26.09.1983 | F | | 1651 | 1657 | Script for Paracetamol with Metoclopramide given | | JADF | |
| 24.06.2008 | 20.06.2006 | F | | 1657 | 1701 | Script for Diprobase cream & Paracetamol suspension given | | SF | |
| 24.06.2008 | 21.12.1935 | M | | 1701 | 1709 | For GTT | | KAR | |
| 24.06.2008 | 05.09.1998 | F | | 1725 | 1730 | Septic insect bit on the neck | Flucloxacillin | EVW | |
| 24.06.2008 | 09.02.1981 | F | URTI | 1703 | 1734 | Sore throat | Amoxycillin | LAD | |
| 24.06.2008 | 06.03.1969 | F | | 1737 | 1754 | Referred to Dermatologist (cancer referral) regarding mole on (L) arm, possibly a melanoma | | KSLC | |
| 24.06.2008 | 21.12.1922 | M | | 1754 | 1801 | Script for Furosemide given | | LD | For serum BNP. |
| 24.06.2008 | 26.05.1996 | M | | 1801 | 1809 | For X-Rays of the (R) foot | | BF | |
| 24.06.2008 | 07.02.1948 | M | RTI | 1816 | 1824 | Chesty cough | Ciprofloxacin | GRC | |
| 25.06.2008 | 16.09.1936 | M | | 947 | 953 | PSA result normal | | LPCE | |
| 25.06.2008 | 02.12.1954 | M | | 953 | 959 | Script for Prochlorperazine given | | OAK | |

Result of a query that lists all consultations from the 22<sup>nd</sup> to the end of June 2008 (ConsultationsSeenFrom22ndTillEndOfJun2008)

| SurgeryDate | DateOfBirth | Sex | Diagnosis | TimeIn | TimeOut | Complaints | Treatments | Initials | Notes |
|---|---|---|---|---|---|---|---|---|---|
| 25.06.2008 | 27.04.1939 | F | | 959 | 1006 | For Chesty X-Rays | | DBS | |
| 25.06.2008 | 12.04.1932 | F | | 1008 | 1022 | Script for Prochlorperazine given | | JMA | |
| 25.06.2008 | 28.07.1946 | M | | 1024 | 1028 | Script for Flucloxacillin given | | PWD | |
| 25.06.2008 | 06.06.1947 | M | | 1028 | 1033 | Script for Ciprofloxacin given | | TLS | |
| 25.06.2008 | 10.04.1937 | F | | 1038 | 1048 | Script for Loratadine given | | MC | Referred to Dermatologist regarding itching on arms & upper chest. |
| 25.06.2008 | 08.04.1961 | F | S/Leave | 1048 | 1101 | (R) shoulder pain - Med. 5 | | STS | Referred to Rheumatologist (BUPA) regarding (R) shoulder pain. |
| 25.06.2008 | 01.08.1947 | F | S/Leave | 1101 | 1109 | Chest Infection | | JLC | |
| 25.06.2008 | 21.01.1962 | F | | 1101 | 1109 | Script for Levothyroxine given | | JCC | For USScan of the neck & for Thyroid antibodies. |
| 25.06.2008 | 28.09.1937 | F | | 1145 | 1203 | Referred to Gynaecologist regarding large cystocele | | MR | For MSU. |

Result of a query that lists all consultations from the 22nd to the end of June 2008 (ConsultationsSeenFrom22ndTillEndOfJun2008)

| SurgeryDate | DateOfBirth | Sex | Diagnosis | TimeIn | TimeOut | Complaints | Treatments | Initials | Notes |
|---|---|---|---|---|---|---|---|---|---|
| 25.06.2008 | 14.01.1951 | F | | 1645 | 1657 | Script for Fexofenadine, Macrogol compound npf oral powder, Prednisolone with cinchocaine ointment & suppository | | RD | |
| 25.06.2008 | 08.07.1952 | F | S/Leave | 1657 | 1707 | Back Pain | | PMA | Referred to Orthopaedic Surgeon regarding the back pain |
| 25.06.2008 | 17.04.1945 | F | RTI | 1707 | 1712 | Chesty cough | Erythromycin | MC | Penicillin allergy. |
| 25.06.2008 | 07.05.1965 | F | | 1712 | 1721 | Referred to ENT Surgeon regarding her recurrent imbalance | | SAM | |
| 25.06.2008 | 28.02.1986 | F | | 1721 | 1725 | Pregnancy test positive | | JEM | |
| 25.06.2008 | 01.01.1951 | F | | 1725 | 1731 | Her UTI symptoms have improved with the antibiotics | | CR | |
| 25.06.2008 | 27.08.1952 | F | | 1731 | 1738 | Script for Otomize ear spray given | | KLB | |
| 25.06.2008 | 31.10.1920 | F | | 1740 | 1749 | Medication Review done | | NMB | |
| 25.06.2008 | 20.07.1956 | M | | 1759 | 1807 | For X-Rays of the (R) knee | | MDJ | |
| 25.06.2008 | 01.03.1994 | M | | 1808 | 1812 | Script for Levocetirizine given | | JAZ | |
| 26.06.2008 | 14.11.1949 | F | | 944 | 951 | Medication Review done | | CBL | |

457

Result of a query that lists all consultations from the 22nd to the end of June 2008 (ConsultationsSeenFrom22ndTillEndOfJun2008)

| SurgeryDate | DateOfBirth | Sex | Diagnosis | TimeIn | TimeOut | Complaints | Treatments | Initials | Notes |
|---|---|---|---|---|---|---|---|---|---|
| 26.06.2008 | 10.01.1924 | M | | 1012 | 1018 | Referred to Audiology clinic regarding bilateral hearing loss | | HAJB | |
| 26.06.2008 | 01.05.1974 | F | | 1018 | 1027 | Referred to Ophthalmologist regarding the persistent blurred vision in the (L) eye | | SAR | Script for Co-codamol & Diclofenac e/c given. |
| 26.06.2008 | 30.04.1943 | M | | 1027 | 1037 | Script for Dihydrocodeine & Tramadol given | | KL | |
| 26.06.2008 | 15.12.1939 | M | | 1037 | 1044 | Script for Fusidic acid with Hydrocortisone cream given | | ERC | |
| 26.06.2008 | 22.02.1936 | F | | 1046 | 1102 | Referred to Chest Physician regarding her breathlessness | | RPM | Script for Tiotropium given. |
| 26.06.2008 | 10.12.1941 | F | | 1102 | 1110 | Medication Review done | | PT | |
| 26.06.2008 | 25.06.1938 | F | | 1110 | 1126 | Referred to Neurologist regarding the pins & needles in her legs | | JEL | |
| 26.06.2008 | 11.04.1968 | F | | 1126 | 1129 | Seen by the nurse for 6 weeks post-natal check | | TVC | Baby in SCBU. |
| 26.06.2008 | 29.05.1994 | F | | 1138 | 1144 | Septic wound on the (L) foot | Flucloxacillin | CB | |

Result of a query that lists all consultations from the 22nd to the end of June 2008 (ConsultationsSeenFrom22ndTillEndOfJun2008)

| SurgeryDate | DateOfBirth | Sex | Diagnosis | TimeIn | TimeOut | Complaints | Treatments | Initials | Notes |
|---|---|---|---|---|---|---|---|---|---|
| 26.06.2008 | 13.03.1944 | F | | 1643 | 1654 | Medication Review done | | BCO | |
| 26.06.2008 | 17.07.1997 | M | | 1654 | 1705 | Referred to Dermatologist regarding spot on the abdomen with a halo around it | | JJL | Script for Salbutamol inhaler given. |
| 26.06.2008 | 16.06.1967 | M | | 1705 | 1717 | Script for Flucloxacillin given | | PBK | |
| 26.06.2008 | 08.12.1962 | F | Pain | 1717 | 1725 | (L) tennis elbow | Co-codamol & Diclofenac e/c | BJM | |
| 26.06.2008 | 23.12.1952 | F | RTI | 1725 | 1735 | Chesty cough | Amoxycillin | GCB | |
| 26.06.2008 | 04.06.1958 | F | | 1734 | 1744 | Script for Amoxycillin given | | JDC | |
| 26.06.2008 | 12.11.1968 | F | | 1744 | 1753 | Script for Metformin m/r given | | SEL | |
| 26.06.2008 | 13.01.1940 | M | | 1753 | 1803 | BP 158/71 | | JWW | |
| 26.06.2008 | 21.08.1997 | M | | 1803 | 1812 | In growing toe nail | Flucloxacillin | FJF | Referred to Dermatologist on scalp which has changed colour. |
| 26.06.2008 | 28.01.1980 | F | | 1812 | 1834 | Copies of letters from Gynaecologist given to the patient at her request | | JLD | |
| 26.06.2008 | 09.05.1973 | M | RTI | 1834 | 1839 | Chesty cough | Erythromycin | MPC | |
| 26.06.2008 | 08.06.1989 | M | | 1839 | 1843 | Stool for C&S | | AJS | Penicillin allergy. |

Result of a query that lists all consultations from the 22nd to the end of June 2008 (ConsultationsSeenFrom22ndTillEndOfJun2008)

| SurgeryDate | DateOfBirth | Sex | Diagnosis | TimeIn | TimeOut | Complaints | Treatments | Initials | Notes |
|---|---|---|---|---|---|---|---|---|---|
| 27.06.2008 | 13.10.1989 | F | URTI | 935 | 943 | Painful & discharging (L) ear | Amoxycillin & Sofradex ear drops | RLB | |
| 27.06.2008 | 26.11.1954 | M | | 951 | 1005 | Private script for Viagra given | | PHM | |
| 27.06.2008 | 25.06.1934 | F | | 1005 | 1022 | Script for GTN spray given | | EW | Referred to Cardiologist regarding chest tightness with pains going into the jaw & down the (L) arm. |
| 27.06.2008 | 22.05.1931 | F | | 1022 | 1038 | Medication Review Done | | DK | |
| 27.06.2008 | 22.05.1920 | F | | 1038 | 1050 | Medication Review Done | | JHC | |
| 27.06.2008 | 23.10.1971 | F | | 1050 | 1057 | Medication Review Done | | JLE | |
| 27.06.2008 | 14.01.1964 | F | Pain | 1057 | 1106 | (R) shoulder pain | Ibuprofen | LJP | |
| 27.06.2008 | 10.09.1936 | M | | 1106 | 1112 | Script for Metformin given | | BBB | |
| 27.06.2008 | 07.09.1984 | F | | 1112 | 1118 | Urine Pregnancy test positive | | JLG | |
| 27.06.2008 | 06.06.1936 | F | | 1118 | 1128 | Script for Candesartan given | | AJW | |
| 27.06.2008 | 19.09.1925 | F | | 1128 | 1140 | Script for Dihydrocodeine given | | JME | |
| 27.06.2008 | 21.10.1929 | F | URTI | 1140 | 1147 | Sore throat | Erythromycin | PMJ | Penicillin allergy. |

Result of a query that lists all consultations from the 22nd to the end of June 2009 (ConsultationsSeenFrom22ndTillEndOfJun2009)

| SurgeryDate | DateOfBirth | Sex | Diagnosis | TimeIn | TimeOut | Complaints | Treatments | Initials | Notes |
|---|---|---|---|---|---|---|---|---|---|
| 22.06.2009 | 09.05.1937 | F | | 950 | 1000 | Script for Fusidic acid with Betamethasone cream given | | KMN | |
| 22.06.2009 | 20.05.1938 | F | | 1000 | 1006 | Script for Amoxycillin given | | DSMS | |
| 22.06.2009 | 19.06.1927 | F | | 1006 | 1020 | Script for Atorvastatin given | | GEG | |
| 22.06.2009 | 05.12.1973 | F | | 1020 | 1026 | Referred for Endoscopy regarding her bowels problems | | VNB | |
| 22.06.2009 | 29.07.1969 | M | | 1026 | 1035 | Script for Lisinopril given | | AKL | |
| 22.06.2009 | 07.11.1988 | F | | 1049 | 1107 | Script for Clindamycin gel given | | ECC | |
| 22.06.2009 | 31.07.1923 | M | | 1107 | 1114 | Referred to Dermatologist regarding the BCC-like lesion on the (R) fore-arm | | HO | |
| 22.06.2009 | 21.02.1916 | F | | 1121 | 1133 | The Parking Badge Scheme for Disabled People Medical Practitioner Report form (ESS208B) completed with the patient | | EFH | Script for Qvar inhaler given. Penicillin allergy. |
| 22.06.2009 | 01.03.1994 | M | | 1645 | 1650 | Hay fever | Levocetirizine | JAZ | |

461

Result of a query that lists all consultations from the 22nd to the end of June 2009 (ConsultationsSeenFrom22ndTillEndOfJun2009)

| SurgeryDate | DateOfBirth | Sex | Diagnosis | TimeIn | TimeOut | Complaints | Treatments | Initials | Notes |
|---|---|---|---|---|---|---|---|---|---|
| 22.06.2009 | 14.08.1936 | M | | 1658 | 1705 | Script for Amoxycillin & Sofradex ear drops given | | ECM | |
| 22.06.2009 | 13.03.1963 | F | | 1705 | 1715 | For X-Rays of the (R) knee | | VN | |
| 22.06.2009 | 28.12.2004 | M | URTI | 1715 | 1722 | Sore throat | Amoxycillin | CAW | |
| 22.06.2009 | 09.01.1949 | F | | 1722 | 1731 | BP 158/105 | | DFH | |
| 22.06.2009 | 02.05.1949 | M | | 1731 | 1740 | Medication Review Done | | RB | |
| 22.06.2009 | 03.02.2008 | F | | 1745 | 1750 | Sleepy & unwell | Amoxycillin | AAL | |
| 22.06.2009 | 21.09.1983 | M | | 1750 | 1756 | Script for Lansoprazole given | | JH | |
| 22.06.2009 | 28.04.2008 | M | | 1756 | 1804 | Script for Paracetamol & Calamine lotion | | TJW | |
| 22.06.2009 | 14.04.1946 | F | URTI | 1804 | 1808 | Sore throat | Amoxycillin | VBB | |
| 22.06.2009 | 13.11.1949 | M | | 1808 | 1848 | Referred to Urologist to expedite his bladder operation date | | BEP | |
| 23.06.2009 | 13.03.1944 | F | | 948 | 954 | Medication Review Done | | BCO | |
| 23.06.2009 | 02.01.1956 | M | | 956 | 1011 | Referred to Breast Surgeon regarding lump under (R) nipple | | LAW | For Chest X-Rays. |
| 23.06.2009 | 31.10.1950 | F | | 1011 | 1028 | Script for Amitriptyline given | | WG | |
| 23.06.2009 | 16.08.1927 | F | | 1028 | 1036 | Medication Review Done | | GC | |

Result of a query that lists all consultations from the 22nd to the end of June 2009 (ConsultationsSeenFrom22ndTillEndOfJun2009)

| SurgeryDate | DateOfBirth | Sex | Diagnosis | TimeIn | TimeOut | Complaints | Treatments | Initials | Notes |
|---|---|---|---|---|---|---|---|---|---|
| 23.06.2009 | 19.05.1935 | F | | 1036 | 1043 | Script for Atenolol given | | SMK | |
| 23.06.2009 | 14.11.1949 | F | URTI | 1043 | 1052 | Pain in the sinuses | Amoxycillin | CBL | |
| 23.06.2009 | 29.08.1939 | M | | 1052 | 1111 | Referred to Physiotherapist regarding his bad back | | JFP | |
| 23.06.2009 | 03.05.1977 | M | | 1111 | 1122 | Script for Fusidic acid with Hydrocortisone cream given | | CC | |
| 23.06.2009 | 07.12.1947 | M | | 1122 | 1146 | Script for Omeprazole given | | PJB | |
| 23.06.2009 | 28.09.1924 | F | RTI | 1451 | 1301 | Chesty cough | Amoxycillin | VMG | Home visit. Macrodantin allergy. |
| 23.06.2009 | 23.07.1976 | M | | 1647 | 1653 | Hay fever | Fexofenadine | BJW | |
| 23.06.2009 | 23.10.1994 | F | | 1653 | 1700 | Hay fever | Acrivastine | KAR | |
| 23.06.2009 | 01.05.1974 | F | | 1700 | 1706 | Hay fever | Cetirizine | SAR | |
| 23.06.2009 | 16.09.1936 | M | | 1710 | 1719 | Referred to Dermatologist as he missed his earlier appointment | | LPCE | Private script for Viagra given. |
| 23.06.2009 | 03.02.1951 | M | | 1719 | 1726 | Referred to ENT Surgeon regarding persistent nasal congestion | | FRH | |
| 23.06.2009 | 07.03.1955 | F | RTI | 1726 | 1733 | Chesty cough | Amoxycillin | DN | |
| 23.06.2009 | 17.05.2007 | F | RTI | 1733 | 1737 | Chesty cough | Amoxycillin | GJA | |

Result of a query that lists all consultations from the 22$^{nd}$ to the end of June 2009 (ConsultationsSeenFrom22ndTillEndOfJun2009)

| SurgeryDate | DateOfBirth | Sex | Diagnosis | TimeIn | TimeOut | Complaints | Treatments | Initials | Notes |
|---|---|---|---|---|---|---|---|---|---|
| 23.06.2009 | 27.10.1931 | F | | 1739 | 1806 | Script for Seretide Accuhaler & Trimethoprim given | | JEID | |
| 23.06.2009 | 18.01.1958 | F | | 1806 | 1815 | Referred to Orthopaedic Surgeon regarding lump, possible ganglion, on the (L) wrist | | LRG | |
| 23.06.2009 | 24.12.1989 | F | | 1819 | 1829 | Referred to ENT Surgeon regarding her epistaxes | | AJR | |
| 24.06.2009 | 22.04.1975 | F | | 942 | 950 | For X-Rays of the (R) ankle & (R) foot | | SAG | |
| 24.06.2009 | 27.03.1935 | M | | 950 | 1007 | He is aware that he needs to increase his daily Hydrocortisone intake | | RH | |
| 24.06.2009 | 16.08.1983 | F | | 1007 | 1017 | Script for Amoxycillin, Fluoxetine & Betamethasone scalp application given | | CEC | |
| 24.06.2009 | 20.01.1941 | F | | 1017 | 1024 | Referred to Orthopaedic Surgeon regarding her bilateral osteo-arthritic knees pain | | BDD | |

Result of a query that lists all consultations from the 22nd to the end of June 2009 (ConsultationsSeenFrom22ndTillEndOfJun2009)

| SurgeryDate | DateOfBirth | Sex | Diagnosis | TimeIn | TimeOut | Complaints | Treatments | Initials | Notes |
|---|---|---|---|---|---|---|---|---|---|
| 24.06.2009 | 05.03.1943 | M |  | 1024 | 1030 | Referred to Dermatologist regarding psoriasis on his elbow |  | HTB |  |
| 24.06.2009 | 08.10.1938 | M |  | 1030 | 1040 | Medication Review Done |  | TAC |  |
| 24.06.2009 | 23.11.1975 | F | RTI | 1040 | 1049 | Chesty cough | Amoxycillin | TRHS | Script for Norethisterone given. |
| 24.06.2009 | 20.02.1953 | F |  | 1049 | 1056 | For X-Rays of the (R) knee & (R) wrist |  | SLF |  |
| 24.06.2009 | 08.11.1921 | F |  | 1056 | 1115 | Referred to Oral Surgeon regarding her darkish tongue |  | JW | Script for Nystatin oral suspension given. |
| 24.06.2009 | 25.07.1988 | F |  | 1115 | 1125 | For Pregnancy test |  | MPI | Referred for T.O.P. |
| 24.06.2009 | 16.06.1915 | M |  | 1328 | 1344 | Script for Paracetamol given |  | LB | Home visit. |
| 24.06.2009 | 21.03.1973 | M |  | 1642 | 1654 | Script for Adcal-D3 given |  | DRK |  |
| 24.06.2009 | 14.12.1954 | F |  | 1654 | 1702 | Script for Dixarit given |  | SAH | Referred to Dermatologist regarding mole on the medial aspect of the (R) thigh. |
| 24.06.2009 | 18.06.2003 | F | RTI | 1702 | 1710 | Chesty cough | Amoxycillin | FLR |  |
| 24.06.2009 | 21.09.1947 | M |  | 1710 | 1720 | Medication Review Done |  | DL |  |

465

Result of a query that lists all consultations from the 22nd to the end of June 2009 (ConsultationsSeenFrom22ndTillEndOfJun2009)

| SurgeryDate | DateOfBirth | Sex | Diagnosis | TimeIn | TimeOut | Complaints | Treatments | Initials | Notes |
|---|---|---|---|---|---|---|---|---|---|
| 24.06.2009 | 27.03.1931 | F | URTI | 1720 | 1727 | Sore throat | Erythromycin & Codeine linctus | MMA | |
| 24.06.2009 | 31.03.1956 | F | | 1731 | 1743 | Script for Amoxycillin given | | SD | For FBC, U/Es & MSU. |
| 24.06.2009 | 20.02.2003 | F | Rash | 1751 | 1758 | Impetigo-like rash on buttock | Flucloxacillin | CH | Erythromycin allergy. |
| 24.06.2009 | 06.09.2004 | F | | 1811 | 1818 | To apply own calamine lotion to her possible viral rash | | PLB | |
| 25.06.2009 | 19.09.1925 | F | | 942 | 1000 | For X-Rays of the (L) knee | | JME | |
| 25.06.2009 | 25.07.1939 | F | | 1004 | 1010 | Script for Spironolactone given | | JLB | |
| 25.06.2009 | 06.08.1930 | F | | 1010 | 1018 | The Parking Badge Scheme for Disabled People Medical Practitioner Report form ESS208B completed with the patient in the Surgery | | LP | |
| 25.06.2009 | 06.06.1940 | M | | 1018 | 1025 | Script for Trimethoprim given | | CJH | |
| 25.06.2009 | 14.05.1923 | M | | 1025 | 1031 | Injection Zoladex 10.8mg given sc. | | AM | |
| 25.06.2009 | 12.02.1996 | M | | 1031 | 1040 | Script for Amoxycillin & Cetirizine given | | JW | |
| 25.06.2009 | 23.03.1967 | F | | 1040 | 1048 | Script for Amoxycillin & Prochlorperazine given | | TPW | |

## Result of a query that lists all consultations from the 22nd to the end of June 2009 (ConsultationsSeenFrom22ndTillEndOfJun2009)

| SurgeryDate | DateOfBirth | Sex | Diagnosis | TimeIn | TimeOut | Complaints | Treatments | Initials | Notes |
|---|---|---|---|---|---|---|---|---|---|
| 25.06.2009 | 23.02.1985 | F | | 1058 | 1109 | 6 weeks post-natal check done | | SJL | |
| 25.06.2009 | 24.01.1992 | F | | 1058 | 1109 | 6 weeks post-natal check done | | RFC | For Pregnancy test. |
| 25.06.2009 | 21.11.1923 | M | | 1132 | 1139 | Injection Zoladex 10.8mg given sc | | RU | |
| 25.06.2009 | 09.04.1997 | F | URTI | 1642 | 1652 | Sore throat | Amoxycillin | HBS | |
| 25.06.2009 | 22.07.1961 | M | | 1655 | 1700 | (L) Eye infection | Chloramphenicol eye ointment | PWL | |
| 25.06.2009 | 09.10.1924 | F | | 1700 | 1712 | Script for Amoxycillin, Beconase Aqueous nasal spray, Montelukast & Prednisolone e/c given | | NOM | |
| 25.06.2009 | 21.02.1976 | F | S/Leave | 1712 | 1718 | Dizziness in Pregnancy | | FPT | |
| 25.06.2009 | 25.01.1939 | F | | 1718 | 1737 | Medication Review Done | | PMC | |
| 25.06.2009 | 04.10.1968 | F | | 1747 | 1757 | Script for Citalopram given | | AW | |
| 25.06.2009 | 08.10.1940 | M | | 1757 | 1809 | Script for Amitriptyline & Dihydrocodeine given | | GAFM | Referred to Dermatologist regarding his (R) sided T.10 shingles rash with swelling. |

Result of a query that lists all consultations from the 22nd to the end of June 2009 (ConsultationsSeenFrom22ndTillEndOfJun2009)

| SurgeryDate | DateOfBirth | Sex | Diagnosis | TimeIn | TimeOut | Complaints | Treatments | Initials | Notes |
|---|---|---|---|---|---|---|---|---|---|
| 26.06.2009 | 22.10.1966 | M | | 928 | 934 | Referred to Physiotherapist regarding his persistent back & (L) hip pain | | JS | Penicillin allergy. |
| 26.06.2009 | 21.09.1947 | M | S/Leave | 938 | 953 | Operation on the (L) thumb | | DL | |
| 26.06.2009 | 28.06.1959 | F | | 953 | 1003 | Script for Amoxycillin given | | PIS | For Chest X-Rays. |
| 26.06.2009 | 14.12.1971 | F | | 1003 | 1016 | Script for Co-codamol given | | JCH | Referred to Cardiologist regarding hole in her heart, chest & arms ache on exertion. |
| 26.06.2009 | 26.03.1935 | F | | 1016 | 1030 | Script for Ferrous Sulphate given | | RJ | |
| 26.06.2009 | 29.12.1983 | M | Rash | 1030 | 1039 | Folliculitis widespread | Tetracycline | LDS | For FBC, U/Es & Fasting Glucose. |
| 26.06.2009 | 25.08.1933 | F | | 1039 | 1044 | Medication Review Done | | PCH | |
| 26.06.2009 | 19.06.1944 | F | | 1044 | 1050 | Script for Levothyroxine given | | PJL | |
| 26.06.2009 | 23.02.1969 | M | | 1050 | 1106 | Medication Review Done | | DJP | |
| 26.06.2009 | 09.06.1934 | M | RTI | 1106 | 1110 | Chesty cough | Trimethoprim | MKC | Penicillin allergy. |
| 26.06.2009 | 14.08.1935 | M | | 1110 | 1120 | Vertigo | Prochlorperazine | RAT | |

Result of a query that lists all consultations from the 22nd to the end of June 2009 (ConsultationsSeenFrom22ndTillEndOfJun2009)

| SurgeryDate | DateOfBirth | Sex | Diagnosis | TimeIn | TimeOut | Complaints | Treatments | Initials | Notes |
|---|---|---|---|---|---|---|---|---|---|
| 26.06.2009 | 08.05.1939 | R | URTI | 1125 | 1131 | (L) ear ache | Amoxycillin & Otomize ear spray | JCH | |
| 26.06.2009 | 03.04.1918 | F | | 1416 | 1426 | Patient is to be referred to DAU, SGH, regarding poor appetite, frequent falls & generally feeling unwell | | JMR | |
| 29.06.2009 | 06.09.1974 | M | URTI | 945 | 958 | Congested sinuses | Amoxycillin | DGH | Script for Cetirizine given. |
| 29.06.2009 | 09.05.1937 | F | | 958 | 1003 | Medication Review Done | | KMN | |
| 29.06.2009 | 29.04.1935 | F | | 1005 | 1020 | Medication Review Done | | CM | |
| 29.06.2009 | 24.04.1986 | M | | 1020 | 1032 | Referred to ENT Surgeon (Benenden) regarding epistaxes from the (L) nostril | | RRB | Referred to Neurologist (Benenden) regarding his persistent headaches. |
| 29.06.2009 | 17.03.1958 | M | | 1032 | 1044 | Referred to Colorectal Surgeon regarding anal soilage and leakage | | KEW | Referred to Dermatologist regarding multiple skin tags all over his body. |
| 29.06.2009 | 19.05.1944 | F | | 1044 | 1058 | Medication Review Done | | AWB | |

Result of a query that lists all consultations from the 22nd to the end of June 2009 (ConsultationsSeenFrom22ndTillEndOfJun2009)

| SurgeryDate | DateOfBirth | Sex | Diagnosis | TimeIn | TimeOut | Complaints | Treatments | Initials | Notes |
|---|---|---|---|---|---|---|---|---|---|
| 29.06.2009 | 28.07.1971 | F | | 1104 | 1115 | Referred to Endocrinologist regarding her weight gain, spotty skin & hirsutism as apparently advised by the Gynaecologists | | ALB | |
| 29.06.2009 | 15.05.1945 | M | UTI | 1115 | 1126 | Back Pain & frequency of micturition | Trimethoprim | VCC | For MSU. |
| 29.06.2009 | 01.07.1927 | F | | 1126 | 1146 | Script for Macrogol compound half-strength & Lisinopril given | | DMSG | For USScan of the abdomen. |
| 29.06.2009 | 06.05.1932 | F | RTI | 1424 | 1434 | Chesty cough | Amoxycillin | RRT | Home visit. |
| 29.06.2009 | 14.01.1934 | F | | 1436 | 1445 | General condition not too bad | | MRP | Home visit. She is not suitable for 2 weekly visits at present. |
| 29.06.2009 | 04.05.1937 | F | | 1647 | 1656 | Script for Dihydrocodeine given | | DMB | Referred to Physiotherapist regarding her (R) shoulder, neck & back pain. |
| 29.06.2009 | 21.08.1934 | F | | 1656 | 1717 | Script for Metformin m/r & Rosiglitazone given | | IEW | |
| 29.06.2009 | 01.11.1990 | M | Rash | 1717 | 1726 | Impetigo-like rash on face | Flucloxacillin & Fusidic acid cream | JN | |

470

Result of a query that lists all consultations from the 22nd to the end of June 2009 (ConsultationsSeenFrom22ndTillEndOfJun2009)

| SurgeryDate | DateOfBirth | Sex | Diagnosis | TimeIn | TimeOut | Complaints | Treatments | Initials | Notes |
|---|---|---|---|---|---|---|---|---|---|
| 29.06.2009 | 09.11.1990 | M | | 1726 | 1731 | For FBC, U/Es, Fasting Glucose & TFTs | | DAW | |
| 29.06.2009 | 06.01.1955 | M | UTI | 1731 | 1741 | Dysuria | Trimethoprim | MAS | |
| 29.06.2009 | 06.11.1935 | F | | 1743 | 1753 | Script for Quinine Sulphate given | | SRB | For X-Rays of the hips. |
| 29.06.2009 | 26.11.2003 | F | | 1753 | 1758 | Referred to Dermatologist regarding her bad eczema in her popliteal fossae | | CSIB | |
| 29.06.2009 | 04.07.1959 | F | | 1807 | 1845 | Medication Review Done | | SAB | Her husband came to the Surgery. |

Result of a query that lists all consultations from the 22nd to the end of June 2010 (ConsultationsSeenFrom22ndTillEndOfJun2010)

| SurgeryDate | DateOfBirth | Sex | Diagnosis | TimeIn | TimeOut | Complaints | Treatments | Initials | Notes |
|---|---|---|---|---|---|---|---|---|---|
| 22.06.2010 | 12.08.1936 | M | | 943 | 953 | Patient has not got Diabetes after checking fasting Glucose | | RHP | |
| 22.06.2010 | 12.05.1949 | F | | 953 | 1004 | Script for Diazepam given | | MK | |
| 22.06.2010 | 25.01.1944 | F | Pain | 1004 | 1012 | (L) knee pain | Diclofenac e/c, Dihydrocodeine & Omeprazole | HPS | |

Result of a query that lists all consultations from the 22ⁿᵈ to the end of June 2010 (ConsultationsSeenFrom22ndTillEndOfJun2010)

| SurgeryDate | DateOfBirth | Sex | Diagnosis | TimeIn | TimeOut | Complaints | Treatments | Initials | Notes |
|---|---|---|---|---|---|---|---|---|---|
| 22.06.2010 | 29.08.1939 | M | | 1012 | 1030 | Medication Review Done | | JFP | |
| 22.06.2010 | 29.08.1976 | M | | 1030 | 1038 | Script for Pentasa m/r granules given | | PLC | |
| 22.06.2010 | 07.10.1933 | M | | 1038 | 1046 | Script for Co-codamol & Ferrous Sulphate given | | FDF | For MSU. |
| 22.06.2010 | 10.04.1937 | F | | 1046 | 1053 | Advised to discuss with SGH Rheumatologist why she was told after DEXA scan that she has no osteoporosis even though she was told at Basildon hospital that she had it | | MC | |
| 22.06.2010 | 09.06.1934 | M | | 1053 | 11010 | Cramps | Quinine Sulphate | MKC | |
| 22.06.2010 | 06.12.2006 | F | | 1101 | 1105 | Medication Review Done | | ALS | |
| 22.06.2010 | 20.04.1965 | F | | 1105 | 1113 | Script for Omeprazole given | | KCY | |
| 22.06.2010 | 23.01.1999 | F | URTI | 1113 | 1118 | (R) ear ache | Erythromycin | LG | |
| 22.06.2010 | 24.05.1909 | F | | 1333 | 1350 | Script for Erythromycin & Paracetamol given | | HMP | Penicillin allergy. Home visit. |

Result of a query that lists all consultations from the 22nd to the end of June 2010 (ConsultationsSeenFrom22ndTillEndOfJun2010)

| SurgeryDate | DateOfBirth | Sex | Diagnosis | TimeIn | TimeOut | Complaints | Treatments | Initials | Notes |
|---|---|---|---|---|---|---|---|---|---|
| 22.06.2010 | 28.09.1924 | F | | 1401 | 1415 | District Nurse to arrange for tissue viability nurses to assess the wounds on her legs before possible referral to Vascular Surgeon | | VMG | Home visit. Macrodantin allergy. |
| 22.06.2010 | 15.01.1927 | M | | 1422 | 1432 | Lipoma on the sacral area | | HD | Home visit. |
| 22.06.2010 | 11.01.1960 | F | | 1643 | 1655 | Script for Co-codamol, Diclofenac e/c & Omeprazole given | | FN | |
| 22.06.2010 | 30.03.1956 | F | URTI | 1655 | 1659 | (R) ear ache | Erythromycin & Otomize ear spray | JAF | Penicillin allergy. |
| 22.06.2010 | 16.03.1978 | M | S/Leave | 1659 | 1712 | Chest Infection - Private | | JWPS | Script for Amoxycillin given. |
| 22.06.2010 | 17.02.1958 | M | S/Leave | 1712 | 1722 | Med. 3 04/10 given for Diarrhoea & Vomiting from 22.06.10 until 24.06.10 | | RFFA | |
| 22.06.2010 | 18.06.1960 | F | S/Leave | 1722 | 1734 | Med. 3 04/10 given for Laparoscopic Cholecystectomy for 2 weeks from 22.06.10 | | AMF | Script for Flucloxacillin & Metoclopramide given |

473

Result of a query that lists all consultations from the 22nd to the end of June 2010 (ConsultationsSeenFrom22ndTillEndOfJun2010)

| SurgeryDate | DateOfBirth | Sex | Diagnosis | TimeIn | TimeOut | Complaints | Treatments | Initials | Notes |
|---|---|---|---|---|---|---|---|---|---|
| 22.06.2010 | 06.06.1961 | M | S/Leave | 1734 | 1743 | Med. 3 04/10 given for Stress from 21.06.10 for one month | | LG | Script for Citalopram given. |
| 22.06.2010 | 31.01.2006 | M | | 1743 | 1750 | Medication Review Done | | HEWD | |
| 22.06.2010 | 27.05.1968 | M | S/Leave | 1750 | 1803 | Med. 3 04/10 given for Stress from 22.06.10 until 28.09.10 | | LJH | |
| 22.06.2010 | 27.09.1967 | F | | 1803 | 1813 | Script for Salbutamol inhaler given | | JTR | |
| 22.06.2010 | 17.03.1968 | F | | 1813 | 1828 | Script for Lisinopril given | | NJB | |
| 22.06.2010 | 20.02.2004 | M | URTI | 1828 | 1832 | Sore throat | Amoxycillin | BJW | |
| 23.06.2010 | 06.12.1940 | F | | 949 | 954 | Script for Dihydrocodeine given | | MC | |
| 23.06.2010 | 02.04.1976 | F | | 954 | 1002 | Script for Co-codamol given | | SLH | Referred to Rheumatologist (BUPA) regarding worsening pain in the (L) shoulder. |
| 23.06.2010 | 29.02.1941 | F | | 1002 | 1015 | Script for Metformin 1g m/r tablets given | | SJW | |
| 23.06.2010 | 09.12.1945 | F | | 1015 | 1028 | Script for Flucloxacillin given | | AML | |
| 23.06.2010 | 26.11.1929 | F | | 1028 | 1036 | Script for Betahistine given | | DEG | |

Result of a query that lists all consultations from the 22nd to the end of June 2010 (ConsultationsSeenFrom22ndTillEndOfJun2010)

| SurgeryDate | DateOfBirth | Sex | Diagnosis | TimeIn | TimeOut | Complaints | Treatments | Initials | Notes |
|---|---|---|---|---|---|---|---|---|---|
| 23.06.2010 | 02.03.1948 | M | | 1036 | 1047 | Medication Review Done | | JHH | |
| 23.06.2010 | 20.02.1930 | M | | 1047 | 1051 | Script for Loratadine given | | AL | |
| 23.06.2010 | 18.02.1968 | F | S/Leave | 1054 | 1106 | Med. 3 04/10 given for Abdominal Wound Infection from 2206.10 for one month | | PAC | Script for Metoclopramide & Tramadol capsules given. |
| 23.06.2010 | 26.09.1937 | M | | 1644 | 1654 | Medication Review Done | | DJD | |
| 23.06.2010 | 07.06.1997 | F | | 1654 | 1700 | Script for Fucibet cream given | | RAW | |
| 23.06.2010 | 12.05.1990 | M | | 1702 | 1708 | Script for Budesonide nasal spray, Cetirizine & Sodium Cromoglicate eye drops given | | APS | |
| 23.06.2010 | 13.03.1973 | F | | 1708 | 1717 | Script for Budesonide nasal spray, Cetirizine & Sodium Cromoglicate eye drops given | | LNS | |
| 23.06.2010 | 23.01.1968 | F | | 1717 | 1720 | She will observe the lipoma on her (L) chest for now | | KS | |
| 23.06.2010 | 01.10.1937 | F | | 1720 | 1724 | To see the nurse in about 4 months for repeat Clotting screen | | SGE | |

Result of a query that lists all consultations from the 22nd to the end of June 2010 (ConsultationsSeenFrom22ndTillEndOfJun2010)

| SurgeryDate | DateOfBirth | Sex | Diagnosis | TimeIn | TimeOut | Complaints | Treatments | Initials | Notes |
|---|---|---|---|---|---|---|---|---|---|
| 23.06.2010 | 06.08.1944 | M | | 1724 | 1728 | Medication Review Done | | CHL | |
| 23.06.2010 | 02.02.1949 | F | | 1742 | 1748 | Script for co-codamol given | | LL | |
| 23.06.2010 | 20.10.1983 | F | | 1751 | 1757 | Script for Chlorphenamine tablets & Prednisolone e/c tablets given | | ARS | |
| 23.06.2010 | 02.09.1977 | F | | 1801 | 1817 | Script for Loratadine & Sodium Cromoglicate eye drops given | | RMS | Referred to Physiotherapist regarding her back pain. |
| 24.06.2010 | 04.04.1979 | M | | 944 | 956 | Script for Ferrous Sulphate & Lansoprazole given | | BBG | |
| 24.06.2010 | 16.09.1936 | M | | 956 | 1000 | Private script for Viagra given | | LPCE | |
| 24.06.2010 | 16.06.1967 | M | | 1000 | 1012 | Script for Atorvastatin given | | PBK | |
| 24.06.2010 | 10.04.1986 | F | RTI | 1020 | 1029 | Chesty cough | Amoxycillin | AJL | |
| 24.06.2010 | 15.09.1939 | M | | 1029 | 1038 | Medication Review Done | | WJS | |
| 24.06.2010 | 05.03.1934 | M | | 1038 | 1048 | For PSA & MSU | | CHD | |
| 24.06.2010 | 06.07.1946 | F | | 1048 | 1101 | Script for Atenolol given | | MEF | Script for Microgynon 30 given. |

476

Result of a query that lists all consultations from the 22nd to the end of June 2010 (ConsultationsSeenFrom22ndTillEndOfJun2010)

| SurgeryDate | DateOfBirth | Sex | Diagnosis | TimeIn | TimeOut | Complaints | Treatments | Initials | Notes |
|---|---|---|---|---|---|---|---|---|---|
| 24.06.2010 | 09.04.1938 | M | | 1101 | 1115 | Script for Perindopril & Bendroflumethiazide given | | NWH | |
| 24.06.2010 | 30.07.1989 | F | | 1115 | 1122 | Script for Co-Amoxiclav given | | CJB | |
| 24.06.2010 | 16.09.1924 | F | | 1332 | 1358 | Script for Trimethoprim given | | GPM | For MSU. Home visit. |
| 24.06.2010 | 22.04.1966 | M | | 1650 | 1702 | For MSU, FBC & U/Es | | CD | |
| 24.06.2010 | 02.12.1954 | M | | 1702 | 1715 | Script for Carbimazole given | | OAK | |
| 24.06.2010 | 02.04.1976 | F | | 1715 | 1719 | For X-Rays of the (L) Shoulder | | SLH | |
| 24.06.2010 | 22.02.1963 | M | | 1719 | 1723 | Script for Cetirizine & Beconase given | | JBD | |
| 24.06.2010 | 22.02.1936 | F | | 1723 | 1727 | For X-Rays of the (L) knee | | RPM | |
| 24.06.2010 | 19.08.1951 | M | | 1727 | 1732 | Script for Co-codamol & Diclofenac e/c given | | KVB | |
| 24.06.2010 | 19.06.1927 | F | | 1732 | 1742 | Medication Review Done | | GEG | |
| 24.06.2010 | 23.04.1950 | F | | 1744 | 1754 | Script for Co-codamol & Diclofenac e/c given | | PEH | Referred to Physiotherapist regarding (R) shoulder pain. |
| 24.06.2010 | 26.08.1999 | M | URTI | 1805 | 1808 | Sore throat | Amoxycillin | JLM | |

477

Result of a query that lists all consultations from the 22nd to the end of June 2010 (ConsultationsSeenFrom22ndTillEndOfJun2010)

| SurgeryDate | DateOfBirth | Sex | Diagnosis | TimeIn | TimeOut | Complaints | Treatments | Initials | Notes |
|---|---|---|---|---|---|---|---|---|---|
| 24.06.2010 | 28.07.1977 | M | | 1808 | 1818 | Referred to Counsellor regarding feeling low since separating from his wife | | CMG | |
| 24.06.2010 | 28.09.1924 | F | | 1818 | 1830 | Script for Citalopram & Ensure Plus given | | VMG | |
| 25.06.2010 | 16.05.1958 | M | | 931 | 939 | Medication Review Done | | SOS | |
| 25.06.2010 | 23.01.1994 | F | | 939 | 942 | Script for Chloramphenicol eye drops & Loratadine given | | WMS | |
| 25.06.2010 | 24.07.1956 | M | | 948 | 958 | Script for Chloramphenicol eye drops, Flucloxacillin & Ketoconazole shampoo given | | SS | |
| 25.06.2010 | 24.03.1973 | M | | 1004 | 1016 | For X-Rays of the (R) foot, FBC, U/Es, Fasting Glucose, TFTs, Fasting Lipids & LFTs | | JCM | |
| 25.06.2010 | 07.01.1987 | F | | 1016 | 1028 | Referred to ENT Clinic regarding her dizziness | | LRB | For FBC, U/Es, Fasting Glucose, serum Ferritin, B12 & Folate. |

478

Result of a query that lists all consultations from the 22nd to the end of June 2010 (ConsultationsSeenFrom22ndTillEndOfJun2010)

| SurgeryDate | DateOfBirth | Sex | Diagnosis | TimeIn | TimeOut | Complaints | Treatments | Initials | Notes |
|---|---|---|---|---|---|---|---|---|---|
| 25.06.2010 | 02.12.1996 | F | | 1028 | 1033 | Referred to Dermatologist regarding the compound mole on the back of her neck | | LEC | |
| 25.06.2010 | 23.02.1941 | M | | 1036 | 1056 | Script for Amoxycillin & Metformin given | | RWM | |
| 25.06.2010 | 27.04.1925 | M | | 1056 | 1107 | Script for Nifedipine m/r capsules given | | RWF | |
| 25.06.2010 | 26.09.1983 | F | | 1107 | 1113 | Script for Flucloxacillin, Beconase Aqueous nasal spray & Loratadine given | | JADF | |
| 28.06.2010 | 01.01.1953 | M | | 948 | 952 | Private script for Cialis given | | TPH | |
| 28.06.2010 | 28.03.1926 | F | | 952 | 1005 | Script for Salicylates with nicotinate cream given | | JD | |
| 28.06.2010 | 11.10.1942 | M | | 1005 | 1019 | Script for Macrogol compound half-strength oral powder sachets NPF given | | RWA | |
| 28.06.2010 | 25.01.1948 | F | | 1019 | 1028 | Referred to Neurologist regarding going backwards when she steps backwards | | JW | |

479

Result of a query that lists all consultations from the 22nd to the end of June 2010 (ConsultationsSeenFrom22ndTillEndOfJun2010)

| SurgeryDate | DateOfBirth | Sex | Diagnosis | TimeIn | TimeOut | Complaints | Treatments | Initials | Notes |
|---|---|---|---|---|---|---|---|---|---|
| 28.06.2010 | 08.04.1945 | M | | 1028 | 1035 | Referred to Physiotherapist regarding (L) shoulder pain | | GTW | |
| 28.06.2010 | 06.11.1981 | F | | 1035 | 1040 | Referred to Ophthalmologist (urgent) regarding her (L) scleritis or episcleritis | | CL | |
| 28.06.2010 | 05.06.1930 | F | | 1040 | 1052 | For Chest X-Rays (urgent) | | JMF | Script for Amoxycillin & Quinine bisulphate given. |
| 28.06.2010 | 24.10.1946 | F | | 1052 | 1056 | Script for Orlistat given | | MW | |
| 28.06.2010 | 15.06.1942 | M | | 1056 | 1100 | Private script for Cialis given | | SJF | |
| 28.06.2010 | 28.09.1959 | F | | 1644 | 1652 | Referred to Rheumatologist about her multiple joints pains | | CAS | |
| 28.06.2010 | 10.01.1995 | F | | 1652 | 1659 | Referred to Podiatrist regarding pain in the sole of her (R) foot | | KNBL | |
| 28.06.2010 | 13.01.1945 | M | | 1659 | 1708 | Medication Review Done | | MPG | |
| 28.06.2010 | 19.01.1964 | F | | 1708 | 1720 | Sinusitis | Amoxycillin | NAB | |
| 28.06.2010 | 29.04.1982 | M | URTI | 1721 | 1728 | For Lumbar Spine X-Rays | | AP | |

480

**Result of a query that lists all consultations from the 22nd to the end of June 2010 (ConsultationsSeenFrom22ndTillEndOfJun2010)**

| SurgeryDate | DateOfBirth | Sex | Diagnosis | TimeIn | TimeOut | Complaints | Treatments | Initials | Notes |
|---|---|---|---|---|---|---|---|---|---|
| 28.06.2010 | 04.01.1967 | F | | 1728 | 1737 | For FBC & TFTs | | MC | |
| 28.06.2010 | 14.11.1963 | F | S/Leave | 1754 | 1806 | Med. 3 04/10 given for Hoarseness & Dysphagia for 2 months from 28.06.10 | | SJK | |

**Result of a query that lists all consultations from the 22nd to the end of June 2011 (ConsultationsSeenFrom22ndTillEndOfJun2011)**

| SurgeryDate | DateOfBirth | Sex | Diagnosis | TimeIn | TimeOut | Complaints | Treatments | Initials | Notes |
|---|---|---|---|---|---|---|---|---|---|
| 22.06.2011 | 03.10.1941 | M | | 946 | 955 | Medication Review Done | | JJD | |
| 22.06.2011 | 24.10.1946 | F | | 955 | 1008 | Medication Review Done | | MW | |
| 22.06.2011 | 09.08.1939 | M | | 1008 | 1021 | Referred to Dermatologist (cancer referral) regarding the possible SCC lesion on his (R) temple | | JL | |
| 22.06.2011 | 27.10.1933 | M | | 1021 | 1028 | Script for Olanzapine given | | FDF | |
| 22.06.2011 | 25.07.1939 | F | | 1028 | 1049 | Script for Pioglitazone given | | JLB | Referred to ENT Surgeon (urgent) regarding possible BCC on her (L) ear lobe. For USScan of the Abdomen/Pelvis. |

Result of a query that lists all consultations from the 22nd to the end of June 2011 (ConsultationsSeenFrom22ndTillEndOfJun2011)

| SurgeryDate | DateOfBirth | Sex | Diagnosis | TimeIn | TimeOut | Complaints | Treatments | Initials | Notes |
|---|---|---|---|---|---|---|---|---|---|
| 22.06.2011 | 22.02.1944 | M | | 1049 | 1059 | Script for Amoxycillin given | | AS | Referred to Orthopaedic Surgeon regarding pain in his (L) hip. |
| 22.06.2011 | 27.11.1949 | M | | 1059 | 1108 | Referred to Cardiologist regarding the prominent ascending aorta shown on his Chest X-Rays | | BPG | |
| 22.06.2011 | 24.04.1948 | F | | 1108 | 1114 | Script for Lansoprazole given | | CSP | |
| 22.06.2011 | 14.11.1916 | F | | 1340 | 1400 | Script for Loratadine & Calamine lotion given | | WAT | Home visit. |
| 22.06.2011 | 22.10.2009 | F | Rash | 1653 | 1659 | Infected eczema in the (R) elbow | Flucloxacillin & Fusidic acid with Hydrocortisone cream | CMGM | |
| 22.06.2011 | 22.01.2006 | F | | 1659 | 1705 | Referred to Dermatologist regarding mole on the (L) buttock | | KEGM | |
| 22.06.2011 | 29.11.1937 | F | | 1710 | 1725 | Referred to Vascular Surgeon regarding her claudication as advised by the orthopaedic Surgeon | | MRS | Referred to Dermatologist regarding her abdominal mole. Referred for Colonoscopy regarding her loose motions. |

Result of a query that lists all consultations from the 22nd to the end of June 2011 (ConsultationsSeenFrom22ndTillEndOfJun2011)

| SurgeryDate | DateOfBirth | Sex | Diagnosis | TimeIn | TimeOut | Complaints | Treatments | Initials | Notes |
|---|---|---|---|---|---|---|---|---|---|
| 22.06.2011 | 20.02.1930 | M | | 1725 | 1734 | Script for Co-codamol given | | AL | For X-Rays. |
| 22.06.2011 | 16.04.1966 | M | | 1734 | 1742 | I explained dot patient that I have no competency to say that he is not fit for work when the DSS has found him fit | | AJDP | |
| 22.06.2011 | 08.12.2000 | F | URTI | 1745 | 1750 | Sore throat | Amoxycillin | EL | |
| 22.06.2011 | 02.05.1949 | M | | 1752 | 1804 | Script for Tamsulosin given | | RB | Referred to Orthopaedic Surgeon regarding the knotty longitudinal lump on his (L) upper arm. |
| 23.06.2011 | 08.01.1972 | M | | 953 | 959 | Referred to Dermatologist regarding his pruritus ani as advised by the surgeons | | EM | |
| 23.06.2011 | 01.06.1937 | M | | 959 | 1018 | Referred to Community Diabetic nurses regarding his inadequately controlled Diabetes | | JNN | |
| 23.06.2011 | 26.03.1958 | F | S/Leave | 1018 | 1029 | Med. 3 04/10 given for Depression for one month from 16.06.11 | | JLS | Script for Hydrocortisone with Miconazole cream given. |

Result of a query that lists all consultations from the 22nd to the end of June 2011 (ConsultationsSeenFrom22ndTillEndOfJun2011)

| SurgeryDate | DateOfBirth | Sex | Diagnosis | TimeIn | TimeOut | Complaints | Treatments | Initials | Notes |
|---|---|---|---|---|---|---|---|---|---|
| 23.06.2011 | 10.03.1936 | M | | 1029 | 1037 | Medication Review Done | | TCC | |
| 23.06.2011 | 07.10.2009 | M | | 1037 | 1043 | Thread worms | Mebendazole | KHS | |
| 23.06.2011 | 03.12.1924 | F | | 1043 | 1052 | Script for Transvasin Heat Rub cream given | | AH | |
| 23.06.2011 | 19.10.1934 | F | | 1109 | 1127 | Script for Ferrous Sulphate & Senna given | | IS | |
| 23.06.2011 | 23.02.1969 | M | | 1646 | 1659 | Referred for ECG regarding his tachycardia | | DJP | |
| 23.06.2011 | 05.03.1954 | F | | 1659 | 1708 | Script for Tramadol given | | PSC | For X-Rays of the Lumbar Spine. |
| 23.06.2011 | 26.03.1965 | F | | 1708 | 1715 | Script for Tramadol & Dihydrocodeine given | | CP | |
| 23.06.2011 | 10.09.1999 | F | | 1715 | 1736 | Script for Amoxycillin, Clarithromycin & Omeprazole given | | EHMK | |
| 23.06.2011 | 02.02.1976 | F | | 1736 | 1749 | Script for Citalopram, Metronidazole & Phenoxymethylpenicillin given | | NBB | |
| 23.06.2011 | 21.02.1963 | F | | 1749 | 1802 | Script for Efexor XL given | | DLG | |
| 23.06.2011 | 22.02.1971 | F | | 1802 | 1811 | For FBC, serum Fasting Glucose, U/Es & Fasting Lipids | | SB | |

Result of a query that lists all consultations from the 22nd to the end of June 2011 (ConsultationsSeenFrom22ndTillEndOfJun2011)

| SurgeryDate | DateOfBirth | Sex | Diagnosis | TimeIn | TimeOut | Complaints | Treatments | Initials | Notes |
|---|---|---|---|---|---|---|---|---|---|
| 23.06.2011 | 28.09.1937 | F | | 1811 | 1818 | Referred to Dermatologist regarding red petechial rash on the legs | | MR | |
| 24.06.2011 | 08.10.1950 | F | | 934 | 944 | Script for Loperamide given | | CAH | |
| 24.06.2011 | 19.07.1925 | F | Rash | 944 | 950 | C8/T1 region shingles | Acyclovir tablets | RMW | |
| 24.06.2011 | 30.08.1979 | F | | 950 | 1000 | Medication Review Done | | JJG | |
| 24.06.2011 | 07.10.2009 | M | | 1000 | 1007 | Mother is happy to give him Vermox even though she knows that it is unlicensed for his age group but recommended in the BNF for children | | KHS | |
| 24.06.2011 | 13.10.2006 | F | URTI | 1017 | 1032 | Sore throat | Amoxycillin | MKT | |
| 24.06.2011 | 27.01.1934 | F | | 1047 | 1107 | Script for Irbesartan given | | JWC | Script for Paracetamol given. Ibuprofen allergy. |
| 27.06.2011 | 11.06.1951 | F | S/Leave | 947 | 1000 | Med. 3 04/10 given for Bunionectomy (L) foot for 5 weeks from 27.06.11 | | PAP | |

485

Result of a query that lists all consultations from the 22$^{nd}$ to the end of June 2011 (ConsultationsSeenFrom22ndTillEndOfJun2011)

| SurgeryDate | DateOfBirth | Sex | Diagnosis | TimeIn | TimeOut | Complaints | Treatments | Initials | Notes |
|---|---|---|---|---|---|---|---|---|---|
| 27.06.2011 | 15.10.1969 | F | | 1000 | 1011 | Referred to Breast Surgeon regarding the persistent whitish discharge from the (L) breast & associated pain in the breast | | MAC | |
| 27.06.2011 | 27.07.1948 | M | | 1011 | 1021 | Script for Lisinopril given | | BAG | |
| 27.06.2011 | 06.12.1947 | M | | 1022 | 1035 | For FBC, U/Es, Fasting Glucose & Chest X-Rays | | BSK | Referred for Colonoscopy regarding his diarrhoea & constipation. |
| 27.06.2011 | 20.11.1992 | F | | 1035 | 1051 | For MSU, FBC, U/Es, KUB & Pelvic USScan | | JLC | |
| 27.06.2011 | 14.09.1962 | M | S/Leave | 1051 | 1118 | Med. 3 04/10 given for Fractured Neck of (R) Femur for 4 months from 09.06.11 | | KMD | Script for Amoxycillin & Otomize ear spray given |
| 27.06.2011 | 06.11.1981 | F | | 1118 | 1130 | Referred to Physiotherapist regarding her (R) shoulder pain | | CL | For Urine Pregnancy test. |
| 27.06.2011 | 31.05.1930 | F | | 1130 | 1143 | Referred to Breast Surgeon (cancer referral) regarding new possibly (R) breast lump | | SAW | |

**Result of a query that lists all consultations from the 22ⁿᵈ to the end of June 2011 (ConsultationsSeenFrom22ndTillEndOfJun2011)**

| SurgeryDate | DateOfBirth | Sex | Diagnosis | TimeIn | TimeOut | Complaints | Treatments | Initials | Notes |
|---|---|---|---|---|---|---|---|---|---|
| 27.06.2011 | 30.09.1925 | M | | 1143 | 1158 | The Medical Report Form Blue Badge Parking Scheme ECC1190 (ESS208B) form completed with his daughter in Surgery | | JCA | His daughter came to the Surgery. |
| 27.06.2011 | 05.08.1936 | F | | 1648 | 1657 | Medication Review Done | | SAMN | |
| 27.06.2011 | 13.11.1949 | M | | 1657 | 1703 | Referred to General Surgeon regarding a lump on his (L) upper back | | BEP | |
| 27.06.2011 | 20.11.1988 | M | | 1703 | 1710 | Script for Flucloxacillin given | | CSB | |
| 27.06.2011 | 17.03.1961 | M | | 1711 | 1736 | Referred to Psychiatrist regarding his anxiety problems & missing his appointment | | LDM | Referred to Gastroenterologist regarding his rectal bleeding. |
| 27.06.2011 | 25.06.1938 | F | | 1736 | 1745 | Referred to Podiatrist regarding her (L) in growing toe nail | | JEL | Referred to Chest Physician regarding her persistent cough. |
| 27.06.2011 | 24.10.1989 | F | URTI | 1745 | 1750 | Sore throat | Amoxycillin | HSI | |
| 27.06.2011 | 18.03.1987 | F | | 1806 | 1817 | Referred to Dermatologist regarding her acne | | LP | Referred to Gynaecologist regarding heavy painful periods. |

Result of a query that lists all consultations from the 22nd to the end of June 2011 (ConsultationsSeenFrom22ndTillEndOfJun2011)

| SurgeryDate | DateOfBirth | Sex | Diagnosis | TimeIn | TimeOut | Complaints | Treatments | Initials | Notes |
|---|---|---|---|---|---|---|---|---|---|
| 28.06.2011 | 22.02.1963 | M | | 948 | 955 | Script for Beconase Aqueous nasal spray & Cetirizine given | | JBP | |
| 28.06.2011 | 12.04.1938 | M | | 955 | 1003 | Script for Atorvastatin given | | MAF | |
| 28.06.2011 | 15.12.1939 | M | | 1003 | 1010 | Medication Review Done | | ERC | |
| 28.06.2011 | 24.03.1935 | F | | 1010 | 1016 | Script for Lansoprazole & Propranolol given | | PW | |
| 28.06.2011 | 01.02.1980 | F | | 1016 | 1022 | Referred to Dermatologist regarding dark spotty moles in her axillae since having her son 14 weeks ago | | LTK | |
| 28.06.2011 | 07.10.2009 | M | | 1030 | 1039 | To give the 2nd dose of worm medicine as recommended | | KHS | |
| 28.06.2011 | 25.04.1935 | M | | 1039 | 1048 | Referred for Gastroscopy regarding his dysphagia | | FCW | |
| 28.06.2011 | 20.11.1946 | M | | 1053 | 1103 | BP 126/83 | | LPH | |
| 28.06.2011 | 08.02.1939 | F | | 1103 | 1120 | Script for Beconase Aqueous nasal spray, Loratadine & Transvasin heat rub cream | | IB | |

## Result of a query that lists all consultations from the 22nd to the end of June 2011 (ConsultationsSeenFrom22ndTillEndOfJun2011)

| SurgeryDate | DateOfBirth | Sex | Diagnosis | TimeIn | TimeOut | Complaints | Treatments | Initials | Notes |
|---|---|---|---|---|---|---|---|---|---|
| 28.06.2011 | 15.01.1948 | F | | 1400 | 1415 | For FBC, U/Es, Fasting Glucose & Chest X-Rays | | EAW | Home visit. |
| 28.06.2011 | 27.08.1922 | M | | 1418 | 1438 | He will rather wait for 2 days until when he is reviewed in the hospital rather than be admitted as an emergency | | AC | Home visit. |
| 28.06.2011 | 05.03.1943 | M | | 1646 | 1657 | Private script for Sildenafil given | | HTB | |
| 28.06.2011 | 14.01.1994 | F | | 1659 | 1711 | Script for E45 cream & Microgynon 30 given | | GJG | Referred to Neurologist regarding her fainting attacks. |
| 28.06.2011 | 05.08.1942 | M | | 1717 | 1725 | Referred to Orthopaedic Surgeon (urgent) regarding his (R) painful knee | | RP | |
| 28.06.2011 | 13.12.1966 | M | | 1725 | 1732 | To use warm olive oil & then sodium bicarbonate ear drops & then to have his ear syringed | | AL | |
| 28.06.2011 | 24.10.1959 | M | | 1756 | 1811 | Script for Flucloxacillin given | | BRH | |
| 29.06.2011 | 07.10.1933 | M | | 943 | 949 | Script for Ferrous Sulphate given | | FDF | |

Result of a query that lists all consultations from the 22nd to the end of June 2011 (ConsultationsSeenFrom22ndTillEndOfJun2011)

| SurgeryDate | DateOfBirth | Sex | Diagnosis | TimeIn | TimeOut | Complaints | Treatments | Initials | Notes |
|---|---|---|---|---|---|---|---|---|---|
| 29.06.2011 | 22.03.1986 | F | URTI | 949 | 954 | Sore throat | Amoxycillin | KAS | |
| 29.06.2011 | 04.10.1968 | F | S/Leave | 954 | 1003 | Med. 3 04/10 given for Stress and Anxiety for one month from 27.06.11 | | AW | |
| 29.06.2011 | 22.02.1936 | F | | 1021 | 1031 | Referred to Oral Surgeon regarding pain & swelling in the (L) lower jaw | | RPM | |
| 29.06.2011 | 05.03.1934 | M | | 1031 | 1045 | Copy of his Taxi Medical form (completed one) given to him as the original one has been misplaced | | CHD | |
| 29.06.2011 | 25.11.1945 | F | | 1045 | 1051 | Script for Aqueous cream given | | CLH | |
| 29.06.2011 | 31.07.1961 | F | | 1106 | 1116 | Script for Macrogol compound half-strength, Norethisterone & Simvastatin given | | CMW | |
| 29.06.2011 | 04.03.1947 | M | | 1320 | 1340 | Script for Amoxycillin & Co-codamol given | | GSB | Home visit. |
| 29.06.2011 | 05.06.1947 | M | | 1647 | 1654 | For FBC, U/Es, serum cholesterol, LFTs & Fasting Glucose | | TLS | |

490

Result of a query that lists all consultations from the 22<sup>nd</sup> to the end of June 2011 (ConsultationsSeenFrom22ndTillEndOfJun2011)

| SurgeryDate | DateOfBirth | Sex | Diagnosis | TimeIn | TimeOut | Complaints | Treatments | Initials | Notes |
|---|---|---|---|---|---|---|---|---|---|
| 29.06.2011 | 31.10.1969 | F | | 1654 | 1704 | Referred to ENT Surgeon regarding her persistent (L) ear ache | | SJY | Script for Otomize ear spray given. |
| 29.06.2011 | 05.12.1956 | M | | 1704 | 1709 | Script for Fexofenadine, Hydrocortisone with Miconazole cream & Omeprazole given | | DTB | |
| 29.06.2011 | 18.12.1959 | M | | 1709 | 1721 | For Chest X-Rays | | DKG | |
| 29.06.2011 | 17.06.1935 | F | | 1722 | 1732 | Script for Dihydrocodeine, Lactulose & Tramadol given | | SWLB | |
| 29.06.2011 | 29.05.1967 | M | | 1750 | 1806 | For FBC, U/Es, TFTs, Fasting Glucose, Fasting Lipids & LFTs | | CRCS | Script for Amitriptyline given. |
| 29.06.2011 | 03.11.1964 | M | S/Leave | 1806 | 1820 | Med. 3 04/10 given for Depression for 3 months from 28.06.11 | | SD | Script for Fluoxetine given. |

Result of a query that lists all consultations from the 22ⁿᵈ to the end of June 2012 (ConsultationsSeenFrom22ndTillEndOfJun2012)

| SurgeryDate | DateOfBirth | Sex | Diagnosis | TimeIn | TimeOut | Complaints | Treatments | Initials | Notes |
|---|---|---|---|---|---|---|---|---|---|
| 22.06.2012 | 29.06.1947 | F | | 943 | 952 | Script for Furosemide given | | SLS | Referred to Physiotherapist regarding pain in her (L) ankle. |
| 22.06.2012 | 11.09.1947 | M | | 952 | 1003 | Script for Codeine tablets & Prednisolone e/c tablets given | | TSN | |
| 22.06.2012 | 18.09.1946 | F | | 1003 | 1016 | For TFTs | | SL | |
| 22.06.2012 | 02.07.1943 | M | | 1016 | 1023 | Script for Lansoprazole given | | RJW | |
| 22.06.2012 | 14.08.1927 | M | | 1023 | 1030 | Script for Amitriptyline & Cetirizine given | | WRW | |
| 22.06.2012 | 29.12.2000 | F | | 1030 | 1035 | Script for Otosporin ear drops given | | MMS | |
| 22.06.2012 | 09.08.1971 | M | RTI | 1036 | 1046 | Chesty cough | Erythromycin | JCW | For Chest X-Rays. Penicillin allergy. |
| 22.06.2012 | 11.12.1944 | F | | 1055 | 1102 | Referred to General Surgeon regarding her multiple hall bladder stones showed on USScan | | GMW | |
| 22.06.2012 | 16.08.1927 | F | | 1102 | 1119 | Referred to the Essex Cardiac & Stroke Network (SGH) regarding possible TIA | | GC | |

Result of a query that lists all consultations from the 22nd to the end of June 2012 (ConsultationsSeenFrom22ndTillEndOfJun2012)

| SurgeryDate | DateOfBirth | Sex | Diagnosis | TimeIn | TimeOut | Complaints | Treatments | Initials | Notes |
|---|---|---|---|---|---|---|---|---|---|
| 25.06.2012 | 08.08.1953 | M | | 945 | 957 | Medication Review Done | | BP | |
| 25.06.2012 | 06.11.1961 | F | S/Leave | 957 | 1011 | Med. 3 04/10 given for Stress from 21.06.12 for 2 months | | DCMF | Referred to Counsellor regarding her stress. Script for Chloramphenicol eye drops given. |
| 25.06.2012 | 12.10.1948 | F | RTI | 1011 | 1021 | Chesty cough | Amoxycillin | SFC | For Chest X-Rays. |
| 25.06.2012 | 03.03.1946 | M | | 1021 | 1028 | For X-Rays of the (L) Ring finger | | SP | |
| 25.06.2012 | 18.06.1951 | M | RTI | 1035 | 1043 | Chesty cough | Amoxycillin | AL | For Chest X-Rays. |
| 25.06.2012 | 24.09.1930 | F | | 1043 | 1100 | I informed the patient that her USScan showed a small incisional hernia | | JMC | |
| 25.06.2012 | 23.09.1951 | F | | 1100 | 1107 | Script for Chloramphenicol eye drops given | | DJS | |
| 25.06.2012 | 28.09.1937 | F | | 1107 | 1113 | Script for Lacri-lube eye ointment & Acetylcysteine 5% eye drops given | | MR | |
| 25.06.2012 | 29.06.1939 | M | | 1345 | 1410 | Script for Prednisolone & Oramorph given | | CRG | Referred to DAU, SGH regarding his body pains. Home visit. |

Result of a query that lists all consultations from the 22nd to the end of June 2012 (ConsultationsSeenFrom22ndTillEndOfJun2012)

| SurgeryDate | DateOfBirth | Sex | Diagnosis | TimeIn | TimeOut | Complaints | Treatments | Initials | Notes |
|---|---|---|---|---|---|---|---|---|---|
| 25.06.2012 | 16.03.1978 | M | | 1646 | 1656 | Script for Amitriptyline & Salbutamol inhaler | | JWPS | Referred for Gastroscopy regarding his haematemesis & vomiting. |
| 25.06.2012 | 21.01.1972 | F | | 1656 | 1722 | Referred to Gastroenterologist following her barium enema studies as suggested by the Colonoscopist | | WKA | |
| 25.06.2012 | 08.04.1942 | M | | 1722 | 1728 | Script for Fexofenadine given | | GFT | |
| 25.06.2012 | 09.09.1993 | M | | 1728 | 1736 | Referred to Counsellor regarding his flashback about his unhappy childhood years due to his parents separation | | MPC | |
| 25.06.2012 | 23.08.1963 | F | | 1736 | 1742 | Script for Flucloxacillin given | | GPB | |
| 25.06.2012 | 16.05.1964 | M | | 1742 | 1749 | Script for Codeine tablets given | | GDC | |
| 25.06.2012 | 25.12.1946 | F | | 1749 | 1754 | Referred to Physiotherapist regarding her (L) arm pain | | AS | |

Result of a query that lists all consultations from the 22nd to the end of June 2012 (ConsultationsSeenFrom22ndTillEndOfJun2012)

| SurgeryDate | DateOfBirth | Sex | Diagnosis | TimeIn | TimeOut | Complaints | Treatments | Initials | Notes |
|---|---|---|---|---|---|---|---|---|---|
| 25.06.2012 | 26.04.1944 | F | | 1754 | 1803 | For B12, Folate, TFTs & Ferritin | | AW | |
| 25.06.2012 | 18.03.1978 | M | | 1803 | 1815 | Script for Acrivastine & Omeprazole given | | TRM | Referred to Orthopaedic Surgeon (BUPA) regarding pain in his (L) knee following a fall. |
| 26.06.2012 | 07.04.1966 | M | S/Leave | 942 | 950 | Med. 3 04/10 given for Back Pain from 25.06.12 for 2 weeks | | SG | |
| 26.06.2012 | 14.08.1927 | M | | 950 | 959 | Script for Amitriptyline & Co-codamol given | | RJW | |
| 26.06.2012 | 05.06.2010 | M | | 959 | 1006 | Balanitis | Trimethoprim | EM | |
| 26.06.2012 | 05.01.2009 | M | Rash | 1006 | 1011 | Bilateral contact dermatitis both palms | Fucidin H cream | JJWI | |
| 26.06.2012 | 24.01.1958 | F | | 1011 | 1022 | Medication Review Done | | JDB | |
| 26.06.2012 | 04.09.1952 | M | RTI | 1022 | 1031 | Chesty cough | Amoxycillin | DJB | |
| 26.06.2012 | 24.03.1935 | F | | 1031 | 1049 | General bowels physiology described to the patient & awaiting barium enema studies result | | PW | |
| 26.06.2012 | 26.11.1929 | F | | 1049 | 1118 | For LFTs, TFTs & serum cholesterol | | DEG | |

495

Result of a query that lists all consultations from the 22nd to the end of June 2012 (ConsultationsSeenFrom22ndTillEndOfJun2012)

| SurgeryDate | DateOfBirth | Sex | Diagnosis | TimeIn | TimeOut | Complaints | Treatments | Initials | Notes |
|---|---|---|---|---|---|---|---|---|---|
| 26.06.2012 | 31.07.1923 | M | | 1118 | 1125 | Referred to Audiology clinic regarding deafness in the (R) ear | | HO | |
| 26.06.2012 | 08.10.1924 | F | | 1125 | 1137 | Script for Clarithromycin, Flucloxacillin & Furosemide given | | GVR | For BNF, U/Es, LFTs, FBC & serum cholesterol. |
| 26.06.2012 | 31.07.1923 | M | | 1645 | 1652 | Cryotherapy blasts applied to scalp seborrheic warts | | HO | |
| 26.06.2012 | 08.04.1945 | M | | 1652 | 1702 | Cryotherapy blasts applied to warts on (R) ring finger | | GTW | |
| 26.06.2012 | 19.12.1945 | F | | 1702 | 1715 | Script for Trimethoprim given | | JMB | For FBC, U/Es, TFTs, Fasting Glucose, LFTs & MSU. |
| 26.06.2012 | 18.04.1930 | F | | 1715 | 1737 | Medication Review Done | | IDB | |
| 26.06.2012 | 24.12.1989 | F | | 1737 | 1746 | Injection Hydroxocobalamin given to (R) arm | | AJR | |
| 26.06.2012 | 09.03.2006 | F | URTI | 1746 | 1751 | Sore throat | Amoxycillin | IKR | |
| 26.06.2012 | 27.11.1955 | F | | 1751 | 1800 | For FBC, U/Es, Fasting Glucose, TFTs & LFTs | | JVH | |
| 26.06.2012 | 21.12.2004 | F | | 1800 | 1810 | Script for Ibuprofen & Paracetamol given | | JAJO | |

Result of a query that lists all consultations from the 22nd to the end of June 2012 (ConsultationsSeenFrom22ndTillEndOfJun2012)

| SurgeryDate | DateOfBirth | Sex | Diagnosis | TimeIn | TimeOut | Complaints | Treatments | Initials | Notes |
|---|---|---|---|---|---|---|---|---|---|
| 26.06.2012 | 06.11.1961 | F | | 1810 | 1850 | Fostering Medical Examination done for the patient | | BSM | |
| 26.06.2012 | 09.05.1973 | M | S/Leave | 1850 | 1858 | Med. 3 04/10 given for Back Pain from 25.06.12 for 2 weeks | | MPC | Script for Citalopram, Dihydrocodeine, Amitripyline & Oramorph given. |
| 27.06.2012 | 01.09.1946 | M | | 945 | 1002 | Script for Bisoprolol given | | PAH | Referred to Chest Physician for sleep studies as requested from the Cardiology clinic. |
| 27.06.2012 | 16.03.1956 | F | | 1002 | 1010 | She will come back later for extension of her sick leave | | SPD | |
| 27.06.2012 | 18.07.1929 | F | | 1010 | 1018 | Script for Diprobase cream & Erythromycin given | | JMMG | |
| 27.06.2012 | 09.04.1938 | M | | 1018 | 1027 | Script for Amoxycillin given | | NWH | For FBC, U/Es, TFTs, LFTs, Cholesterol, B12, Folate & Ferritin. |
| 27.06.2012 | 10.04.1984 | M | | 1027 | 1036 | To come in for cryotherapy to his plantar warts | | BM | |

Result of a query that lists all consultations from the 22nd to the end of June 2012 (ConsultationsSeenFrom22ndTillEndOfJun2012)

| SurgeryDate | DateOfBirth | Sex | Diagnosis | TimeIn | TimeOut | Complaints | Treatments | Initials | Notes |
|---|---|---|---|---|---|---|---|---|---|
| 27.06.2012 | 09.11.1972 | F | | 1042 | 1054 | Referred to ENT Surgeon as requested by Haematologist for pains in her ears & pressure on her nose | | LSS | |
| 27.06.2012 | 27.10.1960 | F | | 1054 | 1113 | Script for Cetraben & Fucibet cream given | | DLK | Referred to Orthopaedic Surgeon regarding his worsening back pain for consideration for a re-do back operation. |
| 27.06.2012 | 10.08.1931 | M | | 1113 | 1120 | Medication Review Done | | REW | |
| 27.06.2012 | 10.04.1971 | F | | 1641 | 1651 | Script for Adcal-D3 & Alendronic acid given | | KS | |
| 27.06.2012 | 18.09.1946 | F | | 1651 | 1705 | Referred to Neck Surgeon regarding her goitre in view of her past history of (L) breast cancer | | SL | |
| 27.06.2012 | 11.11.1969 | F | | 1705 | 1715 | Script for Qvar & Salbutamol inhalers given | | TLP | |
| 27.06.2012 | 27.02.1992 | M | | 1715 | 1721 | Script for Cetirizine given | | CPH | |
| 27.06.2012 | 05.03.1934 | M | | 1721 | 1731 | Medication Review Done | | CHD | |

Result of a query that lists all consultations from the 22nd to the end of June 2012 (ConsultationsSeenFrom22ndTillEndOfJun2012)

| SurgeryDate | DateOfBirth | Sex | Diagnosis | TimeIn | TimeOut | Complaints | Treatments | Initials | Notes |
|---|---|---|---|---|---|---|---|---|---|
| 27.06.2012 | 20.02.1990 | M |  | 1731 | 1746 | Referred for Gastroscopy regarding his haematemesis |  | JLG |  |
| 27.06.2012 | 02.04.1959 | F |  | 1746 | 1752 | Referred to Dermatologist regarding the raised lesion on her (R) upper eye lid |  | JW |  |
| 27.06.2012 | 08.10.1940 | M |  | 1752 | 1800 | For HbA1c & Fasting Glucose |  | GAFM |  |
| 27.06.2012 | 18.03.1987 | F | S/Leave | 1800 | 1806 | Med. 3 04/10 given for Back Pain from 27.06.12 for 1 week |  | LP |  |
| 27.06.2012 | 08.01.1998 | F |  | 1818 | 1826 | She may come back in about 2 months to be referred to a shoulder specialist if the swelling on the (L) side of the neck persists |  | ELB |  |
| 28.06.2012 | 05.10.1999 | F |  | 942 | 952 | Script for Erythromycin, Fostair inhaler & Prednisolone |  | MMCC |  |
| 28.06.2012 | 19.01.1964 | F | S/Leave | 952 | 1003 | Med. 3 04/10 given for Pain in the neck after operation from 24.06.12 for 3 months |  | NAB | Script for Carbamazepine given |

Result of a query that lists all consultations from the 22nd to the end of June 2012 (ConsultationsSeenFrom22ndTillEndOfJun2012)

| SurgeryDate | DateOfBirth | Sex | Diagnosis | TimeIn | TimeOut | Complaints | Treatments | Initials | Notes |
|---|---|---|---|---|---|---|---|---|---|
| 28.06.2012 | 13.10.1989 | F | S/Leave | 1003 | 1011 | Med. 3 04/10 given for Operation on the (L) ear from 05.06.12 for 1 month | | RLB | Script for Flucloxacillin given. |
| 28.06.2012 | 04.08.1936 | M | URTI | 1011 | 1020 | Sore throat | Erythromycin | ECM | |
| 28.06.2012 | 27.08.1961 | M | | 1020 | 1028 | For X-Rays of the (R) knee | | SRP | |
| 28.06.2012 | 24.03.1971 | M | S/Leave | 1028 | 1036 | Private sick leave given for Pain in the (R) foot from 25.06.12 for one week | | JCM | |
| 28.06.2012 | 08.11.2007 | F | | 1054 | 1100 | Referred to Paediatric Dr. on call, Southend hospital regarding poor appetite & weight loss | | OTA | |
| 28.06.2012 | 29.01.1956 | M | | 1100 | 1107 | Script for Amitriptyline given | | AJH | |
| 28.06.2012 | 17.02.2009 | F | | 1119 | 1128 | Script for Calamine lotion & Cetirizine given | | IEA | |
| 28.06.2012 | 07.02.2011 | M | | 1659 | 1716 | Private script for Mefloquine given | | NDM | Script for Aqueous cream given. |
| 28.06.2012 | 31.08.1999 | M | | 1716 | 1722 | Private script for Mefloquine given | | ETEM | |

Result of a query that lists all consultations from the 22nd to the end of June 2012 (ConsultationsSeenFrom22ndTillEndOfJun2012)

| SurgeryDate | DateOfBirth | Sex | Diagnosis | TimeIn | TimeOut | Complaints | Treatments | Initials | Notes |
|---|---|---|---|---|---|---|---|---|---|
| 28.06.2012 | 15.04.2003 | F | | 1722 | 1728 | Script for Salbutamol inhaler given | | LMC | Referred to Paediatrician regarding her persistent cough. |
| 28.06.2012 | 05.10.1974 | M | | 1730 | 1740 | Referred to Physiotherapist regarding his back pain | | SMG | |
| 28.06.2012 | 13.11.1949 | M | | 1745 | 1758 | Referred to Rheumatologist regarding his gout pain in the feet | | BEP | Script for Codeine tablets given. For Uric acid & U/Es. |
| 28.06.2012 | 16.06.1967 | M | | 1758 | 1806 | Script for Vardenafil given | | PBK | |
| 29.06.2012 | 20.09.1965 | M | | 941 | 958 | Script for Levothyroxine & Omeprazole given | | VJC | |
| 29.06.2012 | 09.10.1926 | M | | 958 | 1008 | For repeat serum B12& Folate level in 3 to 6 months with the nurse | | RAC | |
| 29.06.2012 | 05.04.1952 | M | S/Leave | 1008 | 1024 | Med. 3 04/10 given for Myocardial Infarction from 29.06.12 for 2 months | | LFC | Referred to Counsellor regarding his panic attacks. Script for Amitriptyline given. |

501

Result of a query that lists all consultations from the 22$^{nd}$ to the end of June 2012 (ConsultationsSeenFrom22ndTillEndOfJun2012)

| SurgeryDate | DateOfBirth | Sex | Diagnosis | TimeIn | TimeOut | Complaints | Treatments | Initials | Notes |
|---|---|---|---|---|---|---|---|---|---|
| 29.06.2012 | 13.01.1966 | M |  | 1024 | 1030 | Referred to Dermatologist regarding red spotty rash on his lower legs |  | PJB |  |
| 29.06.2012 | 04.11.1966 | F |  | 1030 | 1035 | To come in later for Cryotherapy to the wart on her lower (R) thigh |  | SJOB |  |
| 29.06.2012 | 04.07.1929 | M |  | 1035 | 1043 | For USScan of the abdomen, TFTs & Urine Albumin:Creatinine ratio |  | RMC |  |
| 29.06.2012 | 25.08.1957 | M | S/Leave | 1045 | 1054 | Med. 3 04/10 given for (R) ankle lateral Ligament Injury from 29.06.12 for 1 month |  | GC |  |
| 29.06.2012 | 02.08.1948 | M |  | 1057 | 1135 | Script for Atorvastatin, Co-codamol, Flucloxacillin & Naproxen given |  | KT | For Chest X-Rays & X-Rays of (R) knee. For Uric acid, LFTs, Cholesterol, U/Es & FBC. |
| 29.06.2012 | 11.10.1942 | M |  | 1357 | 1405 | Patient reassured about the divarification of his epigastric region |  | RWA | Home visit. |

Result of a query that lists all consultations from the 22nd to the end of June 2013 (ConsultationsSeenFrom22ndTillEndOfJun2013)

| SurgeryDate | DateOfBirth | Sex | Diagnosis | TimeIn | TimeOut | Complaints | Treatments | Initials | Notes |
|---|---|---|---|---|---|---|---|---|---|
| 24.06.2013 | 07.05.1938 | F | | 945 | 950 | Script for Salbutamol inhaler given | | ILB | |
| 24.06.2013 | 27.05.1954 | F | | 950 | 1001 | Referred to General Surgeon regarding her solitary thyroid nodule | | CAA | For TFTs, FBC, U/Es & serum cholesterol. |
| 24.06.2013 | 06.02.1946 | F | | 1001 | 1007 | Script for Omeprazole given | | KMT | |
| 24.06.2013 | 06.12.1947 | M | | 1013 | 1023 | Script for Indapamide given | | BSK | |
| 24.06.2013 | 18.09.1946 | F | | 1023 | 1029 | Script for Omeprazole given | | SL | |
| 24.06.2013 | 24.03.2013 | F | | 1029 | 1035 | Mum reassured regarding the (R) breast lump which is improving | | MJP | |
| 24.06.2013 | 15.06.1935 | F | | 1036 | 1046 | Medication Review Done | | SWLB | |
| 24.06.2013 | 29.12.1954 | F | | 1046 | 1056 | Script for Propranolol given | | PAK | |
| 24.06.2013 | 20.11.1946 | M | | 1056 | 1104 | Script for Salbutamol inhaler given | | LPH | |
| 24.06.2013 | 27.01.1934 | F | | 1104 | 1114 | Script for Amlodipine given | | JWC | |
| 24.06.2013 | 27.05.2008 | F | | 1114 | 1122 | Script for Co-Amoxiclav & Fucidin 2% cream given | | HCJN | |

Result of a query that lists all consultations from the 22nd to the end of June 2013 (ConsultationsSeenFrom22ndTillEndOfJun2013)

| SurgeryDate | DateOfBirth | Sex | Diagnosis | TimeIn | TimeOut | Complaints | Treatments | Initials | Notes |
|---|---|---|---|---|---|---|---|---|---|
| 24.06.2013 | 05.06.1924 | M | | 1227 | 1245 | Script for Complan shake, Dexamethasone & Co-codamol given | | DAC | Home visit. |
| 24.06.2013 | 23.06.1962 | M | | 1645 | 1654 | Medication Review Done | | MD | |
| 24.06.2013 | 27.12.1959 | F | | 1655 | 1700 | Script for Cetirizine tablets given | | KDI | |
| 24.06.2013 | 15.10.1969 | F | | 1706 | 1714 | Script for Mebeverine given | | MAC | |
| 24.06.2013 | 29.11.1962 | M | | 1714 | 1721 | He will observe his abdominal pain which is settling down for now | | SP | |
| 24.06.2013 | 22.07.1961 | M | | 1726 | 1733 | Script for Amorolfine 5% medicated nail lacquer & Canesten HC cream given | | PWL | |
| 24.06.2013 | 28.02.1941 | F | | 1733 | 1743 | Script for Pentasa given | | SJW | Septrin allergy. |
| 24.06.2013 | 16.07.1969 | F | | 1743 | 1750 | Script for Amoxycillin & Otosporin given | | NB | |
| 24.06.2013 | 15.10.1965 | M | | 1755 | 1806 | Private script for Viagra given | | SJH | For USScan of the testicles (urgent). |
| 25.06.2013 | 21.05.1958 | F | | 944 | 951 | Script for Omeprazole given | | SB | |

Result of a query that lists all consultations from the 22nd to the end of June 2013 (ConsultationsSeenFrom22ndTillEndOfJun2013)

| SurgeryDate | DateOfBirth | Sex | Diagnosis | TimeIn | TimeOut | Complaints | Treatments | Initials | Notes |
|---|---|---|---|---|---|---|---|---|---|
| 25.06.2013 | 18.04.1965 | M | | 953 | 1010 | For FBC, U/Es, LFTs, Cholesterol, HbA1c & urine microalbumin screen | | MGF | |
| 25.06.2013 | 05.02.2013 | M | | 1010 | 1018 | Script for Fucidin H cream given | | TWNH | |
| 25.06.2013 | 01.02.1980 | F | | 1030 | 1044 | Script for Co-codamol & Senna given | | LTB | |
| 25.06.2013 | 18.12.1925 | F | | 1044 | 1057 | Script for Transvasin Heat Rub cream given | | MAL | |
| 25.06.2013 | 27.01.1940 | F | | 1057 | 1103 | For X-Rays of the (R) wrist & (R) Ulnar (urgent) | | JD | |
| 25.06.2013 | 15.04.1927 | M | | 1103 | 1122 | For FBC, U/Es, B12, Folate & Ferritin | | JB | |
| 25.06.2013 | 09.09.1945 | F | | 1122 | 1136 | script for Fluconazole & Loratadine given | | AML | Referred to ENT Surgeon regarding the possibility of the oesophageal web growing back again. |
| 25.06.2013 | 23.08.1968 | F | | 1136 | 1142 | script for EpiPen injection given | | DBW | |
| 25.06.2013 | 22.05.1931 | F | | 1142 | 1200 | Referred to Gynaecologist (urgent) regarding her post-menopausal bleeding | | DK | For Pelvic USScan. |

## Result of a query that lists all consultations from the 22nd to the end of June 2013 (ConsultationsSeenFrom22ndTillEndOfJun2013)

| SurgeryDate | DateOfBirth | Sex | Diagnosis | TimeIn | TimeOut | Complaints | Treatments | Initials | Notes |
|---|---|---|---|---|---|---|---|---|---|
| 25.06.2013 | 16.07.1936 | F | | 1342 | 1353 | Script for Ciprofloxacin given | | EG | Home visit. |
| 25.06.2013 | 07.07.1961 | F | | 1640 | 1653 | Cryotherapy blasts x 2 applied to skin tag in (L) axillary region | | SSA | Script for Erythromycin given. Penicillin allergy. |
| 25.06.2013 | 27.09.1931 | M | | 1653 | 1700 | Cryotherapy blasts x 2 applied to itchy seborrheic wart on chest | | JJ | |
| 25.06.2013 | 28.09.1978 | F | | 1700 | 1707 | For X-Rays of the Lumbar spine | | TLJ | |
| 25.06.2013 | 21.09.1947 | M | S/Leave | 1707 | 1717 | Med. 3 04/10 given for Stress for 2 weeks from 25.06.13 | | DL | |
| 25.06.2013 | 15.09.1939 | M | | 1717 | 1735 | Script for Finasteride given | | WJS | |
| 25.06.2013 | 12.08.1980 | M | | 1735 | 1742 | Script for Transvasin Heat Rub cream given | | MM | |
| 25.06.2013 | 04.09.1963 | F | | 1744 | 1752 | Her impaired GTT result was explained to her | | AR | |
| 25.06.2013 | 18.01.1977 | F | | 1752 | 1801 | She came in for me to document her fight & bruises with her ex-boyfriend she had last Saturday night | | MP | |

Result of a query that lists all consultations from the 22nd to the end of June 2013 (ConsultationsSeenFrom22ndTillEndOfJun2013)

| SurgeryDate | DateOfBirth | Sex | Diagnosis | TimeIn | TimeOut | Complaints | Treatments | Initials | Notes |
|---|---|---|---|---|---|---|---|---|---|
| 25.06.2013 | 06.08.1941 | M | | 1801 | 1817 | Referred to Chest Physician regarding nodules showed on his chest X-Rays 3 months ago | | AJM | For Chest X-Rays. |
| 25.06.2013 | 15.03.1967 | F | | 1817 | 1827 | For X-Rays of the (L) knee, FBC, TFTs & Fasting Glucose | | MP | |
| 26.06.2013 | 20.09.1965 | M | S/Leave | 944 | 1014 | Med. 3 04/10 given for Bladder infection for 2 weeks from 26.06.13 | | VJC | Script for Ciprofloxacin given. |
| 26.06.2013 | 09.09.1949 | M | | 1014 | 1019 | Medications Review Done | | CSM | |
| 26.06.2013 | 03.02.1949 | F | | 1019 | 1031 | Script for Penicillin V given | | DPH | |
| 26.06.2013 | 17.10.1987 | F | | 1031 | 1050 | Referred to Dermatologist regarding the moles on her thigh & back which are very sore | | JQ | |
| 26.06.2013 | 03.07.1940 | F | | 1050 | 1101 | Script for Codeine tablets, Naproxen & Omeprazole given | | JMM | |
| 26.06.2013 | 08.06.1961 | M | | 1101 | 1107 | Script for Diclofenac e/c given | | MPB | |
| 26.06.2013 | 31.05.1967 | M | | 1107 | 1114 | Medications Review Done | | GKP | |

Result of a query that lists all consultations from the 22nd to the end of June 2013 (ConsultationsSeenFrom22ndTillEndOfJun2013)

| SurgeryDate | DateOfBirth | Sex | Diagnosis | TimeIn | TimeOut | Complaints | Treatments | Initials | Notes |
|---|---|---|---|---|---|---|---|---|---|
| 26.06.2013 | 22.02.1963 | M | | 1114 | 1119 | Script for Cetirizine & Beconase nasal spray given | | JBP | |
| 26.06.2013 | 14.08.1985 | F | | 1119 | 1126 | Referred to Physiotherapist regarding her back & pelvic pains | | CR | |
| 26.06.2013 | 28.02.1941 | F | | 1126 | 1136 | Referred to Gynaecologist regarding her vaginal prolapse | | SJW | |
| 26.06.2013 | 17.08.1912 | F | RTI | 1143 | 1153 | Chesty cough | Co-Amoxiclav & Prednisolone tablets | IAA | For Chest X-Rays. |
| 26.06.2013 | 06.03.1966 | F | | 1645 | 1659 | For USScan of the lower abdomen & pelvis | | JLL | |
| 26.06.2013 | 18.01.1958 | F | | 1659 | 1708 | For FBC, U/Es, Fasting Glucose, TFTs & serum Ferritin | | LRG | |
| 26.06.2013 | 27.07.1995 | F | RTI | 1709 | 1717 | Chesty cough | Paracetamol & Amoxycillin | BM | |
| 26.06.2013 | 08.10.1981 | F | | 1718 | 1729 | Patient informed that her GTT was essentially normal | | SG | |

Result of a query that lists all consultations from the 22nd to the end of June 2013 (ConsultationsSeenFrom22ndTillEndOfJun2013)

| SurgeryDate | DateOfBirth | Sex | Diagnosis | TimeIn | TimeOut | Complaints | Treatments | Initials | Notes |
|---|---|---|---|---|---|---|---|---|---|
| 26.06.2013 | 08.05.1968 | M | | 1740 | 1750 | The result of his recent echocardiogram which was essentially normal was explained to him | | BGV | |
| 26.06.2013 | 04.07.1944 | M | | 1750 | 1759 | Script for Atorvastatin & Metformin/ Sitagliptin given | | JW | |
| 26.06.2013 | 04.01.1967 | F | | 1759 | 1810 | Referred to Orthopaedic Surgeon (foot & ankle Surgeon) regarding her Achilles tendinitis as advised by the Podiatrist | | MC | |
| 27.06.2013 | 29.09.1992 | M | | 943 | 952 | To contact local GUM clinic as he is worried about contacting STD | | EGC | |
| 27.06.2013 | 20.08.1939 | F | | 952 | 1002 | Script for Fucithalmic eye drops given | | SLT | |
| 27.06.2013 | 04.01.1932 | F | | 1002 | 1011 | Script for Amoxycillin & Otosporin ear drops given | | EAC | |
| 27.06.2013 | 22.07.1968 | F | | 1011 | 1021 | Script for Amoxycillin & Codeine Linctus given | | RG | |

509

Result of a query that lists all consultations from the 22nd to the end of June 2013 (ConsultationsSeenFrom22ndTillEndOfJun2013)

| SurgeryDate | DateOfBirth | Sex | Diagnosis | TimeIn | TimeOut | Complaints | Treatments | Initials | Notes |
|---|---|---|---|---|---|---|---|---|---|
| 27.06.2013 | 01.01.1924 | M | | 1021 | 1027 | Script for Nitrolingual spray given | | HAJB | |
| 27.06.2013 | 21.04.1949 | M | | 1027 | 1035 | Script for Transvasin Heat Rub cream given | | RL | For X-Rays of the (R) shoulder |
| 27.06.2013 | 10.11.1969 | F | | 1035 | 1041 | Referred to ENT Surgeon regarding the puffiness under her (L) eye as suggested from the eye clinic | | PS | |
| 27.06.2013 | 09.10.1926 | M | | 1051 | 1109 | Script for BuTrans patch given | | RAC | |
| 27.06.2013 | 29.09.1932 | F | | 1109 | 1126 | Script for Clexane injection given | | SMD | For Fasting Glucose, TFTs, FBC, U/Es, LFTs & Fasting Lipids. |
| 27.06.2013 | 25.12.1948 | M | | 1126 | 1139 | Script for Co-codamol & Metformin given | | CGB | |
| 27.06.2013 | 20.12.1922 | F | | 1340 | 1350 | Script for Furosemide given | | DEA | Home visit. Penicillin allergy. |
| 27.06.2013 | 06.03.1957 | F | | 1645 | 1704 | Referred to Neurologist regarding the epileptic fit which she possibly had in her sleep | | CMT | for ESR & CRP. |
| 27.06.2013 | 22.06.1955 | M | | 1704 | 1720 | His life live screening test result was discussed with him | | MT | |

Result of a query that lists all consultations from the 22nd to the end of June 2013 (ConsultationsSeenFrom22ndTillEndOfJun2013)

| SurgeryDate | DateOfBirth | Sex | Diagnosis | TimeIn | TimeOut | Complaints | Treatments | Initials | Notes |
|---|---|---|---|---|---|---|---|---|---|
| 27.06.2013 | 11.06.1987 | M | | 1720 | 1727 | For FBC, U/Es, Fasting Glucose & ESR | | DP | |
| 27.06.2013 | 08.03.1946 | F | | 1727 | 1733 | For FBC, U/Es, Fasting Lipids, LFTs & X-Rays of the (L) foot | | GRC | |
| 27.06.2013 | 02.01.1988 | M | | 1733 | 1741 | Script for Codeine tablets, Amoxycillin & cetraben cream | | AHK | |
| 27.06.2013 | 18.03.1967 | F | | 1741 | 1749 | Script for Norethisterone given | | SO | |
| 27.06.2013 | 11.07.1962 | M | | 1749 | 1756 | Script for Bendroflumethiazide given | | JEG | |
| 27.06.2013 | 10.12.1971 | M | | 1756 | 1803 | Script for Amitriptyline given | | PT | |
| 27.06.2013 | 11.11.1961 | M | | 1808 | 1820 | For FBC, HbA1c, TFTs & U/Es | | AMP | |
| 28.06.2013 | 08.10.1963 | M | | 941 | 953 | BP 131/82 | | RBA | |
| 28.06.2013 | 28.04.1934 | F | | 953 | 1001 | Script for Nasonex nasal spray given | | JSB | |
| 28.06.2013 | 23.02.1969 | M | | 1001 | 1027 | Referred to Sleep clinic regarding ?falling asleep whilst driving the underground train | | DJP | For TFTs, FBC, U/Es, Cholesterol & HbA1c |

Result of a query that lists all consultations from the 22nd to the end of June 2013 (ConsultationsSeenFrom22ndTillEndOfJun2013)

| SurgeryDate | DateOfBirth | Sex | Diagnosis | TimeIn | TimeOut | Complaints | Treatments | Initials | Notes |
|---|---|---|---|---|---|---|---|---|---|
| 28.06.2013 | 09.04.1975 | F | | 1027 | 1033 | Referred to Breast Surgeon for genetic counselling as she has a very strong family history of breast cancer | | KLS | |
| 28.06.2013 | 20.02.1953 | F | | 1033 | 1041 | She will come back later to have her skin tags treated by cryotherapy | | SLF | |
| 28.06.2013 | 31.05.1947 | F | | 1043 | 1049 | Script for Verrugon complete 50% ointment given | | BJD | |
| 28.06.2013 | 08.01.2009 | M | RTI | 1049 | 1054 | Chesty cough | Amoxycillin | CNC | |
| 28.06.2013 | 19.08.1939 | F | | 1054 | 1109 | Medications Review Done | | JEN | |
| 28.06.2013 | 01.11.1939 | M | | 1109 | 1119 | Medications Review Done | | JN | |
| 28.06.2013 | 30.10.1927 | F | | 1325 | 1340 | DNAR form completed for the patient & signed | | VFL | Home visit. |
| 28.06.2013 | 07.02.1952 | M | | 1340 | 1355 | Script for Lorazepam & Trimethoprim given | | GAH | Home visit. |

Result of a query that lists all consultations from the 22nd to the end of June 2014 (ConsultationsSeenFrom22ndTillEndOfJun2014)

| SurgeryDate | DateOfBirth | Sex | Diagnosis | TimeIn | TimeOut | Complaints | Treatments | Initials | Notes |
|---|---|---|---|---|---|---|---|---|---|
| 23.06.2014 | 17.06.1965 | F | | 943 | 959 | Script for Laxido orange oral powder sachets & Duloxetine given | | JLP | |
| 23.06.2014 | 08.10.1940 | M | | 959 | 1021 | For Folate & Ferritin | | GAFM | |
| 23.06.2014 | 28.07.1939 | F | | 1021 | 1046 | Script for Forxiga, Paracetamol & Sodium Feredetate given | | RMM | For B12 & TFTs. |
| 23.06.2014 | 25.01.1939 | F | | 1046 | 1055 | Script for Furosemide given | | PMC | |
| 23.06.2014 | 17.07.1981 | M | | 1055 | 1101 | Script for Doxycycline given | | BLW | |
| 23.06.2014 | 04.12.1957 | F | | 1101 | 1109 | Script for Naproxen tablets given | | TA | |
| 23.06.2014 | 13.12.1934 | F | | 1109 | 1123 | Script for Metformin given | | SDH | |
| 23.06.2014 | 23.04.1950 | F | | 1123 | 1147 | Script for Fucidin H cream & Cetraben emollient cream given | | PEH | Injection Depo-Medrone with Lidocaine 2mls given to the (R) shoulder (posterior approach). |
| 23.06.2014 | 25.12.1948 | M | | 1646 | 1700 | Script for Naproxen, Omeprazole, Betahistine & Sildenafil given to the patient | | CGB | |

513

Result of a query that lists all consultations from the 22nd to the end of June 2014 (ConsultationsSeenFrom22ndTillEndOfJun2014)

| SurgeryDate | DateOfBirth | Sex | Diagnosis | TimeIn | TimeOut | Complaints | Treatments | Initials | Notes |
|---|---|---|---|---|---|---|---|---|---|
| 23.06.2014 | 06.06.1945 | M | | 1700 | 1734 | The issues surrounding the completion of Section 1 of the Taxi Medical examination - Eye test section sorted out for him | | LJB | |
| 23.06.2014 | 22.10.2009 | F | | 1734 | 1742 | For repeat MSU in one month, form given to the patient | | CMGM | |
| 23.06.2014 | 16.09.1997 | F | | 1742 | 1752 | For FBC, U/Es, Fasting Glucose & Pregnancy test | | GJJ | |
| 23.06.2014 | 05.10.1974 | M | | 1752 | 1800 | Script for Permethrin 5% cream given | | SMG | |
| 23.06.2014 | 03.07.1989 | M | | 1817 | 1820 | Reassured about his enlarged (R) breast, being seen privately was discussed | | WDH | |
| 23.06.2014 | 06.11.1968 | M | | 1817 | 1820 | Reassured about the 4mm epididymal cyst noted on the USScan of his testicles | | ARP | |
| 23.06.2014 | 18.03.1978 | M | | 1820 | 1823 | script for Acrivastine & Omeprazole given | | TRM | |
| 23.06.2014 | 20.04.1938 | M | | 1823 | 1829 | To see me in one month for repeat MSU, PSA & rectal examination | | DAD | |

Result of a query that lists all consultations from the 22nd to the end of June 2014 (ConsultationsSeenFrom22ndTillEndOfJun2014)

| SurgeryDate | DateOfBirth | Sex | Diagnosis | TimeIn | TimeOut | Complaints | Treatments | Initials | Notes |
|---|---|---|---|---|---|---|---|---|---|
| 23.06.2014 | 17.02.1987 | F | | 1829 | 1845 | script for Co-codamol, Trimethoprim & Metoclopramide given | | KMT | |
| 24.06.2014 | 02.09.1941 | F | | 947 | 1000 | Script for Simvastatin given | | MS | |
| 24.06.2014 | 07.05.1938 | F | | 1000 | 1010 | Script for Betahistine given | | IB | |
| 24.06.2014 | 20.02.1930 | M | | 1010 | 1022 | Medications Review Done | | AL | |
| 24.06.2014 | 22.09.1967 | F | | 1022 | 1032 | Script for Diazepam, Naproxen & Transvasin cream given | | SG | |
| 24.06.2014 | 17.12.1956 | M | | 1032 | 1050 | Script for Doxycycline given | | PAE | For FBC, U/Es, Fasting Lipids, LFTs & Fasting Glucose. |
| 24.06.2014 | 04.03.1982 | F | | 1050 | 1055 | Referred to Dermatologist (community) regarding mole on the (L) side of her neck | | GV | |
| 24.06.2014 | 27.03.1996 | M | | 1055 | 1105 | For MSU, FBC, U/Es, HbA1c, urine microalbumin screen, LFTs & Cholesterol | | HAJS | |

515

Result of a query that lists all consultations from the 22nd to the end of June 2014 (ConsultationsSeenFrom22ndTillEndOfJun2014)

| SurgeryDate | DateOfBirth | Sex | Diagnosis | TimeIn | TimeOut | Complaints | Treatments | Initials | Notes |
|---|---|---|---|---|---|---|---|---|---|
| 24.06.2014 | 03.05.1938 | F | | 1105 | 1115 | For B12, Folate & Ferritin in 3 months, form given to the patient | | MFB | |
| 24.06.2014 | 22.01.2006 | F | RTI | 1115 | 1121 | Chesty cough | Amoxycillin | KEGM | |
| 24.06.2014 | 18.05.1979 | F | | 1132 | 1140 | Script for Co-Amoxiclav given | | MJH | |
| 24.06.2014 | 27.09.1931 | M | | 1645 | 1657 | Script for Clarithromycin given | | JJ | |
| 24.06.2014 | 21.06.1942 | M | | 1657 | 1702 | To see me in 6 months for repeat PSA | | WJB | |
| 24.06.2014 | 14.05.1971 | M | | 1702 | 1710 | Script for Ibuprofen & Transvasin Heat Rub cream given | | NJF | |
| 24.06.2014 | 02.06.1994 | F | | 1710 | 1715 | Referred to Podiatrist regarding the painful bunion on her (R) foot | | EPB | |
| 24.06.2014 | 19.09.1962 | M | RTI | 1720 | 1727 | Chesty cough | Doxycycline | KPW | |
| 24.06.2014 | 23.01.1961 | F | | 1810 | 1903 | For AH Adult Health Report Medical examination and fostering form completed for the patient | | JJH | |

Result of a query that lists all consultations from the 22nd to the end of June 2014 (ConsultationsSeenFrom22ndTillEndOfJun2014)

| SurgeryDate | DateOfBirth | Sex | Diagnosis | TimeIn | TimeOut | Complaints | Treatments | Initials | Notes |
|---|---|---|---|---|---|---|---|---|---|
| 25.06.2014 | 17.03.1985 | F | | 943 | 951 | Script for Doxycycline & Fucidin cream given | | KAB | |
| 25.06.2014 | 25.08.1933 | F | | 951 | 1012 | Script for Doxycycline & Transvasin Heat Rub cream given | | PCH | Referred to Orthopaedic Surgeon regarding persistent pain in the (R) shoulder. |
| 25.06.2014 | 30.01.1999 | F | | 1012 | 1029 | To go on cholecalciferol maintenance dose | | ALCJ | |
| 25.06.2014 | 19.08.1951 | M | | 1029 | 1035 | Medications Review Done | | KVB | |
| 25.06.2014 | 26.06.1990 | M | | 1035 | 1041 | For Chest X-Rays | | KSH | |
| 25.06.2014 | 17.04.1936 | M | | 1041 | 1052 | Medications Review Done | | RB | |
| 25.06.2014 | 20.01.1941 | F | | 1052 | 1103 | Script for Transvasin Heat Rub cream given | | BDD | For Fasting Glucose, FBC, U/Es, Cholesterol, LFTs, Ferritin & TFTs. |
| 25.06.2014 | 06.11.1929 | M | | 1103 | 1119 | For FBC, U/Es, Fasting Glucose, B12, Folate, Ferritin, PSA, LFTs, Cholesterol & urine microalbumin screen | | FAD | |

Result of a query that lists all consultations from the 22nd to the end of June 2014 (ConsultationsSeenFrom22ndTillEndOfJun2014)

| SurgeryDate | DateOfBirth | Sex | Diagnosis | TimeIn | TimeOut | Complaints | Treatments | Initials | Notes |
|---|---|---|---|---|---|---|---|---|---|
| 25.06.2014 | 01.12.1993 | F | | 1119 | 1130 | Her baby is having her 6 weeks post-natal check with their new GP tomorrow | | LFC | |
| 25.06.2014 | 23.08.1975 | M | | 1645 | 1659 | For FBC, U/Es, Fasting Glucose, Fasting Lipids & TFTs | | IMER | |
| 25.06.2014 | 06.02.1946 | F | | 1659 | 1705 | Script for Prochlorperazine given | | KMT | |
| 25.06.2014 | 30.04.2005 | M | | 1705 | 1721 | He is under the care of specialists for his congenital heart problem | | TJES | |
| 25.06.2014 | 10.09.1968 | M | | 1721 | 1730 | To put in a self-certificate for the first week | | KRH | |
| 25.06.2014 | 06.07.1936 | F | | 1730 | 1739 | Medications Review Done | | MLW | |
| 25.06.2014 | 25.04.2007 | F | | 1739 | 1745 | Script for Amoxycillin given | | BADS | |
| 25.06.2014 | 08.01.1942 | F | | 1745 | 1753 | Script for Clarithromycin given | | SM | |
| 25.06.2014 | 22.07.1961 | M | | 1757 | 1809 | Script for Co-Amoxiclav, Codeine Linctus & Ventolin inhaler given | | PWL | |

## Result of a query that lists all consultations from the 22$^{nd}$ to the end of June 2014 (ConsultationsSeenFrom22ndTillEndOfJun2014)

| SurgeryDate | DateOfBirth | Sex | Diagnosis | TimeIn | TimeOut | Complaints | Treatments | Initials | Notes |
|---|---|---|---|---|---|---|---|---|---|
| 25.06.2014 | 06.08.1941 | M | | 1809 | 1818 | Script for Forxiga given | | AJM | |
| 26.06.2014 | 18.10.1949 | M | | 944 | 1002 | Script for Colchicine tablets given | | BJG | |
| 26.06.2014 | 06.11.1961 | F | | 1002 | 1014 | Script for Doxycycline & Prednisolone given | | BSM | For TFTs, U/Es, LFTs, Fasting Glucose & Fasting Lipids. |
| 26.06.2014 | 13.01.1979 | M | | 1014 | 1022 | Script for Transvasin Heat Rub cream given | | CAW | |
| 26.06.2014 | 22.02.1944 | M | | 1022 | 1030 | For FBC, CRP & ESR | | AS | |
| 26.06.2014 | 28.07.1939 | F | | 1030 | 1048 | Script for Atorvastatin given | | RMM | |
| 26.06.2014 | 08.10.1940 | M | | 1048 | 1058 | Script for Ferrous Fumarate given | | GAFM | |
| 26.06.2014 | 11.01.1960 | F | | 1058 | 1111 | For FBC, ESR, U/Es & CRP | | FN | |
| 26.06.2014 | 22.02.1936 | F | | 1111 | 1124 | Script for Laxido Orange oral powder sachets given | | RPM | For FBC, U/Es, Cholesterol, LFTs, HbA1c & urine microalbumin screen. |
| 26.06.2014 | 27.01.1934 | F | | 1124 | 1130 | Script for Doxycycline & Chloramphenicol eye drops given | | JWC | |

Result of a query that lists all consultations from the 22nd to the end of June 2014 (ConsultationsSeenFrom22ndTillEndOfJun2014)

| SurgeryDate | DateOfBirth | Sex | Diagnosis | TimeIn | TimeOut | Complaints | Treatments | Initials | Notes |
|---|---|---|---|---|---|---|---|---|---|
| 26.06.2014 | 28.09.1937 | F | | 1645 | 1653 | Cryotherapy bursts x2 applied to seborrheic wart in the (L) groin | | MR | |
| 26.06.2014 | 20.08.1939 | F | | 1653 | 1659 | Script for Cetraben cream given | | SLT | |
| 26.06.2014 | 14.10.1969 | F | | 1659 | 1712 | Script for Naproxen & Co-codamol given | | LB | |
| 26.06.2014 | 28.02.1941 | F | | 1712 | 1722 | Referred to Urologist (Haematuria clinic - urgent) regarding her painless frank haematuria | | SJW | |
| 26.06.2014 | 29.11.1946 | F | | 1722 | 1734 | Script for Doxycycline & Prednisolone given | | PW | For FBC, U/Es & Malarial screening. |
| 26.06.2014 | 11.09.1947 | M | | 1739 | 1747 | Script for Doxycycline given | | TSN | |
| 26.06.2014 | 03.11.1994 | F | | 1747 | 1752 | To see the nurse in 6 months for repeat U/Es | | SMB | |
| 26.06.2014 | 22.02.1971 | M | | 1752 | 1802 | Script for Doxycycline & Tramadol given | | SB | |
| 27.06.2014 | 17.09.1965 | F | | 943 | 950 | Script for Doxycycline & Prednisolone tablets given | | PAE | |
| 27.06.2014 | 17.04.1923 | M | | 950 | 1004 | Script for Doxycycline given | | JWD | |
| 27.06.2014 | 22.04.1975 | F | | 1004 | 1010 | Script for Amoxycillin given | | SAG | |

Result of a query that lists all consultations from the 22nd to the end of June 2014 (ConsultationsSeenFrom22ndTillEndOfJun2014)

| SurgeryDate | DateOfBirth | Sex | Diagnosis | TimeIn | TimeOut | Complaints | Treatments | Initials | Notes |
|---|---|---|---|---|---|---|---|---|---|
| 27.06.2014 | 03.07.1940 | F | | 1020 | 1033 | Script for Doxycycline & Gabapentin given | | JMM | Penicillin allergy. |
| 27.06.2014 | 06.02.1944 | M | | 1033 | 1042 | Referred to Vascular Surgeon regarding his bilateral varicose veins | | AMC | |
| 27.06.2014 | 31.05.1967 | M | | 1103 | 1114 | Referred to Dermatologist (Community) regarding small fibroadenoma on (R) side of his neck | | GKP | |
| 27.06.2014 | 04.07.1929 | M | | 1125 | 1133 | Eprex 2000iu/0.5ml given in (L) Deltoid | | RMC | |

Result of a query that lists all consultations from the 22nd to the end of June 2015 (ConsultationsSeenFrom22ndTillEndOfJun2015)

| SurgeryDate | DateOfBirth | Sex | Diagnosis | TimeIn | TimeOut | Complaints | Treatments | Initials | Notes |
|---|---|---|---|---|---|---|---|---|---|
| 22.06.2015 | 17.03.1958 | M | | 945 | 956 | Medications Review Done | | JDP | |
| 22.06.2015 | 17.08.1997 | M | | 957 | 1003 | Script for Duac Once Daily gel given | | BLMS | |
| 22.06.2015 | 31.05.1930 | F | | 1009 | 1025 | Referred to Gastroenterologist (urgent) regarding her bloated abdomen & changing bowel habits | | SAW | |

Result of a query that lists all consultations from the 22nd to the end of June 2015 (ConsultationsSeenFrom22ndTillEndOfJun2015)

| SurgeryDate | DateOfBirth | Sex | Diagnosis | TimeIn | TimeOut | Complaints | Treatments | Initials | Notes |
|---|---|---|---|---|---|---|---|---|---|
| 22.06.2015 | 11.11.1934 | M | | 1025 | 1039 | Referred to Chest Physician regarding his increasing breathlessness | | VRB | |
| 22.06.2015 | 29.03.1947 | F | S/Leave | 1045 | 1055 | Med. 3 04/10 given for Back Pain for 1 month from 22.06.15 | | GJP | |
| 22.06.2015 | 03.07.1940 | F | | 1225 | 1320 | Script for BuTrans patches, Hirudoid cream, Co-codamol & Indapamide given | | JMM | Home visit. Penicillin allergy. |
| 22.06.2015 | 30.03.1961 | F | S/Leave | 1647 | 1658 | Med. 3 04/10 given for Depression for 1 month from 21.06.15 | | JEW | |
| 22.06.2015 | 22.06.1973 | F | | 1701 | 1711 | The Managing Neck and Back Pain booklet & The STarT Back Musculoskeletal Screening Tool leaflet given to the patient | | JAP | |
| 22.06.2015 | 07.11.1968 | F | | 1711 | 1717 | Script for Amoxycillin given | | RGG | |
| 22.06.2015 | 27.02.1992 | M | | 1721 | 1732 | Script for Calamine lotion & Fexofenadine given | | CPH | |

Result of a query that lists all consultations from the 22nd to the end of June 2015 (ConsultationsSeenFrom22ndTillEndOfJun2015)

| SurgeryDate | DateOfBirth | Sex | Diagnosis | TimeIn | TimeOut | Complaints | Treatments | Initials | Notes |
|---|---|---|---|---|---|---|---|---|---|
| 22.06.2015 | 12.08.1980 | M | | 1732 | 1742 | Script for Codeine tablets & Naproxen given | | MM | The Managing Neck and Back Pain booklet & The STarT Back Musculoskeletal Screening Tool leaflet given to the patient. |
| 22.06.2015 | 28.07.1943 | F | | 1742 | 1802 | Referred to Neurologist (urgent) regarding recurrent episodes of confusion after banging her head badly against a car door about 5 weeks ago | | BS | For TFTs, LFTs, FBC & U/Es. |
| 22.06.2015 | 15.04.2003 | F | | 1802 | 1812 | Script for Amoxycillin given | | LMC | |
| 22.06.2015 | 08.03.1961 | M | | 1812 | 1822 | Script for Fenbid 5% gel given | | RAB | Referred to Orthopaedic Surgeon (Mr. Gree) regarding osteoarthritis in his (R) knee which has deteriorated. |
| 23.06.2015 | 04.07.1929 | M | | 946 | 955 | For FBC & U/Es | | RMC | Penicillin allergy. |
| 23.06.2015 | 17.05.1939 | M | | 955 | 1002 | For X-Rays of the (R) Shoulder & the (R) knee | | JTN | |

Result of a query that lists all consultations from the 22nd to the end of June 2015 (ConsultationsSeenFrom22ndTillEndOfJun2015)

| SurgeryDate | DateOfBirth | Sex | Diagnosis | TimeIn | TimeOut | Complaints | Treatments | Initials | Notes |
|---|---|---|---|---|---|---|---|---|---|
| 23.06.2015 | 04.12.1971 | M | | 1002 | 1010 | For X-Rays of the (R) Shoulder | | PDB | Referred to Dermatologist (Community) regarding moles on his back. |
| 23.06.2015 | 25.01.1948 | F | | 1010 | 1020 | Script for Indapamide given | | JW | |
| 23.06.2015 | 21.11.2006 | F | | 1020 | 1030 | Script for Calamine lotion & Paracetamol given | | EGH | |
| 23.06.2015 | 19.01.1965 | F | | 1030 | 1039 | BP 143/77 | | MJD | |
| 23.06.2015 | 04.11.1977 | F | | 1039 | 1050 | For Urine Pregnancy test | | KOH | |
| 23.06.2015 | 11.07.1962 | M | | 1050 | 1100 | Script for Doxazosin, Indapamide m/r & Lisinopril given | | JEG | |
| 23.06.2015 | 02.07.1943 | M | | 1100 | 1110 | Medications Review Done | | WRW | Referred to Ulcer clinic regarding ulcer on the (L) lower leg. |
| 23.06.2015 | 09.10.1926 | M | | 1110 | 1120 | Script for Mepore dressings given | | RAC | |
| 23.06.2015 | 09.05.1964 | F | | 1648 | 1658 | To see me in December for FBC & serum Ferritin | | CAC | |
| 23.06.2015 | 31.01.1969 | F | | 1658 | 1708 | Referral to General Surgeon regarding her gall bladder stone & abdominal pain | | JP | Script for Co-codamol given. |

Result of a query that lists all consultations from the 22nd to the end of June 2015 (ConsultationsSeenFrom22ndTillEndOfJun2015)

| SurgeryDate | DateOfBirth | Sex | Diagnosis | TimeIn | TimeOut | Complaints | Treatments | Initials | Notes |
|---|---|---|---|---|---|---|---|---|---|
| 23.06.2015 | 31.01.1957 | M | | 1708 | 1718 | Script for Lyrica given | | GKP | For Fasting Glucose, U/Es, FBC, LFTs & Cholesterol. |
| 23.06.2015 | 10.05.2002 | M | | 1718 | 1730 | Script for Duac Once Daily gel prescribed | | KLC | Referred to Dermatologist regarding his acne spots on the face. |
| 23.06.2015 | 14.03.1984 | F | | 1730 | 1739 | Script for Lansoprazole given | | MJW | |
| 23.06.2015 | 20.10.1955 | M | | 1739 | 1749 | To take own Paracetamol & Nurofen for the pain of his Peyronie's disease whilst waiting to contact Urologist | | FSW | |
| 23.06.2015 | 01.12.1989 | F | S/Leave | 1749 | 1803 | Med. 3 04/10 given for Vomiting in Pregnancy for 2 weeks from 23.06.15 | | PB | |
| 23.06.2015 | 18.06.1981 | M | | 1803 | 1812 | Script for Erythromycin given | | SCJ | |
| 23.06.2015 | 22.05.2015 | M | | 1812 | 1822 | Script for Nystan oral suspension & Chloramphenicol eye drops | | OSM | |
| 24.06.2015 | 19.03.1952 | M | | 944 | 956 | BP 147/85 | | RJB | |

Result of a query that lists all consultations from the 22nd to the end of June 2015 (ConsultationsSeenFrom22ndTillEndOfJun2015)

| SurgeryDate | DateOfBirth | Sex | Diagnosis | TimeIn | TimeOut | Complaints | Treatments | Initials | Notes |
|---|---|---|---|---|---|---|---|---|---|
| 24.06.2015 | 04.05.2015 | M | | 956 | 1002 | To take own Calpol & Normal Saline nasal drops | | PR | |
| 24.06.2015 | 31.12.1953 | F | | 1002 | 1011 | Script for Codeine Linctus, Doxycycline & Ranitidine given | | JWH | |
| 24.06.2015 | 10.11.1957 | F | | 1011 | 1019 | Script for Trimethoprim given | | CMH | For MSU. |
| 24.06.2015 | 29.08.1939 | M | | 1019 | 1036 | Script for Diazepam & Co-codamol given | | JFP | For Cervical spine X-Rays. |
| 24.06.2015 | 27.01.1934 | F | | 1036 | 1047 | Script for Chloramphenicol eye drops given | | JWC | For FBC, U/Es, TFTs, LFTs & Cholesterol. |
| 24.06.2015 | 25.07.1939 | F | | 1047 | 1055 | Referred to Community Diabetic specialist nurses regarding her very high HbA1c | | JLB | |
| 24.06.2015 | 31.01.1933 | M | | 1055 | 1103 | Medications Review Done | | MPB | |
| 24.06.2015 | 20.09.1934 | M | | 1103 | 1113 | Script for Doxycycline & Laxido Orange oral powder sachets given | | EWM | |
| 24.06.2015 | 07.02.1997 | M | | 1113 | 1120 | Script for Amoxycillin given | | JAW | |
| 24.06.2015 | 07.04.1922 | M | | 1307 | 1325 | Script for Zopiclone given | | JM | Home visit. |

Result of a query that lists all consultations from the 22nd to the end of June 2015 (ConsultationsSeenFrom22ndTillEndOfJun2015)

| SurgeryDate | DateOfBirth | Sex | Diagnosis | TimeIn | TimeOut | Complaints | Treatments | Initials | Notes |
|---|---|---|---|---|---|---|---|---|---|
| 24.06.2015 | 07.08.1971 | F | | 1643 | 1656 | Medications Review Done | | LPH | |
| 24.06.2015 | 25.06.1938 | F | | 1656 | 1708 | Script for Canesten 1% cream & Doxycycline given | | JEL | |
| 24.06.2015 | 13.05.1992 | F | | 1708 | 1717 | Script for Fucidin H cream given | | ZLB | For Faecal Calprotectin. |
| 24.06.2015 | 21.09.2011 | F | | 1717 | 1724 | Script for Flucloxacillin & Fucidin 2% cream given | | LAL | |
| 24.06.2015 | 11.09.1947 | M | | 1724 | 1736 | Referred to Urologist (BUPA- Mr. Lodg) regarding his phimosis which is getting worse | | TSN | |
| 24.06.2015 | 30.10.1958 | M | | 1736 | 1745 | Patient informed that he has been referred to Dr. Idre regarding problems with his eyes | | MSE | |
| 24.06.2015 | 11.08.1943 | F | | 1755 | 1805 | Script for Flucloxacillin & Acyclovir tablets given | | JMEH | |
| 24.06.2015 | 06.08.1941 | M | | 1813 | 1823 | Script for Metformin given | | AJM | |
| 25.06.2015 | 28.02.1975 | M | | 943 | 954 | Referred to Orthopaedic Surgeon (knee Surgeon) regarding the recurrent pain in his (L) knee | | SN | |

Result of a query that lists all consultations from the 22nd to the end of June 2015 (ConsultationsSeenFrom22ndTillEndOfJun2015)

| SurgeryDate | DateOfBirth | Sex | Diagnosis | TimeIn | TimeOut | Complaints | Treatments | Initials | Notes |
|---|---|---|---|---|---|---|---|---|---|
| 25.06.2015 | 06.11.1961 | F | S/Leave | 954 | 1006 | Med. 3 04/10 given for Chest Infection for 3 weeks from 22.06.15 | | BSM | Penicillin allergy. |
| 25.06.2015 | 23.01.1950 | F | | 1006 | 1018 | Script for Codeine tablets & Fenbid Forte 10% gel given | | SM | |
| 25.06.2015 | 31.12.1965 | F | | 1018 | 1028 | Script for Doxycycline & Otomize ear spray given | | BV | |
| 25.06.2015 | 25.02.1948 | M | | 1028 | 1036 | Script for Atorvastatin given | | TPB | For FBC, U/Es, LFTs, Cholesterol. |
| 25.06.2015 | 06.03.1966 | F | | 1036 | 1051 | Script for Citalopram given | | JLL | |
| 25.06.2015 | 23.05.1927 | M | | 1054 | 1114 | Script for Bactroban 2% ointment, Clarithromycin, Fenbid 5% gel & Metronidazole tablets given | | JM | For FBC, U/Es, LFTs, Cholesterol, HbA1c & Urine microalbumin screen. |
| 25.06.2015 | 02.01.2010 | M | | 1114 | 1121 | Script for Paracetamol & Calamine lotion given | | BLS | |
| 25.06.2015 | 02.08.1948 | M | | 1121 | 1129 | Script for Chloramphenicol eye drops given | | KT | |
| 25.06.2015 | 27.10.1988 | F | | 1646 | 1656 | Script for Co-Amoxiclav given | | RC | |

Result of a query that lists all consultations from the 22nd to the end of June 2015 (ConsultationsSeenFrom22ndTillEndOfJun2015)

| SurgeryDate | DateOfBirth | Sex | Diagnosis | TimeIn | TimeOut | Complaints | Treatments | Initials | Notes |
|---|---|---|---|---|---|---|---|---|---|
| 25.06.2015 | 09.08.1954 | M | | 1656 | 1706 | Quite well in himself | | TPA | |
| 25.06.2015 | 22.03.1933 | F | | 1706 | 1714 | Script for Paracetamol given | | LLW | |
| 25.06.2015 | 20.04.1982 | M | | 1714 | 1723 | Script for Acyclovir tablets given | | NAP | For FBC, U/Es, TFTs, LFTs, Fasting Glucose & Fasting Lipids. |
| 25.06.2015 | 06.04.1950 | M | | 1723 | 1733 | Script for Betamethasone cream, Co-codamol, Fenbid Forte 10% gel & Salamol inhaler given | | PAD | |
| 25.06.2015 | 30.01.1999 | F | | 1733 | 1740 | Mum says that hospital will contact her directly for the repeat echocardiogram in 5 years | | ALCJ | |
| 25.06.2015 | 19.08.1939 | F | | 1740 | 1749 | Medications Review Done | | JEN | |
| 25.06.2015 | 02.05.1959 | M | | 1749 | 1757 | For FBC, U/Es, TFTs, LFTs, Fasting Glucose & Fasting Lipids | | MGM | |
| 26.06.2015 | 18.09.1947 | M | | 944 | 955 | Script for Lansoprazole given | | RVM | Referred for Gastroscopy regarding his indigestion. |

Result of a query that lists all consultations from the 22nd to the end of June 2015 (ConsultationsSeenFrom22ndTillEndOfJun2015)

| SurgeryDate | DateOfBirth | Sex | Diagnosis | TimeIn | TimeOut | Complaints | Treatments | Initials | Notes |
|---|---|---|---|---|---|---|---|---|---|
| 26.06.2015 | 12.08.1936 | M | | 956 | 1005 | Script for Indapamide m/r given | | RHP | For MSU. |
| 26.06.2015 | 02.01.1955 | M | | 1005 | 1012 | Referred to ENT Surgeon regarding persistent problem with hearing in the (R) ear | | TRE | |
| 26.06.2015 | 23.06.1994 | M | | 1015 | 1024 | For FBC, U/Es, Bone profile, TFTs, Fasting Glucose, Fasting Lipids & LFTs | | KCDA | |
| 26.06.2015 | 29.09.2006 | M | | 1042 | 1049 | Script for Amoxycillin & Paracetamol given | | ODA | |
| 26.06.2015 | 16.04.1971 | M | | 1049 | 1056 | Reassured about the 2mm (R) epididymal simple cyst seen on the USScan | | DO | |
| 26.06.2015 | 04.08.1936 | M | | 1056 | 1120 | Script for Praxilene & Ferrous Fumarate given | | ECM | |
| 29.06.2015 | 14.11.1949 | F | | 942 | 954 | Referred to Gynaecologist regarding recurrent vulvar-vaginal irritation | | CBL | |
| 29.06.2015 | 09.10.1926 | M | | 954 | 1004 | Script for Clarithromycin & Metronidazole given | | RAC | |

Result of a query that lists all consultations from the 22nd to the end of June 2015 (ConsultationsSeenFrom22ndTillEndOfJun2015)

| SurgeryDate | DateOfBirth | Sex | Diagnosis | TimeIn | TimeOut | Complaints | Treatments | Initials | Notes |
|---|---|---|---|---|---|---|---|---|---|
| 29.06.2015 | 09.08.1987 | F |  | 1010 | 1022 | Script for Laxido Orange oral powder sachets & Fluconazole given |  | RJM | Penicillin allergy. |
| 29.06.2015 | 17.04.1930 | M |  | 1022 | 1030 | Script for Ferrous Fumarate given |  | FL |  |
| 29.06.2015 | 03.10.1941 | M |  | 1030 | 1043 | Script for Laxido Orange oral powder sachets & Prochlorperazine given |  | JJD |  |
| 29.06.2015 | 12.09.1986 | F |  | 1103 | 1120 | Script for Scheriproct ointment suppositories given |  | OK | Routine 6 weeks post-natal check done. |
| 29.06.2015 | 20.04.1938 | M |  | 1639 | 1656 | Referred to Memory clinic regarding his worsening memory problem |  | DAD |  |
| 29.06.2015 | 03.12.1955 | F |  | 1656 | 1703 | She will observe the pain in her (L) fore-arm for now |  | CAD |  |
| 29.06.2015 | 24.04.1966 | M |  | 1703 | 1712 | Script for Lansoprazole given |  | BSE |  |
| 29.06.2015 | 16.03.1956 | F |  | 1712 | 1723 | Script for Canesten HC cream given |  | SPD | Referred to ENT Surgeon regarding her epistaxes due & due to her intranasal septal defect. |

Result of a query that lists all consultations from the 22$^{nd}$ to the end of June 2015 (ConsultationsSeenFrom22ndTillEndOfJun2015)

| SurgeryDate | DateOfBirth | Sex | Diagnosis | TimeIn | TimeOut | Complaints | Treatments | Initials | Notes |
|---|---|---|---|---|---|---|---|---|---|
| 29.06.2015 | 07.02.2011 | M | | 1723 | 1733 | Script for | | NDM | Referred to Paediatrician regarding the persistent pain in his ankles. |
| 29.06.2015 | 08.09.1957 | M | | 1733 | 1745 | We will try to get the bone scan result from Princess Alexandra Hospital Harlow | | TJG | |
| 29.06.2015 | 10.09.1962 | F | | 1745 | 1752 | Referred for Colonoscopy regarding her changing bowel habits | | PL | |
| 29.06.2015 | 03.12.1960 | M | | 1756 | 1806 | Script for Co-Amoxiclav & Otomize ear spray given | | GTR | |

# RESULTS OF QUERIES THAT LIST ALL CONSULTATIONS FROM THE 22ND TO THE END OF JULY 1997 TO JULY 2015

Result of a query that lists all consultations from the 22nd to the end of July 1997 (ConsultationsSeenFrom22ndTillEndOfJul1997)

| SurgeryDate | DateOfBirth | Sex | Diagnosis | TimeIn | TimeOut | Complaints | Treatments | NumbersID | Notes |
|---|---|---|---|---|---|---|---|---|---|
| 31.07.97 | 20.07.56 | M | URTI | 1819 | 1823 | Sore throat | Amoxycillin | 1126 | He also has stye in the (L) eye, Rx. Chloramphenicol eye ointment. |
| 28.07.97 | 10.02.41 | M | Lump | 936 | 943 | Skin fibroma (R) buttock | For excision | 1158 | |
| 22.07.97 | 19.06.59 | M | S/Leave | 1728 | 1731 | Anxiety state | | 1191 | |
| 25.07.97 | 04.09.67 | M | Pain | 910 | 915 | Lower abdominal pain | Buscopan | 1429 | He is also constipated, Rx. Senna tablets. |
| 31.07.97 | 13.09.48 | F | | 1759 | 1806 | Dry hands, on Thyroxine | For TFTs & FBC | 1577 | She also has heavy periods over the past 3 months. |
| 26.07.97 | 27.02.39 | M | | 1035 | 1041 | On too much Diuretics | To leave off Frumil & continue only with the Frusemide | 1666 | |
| 26.07.97 | 16.10.42 | F | Rash | 1030 | 1034 | Itchy rash in groins | Canesten-H cream | 1667 | |
| 25.07.97 | 05.06.47 | M | S/Leave | 1736 | 1740 | (L) middle finger amputation | | 1770 | |
| 31.07.97 | 07.08.85 | M | Revisit | 916 | 926 | Chesty cough again | Augmentin-Duo | 191 | |
| 25.07.97 | 22.10.66 | M | S/Leave | 1809 | 1817 | (R) testicular cancer -Med 5 | | 1990 | |
| 29.07.97 | 12.09.42 | F | Rash | 1644 | 1652 | Lichen planus rash | To Dermatologist | 20 | She wants to be referred to the Dermatologist. |

Result of a query that lists all consultations from the 22nd to the end of July 1997 (ConsultationsSeenFrom22ndTillEndOfJul1997)

| SurgeryDate | DateOfBirth | Sex | Diagnosis | TimeIn | TimeOut | Complaints | Treatments | NumbersID | Notes |
|---|---|---|---|---|---|---|---|---|---|
| 29.07.97 | 05.09.33 | F | Rash | 1755 | 1800 | Itchy red rash on face | Tetracycline & Zirtek | 2007 | Penicillin allergy. |
| 22.07.97 | 13.12.06 | F | | 1855 | 1915 | Giddiness & vomiting | Buccastem & Rehidrat | 2039 | Home visit. |
| 22.07.97 | 11.02.45 | F | UTI | 1803 | 1808 | Dysuria | Trimethoprim | 2112 | For MSU. |
| 29.07.97 | 11.02.45 | F | | 1712 | 1722 | For repeat MSU in one week | | 2112 | |
| 28.07.97 | 01.04.22 | M | Pain | 1725 | 1732 | Stomach pain | Omeprazole & Buscopan | 2127 | Letter to Gastroenterologist. |
| 28.07.97 | 21.11.88 | F | Revisit | 1711 | 1718 | D&V persists | To Paediatrician | 2507 | |
| 22.07.97 | 07.09.50 | F | | 902 | 907 | For repeat FBC & ESR in 3/12 | | 2528 | |
| 29.07.97 | 27.01.74 | F | | 932 | 946 | Infected burn to back | Erymax & Flamazine | 2590 | Penicillin allergy. FP1001 (GMS4) form signed. |
| 28.07.97 | 08.06.84 | M | | 1014 | 1018 | Tiredness | For FBC | 2670 | His dad wants him checked for anaemia. |
| 23.07.97 | 13.12.89 | M | | 938 | 952 | Penile discharge | Amoxycillin | 2713 | Penile discharge for C&S. Eczema rash around the mouth, Rx. Aqueous cream. |
| 22.07.97 | 26.03.65 | F | Pain | 1748 | 1756 | Painful perineum | Paracetamol | 2714 | |
| 25.07.97 | 27.01.86 | M | Rash | 1713 | 1718 | Itchy rash all over | Zirtek & Calamine lotion | 2717 | |

Result of a query that lists all consultations from the 22nd to the end of July 1997 (ConsultationsSeenFrom22ndTillEndOfJul1997)

| SurgeryDate | DateOfBirth | Sex | Diagnosis | TimeIn | TimeOut | Complaints | Treatments | NumbersID | Notes |
|---|---|---|---|---|---|---|---|---|---|
| 25.07.97 | 23.02.45 | M |  | 1701 | 1708 | BM stix high | For FBC, U/Es, Glucose & HBA1c | 2750 | He also has ?balanitis, Rx. Amoxycillin. |
| 31.07.97 | 27.11.47 | F | Pain | 1726 | 1733 | Pain (R) arm following RTA | Co-dydramol & Movelat gel | 2831 |  |
| 31.07.97 | 22.12.79 | F | Thrush | 1807 | 1811 | Itchy vaginal discharge | Canesten pessary | 2851 |  |
| 22.07.97 | 27.06.59 | F |  | 922 | 938 | Loestrin 20 script |  | 2869 | FP1001 (GMS4) form signed. |
| 22.07.97 | 21.09.19 | M |  | 1020 | 1036 | Infected sebaceous cyst (L) abdomen | Flucloxacillin | 2917 |  |
| 28.07.97 | 22.07.87 | F | URTI | 1733 | 1741 | Sore throat | Augmentin-Duo & Junifen | 293 |  |
| 22.07.97 | 25.07.38 | F | S/Leave | 957 | 1004 | Cancer of the bowel, anterior resection |  | 2964 | She also has warty lesions on her (L) arm & (L) leg, getting bigger. Referred to Dermatologist. |
| 25.07.97 | 29.08.58 | F | Rash | 1719 | 1722 | Itchy rash all over | Zirtek | 2991 |  |
| 30.07.97 | 15.02.32 | F | Pain | 906 | 921 | Abdominal pain | Omeprazole | 3043 | Repeat script for Lentizol. |
| 22.07.97 | 01.03.34 | F | Pain | 1048 | 1053 | (L) abdominal pain | Co-dydramol | 3114 |  |
| 25.07.97 | 10.02.83 | F | URTI | 1750 | 1755 | Sore throat | Erymax | 3150 | Piriton also prescribed. |
| 28.07.97 | 22.02.91 | M |  | 1034 | 1037 | Buzzing in the ears | To use own Olive oil | 3196 |  |

## Result of a query that lists all consultations from the 22nd to the end of July 1997 (ConsultationsSeenFrom22ndTillEndOfJul1997)

| SurgeryDate | DateOfBirth | Sex | Diagnosis | TimeIn | TimeOut | Complaints | Treatments | NumbersID | Notes |
|---|---|---|---|---|---|---|---|---|---|
| 31.07.97 | 17.07.42 | M | S/Leave | 939 | 952 | Back pain | | 3244 | Meptazinol script also given. |
| 31.07.97 | 20.08.31 | F | URTI | 927 | 930 | Sore throat | Suprax | 3266 | Patient prefers Suprax. |
| 22.07.97 | 10.12.30 | M | | 908 | 914 | Squamous carcinoma, fore arm lesion | To Dermatologist | 328 | |
| 30.07.97 | 26.03.58 | F | | 922 | 929 | Infected insect bite on leg | Flucloxacillin & Zirtek | 335 | |
| 26.07.97 | 01.07.79 | M | | 1009 | 1014 | Passing blood PR & diarrhoea | For FBC | 3369 | Stool for C&S. |
| 29.07.97 | 07.10.46 | M | S/Leave | 903 | 913 | Burn to (L) hand & (L) wrist | | 339 | |
| 23.07.97 | 19.07.52 | M | RTI | 918 | 922 | Cough | Amoxycillin | 3430 | |
| 25.07.97 | 05.12.64 | M | RTI | 1832 | 8137 | Cough | Amoxycillin | 3450 | Clarityn also prescribed. |
| 29.07.97 | 09.04.80 | M | | 1749 | 1754 | Drill went through (R) middle finger | Augmentin | 3518 | Advised to go to A/E. |
| 28.07.97 | 23.03.67 | F | URTI | 1830 | 1835 | Sore throat | Penicillin V | 3529 | She also feels tired & drained. For FBC & TFTs. |
| 22.07.97 | 08.04.71 | F | URTI | 939 | 947 | Sore throat | Penicillin V | 3633 | Cilest script also given. FP1001 (GMS4) form signed. |
| 28.07.97 | 14.02.24 | M | Pain | 1704 | 1710 | Headaches again | To Neurologist at Basildon | 3718 | |
| 24.07.97 | 08.01.22 | M | RTI | 957 | 1006 | Cough | Ciprofloxacin | 373 | |

Result of a query that lists all consultations from the 22$^{nd}$ to the end of July 1997 (ConsultationsSeenFrom22ndTillEndOfJul1997)

| SurgeryDate | DateOfBirth | Sex | Diagnosis | TimeIn | TimeOut | Complaints | Treatments | NumbersID | Notes |
|---|---|---|---|---|---|---|---|---|---|
| 24.07.97 | 02.11.20 | F | | 1007 | 1020 | To reduce Amiriptyline dose | | 3789 | |
| 28.07.97 | 02.08.63 | F | | 1200 | 1215 | Routine P/Natal visit | | 3796 | Home visit. |
| 24.07.97 | 17.03.57 | F | | 1714 | 1735 | Wife takes alcohol ++ | To contact Alcoholic anonymous/Open door Benfleet | 3873 | She is denying this & not interested in any help. Husband came to surgery. |
| 23.07.97 | 31.01.93 | M | | 1024 | 1036 | Pre-School Health Examination | | 3879 | (L) testicle undescended, for review in 3/12. |
| 22.07.97 | 21.05.71 | F | Pain | 1756 | 1802 | Pain (R) knee | For X-Ray (R) knee | 39 | FP1001 (GMS4) form signed. |
| 22.07.97 | 21.05.74 | M | | 1823 | 1823 | DNA | | 3911 | |
| 29.07.97 | 18.01.67 | M | | 1732 | 1742 | ?Verruca (R) sole of foot, infected | Salactol & Flucloxacillin | 3942 | |
| 30.07.97 | 02.02.93 | F | | 930 | 938 | Pre-School Health Examination | | 3973 | |
| 25.07.97 | 03.08.92 | M | URTI | 1827 | 1831 | Sore throat | Penicillin V | 3989 | |
| 25.07.97 | 06.09.64 | F | | 1818 | 1826 | Toe nails infection | Sporanox pulse | 3991 | To see Chiropodist. |
| 31.07.97 | 06.05.93 | F | | 1722 | 1725 | Nightmares following RTA | To observe | 4040 | |
| 31.07.97 | 29.01.73 | F | Pain | 1734 | 1739 | Back pain following RTA | Co-dydramol | 4063 | |
| 28.07.97 | 22.03.91 | M | | 1108 | 1113 | Infected insect bites on arm | Clariryn & Flucloxacillin | 4190 | |
| 29.07.97 | 16.11.65 | F | Pain | 1723 | 1731 | Pain (L) labium majus | To use own Paracetamol | 427 | 11 weeks gestation. |

Result of a query that lists all consultations from the 22nd to the end of July 1997 (ConsultationsSeenFrom22ndTillEndOfJul1997)

| SurgeryDate | DateOfBirth | Sex | Diagnosis | TimeIn | TimeOut | Complaints | Treatments | NumbersID | Notes |
|---|---|---|---|---|---|---|---|---|---|
| 25.07.97 | 16.06.55 | F | S/Leave | 1654 | 1700 | Chronic idiopathic fatigue syndrome & Migraine - Med 4 | | 4284 | |
| 24.07.97 | 31.05.86 | F | | 1021 | 1031 | Worms | Vermox | 4369 | |
| 25.07.97 | 01.08.59 | F | | 925 | 945 | Came to discuss triple test result - normal | | 4423 | |
| 25.07.97 | 16.04.94 | M | URTI | 1011 | 1021 | (L) ear ache | Amoxycillin & Junifen | 44409 | |
| 28.07.97 | 08.04.44 | F | Pain | 1742 | 1746 | Low back pain | Co-dydramol | 4465 | |
| 25.07.97 | 10.04.71 | F | | 1000 | 1010 | No periods yet | For Pregnancy test | 4601 | 11 weeks post-natal. |
| 29.07.97 | 30.03.63 | F | Pain | 947 | 957 | Back pain | Kapake | 4622 | |
| 29.07.97 | 12.10.57 | F | RTI | 1743 | 1747 | Cough | Erymax | 4630 | Penicillin allergy. FP1001 (GMS4) form signed. |
| 22.07.97 | 26.01.69 | M | S/Leave | 1037 | 1047 | Kidney infection | | 4646 | |
| 25.07.97 | 06.12.66 | F | RTI | 1642 | 1645 | Cough | Amoxycillin | 4679 | |
| 24.07.97 | 04.10.34 | M | S/Leave | 1709 | 1713 | Pneumonia | | 4720 | |
| 31.07.97 | 04.10.34 | M | S/Leave | 1658 | 1702 | Pneumonia | | 4720 | |
| 24.07.97 | 04.04.82 | M | URTI | 1657 | 1707 | Sore throat | Penicillin V | 4722 | His nasal discharge is worse, letter to ENT Surgeon to bring operation date forward. |

Result of a query that lists all consultations from the 22nd to the end of July 1997 (ConsultationsSeenFrom22ndTillEndOfJul1997)

| SurgeryDate | DateOfBirth | Sex | Diagnosis | TimeIn | TimeOut | Complaints | Treatments | NumbersID | Notes |
|---|---|---|---|---|---|---|---|---|---|
| 24.07.97 | 02.07.11 | F | RTI | 1032 | 1053 | Cough | Erymax | 4727 | Penicillin allergy. She also has epistaxes, Rx. Zestril & Bactroban. For FBC & U/Es. |
| 30.07.97 | 24.10.74 | F | | 1026 | 1030 | Microgynon script | | 4738 | |
| 24.07.97 | 09.10.32 | F | URTI | 913 | 916 | Sore throat | Penicillin V | 4756 | |
| 29.07.97 | 29.08.29 | F | | 1135 | 1205 | Routine home visit | | 4775 | Home visit. |
| 29.07.97 | 15.04.21 | M | | 1205 | 1220 | Routine home visit | | 4793 | Home visit. |
| 29.07.97 | 28.02.27 | M | Revisit | 921 | 928 | Tinnitus is no better | Dose of Serc is to be increased | 4838 | |
| 23.07.97 | 09.07.95 | M | Pain | 1038 | 1046 | Fell & banged head | Paracetamol | 4924 | Advised to go to A/E. |
| 22.07.97 | 12.06.63 | F | | 1731 | 1735 | Assaulted by her own husband | To use own Paracetamol | 4953 | |
| 31.07.97 | 08.11.47 | M | | 1648 | 1657 | Palpitations over the past 7 months | To Cardiologist | 4955 | For FBC, U/Es & TFTs. |
| 29.07.97 | 15.03.33 | F | Rash | 1705 | 1711 | Infected insect bite (L) lower leg | Flucloxacillin & Clarityn | 4971 | |
| 22.07.97 | 05.10.60 | F | Pain | 948 | 956 | Back pain | Co-dydramol & Transvasin cream | 4978 | |
| 22.07.97 | 03.08.57 | F | | 1634 | 1648 | Warfarin & Sanomigran script | | 5009 | |
| 22.07.97 | 15.06.88 | M | RTI | 1649 | 1653 | Cough | Amoxycillin | 5012 | |
| 25.07.97 | 16.03.78 | M | | 1757 | 1808 | Nail puncure (L) palm | Erymax | 5202 | ATT booster given. Advised to go to A/E. |

Result of a query that lists all consultations from the 22nd to the end of July 1997 (ConsultationsSeenFrom22ndTillEndOfJul1997)

| SurgeryDate | DateOfBirth | Sex | Diagnosis | TimeIn | TimeOut | Complaints | Treatments | NumbersID | Notes |
|---|---|---|---|---|---|---|---|---|---|
| 24.07.97 | 17.04.45 | F | | 1705 | 1709 | Epistaxes again | Naseptin cream | 5207 | |
| 22.07.97 | 29.08.76 | M | URTI | 1711 | 1718 | Sore throat | Erymax | 522 | Penicillin allergy. For FBC. |
| 22.07.97 | 11.11.59 | F | | 1700 | 1704 | Painful piles | Proctosedyl suppositories | 5252 | |
| 28.07.97 | 11.11.59 | F | S/Leave | 1644 | 1649 | Painful haemorrhoids | | 5252 | |
| 29.07.97 | 24.11.20 | F | | 1532 | 1644 | (R) leg swollen | Augmentin & Frusemide | 5256 | |
| 28.07.97 | 26.12.79 | F | Rash | 1807 | 1819 | Warts on arm | Salactol gel | 5270 | She also has acne on her back, Rx. Acne gel. |
| 23.07.97 | 11.11.30 | F | | 913 | 917 | Dizziness & vertigo | Stemetil | 5275 | |
| 28.07.97 | 11.10.58 | F | | 1803 | 1806 | Late period | For Pregnancy test | 5283 | |
| 31.07.97 | 11.10.58 | F | | 1747 | 1758 | Positive pregnancy test | | 5283 | |
| 25.07.97 | 04.12.57 | F | Pain | 1635 | 1641 | Back pain | Physiotherapy | 5288 | |
| 30.07.97 | 30.07.97 | F | URTI | 1019 | 1026 | Fever | Amoxycillin & Paracetamol | 5289 | |
| 31.07.97 | 25.05.96 | F | Revisit | 1510 | 1520 | Fever & Rash | Junifen | 5289 | To continue antibiotics & Paracetamol. Home visit. |

Result of a query that lists all consultations from the 22nd to the end of July 1997 (ConsultationsSeenFrom22ndTillEndOfJul1997)

| SurgeryDate | DateOfBirth | Sex | Diagnosis | TimeIn | TimeOut | Complaints | Treatments | NumbersID | Notes |
|---|---|---|---|---|---|---|---|---|---|
| 31.07.97 | 01.06.93 | M | URTI | 953 | 1003 | Stye (L) upper eye lid | Fucithalmic eye droops | 5318 | He also has sore throat, Rx. Augmentin-Duo. He also has enlarged tonsils & frequent sore throats, hence referred to ENT Surgeon. |
| 24.07.97 | 07.04.66 | M | | 1746 | 1758 | Abscess anterior abdominal wall | Flucloxacillin & Amoxycillin | 5346 | Fucidin also prescribed. |
| 31.07.97 | 30.06.73 | M | S/Leave | 1812 | 1815 | Fracture shaft of (R) Tibia | | 5408 | |
| 23.07.97 | 18.04.63 | F | Pain | 1005 | 1013 | Pain & heaviness (L) side of the fore-head | Co-dydramol | 5415 | ESR requested. Migraine pink also prescribed. |
| 25.07.97 | 18.04.63 | F | Revisit | 1838 | 1846 | Still has pain (L) fore-head | To Neurologist | 5415 | |
| 28.07.97 | 14.10.53 | M | Rash | 1000 | 1010 | Itchy rash on foot | Canesten HC cream | 5452 | 1% OH Cortisone cream & Rhinocort nasal spray also prescribed. |
| 31.07.97 | 02.12.93 | M | Revisit | 931 | 937 | Itchy rash on back of leg is no better | Canesten-HC cream & Aqueous cream | 5569 | |
| 24.07.97 | 26.08.25 | M | Pain | 1637 | 1643 | Hip pain | Co-dydramol & Senna tablets | 5581 | On waiting list for hip operation. |
| 31.07.97 | 07.07.59 | M | | 1632 | 1638 | Bendrofluazide script | | 5584 | |

Result of a query that lists all consultations from the 22nd to the end of July 1997 (ConsultationsSeenFrom22ndTillEndOfJul1997)

| SurgeryDate | DateOfBirth | Sex | Diagnosis | TimeIn | TimeOut | Complaints | Treatments | NumbersID | Notes |
|---|---|---|---|---|---|---|---|---|---|
| 28.07.97 | 27.12.59 | F | URTI | 1650 | 1703 | Sore throat | Cephalexin | 5609 | Penicillin allergy. |
| 28.07.97 | 05.10.36 | M | RTI | 1719 | 1724 | Recurrent cough | Augmentin | 5653 | For CXR. |
| 26.07.97 | 01.07.97 | F | | 1022 | 1028 | Sniffly | To give fluids | 5656 | |
| 26.07.97 | 14.05.80 | F | | 1120 | 1127 | Corneal abrasion (R) eye | Chloramphenicol eye ointment | 571 | |
| 24.07.97 | 26.08.49 | F | S/Leave | 930 | 943 | Thrombosis (R) leg | | 610 | |
| 25.07.97 | 20.09.28 | F | URTI | 903 | 909 | Sore throat | Penicillin V | 663 | |
| 31.07.97 | 24.04.66 | M | | 1703 | 1722 | Frusemide & Senna tablets script | | 669 | |
| 22.07.97 | 27.02.41 | M | RTI | 1810 | 1813 | Cough | Ciprofloxacin | 675 | |
| 22.07.97 | 24.03.60 | M | URTI | 1813 | 1816 | Sore throat | Penicillin V | 675 | |
| 26.07.97 | 28.08.64 | M | Rash | 1153 | 1200 | Fungal scalp rash | Nizoral shampoo | 846 | |
| 30.07.97 | 20.09.45 | M | Revisit | 1004 | 1010 | Tickly cough again | Augmentin | 89 | Snores a lot, sleeps with his mouth open. Referred to ENT Surgeon. |
| 29.07.97 | 15.03.75 | F | | 1659 | 1704 | (R) peri-orbital oedema | Zirtek & Fucithalmic eye drops | 934 | |
| 28.07.97 | 06.04.37 | M | Lump | 908 | 915 | Lipoma (R) side of face | To Surgeon at Basildon Hosp | 988 | |
| 31.07.97 | 26.10.62 | M | Rash | 1639 | 1647 | Red rash on arms & legs | Tetracycline & Fucidin cream | NP | |
| 24.07.97 | 14.08.96 | M | URTI | 906 | 912 | (R) ear infection | Amoxycillin & Paracetamol | Temp | |
| 29.07.97 | 02.12.58 | F | | 1033 | 1040 | Infected wound (R) middle finger | Flucloxacillin | Temp | Tetanus toxoid booster given. |

Result of a query that lists all consultations from the 22nd to the end of July 1997 (ConsultationsSeenFrom22ndTillEndOfJul1997)

| SurgeryDate | DateOfBirth | Sex | Diagnosis | TimeIn | TimeOut | Complaints | Treatments | NumbersID | Notes |
|---|---|---|---|---|---|---|---|---|---|
| 29.07.97 | 20.12.78 | F | | 1040 | 1044 | Ventolin & Becotide inhalers script given | | Temp | |
| 30.07.97 | 14.02.60 | F | | 1030 | 1033 | Urticarial rash | Zirtek & Calamine lotion | Temp | |

Result of a query that lists all consultations from the 22nd to the end of July 1998 (ConsultationsSeenFrom22ndTillEndOfJul1998)

| SurgeryDate | DateOfBirth | Sex | Diagnosis | TimeIn | TimeOut | Complaints | Treatments | NumbersID | Notes |
|---|---|---|---|---|---|---|---|---|---|
| 22.07.98 | 20.09.84 | F | Rash | 1112 | 1115 | Itchy rash on abdomen | Canesten-HC cream | Temp | |
| 23.07.98 | 28.04.73 | F | | 1725 | 1730 | Script for Human Insulartard penfil & Human Actrapid penfil | | Temp | |
| 23.07.98 | 19.06.75 | F | URTI | 1753 | 1805 | Bunged up & fever | Amoxycillin | Temp | Microgynon 30 script also given. |
| 24.07.98 | 04.06.69 | F | | 1819 | 1931 | Pregnancy test positive | | NP | |
| 25.07.98 | 25.09.64 | F | | 1035 | 1045 | Abdominal pain | Colpermin & Buscopan | Temp | |
| 28.07.98 | 06.10.66 | F | | 1635 | 1644 | Late period | For Pregnancy test | Temp | |
| 27.07.98 | 23.09.54 | M | | 908 | 916 | Prozac script | | 1017 | |
| 22.07.98 | 16.03.47 | F | | 1745 | 1755 | CXR - (L) basal effusion | For repeat CXR in 6 months | 107 | |

Result of a query that lists all consultations from the 22nd to the end of July 1998 (ConsultationsSeenFrom22ndTillEndOfJul1998)

| SurgeryDate | DateOfBirth | Sex | Diagnosis | TimeIn | TimeOut | Complaints | Treatments | NumbersID | Notes |
|---|---|---|---|---|---|---|---|---|---|
| 23.07.98 | 25.09.30 | M | RTI | 931 | 942 | Cough | Amoxycillin | 122 | New patient check done. BP 180/120. For FBC, U/Es, LFTs & Cholesterol. |
| 28.07.98 | 22.08.63 | M | | 905 | 920 | Blistery rash on his (R) foot | Fucidin-H cream & Oxytetracycline | 1370 | New patient check done. |
| 28.07.98 | 08.02.74 | F | | 1821 | 1830 | D&V | Electrolade | 1469 | New patient check done. Stool sent for C&S. |
| 27.07.98 | 09.03.47 | F | | 1741 | 1746 | Imigran script given | | 1500 | New patient check done. |
| 22.07.98 | 25.05.79 | F | S/leave | 1043 | 1050 | Chest pain - Med 5 | | 152 | She also has vomiting, Rx. Metoclopramide. |
| 27.07.98 | 25.05.79 | F | S/leave | 954 | 957 | Chest pain | | 152 | |
| 22.07.98 | 14.12.24 | M | Revisit | 1725 | 1730 | Still chesty | Co-Amoxiclav | 1586 | |
| 22.07.98 | 06.04.37 | F | S/leave | 904 | 914 | Shingles | | 1604 | |
| 23.07.98 | 03.05.51 | F | | 1044 | 1054 | Swollen upper lip | Telfast & Oxytetracycline | 162 | New patient check done. |
| 22.07.98 | 22.01.57 | M | | 1720 | 1725 | Palpitations | Referred to Cardiologist | 1672 | New patient check done. For FBC & TFTs. |
| 23.07.98 | 19.11.53 | M | | 926 | 931 | Wax in both ears | Cerumol ear drops | 1729 | New patient check done. For ear syringing. |

Result of a query that lists all consultations from the 22nd to the end of July 1998 (ConsultationsSeenFrom22ndTillEndOfJul1998)

| SurgeryDate | DateOfBirth | Sex | Diagnosis | TimeIn | TimeOut | Complaints | Treatments | NumbersID | Notes |
|---|---|---|---|---|---|---|---|---|---|
| 27.07.98 | 30.04.17 | M | Pain | 936 | 945 | Pain & swelling (R) ankle | Diclofenac enteric coated & Flucloxacillin | 1733 | New patient check done. |
| 23.07.98 | 30.10.35 | M |  | 1745 | 1753 | (R) jaw clicks | Paracetamol | 1790 |  |
| 23.07.98 | 30.08.66 | M |  | 1809 | 1816 | To come back for ear syringing |  | 1804 |  |
| 28.07.98 | 20.09.46 | F |  | 1747 | 1756 | ?Rheumatoid Arthritis | For RA-Latex test | 1973 |  |
| 22.07.98 | 21.11.54 | M |  | 1810 | 1814 | Still getting coughing fits | Co-Amoxiclav | 2018 |  |
| 23.07.98 | 11.04.30 | F | Pain | 900 | 915 | Pain (R) knee | Co-Proxamol & Inj. Depo-Medrone with Lidocaine | 2113 | New patient check done. |
| 22.07.98 | 25.04.62 | M | Revisit | 920 | 929 | His hay fever is still quite bad | Inj. Kenalog | 2142 | He is already on Loratadine. |
| 22.07.98 | 22.03.33 | F | Pain | 1707 | 1715 | Pain at the back of the neck & dizziness | Ibuprofen & Stemetil | 2179 | New patient check done. For FBC. |
| 24.07.98 | 17.02.22 | F |  | 1746 | 1755 | ROC cream script given |  | 2285 | New patient check done. |
| 27.07.98 | 28.12.62 | M | Rash | 1648 | 1658 | Itchy red rash on (R) leg | Flucloxacillin & Telfast | 2354 | New patient check done. |
| 24.07.98 | 02.12.48 | M |  | 900 | 913 | Hypercholesterolaemia | Atorvastatin | 2380 |  |
| 28.07.98 | 01.10.20 | M | Pain | 1700 | 1705 | Pain (R) foot | For X-Ray (R) foot | 2463 |  |
| 28.07.98 | 07.09.80 | F |  | 942 | 946 | Microgynon-30 script given |  | 2577 | New patient check done. |

Result of a query that lists all consultations from the 22nd to the end of July 1998 (ConsultationsSeenFrom22ndTillEndOfJul1998)

| SurgeryDate | DateOfBirth | Sex | Diagnosis | TimeIn | TimeOut | Complaints | Treatments | NumbersID | Notes |
|---|---|---|---|---|---|---|---|---|---|
| 28.07.98 | 07.02.76 | M | Lump | 1815 | 1821 | Cystic lump in (L) buttock close to the midline | Referred to Surgeon | 2592 | New patient check done. |
| 22.07.98 | 06.01.93 | F | Revisit | 1633 | 1646 | Still has back pain | Zydol SR & Diclofenac SR | 2642 | She also has hypertension, BP 220/130. Rx. Atenolol & Adalat LA 30. |
| 24.07.98 | 06.01.43 | F | S/leave | 1015 | 1030 | Back pain | | 2642 | Referred to Orthopaedic Surgeon (Basildon) - BUPA. |
| 27.07.98 | 30.01.46 | F | URTI | 1030 | 1045 | Sore throat | Amoxycillin | 290 | New patient check done. |
| 22.07.98 | 18.10.87 | F | Pain | 1034 | 1043 | Abdominal pain | Lactulose | 2960 | She also has vomiting, Rx. Metoclopramide. New patient check done. |
| 22.07.98 | 06.04.68 | M | URTI | 1734 | 1739 | Sore throat | Amoxycillin & Co-dydramol | 3088 | New patient check done. |
| 22.07.98 | 13.11.53 | M | S/leave | 1715 | 1720 | Back pain | | 3119 | New patient check done. |
| 27.07.98 | 01.11.59 | M | S/leave | 1729 | 1734 | (R) Myringoplasty | | 3179 | New patient check done. |
| 22.07.98 | 30.04.85 | M | Rash | 1803 | 1810 | ?Viral rash, itchy | Clarityn | 318 | New patient check done. |
| 27.07.98 | 15.04.29 | M | | 1746 | 1755 | Doralese script | | 327 | New patient check done. |

Result of a query that lists all consultations from the 22nd to the end of July 1998 (ConsultationsSeenFrom22ndTillEndOfJul1998)

| SurgeryDate | DateOfBirth | Sex | Diagnosis | TimeIn | TimeOut | Complaints | Treatments | NumbersID | Notes |
|---|---|---|---|---|---|---|---|---|---|
| 28.07.98 | 30.03.62 | M | | 1713 | 1721 | H. pylori positive | Amoxycillin, Metronidazole & Omeprazole | 3281 | |
| 22.07.98 | 30.09.61 | F | Pain | 939 | 955 | Pain (R) wrist | Co-dydramol & Transvasin cream | 3397 | New patient check done. FP1001 (GMS4) form signed. She is worried about the moles on her back and her shoulder, referred to Dermatologist - BUPA. |
| 23.07.98 | 12.04.68 | F | | 1245 | 1255 | Routine P/Natal visit | | 3454 | |
| 27.07.98 | 12.04.68 | F | | 1315 | 1320 | Routine P/Natal check | | 3454 | |
| 28.07.98 | 19.06.43 | M | | 946 | 952 | BP 160/100 | | 3487 | |
| 27.07.98 | 26.08.67 | F | | 1635 | 1640 | (L) ear is blocked & sore | Amoxycillin & Otomize spray | 3497 | New patient check done. |
| 27.07.98 | 03.12.44 | F | RTI | 1734 | 1741 | Cough | Ciprofloxacin | 3509 | She also has dizziness & insomnia, Rx. Stemetil & Zopiclone. |
| 24.07.98 | 09.10.48 | F | | 1831 | 1840 | New patient check done. | | 3511 | |
| 24.07.98 | 14.12.38 | F | | 952 | 1003 | Worried about the moles on her abdomen | Referred to Dermatologist | 36 | New patient check done. Tetanus Booster given. |

## Result of a query that lists all consultations from the 22nd to the end of July 1998 (ConsultationsSeenFrom22ndTillEndOfJul1998)

| SurgeryDate | DateOfBirth | Sex | Diagnosis | TimeIn | TimeOut | Complaints | Treatments | NumbersID | Notes |
|---|---|---|---|---|---|---|---|---|---|
| 22.07.98 | 02.05.92 | M | URTI | 1030 | 1034 | Sore throat | Amoxycillin & Paracetamol | 3606 | |
| 22.07.98 | 04.11.66 | F | URTI | 1814 | 1830 | Sore throat | Co-Amoxiclav | 3632 | New patient check done. She had a contact with a man whose son was diagnosed as having meningococcal meningitis 4 days ago, Rifampicin. |
| 24.07.98 | 07.05.61 | F | Pain | 1755 | 1800 | Pain (R) hand | Co-dydramol & Transvasin cream | 3653 | |
| 27.07.98 | 13.07.14 | M | | 1052 | 1102 | (L) leg painful & chesty | Amoxycillin, Salbutamol inhaler & Co-dydramol | 3714 | |
| 27.07.98 | 17.09.26 | F | | 1658 | 1705 | Infection (L) Lacrimal sac | Flucloxacillin & Fucithalmic eye drops | 3719 | New patient check done. |
| 23.07.98 | 07.07.61 | F | Pain | 1111 | 1116 | Pain (R) upper gum | Erythromycin | 3768 | Penicillin allergy. |
| 22.07.98 | 19.03.15 | F | | 1050 | 1112 | Repeat script for Atenolol, Temazepam, Ismo Retard, Co-codamol & Betahistine | | 3888 | |
| 27.07.98 | 04.09.85 | M | Revisit | 1630 | 1635 | Rash on finger is still bad | Fucibet cream | 3959 | |
| 27.07.98 | 14.05.23 | M | Pain | 1000 | 1006 | (R) Otitis ext. | Otomize spray | 4031 | |

## Result of a query that lists all consultations from the 22nd to the end of July 1998 (ConsultationsSeenFrom22ndTillEndOfJul1998)

| SurgeryDate | DateOfBirth | Sex | Diagnosis | TimeIn | TimeOut | Complaints | Treatments | NumbersID | Notes |
|---|---|---|---|---|---|---|---|---|---|
| 22.07.98 | 03.07.93 | M | | 1755 | 1803 | Burns (L) leg | Flucloxacillin & Fucidin cream | 4067 | New patient check done. |
| 28.07.98 | 08.04.61 | F | | 1003 | 1013 | Blurred vision | To see own Optician | 407 | New patient check done. |
| 28.07.98 | 10.04.58 | F | | 1728 | 1740 | Recurrent sinus problems | Referred to ENT Surgeon | 4129 | New patient check done. |
| 23.07.98 | 29.11.62 | M | | 1630 | 1636 | He will come back tomorrow to be signed off | | 4135 | |
| 24.07.98 | 29.11.62 | M | S/leave | 924 | 926 | Labyrinthitis | | 4135 | |
| 27.07.98 | 20.11.38 | M | | 1300 | 1310 | Pedal oedema | Frusemide, Klaricid & Praxilene | 4187 | New patient check done. Home visit. |
| 22.07.98 | 07.05.65 | F | URTI | 914 | 920 | Sore throat & (R) ear ache | Amoxycillin & Sofradex ear drops | 4189 | New patient check done. FP1001 (GMS4) form signed. |
| 22.07.98 | 22.03.11 | F | | 1304 | 1330 | Pedal oedema & red | Klaricid & Bendrofluazide | 4205 | Home visit. |
| 28.07.98 | 25.12.16 | M | Pain | 1740 | 1747 | Pain (L) foot | Co-Proxamol & Movelat cream | 4286 | For X-Ray. Frusemide script also given. |
| 27.07.98 | 24.06.28 | M | | 916 | 930 | Unwell & Insomnia | Amoxycillin & Zopiclone | 4312 | New patient check done. |
| 24.07.98 | 11.01.64 | F | RTI | 1649 | 1654 | Cough | Amoxycillin | 4320 | New patient check done. |
| 24.07.98 | 16.04.93 | F | RTI | 1654 | 1659 | Cough | Amoxycillin | 4327 | New patient check done. |
| 23.07.98 | 21.01.45 | M | | 1038 | 1044 | Wants his repeat script sorted out | | 4329 | New patient check done. |

Result of a query that lists all consultations from the 22nd to the end of July 1998 (ConsultationsSeenFrom22ndTillEndOfJul1998)

| SurgeryDate | DateOfBirth | Sex | Diagnosis | TimeIn | TimeOut | Complaints | Treatments | NumbersID | Notes |
|---|---|---|---|---|---|---|---|---|---|
| 24.07.98 | 12.08.67 | F | | 1034 | 1049 | Requests sterilization | Referred to Gynaecologist | 4402 | New patient check done. |
| 22.07.98 | 24.05.94 | M | URTI | 1646 | 1651 | Sore throat | Amoxycillin | 4469 | |
| 23.07.98 | 24.05.94 | M | | 1026 | 1038 | (L) Gum abscess | Flagyl & Junifen | 4469 | |
| 27.07.98 | 06.11.68 | F | | 1813 | 1821 | Bilateral ingrown toe nail | Erythromycin | 4479 | New patient check done. Penicillin allergy. Referred to Orthopaedic Surgeon. |
| 27.07.98 | 13.01.34 | M | Revisit | 1711 | 1721 | Pain (L) hip is still bad | Zydol SR & Diclofenac SR | 4528 | For X-Ray of the hips. |
| 27.07.98 | 28.08.94 | M | URTI | 945 | 949 | Throat croaky | Amoxycillin | 4546 | |
| 24.07.98 | 22.04.49 | F | | 1635 | 1645 | ?Post-menopausal | For FBC, FSH & LH | 4562 | New patient check done. |
| 23.07.98 | 27.02.62 | F | Pain | 915 | 926 | Breasts are very sore & tender | Referred to Surgeon | 4571 | |
| 22.07.98 | 21.02.76 | F | | 1002 | 1014 | Late period | For Pregnancy test | 4585 | |
| 24.07.98 | 16.11.62 | F | | 1721 | 1735 | Script for Amoxycillin, Gaviscon & Noriday | | 4655 | |
| 27.07.98 | 02.07.43 | M | | 1102 | 1107 | Recurrent infected (L) cheek | Referred to Maxillo-facial surgeon | 4667 | He has implant in (L) cheek. |
| 28.07.98 | 05.06.26 | F | | 928 | 942 | Oesophagitis on endoscopy | Cisapride | 4719 | Her (L) knee is still painful, referred to Orthopaedic Surgeon. |

Result of a query that lists all consultations from the 22nd to the end of July 1998 (ConsultationsSeenFrom22ndTillEndOfJul1998)

| SurgeryDate | DateOfBirth | Sex | Diagnosis | TimeIn | TimeOut | Complaints | Treatments | NumbersID | Notes |
|---|---|---|---|---|---|---|---|---|---|
| 27.07.98 | 17.03.67 | M | S/leave | 930 | 936 | Tenosynovitis (R) wrist | | 4854 | |
| 22.07.98 | 03.008.93 | F | RTI | 1020 | 1024 | Cough | Amoxycillin | 4914 | |
| 22.07.98 | 16.10.63 | F | Depression | 1014 | 1020 | Unable to cope | Referred to CPN | 4916 | New patient check done. |
| 27.07.98 | 12.06.63 | F | RTI | 1045 | 1052 | Cough | Amoxycillin & Salbutamol inhaler | 4953 | New patient check done. FP1001 (GMS4) form signed. |
| 22.07.98 | 15.06.88 | M | Rash | 1739 | 1745 | Rash on trunk & itchy | Unguentum Merck, Loratadine & Oilatum Plus emollient | 5012 | New patient check done. |
| 27.07.98 | 14.03.55 | F | Anaemia | 1803 | 1813 | Hb 11.8 g/dl | Ferrous Sulphate | 5013 | |
| 28.07.98 | 14.05.51 | M | | 1033 | 1039 | Piles & mouth ulcers | Scheriproct suppositories, Scheriproct ointment & Erythromycin | 5031 | New patient check done. Penicillin allergy. |
| 24.07.98 | 26.10.71 | M | RTI | 1735 | 1744 | Cough | Amoxycillin | 5044 | New patient check done. He also gets embarrassing perspiration, referred to Surgeon. To try Driclor OTC. |

552

Result of a query that lists all consultations from the 22nd to the end of July 1998 (ConsultationsSeenFrom22ndTillEndOfJul1998)

| SurgeryDate | DateOfBirth | Sex | Diagnosis | TimeIn | TimeOut | Complaints | Treatments | NumbersID | Notes |
|---|---|---|---|---|---|---|---|---|---|
| 23.07.98 | 01.10.56 | M | | 1805 | 1809 | Mouth ulcers | Erythromycin | 5070 | New patient check done. Penicillin allergy. |
| 24.07.98 | 02.05.85 | F | Rash | 1659 | 1704 | Infected rash with wound between the (L) toes | Lamisil cream & Flucloxacillin | 5114 | New patient check done. |
| 22.07.98 | 17.04.45 | F | | 1024 | 1030 | Script for Rhinocort Aqua nasal spray given | | 5207 | |
| 22.07.98 | 02.04.96 | M | | 955 | 1002 | Spots in the mouth & (L) ear ache | Amoxycillin & Ibuprofen | 5255 | |
| 28.07.98 | 01.06.93 | M | URTI | 1809 | 1815 | Infected rhinorrhoea | Augmentin-Duo | 5318 | |
| 23.07.98 | 11.05.74 | F | | 1006 | 1026 | Going on holidays, wants her period delayed | Norethisterone | 5351 | |
| 22.07.98 | 11.11.69 | F | | 929 | 939 | Headaches & swollen legs | Referred to Gynaecological Dr. on call | 5363 | She is 27 weeks gestation. Her BP is 140/90. She also has flashes of light in front of her eyes. |
| 23.07.98 | 11.11.69 | F | | 1700 | 1710 | Pregaday script given | | 5363 | |
| 22.07.98 | 25.01.23 | M | | 1651 | 1702 | Transvasin script given | | 5370 | New patient check done. |
| 24.07.98 | 10.11.57 | F | Pain | 1709 | 1721 | Loin pains | For MSU | 5385 | New patient check done. |
| 23.07.98 | 29.12.37 | F | Pain | 1645 | 1654 | Pain (L) shoulder | Diclofenac SR & Inj. Depo-Medrone with Lidocaine | 5395 | |

Result of a query that lists all consultations from the 22nd to the end of July 1998 (ConsultationsSeenFrom22ndTillEndOfJul1998)

| SurgeryDate | DateOfBirth | Sex | Diagnosis | TimeIn | TimeOut | Complaints | Treatments | NumbersID | Notes |
|---|---|---|---|---|---|---|---|---|---|
| 28.07.98 | 25.06.21 | M | URTI | 1039 | 1043 | Sore throat | Amoxycillin | 5474 | |
| 28.07.98 | 13.10.93 | F | Pain | 1644 | 1655 | Pain (R) thigh | For X-Ray (R) femur | 5476 | She fell in Tesco & injured her leg. |
| 28.07.98 | 24.02.18 | M | Lump | 1013 | 1033 | Lump on neck is painful at times | Patient will complain | 5490 | Referral letter was sent back by hospital consultant as lipomas are not funded. |
| 27.07.98 | 28.10.36 | M | Pain | 1640 | 1648 | Pain (L) thigh & (L) heel | Movelat cream | 554 | New patient check done. For X-Ray (L) heel. |
| 24.07.98 | 17.04.23 | M | Pain | 913 | 924 | Pain (L) testicle | For USScan testicles | 560 | Nystaform script given. MSU requested. |
| 28.07.98 | 19.12.74 | F | UTI | 1830 | 1835 | Dysuria & frequency | Trimethoprim | 5616 | FP1001 (GMS4) form signed. MSU requested. |
| 28.07.98 | 24.04.33 | F | | 1705 | 1713 | Ponstan script given | | 5666 | |
| 23.07.98 | 09.07.64 | F | | 954 | 1006 | FBC: MCV & MCH are slightly elevated | For repeat FBC in 3 months | 5729 | |
| 23.07.98 | 24.04.35 | F | | 1054 | 1100 | Recurrent ear discharge | Referred to ENT Surgeon | 5770 | |
| 28.07.98 | 15.03.67 | F | Rash | 1801 | 1806 | Weepy blisters on feet | Fucidin-H cream | 5783 | She also has back pain, Rx. Co-dydramol. |
| 28.07.98 | 07.08.96 | F | Rash | 1756 | 1801 | Itchy dry skin & rash on face | Unguentum Merck, Diprobase & Diprobath | 5784 | |

554

### Result of a query that lists all consultations from the 22nd to the end of July 1998 (ConsultationsSeenFrom22ndTillEndOfJul1998)

| SurgeryDate | DateOfBirth | Sex | Diagnosis | TimeIn | TimeOut | Complaints | Treatments | NumbersID | Notes |
|---|---|---|---|---|---|---|---|---|---|
| 23.07.98 | 15.10.96 | F | URTI | 1636 | 1645 | Fever & unwell | Amoxycillin & Ibuprofen | 5874 | |
| 27.07.98 | 23.01.89 | M | RTI | 1705 | 1711 | Cough | Amoxycillin & Bricanyl inhaler | 5894 | |
| 28.07.98 | 12.10.96 | F | Rash | 1630 | 1635 | Nappy rash | Timodine cream | 5904 | |
| 24.07.98 | 31.07.36 | M | | 926 | 938 | Disability benefit application refused | | 5924 | |
| 24.07.98 | 08.01.98 | F | | 1800 | 1812 | Not feeding well | Referred to Paediatric Dr. on call, SGH | 5948 | |
| 23.07.98 | 03.06.83 | F | | 1710 | 1715 | Septic (R) ingrown toe nail | Flucloxacillin | 6032 | |
| 28.07.98 | 16.03.98 | F | URTI | 1655 | 1700 | Infected rhinorrhoea | Amoxycillin | 6038 | |
| 24.07.98 | 23.06.45 | F | Pain | 1006 | 1015 | (L) knee swollen & painful | Diclofenac SR & Co-dydramol | 6040 | |
| 24.07.98 | 18.07.65 | F | Rash | 1812 | 1819 | Contact dermatitis | Fucidin-H cream & Telfast | 6042 | Urticarial rash on the arms & hands over the past 2 days. |
| 28.07.98 | 26.03.53 | F | Anaemia | 1043 | 1055 | Hb 11.7 gm/dl | Ferrous Sulphate | 6049 | |
| 28.07.98 | 27.01.45 | M | S/leave | 1806 | 1809 | Back pain | | 6086 | |
| 22.07.98 | 19.05.98 | M | | 1355 | 1400 | Fever & unwell | His mum has taken him to hospital | 6089 | Home visit. |
| 23.07.98 | 19.05.98 | M | | 1730 | 1735 | Nose blocked | Normal saline nasal drops | 6089 | |

Result of a query that lists all consultations from the 22nd to the end of July 1998 (ConsultationsSeenFrom22ndTillEndOfJul1998)

| SurgeryDate | DateOfBirth | Sex | Diagnosis | TimeIn | TimeOut | Complaints | Treatments | NumbersID | Notes |
|---|---|---|---|---|---|---|---|---|---|
| 24.07.98 | 10.07.81 | M | URTI | 1704 | 1709 | Sore throat | Penicillin V | 616 | New patient check done. |
| 28.07.98 | 10.03.59 | F |  | 1721 | 1728 | DHC & Rhinocort Aqua nasal spray script given |  | 639 | New patient check done. |
| 22.07.98 | 20.09.28 | F | Revisit | 1730 | 1734 | Still chesty | Co-Amoxiclav | 663 |  |
| 28.07.98 | 27.04.25 | M |  | 920 | 928 | Co-dydramol script |  | 751 |  |
| 28.07.98 | 30.06.58 | F |  | 952 | 1003 | Pain (L) arm | Diclofenac enteric coated | 970 | New patient check done. |
| 27.07.98 | 04.11.77 | F | URTI | 1721 | 1729 | Sore throat | Co-Amoxiclav | 990 | New patient check done. |

Result of a query that lists all consultations from the 22nd to the end of July 1999 (ConsultationsSeenFrom22ndTillEndOfJul1999)

| SurgeryDate | DateOfBirth | Sex | Diagnosis | TimeIn | TimeOut | Complaints | Treatments | NumbersID | Notes |
|---|---|---|---|---|---|---|---|---|---|
| 22.07.99 | 31.03.88 | M |  | 1705 | 1709 | Script for Bricanyl turbohaler given |  | Temp |  |
| 22.07.99 | 19.04.77 | F |  | 1808 | 1812 | Script for Microgynon-30 given |  | Temp |  |
| 23.07.99 | 12.03.91 | F |  | 1021 | 1025 | Script for Bricanyl turbohaler given |  | Temp |  |
| 27.07.99 | 16.08.94 | M | URTI | 1635 | 1643 | Sore throat | Amoxycillin, Paracetamol & Ibuprofen suspension | Temp |  |

Result of a query that lists all consultations from the 22nd to the end of July 1999 (ConsultationsSeenFrom22ndTillEndOfJul1999)

| SurgeryDate | DateOfBirth | Sex | Diagnosis | TimeIn | TimeOut | Complaints | Treatments | NumbersID | Notes |
|---|---|---|---|---|---|---|---|---|---|
| 28.07.99 | 01.10.69 | F | | 1714 | 1719 | Late period | For Pregnancy test | Temp | |
| 29.07.99 | 17.06.68 | M | Pain | 1641 | 1648 | Pain (L) testicle | For USScan of the testicles | Temp | |
| 27.07.99 | 18.10.48 | F | | 1823 | 1826 | She saw Oncologist specialist & had brain scan | | 1009 | Her husband came to Surgery. |
| 27.07.99 | 20.11.46 | M | | 1815 | 1823 | Dizziness & vomiting | Prochlorperazine | 1011 | For Physiotherapy. |
| 22.07.99 | 15.11.72 | M | Rash | 1057 | 1102 | Itchy rash on arms & legs, ?Scabies | Lyclear Dermal cream | 1068 | |
| 23.07.99 | 08.02.39 | F | | 1014 | 1021 | X-Ray Pelvis/hips - normal | | 113 | |
| 30.07.99 | 13.03.54 | F | UTI | 1000 | 1008 | Dysuria & frequency | Trimethoprim | 1172 | NP check done. |
| 30.07.99 | 19.04.59 | M | URTI | 1736 | 1740 | Sore throat | Co-Amoxiclav | 1177 | Script for Fucibet ointment given. |
| 28.07.99 | 10.08.27 | M | | 1028 | 1047 | Insomnia | Zopiclone | 1214 | Script for Frusemide was also given. |
| 29.07.99 | 05.02.46 | F | | 1634 | 1641 | Script for Fluconazole, Co-Proxamol & Ibuprofen given | | 1268 | |
| 29.07.99 | 18.08.72 | F | | 927 | 938 | Section 7 of the 'How to apply for access to information held on Police computers form completed | | 1295 | She needs to pay £20. |
| 27.07.99 | 22.01.17 | F | Pain | 1203 | 1220 | Pain (R) side of chest | Co-Amoxiclav | 1320 | Home visit. |

| SurgeryDate | DateOfBirth | Sex | Diagnosis | TimeIn | TimeOut | Complaints | Treatments | NumbersID | Notes |
|---|---|---|---|---|---|---|---|---|---|
| 23.07.99 | 06.06.47 | F | | 1025 | 1034 | Stool culture: Campylobacter species isolated | | 1356 | |
| 29.07.99 | 01.12.34 | F | | 1716 | 1725 | Diarrhoea & abdominal pain | Referred to Physician | 1371 | |
| 27.07.99 | 15.01.26 | F | | 930 | 940 | Didronel PMO tabs put on repeat script | | 1432 | |
| 26.07.99 | 23.06.52 | F | | 1706 | 1719 | Burst condom | Levonorgestrel | 1441 | FP1001 (GMS4) form signed. 25 tablets (750 mcg) of Levonorgestrel & to be repeated 12 hours later. She is a heavy smoker and she 47 years old. |
| 22.07.99 | 05.01.84 | M | S/Leave | 1013 | 1022 | Stress - Private | | 1504 | |
| 22.07.99 | 28.07.36 | M | | 1645 | 1705 | Infected abrasion & wounds on (R) arm | Flucloxacillin | 1508 | Tetanus Toxoid Booster given. Private script for Viagra given. |
| 23.07.99 | 08.08.24 | F | | 1807 | 1817 | To continue own medication | | 1559 | |
| 29.07.99 | 08.08.24 | F | | 1800 | 1819 | She is due to start radiotherapy early next week | | 1559 | |
| 27.07.99 | 27.04.68 | M | S/Leave | 907 | 916 | Fractured (L) thumb & laceration (L) knee - Med 3 & Med 5 | | 1565 | |

Result of a query that lists all consultations from the 22nd to the end of July 1999 (ConsultationsSeenFrom22ndTillEndOfJul1999)

Result of a query that lists all consultations from the 22nd to the end of July 1999 (ConsultationsSeenFrom22ndTillEndOfJul1999)

| SurgeryDate | DateOfBirth | Sex | Diagnosis | TimeIn | TimeOut | Complaints | Treatments | NumbersID | Notes |
|---|---|---|---|---|---|---|---|---|---|
| 29.07.99 | 24.05.29 | M | Revisit | 1226 | 1240 | His tongue is still coated & dry | Glandosane | 1585 | Home visit. He is not keen to be referred to hospital. |
| 27.07.99 | 17.07.70 | F | | 1753 | 1757 | Script for Dianette given | | 1658 | |
| 27.07.99 | 26.06.53 | M | | 1743 | 1747 | (L) knee is inflamed | Flucloxacillin | 1681 | |
| 28.07.99 | 01.08.42 | F | | 1719 | 1726 | Dizziness & tinnitus | Betahistine | 1687 | |
| 28.07.99 | 27.05.41 | F | | 909 | 915 | Stung by a bee on the back of the head | Flucloxacillin | 1785 | |
| 30.07.99 | 14.12.12 | F | | 1815 | 1837 | The Omeprazole & Tildiem LA discontinued & withdrawn as advised by the hospital | | 1805 | Home visit. |
| 26.07.99 | 19.10.36 | F | | 1023 | 1026 | Infected insect bite (L) fore-arm | Flucloxacillin | 1824 | |
| 23.07.99 | 16.09.49 | M | | 1825 | 1828 | Atenolol causes him impotence | Changed to Adalat LA 30 | 1893 | |
| 28.07.99 | 22.02.68 | M | URTI | 1801 | 1807 | Infected rhinorrhoea | Co-Amoxiclav | 205 | |
| 23.07.99 | 23.12.29 | F | | 1743 | 1754 | For Cholesterol, FBC, TFTs, U/Es & Glucose | | 2104 | |
| 28.07.99 | 23.12.29 | F | Pain | 1328 | 1340 | Pain (L) foot | Co-Proxamol & Ibuprofen | 2104 | Scaling rash in her palm & soles, referred to Dermatologist. |
| 26.07.99 | 03.11.57 | F | RTI | 1758 | 1804 | Cough | Amoxycillin | 2210 | FP1001 (GMS4) form signed. |

559

Result of a query that lists all consultations from the 22nd to the end of July 1999 (ConsultationsSeenFrom22ndTillEndOfJul1999)

| SurgeryDate | DateOfBirth | Sex | Diagnosis | TimeIn | TimeOut | Complaints | Treatments | NumbersID | Notes |
|---|---|---|---|---|---|---|---|---|---|
| 26.07.99 | 05.11.83 | F | URTI | 1103 | 1106 | Sore throat | Amoxycillin | 2297 | New Patient check done. |
| 27.07.99 | 02.04.59 | F | | 1655 | 1708 | Hot flushes & night sweats | Dixarit | 2310 | |
| 30.07.99 | 21.06.61 | M | Pain | 912 | 919 | Back pain | Ibuprofen & Co-dydramol | 2343 | |
| 27.07.99 | 06.11.20 | M | Pain | 1802 | 1815 | Chest pain | GTN spray & Imdur | 2423 | |
| 26.07.99 | 23.08.75 | M | | 1646 | 1652 | Abscess (L) upper gum | Amoxycillin & Ibuprofen | 2606 | New Patient check done. |
| 26.07.99 | 12.03.61 | M | URTI | 1652 | 1701 | (L) ear infection | Otosporin ear drops & Amoxycillin | 2606 | He gets recurrent ear infections, referred to ENT Surgeon. |
| 30.07.99 | 27.08.68 | F | | 1008 | 1018 | She would like me to refer her to a super-specialist but omit the statement that she requested it | | 2626 | |
| 26.07.99 | 06.01.43 | F | S/Leave | 935 | 941 | Abdominal pain | | 2642 | |
| 23.07.99 | 16.10.65 | M | | 1758 | 1807 | For repeat MSU | | 2769 | |
| 22.07.99 | 05.09.56 | F | | 1002 | 1013 | Smear: Bacterial vaginosis | Flagyl | 2844 | |
| 26.07.99 | 30.01.46 | F | | 955 | 1001 | ?Phlebitis (R) leg | Flucloxacillin | 290 | |

## Result of a query that lists all consultations from the 22nd to the end of July 1999 (ConsultationsSeenFrom22ndTillEndOfJul1999)

| SurgeryDate | DateOfBirth | Sex | Diagnosis | TimeIn | TimeOut | Complaints | Treatments | NumbersID | Notes |
|---|---|---|---|---|---|---|---|---|---|
| 29.07.99 | 05.01.19 | M | Depression | 904 | 919 | Feels depressed & can't cope | Seroxat suspension | 291 | Wife came to Surgery. His mouth is always dry, Rx. Glandosane. He also has nausea all the time, Rx. Metoclopramide. |
| 29.07.99 | 20.04.85 | F | URTI | 919 | 923 | Otitis ext. | Otomize ear spray & Flucloxacillin | 2918 | |
| 28.07.99 | 01.08.48 | F | S/Leave | 933 | 944 | Dizziness | | 3009 | She also has abdominal pain & T.A.T.T., for MSU, FBC & TFTs. |
| 23.07.99 | 30.09.51 | M | RTI | 1735 | 1743 | Cough | Clarithromycin | 3021 | Penicillin allergy. For CXR. |
| 27.07.99 | 30.03.62 | F | | 1757 | 1802 | Still has epigastric discomfort | | 3112 | |
| 26.07.99 | 06.10.24 | F | Pain | 1001 | 1020 | Pain (L) side of chest | Co-Proxamol & Movelat cream | 312 | Script for Atenolol was also given. |
| 29.07.99 | 06.10.24 | F | | 1733 | 1745 | To continue on the Atenolol | | 312 | |
| 23.07.99 | 18.01.63 | F | | 1002 | 1014 | Burst condom | She has Mirena IUCD in situ | 3177 | |
| 26.07.99 | 13.08.79 | M | URTI | 1754 | 1758 | Sore throat | Co-Amoxiclav | 320 | |
| 22.07.99 | 16.03.25 | M | Revisit | 929 | 943 | He still has diarrhoea | Lomotil, Ciprofloxacin & Electrolade | 3245 | |
| 27.07.99 | 07.09.53 | M | | 1734 | 1743 | Mole on anterior chest wall | Referred to Dermatologist | 3290 | |

Result of a query that lists all consultations from the 22nd to the end of July 1999 (ConsultationsSeenFrom22ndTillEndOfJul1999)

| SurgeryDate | DateOfBirth | Sex | Diagnosis | TimeIn | TimeOut | Complaints | Treatments | NumbersID | Notes |
|---|---|---|---|---|---|---|---|---|---|
| 26.07.99 | 14.08.99 | M | | 906 | 924 | Script for Pravastatin given | | 3353 | For LFTs. |
| 23.07.99 | 24.01.64 | M | | 900 | 924 | Unaware that DSS has found him to be incapable of working | | 3467 | |
| 27.07.99 | 24.01.64 | M | | 1830 | 1846 | The saga about being found unfit continues | To contact Clacton mane | 3467 | |
| 27.07.99 | 06.05.64 | F | Pain | 1826 | 1830 | Headaches & vomiting | Clotam Rapid & Metoclopramide | 3474 | |
| 29.07.99 | 06.12.91 | M | Conjunctivitis | 1648 | 1652 | Sticky & sore (R) blood shot eye | Chloramphenicol eye drops | 3479 | NP check done. |
| 23.07.99 | 01.04.52 | M | | 954 | 1002 | USScan of Aorta is normal | | 3517 | Penicillin allergy. |
| 30.07.99 | 06.06.47 | M | Revisit | 1655 | 1703 | Itchy rash is still present | 0.5% Malathion liquid | 3588 | Referred to Dermatologist. |
| 29.07.99 | 19.06.33 | M | | 1652 | 1713 | Unhappy that the Surgery did not diagnose his Inguinal hernia | | 3648 | |
| 27.07.99 | 31.07.35 | M | | 1643 | 1655 | Poor urinary stream | Referred to Urologist | 3709 | Penicillin allergy. For PSA. |
| 27.07.99 | 29.08.34 | F | | 944 | 953 | She feels panicky & depressed | | 3729 | |
| 23.07.99 | 17.04.56 | M | | 1714 | 1717 | Painful piles | Xyloproct suppositories & Xyloproct ointment | 3773 | |

## Result of a query that lists all consultations from the 22nd to the end of July 1999 (ConsultationsSeenFrom22ndTillEndOfJul1999)

| SurgeryDate | DateOfBirth | Sex | Diagnosis | TimeIn | TimeOut | Complaints | Treatments | NumbersID | Notes |
|---|---|---|---|---|---|---|---|---|---|
| 28.07.99 | 19.01.62 | M | S/Leave | 1649 | 1654 | Stressed, back pain & pain in knees | | 3783 | |
| 23.07.99 | 10.06.28 | F | | 940 | 954 | Script for Doxazosin given | | 3884 | |
| 27.07.99 | 19.03.15 | F | | 1007 | 1026 | Recurrent giddiness & vomiting | Referred to care of the elderly specialist | 3888 | |
| 27.07.99 | 06.03.73 | F | | 925 | 930 | Infected cyst (L) elbow | Flucloxacillin | 3896 | Script for Fluoxetine was also given. |
| 30.07.99 | 19.09.51 | F | S/Leave | 1649 | 1655 | Back pain - Med 5 | | 3910 | She also has D&V, Rx. Electrolade. |
| 27.07.99 | 16.06.66 | F | URTI | 1721 | 1730 | Sinusitis | Co-Amoxiclav & Co-dydramol | 3944 | |
| 28.07.99 | 26.05.57 | M | URTI | 1807 | 1820 | Sore throat | Erythromycin | 3983 | Penicillin allergy. Script for Allopurinol. |
| 22.07.99 | 16.08.29 | M | | 1026 | 1032 | Deafness | Referred to ENT Surgeon | 4009 | |
| 23.07.99 | 18.03.87 | F | | 1754 | 1758 | Skin growing over her little toe nails | Referred to Chiropodist | 4132 | |
| 28.07.99 | 16.06.55 | F | | 1743 | 1801 | Verruca (R) foot | Cuplex gel | 4284 | She also has catarrh in her throat over the past one year, referred to ENT Surgeon. Script for Imigran was also given. |

Result of a query that lists all consultations from the 22nd to the end of July 1999 (ConsultationsSeenFrom22ndTillEndOfJul1999)

| SurgeryDate | DateOfBirth | Sex | Diagnosis | TimeIn | TimeOut | Complaints | Treatments | NumbersID | Notes |
|---|---|---|---|---|---|---|---|---|---|
| 22.07.99 | 24.12.89 | F | | 1638 | 1645 | Infected spot (R) thumb | Flucloxacillin & Fucidin crem | 4328 | |
| 29.07.99 | 10.03.10 | F | | 1150 | 1215 | She feels funny earlier on & now she is better | | 4341 | Home visit. |
| 22.07.99 | 01.09.83 | F | RTI | 1110 | 1121 | Cough & nose bleeds | Amoxycillin & Flixonase nasal spray | 4370 | She is also dizzy & faints, for FBC & Glucose. |
| 28.07.99 | 24.10.86 | M | | 1726 | 1733 | Bed wetting | Desmospray | 438 | NP check done. |
| 22.07.99 | 04.10.28 | F | | 943 | 1002 | USScan of the thyroid gland: solid nodules present in the Thyroid gland | | 4403 | |
| 29.07.99 | 25.04.35 | M | Pain | 1713 | 1716 | Pain (R) hip | For X-Ray (R) hip | 4438 | |
| 22.07.99 | 24.12.91 | M | URTI | 1744 | 1749 | Sore throat | Amoxycillin | 4526 | Script for Loratadine was also given. |
| 27.07.99 | 22.11.66 | M | Depression | 1030 | 1044 | Loss of confidence & aggressive | Referred to CPN | 4602 | |
| 27.07.99 | 29.04.56 | M | | 1846 | 1853 | He wants a copy of report from Orthopaedic Surgeon | Patient is to contact the Orthopaedic Surgeon himself | 466 | I explained to the patient such a letter from the Orthopaedic Surgeon was not received by me. |
| 27.07.99 | 11.08.35 | F | Revisit | 1708 | 1721 | (L) heel is still sore | Referred to Orthopaedic Surgeon | 4670 | Tetanus toxoid Booster given. |
| 27.07.99 | 19.01.24 | F | Rash | 1747 | 1753 | Weepy & itchy rash behind ear lobes | Fucidin-H ointment | 4708 | |

Result of a query that lists all consultations from the 22nd to the end of July 1999 (ConsultationsSeenFrom22ndTillEndOfJul1999)

| SurgeryDate | DateOfBirth | Sex | Diagnosis | TimeIn | TimeOut | Complaints | Treatments | NumbersID | Notes |
|---|---|---|---|---|---|---|---|---|---|
| 28.07.99 | 21.05.35 | M | RTI | 1654 | 1659 | Cough | Amoxycillin | 4788 | |
| 23.07.99 | 14.12.77 | F | S/Leave | 1817 | 1825 | Back pain - Private | | 489 | Script for Co-dydramol was also given. |
| 26.07.99 | 28.10.42 | F | Pain | 942 | 945 | Aches & pain (R) heel | Ibuprofen | 4890 | |
| 30.07.99 | 27.07.95 | F | Rash | 1029 | 1041 | Itchy rash on body, ?Scabies | Lyclear Dermal cream | 4964 | For FBC. She also has PER VAGINA discharge, for Sellotape test. |
| 26.07.99 | 18.09.65 | F | Pain | 1719 | 1747 | Chest pain | Co-dydramol | 4983 | Her LMP was in May, 1999. She is sterilized. For Pregnancy test. |
| 28.07.99 | 18.09.65 | F | | 1659 | 1714 | She wants a letter to whom it may concern regarding housing problems | | 4983 | |
| 30.07.99 | 10.12.43 | M | Pain | 938 | 950 | Stomach ache & weight loss | Buscopan | 5054 | For MSU & USScan of the abdomen. |
| 27.07.99 | 01.10.91 | F | URTI | 1052 | 1027 | Sore throat & fever | Clarithromycin & Paracetamol | 5082 | Penicillin allergy. |
| 23.07.99 | 13.12.27 | F | | 1235 | 1240 | She is already on the way to hospital after being reviewed by the McMillan nurse | | 5118 | Home visit. |

Result of a query that lists all consultations from the 22nd to the end of July 1999 (ConsultationsSeenFrom22ndTillEndOfJul1999)

| SurgeryDate | DateOfBirth | Sex | Diagnosis | TimeIn | TimeOut | Complaints | Treatments | NumbersID | Notes |
|---|---|---|---|---|---|---|---|---|---|
| 22.07.99 | 20.01.60 | M | Depression | 1756 | 1808 | Unable to cope & aggressive | Citalopram | 5119 | New Patient check done. He is also referred to CPN. |
| 22.07.99 | 17.05.86 | F | Lump | 1730 | 1736 | Lumps on the head, ?lymph nodes | | 5135 | |
| 29.07.99 | 09.05.27 | M | | 938 | 957 | Palpitations & irregular heart beats | Referred to Cardiologist | 5162 | His Motens (Lacidipine) was changed to Co-Amilofruse. For U/Es. |
| 29.07.99 | 12.02.96 | M | URTI | 957 | 1004 | Sore throat & fever | Augmentin-Duo & Ibuprofen suspension | 5165 | |
| 28.07.99 | 16.10.75 | F | UTI | 1010 | 1019 | Dysuria | Trimethoprim | 5180 | |
| 23.07.99 | 30.03.56 | F | Conjunctivitis | 1704 | 1709 | Sore & infected upper eye lids | Chloramphenicol eye drops | 5186 | |
| 23.07.99 | 17.04.45 | F | | 931 | 940 | To be on monthly inj. Vit B12 | | 5207 | |
| 28.07.99 | 06.06.78 | F | Pain | 944 | 949 | Chest pain & headaches | Paracetamol | 5232 | She is 14 weeks pregnant. |
| 23.07.99 | 08.12.78 | F | | 1828 | 1831 | Microscopic haematuria on MSU | For repeat MSU in 4 weeks | 5293 | |
| 27.07.99 | 25.09.24 | M | | 1026 | 1030 | Bloated | Mintec | 5367 | |
| 22.07.99 | 16.08.21 | F | Pain | 1325 | 1345 | Pain & cramps in the legs | Nafridrofuryl & Quinine Sulphate | 5406 | Home visit. |
| 22.07.99 | 28.10.95 | F | | 1022 | 1026 | Infected wound (R) thigh | Fucidin ointment & Flucloxacillin | 5536 | |
| 28.07.99 | 06.01.78 | M | Lump | 1019 | 1028 | (L) testicular lump | For USScan of the testicles | 555 | |

Result of a query that lists all consultations from the 22nd to the end of July 1999 (ConsultationsSeenFrom22ndTillEndOfJul1999)

| SurgeryDate | DateOfBirth | Sex | Diagnosis | TimeIn | TimeOut | Complaints | Treatments | NumbersID | Notes |
|---|---|---|---|---|---|---|---|---|---|
| 26.07.99 | 06.03.10 | F | | 1040 | 1054 | Constipated | Co-danthrusate, Colpermin & Fybogel, | 5550 | Script for Frusemide was also given. |
| 23.07.99 | 25.04.97 | F | URTI | 1838 | 1841 | Sore throat | Amoxycillin | 5575 | |
| 22.07.99 | 27.06.50 | M | URTI | 924 | 929 | Sore throat | Co-Amoxiclav | 559 | |
| 26.07.99 | 10.08.40 | F | Rash | 1643 | 1646 | Sweaty & itchy rash under both breasts | Fucidin-H ointment | 5747 | |
| 22.07.99 | 19.11.37 | M | | 1709 | 1712 | FBC normal | | 5776 | |
| 28.07.99 | 28.03.83 | F | Lump | 915 | 924 | Lump (L) lower eye lid | Referred to Ophthalmologist | 580 | New Patient check done. |
| 27.07.99 | 30.05.91 | F | Rash | 953 | 1002 | Itchy, sore & weepy rash on inner thighs | Flucloxacillin & Fucidin-H ointment | 5849 | |
| 26.07.99 | 21.05.74 | M | Lump | 904 | 907 | Inclusion cyst dorsum of (L) elbow | Referred to Surgeon | 5887 | Apparently, he is being using mobile phone a lot, and he complains of pain in the head, referred to Neurologist. |
| 29.07.99 | 12.10.96 | F | RTI | 1757 | 1800 | Cough | Amoxycillin | 5904 | |
| 29.07.99 | 10.08.94 | M | RTI | 1753 | 1757 | Cough | Amoxycillin | 5905 | |
| 29.07.99 | 31.05.62 | F | | 1725 | 1733 | Septic spots on the buttocks | Flucloxacillin & Fucidin cream | 593 | |
| 22.07.99 | 23.02.26 | M | | 1712 | 1722 | Script for Multivitamin given | | 5954 | For MSU, TFTs & PSA. |
| 30.07.99 | 23.03.26 | M | | 919 | 931 | Serum Glucose, TSH & PSA normal | | 5954 | |
| 22.07.99 | 22.02.36 | F | Pain | 1722 | 1730 | Pain in chest | Co-dydramol | 5955 | Penicillin allergy. |

Result of a query that lists all consultations from the 22nd to the end of July 1999 (ConsultationsSeenFrom22ndTillEndOfJul1999)

| SurgeryDate | DateOfBirth | Sex | Diagnosis | TimeIn | TimeOut | Complaints | Treatments | NumbersID | Notes |
|---|---|---|---|---|---|---|---|---|---|
| 23.07.99 | 09.09.64 | F | | 1700 | 1704 | Diarrhoea | Loperamide & Electrolade | 5980 | |
| 23.07.99 | 06.01.87 | F | | 1655 | 1700 | Diarrhoea | Loperamide & Electrolade | 5981 | |
| 23.07.99 | 24.05.29 | M | | 1034 | 1054 | Medications changed to twice daily as far as possible | | 6 | His social worker came to Surgery. |
| 30.07.99 | 13.01.28 | F | | 901 | 912 | She would like Chiropody services | | 6045 | |
| 22.07.99 | 06.04.33 | F | URTI | 1749 | 1756 | Sore throat | Co-Amoxiclav & Paracetamol | 6056 | |
| 27.07.99 | 03.11.60 | F | | 916 | 925 | Diarrhoea | Lomotil, Ciprofloxacin & Electrolade | 6062 | |
| 30.07.99 | 03.11.60 | F | | 1644 | 1649 | Indigestion | Omeprazole | 6062 | |
| 30.07.99 | 05.05.59 | M | | 1703 | 1711 | Superficial phlebitis | Flucloxacillin | 6085 | He also has pain in both knees, Rx. Ibuprofen & Co-dydramol. |
| 26.07.99 | 07.05.38 | F | RTI | 1804 | 1809 | Cough | Amoxycillin | 6122 | |
| 28.07.99 | 03.10.88 | M | Conjunctivitis | 924 | 933 | Sticky (L) eye | Chloramphenicol eye drops | 6135 | Scab in the (L) nostril, Rx. Naseptin cream. |
| 29.07.99 | 22.07.17 | F | | 1004 | 1021 | Painful finger & wrist joints | Referred to Rheumatologist | 6182 | |
| 28.07.99 | 19.11.28 | M | Pain | 1147 | 1105 | Orange badge scheme of parking form completed | | 6233 | |

Result of a query that lists all consultations from the 22nd to the end of July 1999 (ConsultationsSeenFrom22ndTillEndOfJul1999)

| SurgeryDate | DateOfBirth | Sex | Diagnosis | TimeIn | TimeOut | Complaints | Treatments | NumbersID | Notes |
|---|---|---|---|---|---|---|---|---|---|
| 23.07.99 | 03.05.36 | M | Pain | 1831 | 1838 | Chest pain | GTN spray & Aspirin | 6236 | He was seen in Basildon A/E yesterday. Referred to Cardiologist (Basildon hospital). |
| 26.07.99 | 25.02.80 | F | URTI | 1020 | 1023 | Sore throat | Amoxycillin | 6255 | |
| 27.07.99 | 13.10.98 | F | RTI | 1730 | 1734 | Cough | Erythromycin & Ibuprofen suspension | 6258 | Penicillin allergy. For PSA. |
| 22.07.99 | 28.11.84 | F | | 1032 | 1057 | Social services will be contacted by carer to phone me regarding probable referral to child Psychiatrist | | 6294 | |
| 28.07.99 | 05.06.98 | F | Rash | 1739 | 1743 | Nappy rash | Timodine cream | 6318 | |
| 28.07.99 | 12.12.89 | M | | 1733 | 1739 | Regular Epistaxes | Referred to ENT Surgeon | 6326 | |
| 23.07.99 | 06.01.99 | M | | 1649 | 1655 | Diarrhoea | Dioralyte | 6329 | |
| 30.07.99 | 06.01.99 | M | Revisit | 1635 | 1644 | She still has diarrhoea | Rehidrat | 6329 | He also has nappy rash, Rx. Timodine cream. Stool for C&S was also sent. |
| 26.07.99 | 23.01.99 | F | Conjunctivitis | 1635 | 1643 | Yellow discharge from (R) eye | Chloramphenicol eye drops | 6346 | She also has dry patches of skin which bleeds at times, referred to Dermatologist. |

Result of a query that lists all consultations from the 22nd to the end of July 1999 (ConsultationsSeenFrom22ndTillEndOfJul1999)

| SurgeryDate | DateOfBirth | Sex | Diagnosis | TimeIn | TimeOut | Complaints | Treatments | NumbersID | Notes |
|---|---|---|---|---|---|---|---|---|---|
| 26.07.99 | 30.01.46 | M | RTI | 945 | 955 | Cough & haemoptysis | Erythromycin | 6366 | Penicillin allergy. For FBC & CXR. He also has persistent itchy rash in both groins, referred to Dermatologist. |
| 22.07.99 | 05.06.25 | F | Pain | 1102 | 1110 | Pain back of (R) leg | Co-Proxamol | 6403 | She also has mouth ulcer, Rx. Amoxycillin. Script for Ranitidine was also given. |
| 29.07.99 | 05.06.25 | F | Revisit | 923 | 927 | Mouth is still sore | Referred to Oral Surgeon | 6403 | |
| 28.07.99 | 15.12.65 | F | | 1305 | 1325 | Routine P/Natal visit | | 6422 | Home visit. New baby check done. |
| 22.07.99 | 13.06.54 | F | | 908 | 915 | Loss of libido & T.A.T.T. | For LH, FSH & TFTs | 6430 | |
| 28.07.99 | 13.06.54 | F | | 949 | 1007 | LH & FSH levels are raised | Premique cycle | 6430 | For MSU. She is also constipated, Rx. Lactulose. |
| 29.07.99 | 06.03.59 | F | | 1745 | 1753 | Script for Betahistine given | | 644 | |
| 22.07.99 | 16.11.74 | F | | 1736 | 1744 | Pregnancy test positive | For TOP | 6447 | She requests TOP. |
| 26.07.99 | 04.07.76 | M | Revisit | 1054 | 1103 | Persistent diarrhoea | Ciprofloxacin, Lomotil & Electrolade | 6448 | |

Result of a query that lists all consultations from the 22nd to the end of July 1999 (ConsultationsSeenFrom22ndTillEndOfJul1999)

| SurgeryDate | DateOfBirth | Sex | Diagnosis | TimeIn | TimeOut | Complaints | Treatments | NumbersID | Notes |
|---|---|---|---|---|---|---|---|---|---|
| 30.07.99 | 04.07.76 | M | Revisit | 931 | 938 | Diarrhoea has persisted | Referred to Gastro-enterologist | 6448 | |
| 28.07.99 | 25.04.68 | F | Revisit | 1642 | 1649 | Mastalgia is worse | Referred to Surgeon | 6451 | Her (L) eye is watering all the time, Rx. Chloramphenicol eye drops. |
| 26.07.99 | 01.07.99 | F | Rash | 1747 | 1754 | Rash on the neck | Reassured | 6466 | |
| 30.07.99 | 10.11.11 | F | Pain | 1041 | 1049 | Low back pain | Co-codamol effervescent | 6479 | She also has facial rash, Rx. Fucidin-H cream. |
| 23.07.99 | 20.05.26 | M | | 1717 | 1735 | Kitteridge Group claims services Medical Certificate completed | | 666 | His wife came to Surgery. |
| 22.07.99 | 06.06.30 | M | Revisit | 915 | 924 | Swelling over (L) Olecranon process is still present | Referred to Orthopaedic Surgeon | 883 | |
| 23.07.99 | 05.05.49 | M | S/Leave | 924 | 931 | (L) Inguinal hernia | | 910 | |
| 23.07.99 | 01.07.27 | F | | 1709 | 1714 | Pedal oedema | Frusemide | 911 | |
| 23.07.99 | 13.10.79 | M | | 1635 | 1649 | Script for EpiPen script | | 926 | |
| 29.07.99 | 15.03.75 | F | | 1021 | 1037 | Script for Fluoxetine, Lactulose & Microgynon-30 given | | 934 | |

571

## Result of a query that lists all consultations from the 22nd to the end of July 1999 (ConsultationsSeenFrom22ndTillEndOfJul1999)

| SurgeryDate | DateOfBirth | Sex | Diagnosis | TimeIn | TimeOut | Complaints | Treatments | NumbersID | Notes |
|---|---|---|---|---|---|---|---|---|---|
| 30.07.99 | 03.03.29 | F | Pain | 1018 | 1029 | Pain (R) side of the face & neck | Co-Proxamol & Quinine Sulphate | 979 | |
| 26.07.99 | 06.04.37 | M | | 924 | 935 | Letter to whom it may concern that he has high blood pressure | | 988 | |

## Result of a query that lists all consultations from the 22nd to the end of July 2000 (ConsultationsSeenFrom22ndTillEndOfJul2000)

| SurgeryDate | DateOfBirth | Sex | Diagnosis | TimeIn | TimeOut | Complaints | Treatments | NumbersID | Notes |
|---|---|---|---|---|---|---|---|---|---|
| 26.07.2000 | 25.11.1968 | M | | 1806 | 1812 | Headaches & giddiness with itching (R) ear | EarCalm, Prochlorperazine, Diclofenac enteric coated & Erythromycin | Temp | Penicillin allergy. |
| 27.07.2000 | 15.11.1969 | M | URTI | 933 | 942 | Sore throat & dizziness | Prochlorperazine & Amoxycillin | Temp | |
| 28.07.2000 | 25.05.1998 | F | Rash | 1707 | 1714 | Weepy Eczema rash | Diprobase, Alphaderm cream & Elocon cream | Temp | |
| 28.07.2000 | 28.09.1980 | M | | 1745 | 1750 | Script for Diprobase cream, Balneum Plus bath oil & Fuci-bet cream given | | 1012 | |
| 26.07.2000 | 31.10.1969 | F | | 1752 | 1806 | Script for Metronidazole & Penicillin V given | | 1029 | |

Result of a query that lists all consultations from the 22nd to the end of July 2000 (ConsultationsSeenFrom22ndTillEndOfJul2000)

| SurgeryDate | DateOfBirth | Sex | Diagnosis | TimeIn | TimeOut | Complaints | Treatments | NumbersID | Notes |
|---|---|---|---|---|---|---|---|---|---|
| 28.07.2000 | 20.07.1956 | M | | 1803 | 1806 | MFT - No sperms seen | | 1126 | |
| 28.07.2000 | 11.10.1952 | M | Revisit | 945 | 952 | Cystic swelling on (L) knee is still present | Referred to Orthopaedic Surgeon | 1141 | Script for Ibuprofen given. |
| 28.07.2000 | 13.05.1914 | M | Revisit | 1740 | 1745 | Still coughing + | For CXR & Prednisolone enteric coated | 1186 | |
| 25.07.2000 | 03.02.1977 | M | | 1715 | 1722 | Clicking of the neck following injury whilst playing football | For Cervical X-Ray | 1306 | New Patient check done. |
| 26.07.2000 | 07.11.1980 | M | | 1728 | 1733 | Sepsis end of scar | Co-Amoxiclav | 132 | |
| 26.07.2000 | 22.01.1917 | F | | 1302 | 1320 | Breathless & asthmatic | Prednisolone, Amoxycillin & Erythromycin | 1320 | Home visit. |
| 26.07.2000 | 19.10.1965 | F | RTI | 1744 | 1752 | Cough & wheezy attack | Amoxycillin & Prednisolone | 1449 | Erythromycin allergy. Nebulizer given. |
| 24.07.2000 | 18.09.1947 | M | | 902 | 911 | Script for Movelat gel given | | 1456 | |
| 25.07.2000 | 05.08.1942 | M | Revisit | 1754 | 1758 | Rash on legs have persisted | Referred to Dermatologist (Basildon hospital) | 1573 | |
| 26.07.2000 | 14.12.1924 | M | Revisit | 901 | 916 | Cough | Ciprofloxacin & Codeine Linctus | 1586 | Script for Bumetanide given. |

Result of a query that lists all consultations from the 22nd to the end of July 2000 (ConsultationsSeenFrom22ndTillEndOfJul2000)

| SurgeryDate | DateOfBirth | Sex | Diagnosis | TimeIn | TimeOut | Complaints | Treatments | NumbersID | Notes |
|---|---|---|---|---|---|---|---|---|---|
| 25.07.2000 | 27.06.1944 | M | Revisit | 1738 | 1746 | Sore throat persists & mouth ulcers | Difflam spray & Metronidazole | 1673 | For FBC, fasting Glucose & Glandular fever test. |
| 24.07.2000 | 23.08.1971 | M | Revisit | 1744 | 1750 | Low back pain persists | For Physiotherapy | 1770 | |
| 25.07.2000 | 30.10.1935 | M | | 1647 | 1654 | Advised to continue Citalopram | | 1790 | |
| 25.07.2000 | 03.09.1980 | F | Pain | 1654 | 1705 | Headaches & vomiting | Paramax & Ibuprofen | 1901 | FP1001 (GMS4) form signed. T.A.T.T., for FBC & TFTs. Penicillin allergy. |
| 28.07.2000 | 29.11.1929 | F | | 1714 | 1723 | H. pylori positive | Metronidazole, Clarithromycin & Omeprazole | 193 | |
| 26.07.2000 | 19.09.1984 | F | Rash | 1722 | 1728 | Itchy rash on face | Fucidin-H cream | 1978 | Script for Microgynon 30 given. |
| 27.07.2000 | 17.10.1953 | F | URTI | 1012 | 1016 | Sore throat | Co-Amoxiclav | 2020 | |
| 25.07.2000 | 08.04.1948 | M | | 903 | 917 | PR bleeding | Referred to Surgeon | 2062 | |
| 26.07.2000 | 23.04.1950 | F | | 1639 | 1651 | Pain (R) wrist & septic abrasion on chin | Ibuprofen & Flucloxacillin | 2369 | For X-Ray (R) wrist. |
| 25.07.2000 | 28.03.1970 | F | Pain | 1012 | 1022 | Pain (R) wrist | Movelat cream, Kapake & Diclofenac enteric coated | 2375 | Wart on (R), referred to Dermatologist. |

## Result of a query that lists all consultations from the 22nd to the end of July 2000 (ConsultationsSeenFrom22ndTillEndOfJul2000)

| SurgeryDate | DateOfBirth | Sex | Diagnosis | TimeIn | TimeOut | Complaints | Treatments | NumbersID | Notes |
|---|---|---|---|---|---|---|---|---|---|
| 24.07.2000 | 16.03.1927 | F | | 1010 | 1021 | Cholesterol 6.9 mmols/L | Simvastatin | 2415 | |
| 28.07.2000 | 06.06.1957 | F | | 1737 | 1740 | T.A.T.T. | For FBC & TFTs | 2483 | |
| 24.07.2000 | 22.09.1939 | F | | 1750 | 1759 | Indoramin dose increased | | 2510 | |
| 24.07.2000 | 06.01.1943 | F | Rash | 1714 | 1720 | Rash on lower leg | Fucidin-H cream & Co-Amoxiclav | 2642 | |
| 26.07.2000 | 05.02.1933 | F | Revisit | 925 | 930 | She still has (R) shoulder pain | Inj. Depo-Medrone with Lidocaine | 276 | |
| 28.07.2000 | 05.02.1933 | F | | 1030 | 1050 | Inj. Depo-Medrone with Lidocaine given to (R) shoulder | | 276 | |
| 24.07.2000 | 16.07.1938 | M | | 930 | 943 | Cholesterol 6.9 mmols/L | Simvastatin | 2772 | |
| 24.07.2000 | 16.11.1973 | F | URTI | 1025 | 1029 | Sore throat | Amoxycillin | 2836 | FP1001 (GMS4) form signed. |
| 24.07.2000 | 01.06.1969 | F | | 1805 | 1808 | Whitlow improving | Fucidin cream | 2903 | |
| 27.07.2000 | 02.08.1988 | F | | 903 | 918 | Vaginal discharge again | Erythromycin | 2919 | For fasting Glucose. |
| 27.07.2000 | 01.08.1948 | F | Hypertension | 918 | 926 | BP 160/100 | Bendrofluazide | 3009 | |
| 26.07.2000 | 25.02.1986 | F | | 1651 | 1701 | Verrucae (L) foot | Occlusal | 3035 | Heavy periods, Rx. Mefenamic Acid. |
| 28.07.2000 | 16.12.1959 | F | URTI | 1006 | 1014 | Sinusitis | Amoxycillin | 311 | |
| 25.07.2000 | 10.02.1983 | F | URTI | 1641 | 1647 | Sore throat | Clarithromycin | 3150 | Penicillin allergy. |
| 24.07.2000 | 06.12.1945 | M | S/Leave | 1653 | 1706 | Diarrhoea & weakness | | 3198 | Script for Ensure Plus & Enlive given. |

Result of a query that lists all consultations from the 22nd to the end of July 2000 (ConsultationsSeenFrom22ndTillEndOfJul2000)

| SurgeryDate | DateOfBirth | Sex | Diagnosis | TimeIn | TimeOut | Complaints | Treatments | NumbersID | Notes |
|---|---|---|---|---|---|---|---|---|---|
| 25.07.2000 | 19.03.1919 | M | | 939 | 943 | Night cramps (L) leg | Quinine Sulphate | 339 | |
| 26.07.2000 | 12.08.1936 | M | UTI | 1709 | 1722 | Back pain & frequency of micturition | Trimethoprim | 3475 | For MSU. Script for Viagra given. |
| 28.07.2000 | 06.12.1991 | M | Conjunctivitis | 940 | 945 | (R) eye is & watery | Chloramphenicol eye drops | 3476 | |
| 27.07.2000 | 05.12.1937 | M | | 946 | 1002 | Wheezy again | Prednisolone & Budesonide respules | 3646 | |
| 26.07.2000 | 10.03.1946 | F | Revisit | 1044 | 1052 | Chesty cough again | Ciprofloxacin | 3710 | For CXR. |
| 25.07.2000 | 08.11.1931 | F | URTI | 1054 | 1058 | Sore (L) ear, dizziness & nausea | Amoxycillin & Prochlorperazine | 372 | |
| 25.07.2000 | 02.02.1976 | F | RTI | 1034 | 1040 | Cough | Amoxycillin & Simple Linctus | 3762 | |
| 28.07.2000 | 17.03.1957 | F | URTI | 1753 | 1759 | (R) ear ache | Oromize ear spray | 3873 | |
| 27.07.2000 | 10.04.1969 | M | | 1715 | 1719 | Cryotherapy to skin tags (R) side of neck | | 3906 | |
| 27.07.2000 | 19.09.1951 | F | | 1702 | 1715 | Cryotherapy to mole on (R) shoulder & to skin tags (R) side of neck | | 3910 | |
| 25.07.2000 | 02.02.1993 | F | | 1049 | 1054 | Itchy scaly scalp | Nizoral shampoo & Loratadine | 3973 | |
| 28.07.2000 | 18.01.1968 | M | Pain | 1759 | 1803 | Low back pain | Kapake & Diclofenac enteric coated | 3992 | |
| 26.07.2000 | 07.10.1933 | M | | 934 | 941 | Script for Haloperidol & Procyclidine given | | 4055 | |

Result of a query that lists all consultations from the 22nd to the end of July 2000 (ConsultationsSeenFrom22ndTillEndOfJul2000)

| SurgeryDate | DateOfBirth | Sex | Diagnosis | TimeIn | TimeOut | Complaints | Treatments | NumbersID | Notes |
|---|---|---|---|---|---|---|---|---|---|
| 28.07.2000 | 24.09.1983 | F | | 1647 | 1654 | PER VAGINA bleeding & abdominal pain | Mefenamic Acid & Norethisterone | 4196 | She had Depo-Provera injection 2 months ago. |
| 27.07.2000 | 16.05.1938 | M | | 1724 | 1729 | Cryotherapy to 2 moles on (R) side of neck & to skin tags on (R) side of neck | | 4204 | |
| 25.07.2000 | 02.02.1967 | M | Pain | 1004 | 1012 | Pain (R) hip | Co-dydramol | 4235 | Feeling of something stuck in the throat, referred to ENT Surgeon (Basildon hospital) |
| 25.07.2000 | 27.07.1948 | M | Pain | 917 | 927 | Pain (R) shoulder | Transvasin cream | 4254 | Script for Elocon cream & Simple Linctus given. |
| 24.07.2000 | 02.02.1994 | M | | 958 | 1002 | Sepsis (R)IGTN | Flucloxacillin | 4319 | |
| 28.07.2000 | 07.12.1982 | F | Revisit | 958 | 1006 | Pain & swelling (R) wrist is back again | Naprosyn | 4323 | FP1001 (GMS4) form signed. |
| 27.07.2000 | 12.04.1927 | M | | 1002 | 1012 | Script for Simvastatin given | | 4394 | For LFTs. |
| 24.07.2000 | 02.09.1948 | F | URTI | 1759 | 1805 | Sore throat | Erythromycin | 4444 | Penicillin allergy. |
| 25.07.2000 | 23.06.1994 | M | | 1722 | 1738 | (R) ear is sore & bleeding | Referred to ENT clinic, SGH | 4494 | Penicillin allergy. |
| 25.07.2000 | 16.02.1983 | F | URTI | 1040 | 1049 | Sore throat | Amoxicillin | 4596 | |
| 26.07.2000 | 16.02.1983 | F | S/Leave | 1739 | 1744 | Tiredness & Sore throat - Private | | 4596 | |

577

Result of a query that lists all consultations from the 22nd to the end of July 2000 (ConsultationsSeenFrom22ndTillEndOfJul2000)

| SurgeryDate | DateOfBirth | Sex | Diagnosis | TimeIn | TimeOut | Complaints | Treatments | NumbersID | Notes |
|---|---|---|---|---|---|---|---|---|---|
| 26.07.2000 | 03.07.1967 | F | | 941 | 951 | (L) ear ache | EarCalm | 4657 | FP1001 (GMS4) form signed. T.A.T.T, for FBC & TFTs. |
| 28.07.2000 | 10.12.1944 | M | Revisit | 922 | 932 | Pain in (L) groins has persisted | Kapake | 4780 | |
| 25.07.2000 | 22.04.1975 | F | | 1746 | 1751 | Awaiting appointment to see Gastro-enterologist | | 4810 | |
| 25.07.2000 | 18.09.1992 | F | RTI | 1634 | 1639 | Cough | Amoxycillin | 4956 | |
| 25.07.2000 | 27.02.1931 | F | Pain | 927 | 934 | Pain (R) hip | Co-dydramol & Ibuprofen | 5036 | Script for Multivitamins given. |
| 28.07.2000 | 26.08.1913 | F | | 1056 | 1111 | Unable to tolerate Viscotears, her eyes are sore | Referred to Eye clinic, SGH | 5046 | |
| 26.07.2000 | 09.02.1965 | F | URTI | 1733 | 1739 | Sore throat | Penicillin V | 5077 | |
| 24.07.2000 | 11.01.1957 | F | | 1002 | 1010 | Dysuria | Trimethoprim | 5113 | For MSU. |
| 24.07.2000 | 17.09.1975 | F | URTI | 1720 | 1732 | Pain & discharge (R) ear | Flucloxacillin & Otomize ear spray | 5148 | |
| 27.07.2000 | 31.10.1920 | F | | 1637 | 1645 | Cryotherapy to (R) chin | | 5160 | FP1001 (GMS4) form signed. |
| 26.07.2000 | 06.06.1978 | F | Pain | 1836 | 1840 | Toothache & on antibiotics from Dentist | Tylex & Diclofenac enteric coated | 5232 | |
| 26.07.2000 | 17.02.1972 | F | | 1008 | 1015 | Sore throat | Advised to use own Paracetamol | 5279 | |

Result of a query that lists all consultations from the 22nd to the end of July 2000 (ConsultationsSeenFrom22ndTillEndOfJul2000)

| SurgeryDate | DateOfBirth | Sex | Diagnosis | TimeIn | TimeOut | Complaints | Treatments | NumbersID | Notes |
|---|---|---|---|---|---|---|---|---|---|
| 24.07.2000 | 08.12.1978 | F | Rash | 911 | 917 | Weepy, itchy & sore rash on abdomen | Flucloxacillin & Fucidin-H | 5293 | FP1001 (GMS4) form signed. |
| 27.07.2000 | 14.06.1942 | F | S/Leave | 1024 | 1035 | Stressed | | 5303 | |
| 26.07.2000 | 11.11.1969 | F | UTI | 951 | 1008 | (L) loin pain | Co-Amoxiclav | 5363 | For MSU. |
| 27.07.2000 | 25.06.1962 | M | Revisit | 942 | 946 | Still has cough | Ciprofloxacin & Codeine Linctus | 5393 | |
| 28.07.2000 | 05.08.1936 | F | | 1723 | 1737 | Script for Metronidazole & Ciprofloxacin given | | 551 | |
| 24.07.2000 | 01.05.1974 | F | Pain | 1706 | 1714 | Pain (L) lower leg | Co-dydramol | 5556 | |
| 27.07.2000 | 28.09.1921 | F | Pain | 926 | 933 | Pain (L) elbow | Co-dydramol & Ibuprofen | 5597 | |
| 26.07.2000 | 17.04.1923 | M | Rash | 1015 | 1023 | Perineal rash, sore | Fucidin-H cream, Flucloxacillin & Aqueous cream | 560 | |
| 24.07.2000 | 27.12.1941 | F | Pain | 1153 | 1217 | Abdominal pain & vomiting | MST, Sevredol & Buscopan | 5790 | Home visit. |
| 25.07.2000 | 19.04.1984 | F | | 1705 | 1715 | Pregnancy test positive | | 5884 | |
| 27.07.2000 | 20.07.1963 | F | | 1731 | 1735 | Cryotherapy to skin tags on (L) side of neck | | 5892 | |
| 26.07.2000 | 01.11.1966 | M | | 1023 | 1031 | Dribbles urine a lot | For MSU | 5897 | |
| 24.07.2000 | 29.05.1933 | M | | 943 | 958 | Script for Gliclazide & Clinistix | | 5912 | |
| 25.07.2000 | 23.03.1926 | M | | 949 | 1004 | Wax in the ears | Cerumol | 5954 | |
| 25.07.2000 | 29.09.1959 | M | Revisit | 1751 | 1754 | Chest cough again | Ciprofloxacin | 6115 | |

579

## Result of a query that lists all consultations from the 22nd to the end of July 2000 (ConsultationsSeenFrom22ndTillEndOfJul2000)

| SurgeryDate | DateOfBirth | Sex | Diagnosis | TimeIn | TimeOut | Complaints | Treatments | NumbersID | Notes |
|---|---|---|---|---|---|---|---|---|---|
| 28.07.2000 | 20.12.1922 | F | | 1023 | 1030 | Advised to continue Bendrofluazide | | 6237 | |
| 24.07.2000 | 01.07.1999 | F | | 1029 | 1035 | Oral thrush | Nystatin oral suspension | 6466 | |
| 26.07.2000 | 06.11.1968 | M | RTI | 920 | 925 | Cough | Erythromycin | 6490 | Penicillin allergy. |
| 28.07.2000 | 15.08.1999 | M | | 1750 | 1753 | Script for Paracetamol given | | 6521 | |
| 28.07.2000 | 09.04.1944 | F | | 932 | 940 | Pain (R) ear with dizziness | Otomize ear spray & Prochlorperazine | 6592 | |
| 26.07.2000 | 25.06.1953 | M | | 1812 | 1824 | Script for Metformin, Enalapril & Simvastatin given | | 6632 | |
| 25.07.2000 | 06.04.1943 | M | | 1758 | 1801 | Dizziness | Prochlorperazine | 6649 | Tetanus Toxoid allergy. |
| 26.07.2000 | 20.01.2000 | F | | 1824 | 1836 | Fever & screaming | | 6674 | |
| 27.07.2000 | 13.02.1940 | M | | 1630 | 1636 | Cryotherapy to skin tags (L) axilla | | 6704 | |
| 25.07.2000 | 23.07.1968 | M | S/Leave | 1022 | 1034 | Diarrhoea & vomiting - Med. 5 | | 6727 | |
| 28.07.2000 | 11.01.1951 | F | | 1806 | 1826 | Asthma inadequately controlled | Zafirlukast | 6735 | 1st Accolate safety study visit. |
| 28.07.2000 | 10.04.2000 | M | | 1654 | 1707 | Vomiting | Infant Gaviscon | 6761 | Script for Paracetamol given. |
| 24.07.2000 | 21.02.1928 | F | Pain | 1035 | 1050 | Pain (L) hip | Kapake | 6770 | For Hip X-Rays. Cough, Rx. Codeine Linctus. For CXR. |
| 26.07.2000 | 16.05.1967 | M | Pain | 1701 | 1709 | Pain in elbows | Co-dydramol | 6815 | |

Result of a query that lists all consultations from the 22nd to the end of July 2000 (ConsultationsSeenFrom22ndTillEndOfJul2000)

| SurgeryDate | DateOfBirth | Sex | Diagnosis | TimeIn | TimeOut | Complaints | Treatments | NumbersID | Notes |
|---|---|---|---|---|---|---|---|---|---|
| 28.07.2000 | 07.05.1937 | F | | 909 | 922 | (R) ankle oedema | Frusemide | 695 | |
| 26.07.2000 | 10.02.1943 | F | URTI | 916 | 920 | Sore throat | Amoxycillin | 775 | |
| 27.07.2000 | 19.10.1975 | F | | 1158 | 1215 | Routine P/Natal check | | 819 | Home visit. |
| 25.07.2000 | 06.11.1981 | M | Pain | 1801 | 1810 | Shooting pain (R) groin | Co-dydramol & Ibuprofen | 852 | New Patient check done. |
| 27.07.2000 | 06.06.1930 | M | | 1647 | 1702 | Cryotherapy to (R) axilla | | 883 | |
| 24.07.2000 | 04.07.1959 | F | | 1808 | 1816 | Script for Estraderm MX 50 given | | 96 | |
| 28.07.2000 | 03.03.1929 | M | Pain | 1014 | 1023 | Pain (L) knee | Kapake & Flucloxacillin | 979 | |
| 25.07.2000 | 31.12.1930 | F | RTI | 934 | 939 | Cough | Amoxycillin | 989 | |

Result of a query that lists all consultations from the 22nd to the end of July 2001 (ConsultationsSeenFrom22ndTillEndOfJul2001)

| SurgeryDate | DateOfBirth | Sex | Diagnosis | TimeIn | TimeOut | Complaints | Treatments | NumbersID | Notes |
|---|---|---|---|---|---|---|---|---|---|
| 23.07.2001 | 24.12.1929 | F | | 1730 | 1734 | Cystitis again | Trimethoprim & Mist Potassium Citrate | 1059 | Penicillin allergy. |
| 24.07.2001 | 08.02.1939 | F | URTI | 1004 | 1011 | Infected rhinorrhoea | Amoxycillin | 113 | Back pain following a fall, for X-Ray of the Lumbo-Sacral spine. Trimethoprim allergy. |

Result of a query that lists all consultations from the 22nd to the end of July 2001 (ConsultationsSeenFrom22ndTillEndOfJul2001)

| SurgeryDate | DateOfBirth | Sex | Diagnosis | TimeIn | TimeOut | Complaints | Treatments | NumbersID | Notes |
|---|---|---|---|---|---|---|---|---|---|
| 25.07.2001 | 18.05.1949 | M | S/Leave | 1650 | 1655 | Injury (R) shoulder – Med. 5 | | 1160 | |
| 26.07.2001 | 18.11.1946 | F | Pain | 1638 | 1641 | Pain (L) elbow | Diclofenac enteric coated & Dihydrocodeine | 1307 | |
| 23.07.2001 | 08.01.1942 | F | Pain | 1747 | 1752 | Pain in both ears | Amoxycillin, Sofradex ear drops & Co-dydramol | 1435 | |
| 25.07.2001 | 22.07.1939 | F | | 922 | 927 | Septic insect bite (R) thigh | Fucidin cream & Flucloxacillin | 1546 | |
| 23.07.2001 | 17.10.1940 | M | | 1647 | 1702 | Pulse 50/min | Advised to stop Atenolol | 1652 | |
| 27.07.2001 | 28.07.1960 | F | RTI | 959 | 1009 | Cough & painful ribs | Amoxycillin, Co-dydramol & Ibuprofen | 189 | |
| 23.07.2001 | 16.09.1949 | M | Rash | 1023 | 1033 | ?Shingles rash (L) T4 & chest pain | Famciclovir, Co-dydramol & Ibuprofen | 1893 | |
| 24.07.2001 | 19.08.1926 | F | | 1042 | 1049 | Script for Gaviscon tablets given | | 1907 | |
| 24.07.2001 | 23.09.1951 | F | | 1643 | 1651 | Post-menopausal bleeding | Referred to Gynaecologist | 1969 | |
| 26.07.2001 | 20.09.1946 | F | Pain | 1810 | 1817 | Pain (L) leg | Naftidrofuryl | 1973 | Script for Amitriptyline given. |
| 25.07.2001 | 26.08.1987 | F | Revisit | 1732 | 1738 | Facial Acne is getting worse | Zineryt lotion | 2332 | Referred to Dermatologist. |

Result of a query that lists all consultations from the 22nd to the end of July 2001 (ConsultationsSeenFrom22ndTillEndOfJul2001)

| SurgeryDate | DateOfBirth | Sex | Diagnosis | TimeIn | TimeOut | Complaints | Treatments | NumbersID | Notes |
|---|---|---|---|---|---|---|---|---|---|
| 27.07.2001 | 11.05.1959 | F | | 1029 | 1039 | Something coming down vaginally | Referred to Gynaecologist (BUPA) | 2351 | Script for Cefalexin given. Penicillin, Sudafen, Septrin Tetracycline allergy. |
| 23.07.2001 | 28.03.1970 | F | S/Leave | 1708 | 1724 | Pain & numbness in (R) hand | | 2375 | For MSU. |
| 26.07.2001 | 02.12.1948 | M | | 1651 | 1659 | He takes excessive alcohol & will like to stop | Advised to contact the ROCHE Unit | 2380 | |
| 24.07.2001 | 07.02.1921 | M | | 906 | 915 | He wants Insurance claim form completed | | 2381 | |
| 25.07.2001 | 13.11.1970 | F | | 1738 | 1749 | Heavy, painful & prolonged period | Referred to Gynaecologist | 2578 | |
| 24.07.2001 | 05.07.1952 | F | | 1812 | 1823 | Script for Diclofenac enteric coated & Flucloxacillin given | | 2894 | |
| 30.07.2001 | 05.05.1953 | F | Revisit | 917 | 921 | Persistent neck pain | Referred to Orthopaedic Surgeon | 3000 | |
| 27.07.2001 | 26.06.1946 | M | S/Leave | 906 | 918 | Depression | | 3025 | |
| 23.07.2001 | 10.08.1968 | F | | 1033 | 1042 | Intermenstrual bleeding has now stopped | | 3033 | |
| 26.07.2001 | 10.10.1990 | F | | 955 | 959 | Septic bilateral IGTN | Flucloxacillin & Fucidin cream | 3039 | |
| 30.07.2001 | 06.04.1968 | M | | 1703 | 1707 | Script for Salbutamol inhaler given | | 3088 | |

Result of a query that lists all consultations from the 22nd to the end of July 2001 (ConsultationsSeenFrom22ndTillEndOfJul2001)

| SurgeryDate | DateOfBirth | Sex | Diagnosis | TimeIn | TimeOut | Complaints | Treatments | NumbersID | Notes |
|---|---|---|---|---|---|---|---|---|---|
| 26.07.2001 | 01.02.1980 | F | | 942 | 955 | Advised to come back in 10 months if she is still unable to conceive | | 3118 | |
| 25.07.2001 | 06.10.1924 | F | | 1038 | 1043 | Chest pain, getting worse | Advised to go to hospital via Ambulance | 312 | Neighbour came to Surgery. |
| 23.07.2001 | 28.04.1978 | M | | 1737 | 1740 | Moles under (R) arm | For Cryotherapy later | 3167 | |
| 24.07.2001 | 04.07.1929 | M | | 942 | 958 | Enlarged Prostate & elevated PSA | Referred to Urologist (urgent Basildon hospital) | 322 | |
| 26.07.2001 | 12.08.1932 | M | URTI | 1016 | 1019 | Infected rhinorrhoea & mouth ulcers | Amoxycillin | 3344 | |
| 25.07.2001 | 18.07.1978 | F | Pain | 1004 | 1011 | Pain both thighs | Co-dydramol & Lactulose | 337 | Haemorrhoids, Rx. Glyceryl Trinitrate ointment 0.2%. |
| 30.07.2001 | 02.05.1992 | M | | 939 | 948 | Script for Colofac given | | 3606 | |
| 30.07.2001 | 05.12.1937 | M | | 948 | 959 | Wheezy | Prednisolone enteric coated & Fexofenadine | 3646 | |
| 24.07.2001 | 14.06.1957 | F | | 1735 | 1739 | Wants period delayed for holidays | Norethisterone | 3661 | |
| 30.07.2001 | 06.04.1968 | M | | 1717 | 1720 | He is appealing against decision that he is capable of working | | 3684 | |

Result of a query that lists all consultations from the 22nd to the end of July 2001 (ConsultationsSeenFrom22ndTillEndOfJul2001)

| SurgeryDate | DateOfBirth | Sex | Diagnosis | TimeIn | TimeOut | Complaints | Treatments | NumbersID | Notes |
|---|---|---|---|---|---|---|---|---|---|
| 26.07.2001 | 01.10.1954 | M | Mole | 904 | 914 | Sore darkish mole on (L) nipple | Flucloxacillin & Fucidin cream | 3713 | Referred to Dermatologist (Basildon hospital). |
| 26.07.2001 | 23.07.1953 | M | S/Leave | 1748 | 1759 | Cellulitis – Duplicate | | 3725 | Pain (R) shoulder & neck. For X-Ray (R) shoulder & Cervical X-Ray. |
| 27.07.2001 | 24.08.1992 | M | RTI | 1659 | 1702 | Cough | Amoxycillin | 3733 | |
| 24.07.2001 | 24.09.1941 | F | | 1011 | 1018 | Constipated | Lactulose & Senna | 3760 | Wart on face, Rx. Cuplex gel. |
| 23.07.2001 | 02.11.1920 | F | RTI | 1006 | 1012 | Cough | Amoxycillin | 3789 | Erythromycin allergy. |
| 30.07.2001 | 10.06.1928 | F | | 1656 | 1703 | Script for Frusemide given | | 3884 | Penicillin allergy. |
| 30.07.2001 | 06.09.1964 | F | S/Leave | 1720 | 1728 | Agoraphobia (Nervous disability) | | 3991 | |
| 25.07.2001 | 07.04.1964 | F | Conjunctivitis | 1749 | 1754 | Sore & sticky (L) eye | Chloramphenicol eye drops | 4101 | For Fasting Glucose. |
| 30.07.2001 | 21.02.1916 | F | | 959 | 1013 | Script for Ibuprofen, Lansoprazole & inj. Depo-Medrone with Lidocaine given | | 4178 | Penicillin allergy. |
| 30.07.2001 | 19.01.1943 | F | S/Leave | 933 | 939 | (R) knee Arthroscopy | | 4226 | |
| 25.07.2001 | 13.08.1923 | F | RTI | 1000 | 1004 | Cough | Erythromycin | 424 | Penicillin allergy. |
| 23.07.2001 | 19.11.1924 | M | | 911 | 921 | Dizziness & loss of weight | Betahistine | 4264 | For FBC, MSU & CXR. |
| 27.07.2001 | 11.12.1968 | M | Revisit | 1705 | 1711 | (R) sided abdominal/chest pain has persisted | Referred to Pain clinic | 4315 | |

Result of a query that lists all consultations from the 22nd to the end of July 2001 (ConsultationsSeenFrom22ndTillEndOfJul2001)

| SurgeryDate | DateOfBirth | Sex | Diagnosis | TimeIn | TimeOut | Complaints | Treatments | NumbersID | Notes |
|---|---|---|---|---|---|---|---|---|---|
| 27.07.2001 | 30.03.1994 | M | URTI | 1657 | 1659 | Sore throat | Amoxycillin | 4386 | |
| 23.07.2001 | 12.04.1927 | M | | 945 | 1006 | Rectal bleeding | Scheriproct suppositories & Scheriproct ointment | 4394 | Referred to Rectal Surgeon (Very Urgent). |
| 23.07.2001 | 03.05.1946 | F | | 1702 | 1708 | Script for Ibuprofen given | | 4483 | Paracetamol allergy. |
| 23.07.2001 | 27.03.1931 | F | | 1724 | 1730 | (R) sided facial swelling | Amoxycillin | 4618 | |
| 26.07.2001 | 04.10.1934 | M | | 1019 | 1028 | The Parking Badge Scheme for Disabled People Medical Practitioner Report completed | | 4720 | |
| 26.07.2001 | 19.03.1967 | M | | 1659 | 1704 | Reddish warm swelling (R) elbow | Flucloxacillin & Co-dydramol | 4730 | |
| 25.07.2001 | 13.02.1974 | M | | 1754 | 1805 | Requested sleeping tablets | Request declined | 4731 | |
| 27.07.2001 | 10.12.1946 | M | Pain | 918 | 925 | Abdominal pain has persisted | Referred to Gastro-enterologist | 4780 | |
| 26.07.2001 | 28.01.1953 | F | | 1009 | 1016 | Due to have her hysterectomy on 20.08.01 | | 4781 | |
| 25.07.2001 | 02.05.1962 | F | | 1707 | 1717 | Frequency of micturition | Trimethoprim | 4887 | For MSU. |
| 27.07.2001 | 19.05.1981 | F | UTI | 1758 | 1803 | Dysuria & frequency | Trimethoprim | 490 | Penicillin allergy. |

Result of a query that lists all consultations from the 22nd to the end of July 2001 (ConsultationsSeenFrom22ndTillEndOfJul2001)

| SurgeryDate | DateOfBirth | Sex | Diagnosis | TimeIn | TimeOut | Complaints | Treatments | NumbersID | Notes |
|---|---|---|---|---|---|---|---|---|---|
| 23.07.2001 | 14.05.1951 | M | | 1805 | 1812 | Script for Glyceryl Trinitrate ointment given | | 5031 | Penicillin allergy. |
| 26.07.2001 | 09.12.1995 | M | Rash | 930 | 937 | Chicken Pox rah | Paracetamol & Calamine lotion | 5068 | Septic (R) big toe, Rx. Flucloxacillin. |
| 27.07.2001 | 23.05.1978 | F | | 1638 | 1657 | Recurrent pelvic infections | Referred to Gynaecologist | 5204 | |
| 26.07.2001 | 17.02.1972 | F | URTI | 1714 | 1722 | (R) Otitis externa | Otomize ear spray | 5279 | Penicillin allergy. |
| 27.07.2001 | 17.02.1972 | F | Revisit | 1820 | 1824 | (R) ear ache is worse | Erythromycin | 5279 | Penicillin allergy. |
| 25.07.2001 | 03.05.1972 | F | Revisit | 1639 | 1644 | Recurrent vaginal irritation & dyspareunia | Referred to Gynaecologist | 5373 | |
| 23.07.2001 | 03.04.1997 | M | | 921 | 941 | Abdominal pain & fever | Referred to Paediatric Dr. on call, SGH | 5566 | Penicillin allergy. |
| 24.07.2001 | 30.03.1984 | F | | 1634 | 1643 | Late period | For Pregnancy test | 5608 | |
| 27.07.2001 | 09.07.1969 | M | Pain | 1742 | 1758 | Pain (R) groin & (R) testicle | Referred to Surgeon | 563 | For USScan of the testicles. |
| 23.07.2001 | 25.02.1912 | F | | 1042 | 1055 | Poor appetite | Vit. B Co. | 5678 | For FBC. |
| 25.07.2001 | 05.08.1976 | F | | 906 | 915 | Unprotected sexual intercourse | Schering PC4 | 5702 | |
| 26.07.2001 | 18.04.1969 | M | | 914 | 918 | Hay fever | Fexofenadine | 5736 | |
| 25.07.2001 | 10.08.1940 | F | | 1717 | 1727 | Due to see Orthopaedic Surgeon at Old Church hospital | | 5747 | |

## Result of a query that lists all consultations from the 22nd to the end of July 2001 (ConsultationsSeenFrom22ndTillEndOfJul2001)

| SurgeryDate | DateOfBirth | Sex | Diagnosis | TimeIn | TimeOut | Complaints | Treatments | NumbersID | Notes |
|---|---|---|---|---|---|---|---|---|---|
| 30.07.2001 | 21.11.1939 | M | Depression | 907 | 913 | Unable to cope & insomnia since his wife died | Citalopram | 5777 | |
| 24.07.2001 | 06.04.1955 | F | | 958 | 1004 | (L) ear is deaf | Amoxycillin | 579 | |
| 24.07.2001 | 07.03.1942 | M | URTI | 1802 | 1812 | Sore throat | Erythromycin | 5793 | |
| 30.07.2001 | 20.02.1937 | F | | 1641 | 1656 | Script for Co-Proxamol given | | 5798 | |
| 23.07.2001 | 15.07.1936 | M | | 1015 | 1023 | Septic wound (L) shin - old Tibial nail injury | Flucloxacillin | 5881 | For X-Ray (L) Tibia. |
| 26.07.2001 | 25.12.1963 | F | Pain | 1704 | 1714 | Chest pain | GTN spray | 5934 | |
| 24.07.2001 | 23.03.1926 | M | | 1025 | 1042 | He has stopped Pro-Banthine | | 5954 | |
| 25.07.2001 | 17.12.1931 | M | Depression | 915 | 922 | Weepy & unable to cope | Referred to CPN | 5978 | |
| 27.07.2001 | 19.09.1937 | M | RTI | 1702 | 1705 | Cough | Amoxycillin | 6104 | |
| 27.07.2001 | 03.12.1955 | F | | 1731 | 1742 | Hb 9.0 g/dl | For B12, Folate & Ferritin | 614 | |
| 24.07.2001 | 12.04.1952 | M | S/Leave | 1651 | 1655 | Pain (R) hip - Med. 5 | | 6322 | Plaster allergy. |
| 30.07.2001 | 28.03.1945 | M | | 1013 | 1020 | Painful Varicose veins both legs | Referred to Vascular Surgeon (Basildon hospital) | 6357 | Script for Tetracycline given. |
| 24.07.2001 | 29.09.1949 | F | | 1726 | 1735 | Script for Norethisterone given | | 6365 | |
| 27.07.2001 | 21.06.1959 | F | | 1020 | 1029 | May need Physiotherapy locally | | 6458 | |

Result of a query that lists all consultations from the 22nd to the end of July 2001 (ConsultationsSeenFrom22ndTillEndOfJul2001)

| SurgeryDate | DateOfBirth | Sex | Diagnosis | TimeIn | TimeOut | Complaints | Treatments | NumbersID | Notes |
|---|---|---|---|---|---|---|---|---|---|
| 23.07.2001 | 08.05.1939 | F |  | 941 | 945 | The lump on the forehead has disappeared |  | 6643 |  |
| 30.07.2001 | 15.09.1946 | F |  | 1736 | 1742 | Script for Co-dydramol given |  | 6684 |  |
| 24.07.2001 | 08.1.1940 | F |  | 938 | 942 | Sticky & weepy eyes | Chloramphenicol eye drops | 6705 |  |
| 25.07.2001 | 06.07.1969 | M | Pain | 927 | 932 | Back pain | Ibuprofen & Co-dydramol | 6726 |  |
| 24.07.2001 | 27.02.1941 | M |  | 1754 | 1802 | DSS is requesting sick certificate |  | 675 |  |
| 26.07.2001 | 27.02.1941 | M | S/Leave | 959 | 1009 | Emphysema - Med. 5 & Med. 3 |  | 675 |  |
| 25.07.2001 | 10.05.1963 | F |  | 1011 | 1021 | Pregnancy test positive |  | 6852 |  |
| 23.07.2001 | 30.08.1998 | M | Conjunctivitis | 1734 | 1737 | Sticky eyes | Chloramphenicol eye drops | 7041 |  |
| 26.07.2001 | 02.10.1940 | F | Pain | 1726 | 1733 | Low abdominal pain | Dihydrocodeine, Diclofenac enteric coated & Lactulose | 7062 |  |
| 25.07.2001 | 26.05.1949 | M | Pain | 1657 | 1707 | (R) sided abdominal pain | Buscopan & Co-dydramol | 7063 | For CXR & USScan of upper abdomen. |
| 23.07.2001 | 09.10.1976 | F | Lump | 904 | 911 | Fatty lumps on the head | Referred to Surgeon | 7064 |  |
| 23.07.2001 | 02.01.1953 | F |  | 1012 | 1015 | Wants to stop smoking | Smoking cessation visit advised | 7068 |  |

589

Result of a query that lists all consultations from the 22nd to the end of July 2001 (ConsultationsSeenFrom22ndTillEndOfJul2001)

| SurgeryDate | DateOfBirth | Sex | Diagnosis | TimeIn | TimeOut | Complaints | Treatments | NumbersID | Notes |
|---|---|---|---|---|---|---|---|---|---|
| 23.07.2001 | 20.09.1934 | F | | 1752 | 1805 | Script for Doxazosin XL given | | 7069 | Bilateral ankle swelling, on Tildiem LA. Advised to stop the latter. |
| 24.07.2001 | 07.10.1972 | F | | 926 | 938 | Script for Microgynon 30 given | | 7079 | |
| 24.07.2001 | 02.10.1945 | F | URTI | 1659 | 1708 | Sore throat | Amoxycillin | 7087 | |
| 24.07.2001 | 18.10.1920 | F | | 1655 | 1659 | Script for Lansoprazole & Paracetamol given | | 7088 | |
| 24.07.2001 | 11.05.2001 | F | | 1719 | 1726 | Waxy ears | Paracetamol & Amoxycillin | 7129 | |
| 25.07.2001 | 09.06.1924 | F | | 932 | 1000 | History of Bowel carcinoma with metastasis | Referred to Oncologist | 7132 | |
| 26.07.2001 | 23.07.1919 | F | Conjunctivitis | 918 | 930 | Sticky (R) eye | Chloramphenicol eye drops | 750 | For FBC & Fasting Glucose. |
| 26.07.2001 | 10.09.1919 | F | | 1028 | 1039 | Script for Prednisolone enteric coated given | | 823 | |
| 30.07.2001 | 15.04.1973 | F | S/Leave | 1020 | 1027 | Back Pain - Private | | 942 | Script for Co-dydramol given. |
| 27.07.2001 | 20.10.1925 | F | Pain | 1039 | 1054 | Pain & swelling (R) knee | Referred to Orthopaedic Dr. on call, SGH | 952 | Penicillin & Aspirin allergy. |
| 26.07.2001 | 16.07.1983 | F | | 1736 | 1748 | Personality swings | | 967 | Her mother came to Surgery. |

590

Result of a query that lists all consultations from the 22nd to the end of July 2001 (ConsultationsSeenFrom22ndTillEndOfJul2001)

| SurgeryDate | DateOfBirth | Sex | Diagnosis | TimeIn | TimeOut | Complaints | Treatments | NumbersID | Notes |
|---|---|---|---|---|---|---|---|---|---|
| 24.07.2001 | 18.06.2001 | M | | 915 | 926 | Constipated & vomiting | Lactulose & Infant Gaviscon | NP | |
| 25.07.2001 | 20.06.1983 | M | URTI | 1727 | 1732 | Sore throat | Amoxycillin | Temp | |
| 26.07.2001 | 21.11.1992 | F | URTI | 1722 | 1726 | Sore throat | Amoxycillin | Temp | |
| 26.07.2001 | 23.02.1981 | F | | 1759 | 1810 | For Pregnancy test | | Temp | |
| 27.07.2001 | 15.03.1980 | F | RTI | 1011 | 1020 | Cough | Erythromycin | Temp | |
| 27.07.2001 | 29.10.1999 | M | Rash | 1711 | 1719 | Itchy red & sore rash | Fucidin-H cream & Flucloxacillin | Temp | |
| 30.07.2001 | 04.09.1997 | M | | 913 | 917 | Script for Esomeprazole given | | Temp | |

Result of a query that lists all consultations from the 22nd to the end of July 2003 (ConsultationsSeenFrom22ndTillEndOfJul2003)

| SurgeryDate | DateOfBirth | Sex | Diagnosis | TimeIn | TimeOut | Complaints | Treatments | NumbersID | Notes |
|---|---|---|---|---|---|---|---|---|---|
| 24.07.2003 | 28.06.1954 | M | | 1115 | 1127 | Diarrhoea & abdominal pain | Buscopan | Temp | To get OTC Imodium & Dioralyte. Stool for C&S. |
| 29.07.2003 | 31.07.1956 | M | | 918 | 926 | Boils under the arms & the legs | Flucloxacillin | 1027 | For FBC, Fasting Glucose & serum Cholesterol. |
| 25.07.2003 | 30.03.1923 | M | Rash | 1018 | 1025 | Urticarial type rash | Fexofenadine | 1060 | |
| 24.07.2003 | 21.10.1929 | F | | 918 | 929 | Septic insect bites on the legs | Erythromycin & Fusidic Acid cream | 1129 | Script for Thyroxine given. |

Result of a query that lists all consultations from the 22nd to the end of July 2003 (ConsultationsSeenFrom22ndTillEndOfJul2003)

| SurgeryDate | DateOfBirth | Sex | Diagnosis | TimeIn | TimeOut | Complaints | Treatments | NumbersID | Notes |
|---|---|---|---|---|---|---|---|---|---|
| 22.07.2003 | 01.12.1934 | F | | 1005 | 1009 | Script for Simvastatin given | | 1371 | Penicillin & Erythromycin allergy. |
| 22.07.2003 | 28.03.1970 | F | | 1013 | 1020 | Script for Metformin given | | 1371 | |
| 30.07.2003 | 08.04.1961 | F | S/Leave | 908 | 913 | Laparoscopic Cholecystectomy | | 1407 | Itchy vulvo-vaginal region, Rx. Clotrimazole pessary & Clotrimazole 1% + 1% Hydrocortisone cream. |
| 25.07.2003 | 06.08.1941 | M | S/Leave | 909 | 926 | Vomiting - Private | | 1425 | Still vomiting, Referred to Gastro-enterologist. |
| 29.07.2003 | 06.08.1941 | M | S/Leave | 1737 | 1742 | Vomiting | | 1425 | |
| 30.07.2003 | 08.08.1973 | M | | 1733 | 1748 | Script for Rosuvastatin given | | 1454 | |
| 23.07.2003 | 09.10.1924 | F | RTI | 1709 | 1715 | Cough | Amoxycillin | 1477 | |
| 30.07.2003 | 12.05.1963 | F | | 1809 | 1813 | Septic burn area on chest | Flucloxacillin & Fusidic Acid cream | 1506 | |
| 28.07.2003 | 28.01.1920 | F | | 1018 | 1033 | Diabetic Clinic | | 1730 | Script for Atenolol given. |
| 28.07.2003 | 04.04.1939 | M | | 929 | 935 | I explained to his wife that the secretary to Psychogeriatrician will be arranging for urgent OPD appointment for him | | 1845 | |

## Result of a query that lists all consultations from the 22nd to the end of July 2003 (ConsultationsSeenFrom22ndTillEndOfJul2003)

| SurgeryDate | DateOfBirth | Sex | Diagnosis | TimeIn | TimeOut | Complaints | Treatments | NumbersID | Notes |
|---|---|---|---|---|---|---|---|---|---|
| 28.07.2003 | 27.04.1939 | F | | 922 | 929 | Hot sweats | Clonidine | 1846 | |
| 29.07.2003 | 03.05.1981 | F | | 1633 | 1640 | Pregnancy test is positive | | 1902 | |
| 29.07.2003 | 31.08.1982 | F | | 942 | 951 | Sweating heavily in the axillae | Aluminium Chloride 20 % roll on application | 1924 | |
| 28.07.2003 | 29.11.1929 | F | | 1701 | 1707 | Weepy & septic blisters on the legs | Frusemide & Flucloxacillin | 193 | |
| 29.07.2003 | 29.11.1929 | F | Rash | 1721 | 1737 | Itchy rash on chest | Calamine lotion | 193 | |
| 25.07.2003 | 09.07.1940 | M | RTI | 941 | 946 | Chesty cough | Amoxycillin | 2152 | |
| 28.07.2003 | 22.03.1933 | F | Pain | 1636 | 1644 | Injury to (R) knee | For X-Ray | 2179 | Abrasion on the knee, Rx. Flucloxacillin. |
| 24.07.2003 | 18.03.1985 | F | S/Leave | 929 | 935 | Depression - Private | | 2199 | |
| 28.07.2003 | 25.03.1946 | M | Pain | 1631 | 1636 | Pains in his legs | Paracetamol | 2347 | |
| 22.07.2003 | 23.04.1950 | F | S/Leave | 900 | 905 | Prophylactic Laparoscopic BSO | | 2369 | |
| 22.07.2003 | 13.03.1983 | F | Pain | 1820 | 1825 | Dull ache in the (R) knee | For X-Ray | 2388 | |
| 23.07.2003 | 16.03.1927 | F | Depression | 1715 | 1730 | Panic attacks | Amitriptyline | 2415 | |
| 30.07.2003 | 02.06.1955 | F | S/Leave | 1712 | 1715 | Depression & Panic attacks | | 2671 | Penicillin allergy. |
| 23.07.2003 | 30.11.1936 | M | | 913 | 916 | To drink plenty & mobilise when on the plane to his holidays | | 2793 | |

Result of a query that lists all consultations from the 22nd to the end of July 2003 (ConsultationsSeenFrom22ndTillEndOfJul2003)

| SurgeryDate | DateOfBirth | Sex | Diagnosis | TimeIn | TimeOut | Complaints | Treatments | NumbersID | Notes |
|---|---|---|---|---|---|---|---|---|---|
| 29.07.2003 | 25.05.1976 | F |  | 1835 | 1846 | Depressed & unable to cope | Referred to Practice Counsellor | 2797 | Cefaclor allergy. |
| 28.07.2003 | 28.03.1926 | F |  | 952 | 1001 | Septic insect bite on the (R) foot | Flucloxacillin & Fusidic Acid cream | 2837 | Script for Frusemide given. |
| 22.07.2003 | 27.11.1950 | M | Rash | 1714 | 1722 | Itchy red rash both axillae | Clotrimazole 1% + 1% Hydrocortisone cream | 287 |  |
| 28.07.2003 | 21.09.1919 | M |  | 901 | 907 | For repeat U/Es |  | 2917 |  |
| 25.07.2003 | 25.07.1938 | F |  | 1756 | 1803 | Septic abrasion (R) fore-arm | Flucloxacillin & Fusidic Acid cream | 2964 | Script for Rosuvastatin given. |
| 24.07.2003 | 07.07.1983 | F | URTI | 935 | 939 | Sore throat | Amoxycillin | 3085 |  |
| 30.07.2003 | 01.02.1980 | F |  | 922 | 926 | To try OTC thrush medication for her vaginal thrush |  | 3118 |  |
| 22.07.2003 | 13.11.1953 | M | S/Leave | 1722 | 1728 | Multiple joints pain - Med. 5 |  | 3119 | Script for Co-codamol given. |
| 22.07.2003 | 08.06.1961 | M | Revisit | 1655 | 1659 | (L) knee is still sore & keeps giving way | Referred to Orthopaedic Surgeon (Basildon Hospital) | 3154 |  |
| 29.07.2003 | 02.11.1953 | F | Pain | 1715 | 1721 | Neck & (R) arm pain with swelling on fore-arm | Referred to Orthopaedic Surgeon (Basildon Hospital) | 3182 | Penicillin allergy. |

**Result of a query that lists all consultations from the 22nd to the end of July 2003 (ConsultationsSeenFrom22ndTillEndOfJul2003)**

| SurgeryDate | DateOfBirth | Sex | Diagnosis | TimeIn | TimeOut | Complaints | Treatments | NumbersID | Notes |
|---|---|---|---|---|---|---|---|---|---|
| 30.07.2003 | 17.07.1942 | M | Conjunctivitis | 1023 | 1027 | Both eyes are sore, burning, itchy & sticky | Chloramphenicol eye drops | 3244 | Penicillin & Plaster allergy. |
| 29.07.2003 | 15.01.1957 | F | | 1648 | 1656 | Fasting Glucose 13.2 mmols/L | Dietary advice given | 3262 | |
| 30.07.2003 | 28.01.1969 | M | | 926 | 932 | He came to tell me that he is fit to undertake employment | | 3471 | |
| 25.07.2003 | 15.07.1956 | M | | 1739 | 1743 | Script for Kaltostat dressing & Cavilon stick as repeat prescription | | 352 | |
| 25.07.2003 | 29.07.1960 | F | RTI | 956 | 1002 | Cough | Amoxycillin | 3557 | |
| 28.07.2003 | 26.11.1956 | M | Revisit | 1649 | 1657 | (R) ankle still tingles & unable to dorsi-flex the (R) foot | For Physiotherapy | 3644 | |
| 22.07.2003 | 19.06.1933 | M | Pain | 1639 | 1644 | (L) ankle is swollen & painful | Diclofenac enteric coated & Ranitidine | 3648 | For serum Urates. |
| 29.07.2003 | 11.12.1958 | M | Rash | 951 | 956 | Itchy rash on hands | Miconazole 2% + 1% Hydrocortisone cream | 3660 | |
| 30.07.2003 | 30.09.1981 | M | | 1738 | 1748 | Script for Co-codamol given | | 371 | |
| 28.07.2003 | 06.09.1964 | F | S/Leave | 1752 | 1759 | Agoraphobia (Nervous Disability) | | 3991 | |

Result of a query that lists all consultations from the 22nd to the end of July 2003 (ConsultationsSeenFrom22ndTillEndOfJul2003)

| SurgeryDate | DateOfBirth | Sex | Diagnosis | TimeIn | TimeOut | Complaints | Treatments | NumbersID | Notes |
|---|---|---|---|---|---|---|---|---|---|
| 29.07.2003 | 04.12.1974 | F | | 1742 | 1745 | For Fasting Glucose | | 4010 | |
| 23.07.2003 | 07.10.1933 | M | | 936 | 940 | Script for Olanzapine given | | 4055 | |
| 29.07.2003 | 29.01.1973 | F | Conjunctivitis | 1640 | 1646 | (R) lower eye lid area is red | Fusidic Acid eye drops | 4063 | |
| 30.07.2003 | 10.12.1986 | F | | 1631 | 1638 | Hammer 2nd toes both feet | Referred to Orthopaedic Surgeon (Basildon Hospital) | 4130 | FP1001 (GMS4) form signed. |
| 22.07.2003 | 15.09.1964 | F | URTI | 1752 | 1758 | Sore throat | Amoxycillin | 4133 | For FBC & Fasting Glucose. |
| 25.07.2003 | 06.08.1964 | F | URTI | 1750 | 1756 | Sore throat & ear ache | Erythromycin & Otomize ear spray | 4253 | |
| 23.07.2003 | 02.02.1994 | M | Rash | 1739 | 1743 | Possible viral rash | To use own Calamine lotion | 4319 | |
| 30.07.2003 | 09.01.1958 | F | | 1718 | 1724 | Fungal infection of the (L) foot & (L) toes | Terbinafine | 4322 | |
| 30.07.2003 | 06.09.1955 | M | RTI | 1715 | 1718 | Chesty cough | Amoxycillin | 4324 | Septrin allergy. |
| 25.07.2003 | 28.03.1985 | F | | 1703 | 1715 | Pregnancy test is positive | | 4351 | For FBC. |
| 25.07.2003 | 08.04.1944 | F | | 931 | 937 | Script for Mefenamic Acid given | | 4465 | |
| 28.07.2003 | 18.06.1959 | M | | 941 | 952 | Lungs feel tight & as if on fire | Amoxycillin & Prednisolone enteric coated | 4557 | |
| 30.07.2003 | 09.10.1926 | M | | 1005 | 1015 | Dizziness & persistent bilateral ankle oedema | For U/Es, LFTs, FBC & Cholesterol | 4567 | Penicillin allergy. For U/Es, LFTs, FBC & Cholesterol. |

## Result of a query that lists all consultations from the 22nd to the end of July 2003 (ConsultationsSeenFrom22ndTillEndOfJul2003)

| SurgeryDate | DateOfBirth | Sex | Diagnosis | TimeIn | TimeOut | Complaints | Treatments | NumbersID | Notes |
|---|---|---|---|---|---|---|---|---|---|
| 25.07.2003 | 13.03.1932 | M | | 1037 | 1049 | Injection Zoladex given | | 4699 | |
| 23.07.2003 | 24.05.1970 | F | | 923 | 930 | Aching varicose veins in the legs | Referred to Vascular Surgeon (BUPA) | 4921 | |
| 30.07.2003 | 11.03.1961 | M | | 1758 | 1804 | Wax in the ears | Referred to ENT Dept. (Basildon Hospital) for ear syringing | 4954 | |
| 22.07.2003 | 04.12.1995 | M | | 910 | 918 | (R) Shoulder droops down | Referred to Orthopaedic Surgeon (Basildon Hospital) | 5091 | Penicillin allergy. |
| 22.07.2003 | 04.10.1968 | F | | 1706 | 1714 | For repeat USScan of the neck in 3 months | | 511 | |
| 28.07.2003 | 07.04.1949 | F | URTI | 1730 | 1735 | Itchy (R) ear | Otomize ear spray | 513 | |
| 22.07.2003 | 17.05.1986 | F | Revisit | 1737 | 1752 | Still has bilateral lumps in the neck | For TFTs & serum Calcium | 5135 | |
| 29.07.2003 | 19.12.1974 | M | URTI | 1656 | 1704 | (R) ear is sore | Amoxycillin & Otomize ear spray | 5175 | |
| 23.07.2003 | 13.01.1966 | F | S/Leave | 1653 | 1706 | Pneumonia | | 5196 | Abdominal pain, Rx. Buscopan. For USScan of the upper abdomen. |
| 30.07.2003 | 23.05.1948 | F | | 1700 | 1712 | Advised to see the Midwife asap regarding her pregnancy | | 5204 | |

Result of a query that lists all consultations from the 22$^{nd}$ to the end of July 2003 (ConsultationsSeenFrom22ndTillEndOfJul2003)

| SurgeryDate | DateOfBirth | Sex | Diagnosis | TimeIn | TimeOut | Complaints | Treatments | NumbersID | Notes |
|---|---|---|---|---|---|---|---|---|---|
| 28.07.2003 | 09.04.1926 | M | | 1033 | 1046 | Diabetic Clinic | | 5248 | Script for Atenolol given. |
| 23.07.2003 | 04.07.1996 | M | | 958 | 1007 | Diarrhoea & Vomiting | Electrolade | 5312 | Stool for C&S. |
| 29.07.2003 | 08.06.1996 | M | | 1019 | 1022 | Unable to hear properly in the past 4 days | To see Health Visitor | 5324 | |
| 28.07.2003 | 19.12.1981 | F | | 1747 | 1752 | Script for Eugynon 30 given | | 5384 | |
| 24.07.2003 | 23.02.1962 | F | | 901 | 912 | She will come back for Private S/Leave | | 5392 | |
| 30.07.2003 | 16.10.1996 | F | URTI | 1804 | 1809 | Sore throat | Amoxycillin & Paracetamol | 5409 | |
| 25.07.2003 | 06.01.1935 | M | | 1002 | 1010 | Script for Ipratropium inhaler, Salbutamol inhaler & Amoxycillin given | | 5626 | |
| 25.07.2003 | 19.12.1978 | F | URTI | 1010 | 1018 | Sore | Amoxycillin | 5626 | |
| 30.07.2003 | 06.04.1955 | F | S/Leave | 913 | 918 | Arthroscopy (R) knee | | 579 | |
| 22.07.2003 | 19.08.1917 | F | | 1020 | 1033 | Septic insect bite on (R) arm | Flucloxacillin, Fusidic Acid & Fexofenadine | 5822 | Adsorbed Diphtheria & Tetanus vaccine given. |
| 25.07.2003 | 04.07.1973 | F | | 937 | 941 | HVS & Chlamydial swabs normal | | 5950 | |
| 30.07.2003 | 29.07.1951 | M | Rash | 918 | 922 | Fungal infection of the toe nails | Terbinafine | 5958 | |

598

## Result of a query that lists all consultations from the 22nd to the end of July 2003 (ConsultationsSeenFrom22ndTillEndOfJul2003)

| SurgeryDate | DateOfBirth | Sex | Diagnosis | TimeIn | TimeOut | Complaints | Treatments | NumbersID | Notes |
|---|---|---|---|---|---|---|---|---|---|
| 23.07.2003 | 30.01.1931 | F | Pain | 1040 | 1113 | (R) Temporal arteritis | Prednisolone enteric coated | 600 | D/w Medical Dr. on call, SGH. To see in MAU in one week. |
| 29.07.2003 | 20.04.1933 | F | RTI | 1033 | 1040 | Chesty cough | Amoxycillin | 6110 | |
| 28.07.2003 | 25.04.1984 | M | | 1740 | 1747 | Wart on the (L) finger | Occlusal | 6116 | |
| 23.07.2003 | 21.03.1973 | M | | 1743 | 1748 | Hay fever | Fexofenadine | 6142 | Epilim allergy. |
| 28.07.2003 | 09.05.1997 | M | Rash | 1644 | 1649 | Itchy rash on body | Loratadine | 6253 | Septic insect bite wound on the (L) arm, Rx. Flucloxacillin. |
| 25.07.2003 | 10.01.1973 | F | | 1025 | 1037 | Vaginal thrush | Clotrimazole cream & pessary | 6305 | |
| 28.07.2003 | 28.03.1945 | M | S/Leave | 1657 | 1701 | Injury to (L) leg, (L) shoulder & (L) side of face | | 6357 | |
| 29.07.2003 | 21.05.1936 | M | Rash | 956 | 1001 | Itchy rash on arms & buttocks | 1% Hydrocortisone cream & Hydroxyzine | 6396 | |
| 29.07.2003 | 24.03.1960 | M | | 1707 | 1715 | Fungal infection (L) toe nails | Terbinafine | 640 | Script for Atenolol given. |
| 23.07.2003 | 03.01.1958 | F | URTI | 1640 | 1653 | (R) ear ache | Amoxycillin & Otomize ear spray | 6438 | |
| 29.07.2003 | 06.06.1959 | M | | 1755 | 1803 | Rib cage hurts & feels unwell | Amoxycillin | 6461 | Penicillin allergy. |
| 23.07.2003 | 14.04.1978 | F | Lump | 930 | 936 | Lump in the (R) breast | Referred to Breast Surgeon (BUPA) | 6464 | |

Result of a query that lists all consultations from the 22nd to the end of July 2003 (ConsultationsSeenFrom22ndTillEndOfJul2003)

| SurgeryDate | DateOfBirth | Sex | Diagnosis | TimeIn | TimeOut | Complaints | Treatments | NumbersID | Notes |
|---|---|---|---|---|---|---|---|---|---|
| 22.07.2003 | 09.12.1945 | F | Hypertension | 941 | 959 | BP 155/110 | Nifedipine MR 60 mg capsules | 6467 | |
| 30.07.2003 | 27.11.1930 | F | | 1024 | 1046 | To check with the hospital when she will be having the endoscopy | | 6530 | Penicillin allergy. |
| 29.07.2003 | 28.10.1934 | M | | 1745 | 1755 | Constipation | Lactulose | 6581 | Penicillin allergy. For U/Es, ESR, LFTs & Cholesterol. |
| 23.07.2003 | 22.07.1920 | F | Hypertension | 900 | 913 | BP 178/108 | Atenolol & Bendrofluazide | 6599 | Dizziness, Rx. Prochlorperazine. Dysuria, for MSU. |
| 25.07.2003 | 12.02.1959 | F | | 1729 | 1735 | To try Naproxen 500mg tds instead of 250mg tds | | 6602 | |
| 30.07.2003 | 28.02.1960 | F | | 1724 | 1733 | Heavy prolonged period | Norethisterone | 6662 | FP1001 (GMS4) form signed. For FBC, TFTs & Fasting Glucose. |
| 29.07.2003 | 09.06.1973 | M | UTI | 1803 | 1808 | Pain in (L) kidney area | Trimethoprim | 6663 | |
| 29.07.2003 | 23.02.1940 | M | | 1001 | 1019 | Script for Permitab tablets given | | 6704 | For MSU. |
| 25.07.2003 | 05.05.1978 | F | URTI | 926 | 931 | Ear ache | Amoxycillin & Otomize ear spray | 6709 | |
| 28.07.2003 | 14.12.1954 | F | S/Leave | 1759 | 1808 | Back Pain - Med. 5 | | 6851 | |

Result of a query that lists all consultations from the 22nd to the end of July 2003 (ConsultationsSeenFrom22ndTillEndOfJul2003)

| SurgeryDate | DateOfBirth | Sex | Diagnosis | TimeIn | TimeOut | Complaints | Treatments | NumbersID | Notes |
|---|---|---|---|---|---|---|---|---|---|
| 25.07.2003 | 07.07.1980 | M | | 901 | 909 | Script for Orphenadrine given | | 7057 | |
| 28.07.2003 | 26.03.2001 | F | RTI | 914 | 922 | Chesty cough | Amoxycillin | 7058 | |
| 28.07.2003 | 29.07.1983 | M | Pain | 1707 | 1713 | Back Pain following RTA | Dihydrocodeine | 7114 | |
| 23.07.2003 | 21.10.1970 | M | | 1759 | 1804 | To come back if the area od depigmentation gets worse | | 7170 | |
| 29.07.2003 | 09.03.1922 | M | URTI | 1040 | 1048 | Head cold | Amoxycillin | 7171 | Script for Atorvastatin. For Echocardiography. |
| 29.07.2003 | 01.05.1979 | F | | 1152 | 1202 | Routine Post-natal check | | 7193 | Home visit. |
| 25.07.2003 | 05.02.1984 | M | | 1743 | 1747 | Pussy (L)GTN big toe | Flucloxacillin & Fusidic Acid cream | 7208 | |
| 23.07.2003 | 17.03.1940 | F | | 1706 | 1709 | To continue cream for the insect bite on (R) leg | | 7213 | |
| 22.07.2003 | 14.08.1947 | F | S/Leave | 1758 | 1820 | Dislocated (R) shoulder - Private | | 7237 | Referred to Orthopaedic Dr. on call, Basildon Hospital. |
| 28.07.2003 | 27.01.1934 | M | | 935 | 941 | Script for Rosuvastatin given | | 7253 | |

Result of a query that lists all consultations from the 22nd to the end of July 2003 (ConsultationsSeenFrom22ndTillEndOfJul2003)

| SurgeryDate | DateOfBirth | Sex | Diagnosis | TimeIn | TimeOut | Complaints | Treatments | NumbersID | Notes |
|---|---|---|---|---|---|---|---|---|---|
| 28.07.2003 | 28.01.1943 | F | | 1001 | 1009 | Stye (R) lower eye lid | Cefalexin & Co-codamol | 7278 | Penicillin & Erythromycin allergy. |
| 22.07.2003 | 02.03.2002 | F | | 1009 | 1013 | Diarrhoea | Electrolade | 7347 | |
| 22.07.2003 | 25.02.2002 | M | RTI | 959 | 1005 | Still coughing & wheezy | Amoxycillin | 7368 | |
| 30.07.2003 | 28.12.1921 | M | | 1748 | 1758 | Script for Amoxycillin, Erythromycin & Prochlorperazine given | | 7407 | For FBC & Fasting Glucose. |
| 22.07.2003 | 01.06.1937 | M | | 1728 | 1734 | Script for Tadalafil 'SLS' given | | 7425 | |
| 23.07.2003 | 30.09.1923 | M | | 1007 | 1015 | Light-headed | Prochlorperazine | 7457 | For FBC & Fasting Glucose. Ciprofloxacin allergy. |
| 25.07.2003 | 03.07.1950 | F | Rash | 1715 | 1724 | Scalp lesion, bleeds at times | Flucloxacillin & Fusidic Acid cream | 7468 | For FBC. Referred to Dermatologist. |
| 28.07.2003 | 27.09.1969 | F | | 1808 | 1811 | Vaginal thrush | Clotrimazole pessary | 7495 | 6 months pregnant. |
| 29.07.2003 | 25.08.1937 | M | Revisit | 901 | 914 | Still has (L) ear discharge | Otomize ear spray | 7510 | |
| 23.07.2003 | 29.05.1960 | M | | 916 | 923 | To see Practice Counsellor about feeling low & insecure | | 7517 | |
| 25.07.2003 | 20.12.1943 | F | S/Leave | 1724 | 1729 | Pain (R) ankle - DUPLICATE | | 7524 | Penicillin allergy. |

602

## Result of a query that lists all consultations from the 22nd to the end of July 2003 (ConsultationsSeenFrom22ndTillEndOfJul2003)

| SurgeryDate | DateOfBirth | Sex | Diagnosis | TimeIn | TimeOut | Complaints | Treatments | NumbersID | Notes |
|---|---|---|---|---|---|---|---|---|---|
| 22.07.2003 | 25.03.1987 | F | | 918 | 924 | Wart on finger & verrucae on feet | Occlusal | 7558 | |
| 22.07.2003 | 20.02.1953 | F | S/Leave | 924 | 932 | Closed Fracture (L) Hallux | | 7559 | |
| 29.07.2003 | 20.02.1953 | F | S/Leave | 1027 | 1033 | Closed Fracture of the (L) Hallux | | 7559 | |
| 28.07.2003 | 24.02.1952 | F | S/Leave | 1009 | 1018 | Abdominal hysterectomy | | 7567 | |
| 25.07.2003 | 27.10.1966 | M | | 1735 | 1739 | Contact dermatitis (R) hand | 1% Hydrocortisone cream | 7571 | |
| 30.07.2003 | 25.03.1987 | F | URTI | 1638 | 1644 | (L) ear is sore | Amoxycillin | 7588 | FP1001 (GMS4) form signed. |
| 22.07.2003 | 22.06.1974 | F | | 1635 | 1639 | She doesn't want statins for her high Cholesterol | | 7596 | |
| 29.07.2003 | 22.06.1974 | F | | 926 | 934 | Septic bite on (L) foot | Flucloxacillin & Fusidic Acid cream | 7596 | |
| 24.07.2003 | 03.10.1937 | F | Rash | 912 | 918 | Itchy rash both groins | Clotrimazole 1% + 1% Hydrocortisone cream | 7633 | Smelly urine, for MSU. Penicillin allergy. |
| 23.07.2003 | 01.10.1938 | F | | 1015 | 1025 | Script for Ranitidine given | | 7671 | |
| 28.07.2003 | 28.11.1968 | F | Pain | 1713 | 1717 | Pain in the (R) kidney area & tiredness | For FBC, TFTs & MSU | 7687 | |

## Result of a query that lists all consultations from the 22nd to the end of July 2003 (ConsultationsSeenFrom22ndTillEndOfJul2003)

| SurgeryDate | DateOfBirth | Sex | Diagnosis | TimeIn | TimeOut | Complaints | Treatments | NumbersID | Notes |
|---|---|---|---|---|---|---|---|---|---|
| 30.07.2003 | 27.03.1940 | F | | 943 | 1005 | Dry mouth, dry eyes & dry nose | Normal Saline nasal drops, Hypromellose 0.3% eye drops & Glandosane spray | 7692 | T.A.T.T., for FBC, Fasting Glucose & TFTs. |
| 23.07.2003 | 31.05.1930 | F | Pain | 1730 | 1739 | Pain & swelling (L) knee | Referred to Orthopaedic Surgeon (Basildon Hospital) | 7730 | Script for injection MethylPrednisolone 40mg, Lidocaine 10mg/ml 2mls given. |
| 24.07.2003 | 31.05.1930 | F | | 1030 | 1043 | Injection Depo-Medrone with Lidocaine given to the (L) knee | | 7730 | |
| 29.07.2003 | 26.04.1973 | F | Pain | 914 | 918 | Painful split in (R) heel | Flucloxacillin & Fusidic Acid cream | 7752 | |
| 22.07.2003 | 16.04.1944 | F | Hypertension | 1039 | 1051 | BP 153/100 | Bendrofluazide | 7759 | Script for Simvastatin given. |
| 22.07.2003 | 10.12.1941 | F | | 1033 | 1039 | Script for Simvastatin given | | 7775 | |
| 25.07.2003 | 02.01.1939 | F | UTI | 1803 | 1811 | Dysuria & frequency of micturition | Trimethoprim | 7840 | For MSU. |
| 28.07.2003 | 23.08.1944 | F | S/Leave | 907 | 914 | Fractured (R) Humerus | | 7841 | |
| 22.07.2003 | 06.10.1952 | M | RTI | 1650 | 1655 | Cough | Amoxycillin | 7843 | Script for Salbutamol given. |
| 23.07.2003 | 18.05.1935 | M | | 940 | 958 | For PSA & serum Cholesterol | | 83 | |

604

## Result of a query that lists all consultations from the 22nd to the end of July 2003 (ConsultationsSeenFrom22ndTillEndOfJul2003)

| SurgeryDate | DateOfBirth | Sex | Diagnosis | TimeIn | TimeOut | Complaints | Treatments | NumbersID | Notes |
|---|---|---|---|---|---|---|---|---|---|
| 25.07.2003 | 13.09.1918 | M | | 1640 | 1703 | He was referred to SGH but has received a letter to see an Orthopaedic Surgeon at Orsett hospital | | 841 | |
| 25.07.2003 | 28.01.1980 | F | Revisit | 1747 | 1750 | Pain in the 1st (R) MTPJ has persisted | Referred to Podiatrist | 912 | |
| 30.07.2003 | 05.10.1974 | M | | 1813 | 1817 | Septic insect bite on (L) leg | Flucloxacillin & Fusidic Acid cream | 918 | |
| 23.07.2003 | 15.03.1975 | F | | 1025 | 1040 | Painful & bleeding piles | Glyceryl Trinitrate Ointment 0.2% w/w | 934 | |
| 29.07.2003 | 04.07.1959 | F | | 1022 | 1027 | Worried about abdominal lump | For USScan | 96 | Indigestion, Rx. Rabeprazole. |

## Result of a query that lists all consultations from the 22nd to the end of July 2004 (ConsultationsSeenFrom22ndTillEndOfJul2004)

| SurgeryDate | DateOfBirth | Sex | Diagnosis | TimeIn | TimeOut | Complaints | Treatments | NumbersID | Notes |
|---|---|---|---|---|---|---|---|---|---|
| 28.07.2004 | 23.10.1941 | M | | 1735 | 1743 | Enlarged Prostate & high PSA | Referred to Urologist | 1028 | |
| 26.07.2004 | 06.08.1928 | F | | 1003 | 1009 | Wax in the ears | Sodium bicarbonate ear drops | 1074 | Penicillin allergy. |

## Result of a query that lists all consultations from the 22nd to the end of July 2004 (ConsultationsSeenFrom22ndTillEndOfJul2004)

| SurgeryDate | DateOfBirth | Sex | Diagnosis | TimeIn | TimeOut | Complaints | Treatments | NumbersID | Notes |
|---|---|---|---|---|---|---|---|---|---|
| 26.07.2004 | 31.12.1953 | F | Pain | 1009 | 1020 | Pain (L) hip | Co-codamol & Diclofenac enteric coated | 1075 | |
| 30.07.2004 | 31.12.1953 | F | | 907 | 911 | To stop Atenolol for 2 weeks which she thinks is causing her puffy eyes | | 1075 | |
| 28.07.2004 | 08.02.1939 | F | | 957 | 1001 | Script for Fexofenadine given | | 113 | Trimethoprim allergy. |
| 23.07.2004 | 03.03.1984 | M | | 1745 | 1749 | Script for Salbutamol inhaler given | | 1176 | |
| 30.07.2004 | 29.12.1930 | F | | 1038 | 1048 | Persistent rectal bleeding | Referred to Rectal Surgeon | 1188 | Penicillin allergy. |
| 22.07.2004 | 06.06.1947 | F | S/Leave | 939 | 948 | Delorme's procedure | | 1354 | Script for Sodium bicarbonate ear drops given. |
| 26.07.2004 | 26.10.1943 | F | | 920 | 925 | Ankle oedema | Frusemide | 1365 | |
| 29.07.2004 | 21.06.1953 | F | Rash | 1013 | 1026 | Flat rash under breasts | Referred to Dermatologist (Basildon Hospital) | 1505 | Script for Atenolol given. |
| 29.07.2004 | 11.11.1940 | M | | 946 | 951 | Referred to Physiotherapist | | 1611 | |
| 30.07.2004 | 06.05.1984 | F | | 1754 | 1800 | Script for Microgynon-30 given | | 1697 | FP1001 (GMS4) form signed. |
| 30.07.2004 | 03.10.1939 | M | | 1700 | 1708 | Pain & swelling around the (L) big toe has improved | | 1849 | |

## Result of a query that lists all consultations from the 22nd to the end of July 2004 (ConsultationsSeenFrom22ndTillEndOfJul2004)

| SurgeryDate | DateOfBirth | Sex | Diagnosis | TimeIn | TimeOut | Complaints | Treatments | NumbersID | Notes |
|---|---|---|---|---|---|---|---|---|---|
| 26.07.2004 | 19.12.1949 | M | Revisit | 950 | 955 | Recurrent sinus problems | Referred to ENT Surgeon | 216 | |
| 26.07.2004 | 22.03.1933 | F | RTI | 945 | 950 | Chesty cough | Amoxycillin | 2179 | |
| 30.07.2004 | 23.04.1936 | F | Conjunctivitis | 920 | 924 | Sore & pussy (R) eye | | 223 | |
| 26.07.2004 | 06.10.1915 | M | | 1642 | 1650 | Script for Beclomethasone nasal spray & Fusidic Acid cream given | | 229 | |
| 27.07.2004 | 22.03.1936 | F | | 900 | 910 | To try OTC Imodium for her diarrhoea | | 2348 | |
| 26.07.2004 | 07.11.1957 | F | Conjunctivitis | 1718 | 1726 | Blood shot & watery eyes | Chloramphenicol eye drops | 2382 | Penicillin allergy. Script for Atenolol given. |
| 28.07.2004 | 07.11.1957 | F | Revisit | 902 | 919 | Redness in the (R) eye has got worse, ?Episcleritis | Referred to Eye Dr. on call, SGH | 2382 | Penicillin allergy. |
| 22.07.2004 | 17.04.1986 | M | | 1013 | 1023 | Advised to attend the local GUM clinic regarding the spots on his penis | | 2384 | Septrin allergy. |
| 22.07.2004 | 13.03.1983 | F | | 932 | 939 | Script for Co-cyprindiol given | | 2388 | |
| 30.07.2004 | 06.01.1955 | M | | 1714 | 1717 | Private script for Viagra given | | 2556 | |
| 28.07.2004 | 06.01.1943 | F | | 930 | 937 | For BP check with the P/Nurse | | 2642 | |
| 30.07.2004 | 08.03.1920 | M | Rash | 944 | 952 | Weepy seborrheic dermatitis on the (R) ankle | Fusidic Acid with betamethasone cream 2% +.01% | 2738 | |

Result of a query that lists all consultations from the 22nd to the end of July 2004 (ConsultationsSeenFrom22ndTillEndOfJul2004)

| SurgeryDate | DateOfBirth | Sex | Diagnosis | TimeIn | TimeOut | Complaints | Treatments | NumbersID | Notes |
|---|---|---|---|---|---|---|---|---|---|
| 23.07.2004 | 24.03.1973 | M | S/Leave | 906 | 910 | Injury (R) toe | | 2784 | |
| 28.07.2004 | 25.05.1976 | F | | 1706 | 1715 | Sore gums & dizziness | Amoxycillin & Prochlorperazine | 2797 | |
| 30.07.2004 | 09.02.1956 | M | | 1808 | 1816 | Referred to Orthopaedic Surgeon (BUPA) regarding pain at back of the (L) thigh | | 2846 | |
| 30.07.2004 | 25.07.1938 | F | Pain | 1708 | 1714 | Neck pain | Co-codamol | 2964 | |
| 26.07.2004 | 15.12.1939 | M | | 1820 | 1833 | Acute gout attack | Diclofenac e/c | 3272 | 2nd PAR study visit. For Uric Acid. |
| 28.07.2004 | 18.12.1964 | F | Pain | 1024 | 1032 | Her varicose veins on the (R) leg are aching | Referred to Vascular Surgeon | 3282 | |
| 23.07.2004 | 12.08.1932 | M | | 1709 | 1715 | To increase his salt intake | | 3344 | |
| 27.07.2004 | 26.03.1958 | F | | 939 | 948 | Mole on (L) side od face | Referred to Dermatologist (Basildon Hospital) | 335 | |
| 23.07.2004 | 02.03.1948 | M | Rash | 1644 | 1653 | Birth mark on (R) upper shoulder has gone darker recently | Referred to Dermatologist (BUPA) | 3473 | |
| 29.07.2004 | 12.08.1936 | M | | 909 | 918 | Script for Tadalafil given | | 3475 | 3rd EDOS study visit. |
| 30.07.2004 | 17.03.1924 | M | | 1732 | 1738 | For PSA | | 3592 | |
| 26.07.2004 | 31.01.1959 | M | S/Leave | 900 | 904 | Pain in (L) leg | | 3795 | |
| 28.07.2004 | 06.09.1964 | F | S/Leave | 1754 | 1758 | Agoraphobia (Nervous disability) | | 3991 | |

608

Result of a query that lists all consultations from the 22nd to the end of July 2004 (ConsultationsSeenFrom22ndTillEndOfJul2004)

| SurgeryDate | DateOfBirth | Sex | Diagnosis | TimeIn | TimeOut | Complaints | Treatments | NumbersID | Notes |
|---|---|---|---|---|---|---|---|---|---|
| 27.07.2004 | 31.03.1986 | F | Rash | 1014 | 1017 | Itchy rash on arms | 1% Hydrocortisone cream | 4001 | |
| 23.07.2004 | 03.02.1971 | F | | 1749 | 1756 | Referred to Physiotherapist (BUPA) | | 4003 | |
| 28.07.2004 | 27.06.1972 | M | | 1758 | 1802 | Ventral junction of the glans/penile shaft keeps tearing & bleeding during sex | Referred to Urologist | 4012 | |
| 23.07.2004 | 30.10.1969 | F | | 1039 | 1046 | Vaginal lump | Referred to Gynaecologist | 4075 | |
| 22.07.2004 | 13.07.1924 | F | Hypertension | 959 | 1008 | BP 197/106 | Lisinopril | 4244 | Script for Simvastatin given. |
| 30.07.2004 | 30.10.1947 | M | URTI | 1638 | 1654 | Sore throat | Amoxycillin | 431 | Referred to Haematologist. Scoline allergy. |
| 22.07.2004 | 08.04.1944 | F | | 948 | 959 | She will continue with her present HRT | | 4465 | |
| 26.07.2004 | 08.04.1944 | F | | 925 | 934 | Script for Estradiol with norethisterone (continuous combined) tablets 1mg + 0.5mg given | | 4465 | |
| 29.07.2004 | 29.09.1932 | F | Pain | 1000 | 1005 | Pain (L) leg | Dihydrocodeine | 4487 | |
| 27.07.2004 | 09.04.1938 | M | | 948 | 955 | For repeat FBC in 1 year | | 4519 | Tetracycline allergy. |

Result of a query that lists all consultations from the 22nd to the end of July 2004 (ConsultationsSeenFrom22ndTillEndOfJul2004)

| SurgeryDate | DateOfBirth | Sex | Diagnosis | TimeIn | TimeOut | Complaints | Treatments | NumbersID | Notes |
|---|---|---|---|---|---|---|---|---|---|
| 27.07.2004 | 27.08.1922 | M | | 1017 | 1027 | Script for Ranitidine & Co-codamol given | | 4624 | |
| 30.07.2004 | 02.07.1943 | M | | 924 | 931 | For repeat FBC & Cholesterol in 6 months | | 4667 | |
| 27.07.2004 | 21.09.1923 | M | Rash | 1027 | 1034 | Possible lesion on the (L) fore-head | Referred to Dermatologist (Basildon Hospital) | 4692 | |
| 23.07.2004 | 13.03.1932 | M | | 1051 | 1057 | Inj. Zoladex given | | 4699 | |
| 27.07.2004 | 28.02.1927 | M | URTI | 1048 | 1056 | Sore throat | Amoxycillin | 4838 | |
| 28.07.2004 | 03.08.1957 | F | | 1032 | 1038 | Stye on the (L) lower eye lid | Chloramphenicol eye ointment | 5009 | |
| 28.07.2004 | 26.08.1913 | F | | 1630 | 1635 | Liquifilm Tears (Preservative free) required | | 5046 | Daughter came to Surgery. |
| 28.07.2004 | 09.02.1965 | F | Rash | 1001 | 1006 | Mole on (R) chin, aching | Referred to Dermatologist (Basildon) | 5077 | |
| 30.07.2004 | 07.04.1949 | F | | 1654 | 1700 | Advised to go to A/E if she gets chest pain again | | 513 | |
| 26.07.2004 | 20.11.1988 | M | Rash | 1734 | 1739 | Itchy rash on back & front of trunk | Loratadine & Calamine lotion | 5374 | |
| 26.07.2004 | 04.07.1986 | F | | 1712 | 1718 | She will like her period postponed whilst on her holidays | Norethisterone | 5386 | |

610

## Result of a query that lists all consultations from the 22nd to the end of July 2004 (ConsultationsSeenFrom22ndTillEndOfJul2004)

| SurgeryDate | DateOfBirth | Sex | Diagnosis | TimeIn | TimeOut | Complaints | Treatments | NumbersID | Notes |
|---|---|---|---|---|---|---|---|---|---|
| 28.07.2004 | 24.01.1958 | F | Rash | 1038 | 1047 | Brownish patch on (R) cheek | Referred to Dermatologist (Basildon Hospital) | 5396 | Lump on the (L) ear, referred to ENT Surgeon. |
| 30.07.2004 | 24.06.1937 | M | RTI | 1020 | 1024 | Cough | Amoxycillin | 5437 | |
| 28.07.2004 | 12.01.1992 | F | Conjunctivitis | 1655 | 1706 | Sore sticky & red eye | Chloramphenicol eye drops | 5487 | |
| 28.07.2004 | 22.06.1973 | F | | 1644 | 1648 | Dysuria | Amoxycillin | 5488 | For MSU. |
| 26.07.2004 | 06.01.1978 | M | | 1650 | 1704 | Referred to Physiotherapy (BUPA) regarding his bad back | | 555 | |
| 28.07.2004 | 09.02.1963 | F | Revisit | 937 | 952 | She still feels depressed | Fluoxetine | 5567 | |
| 28.07.2004 | 12.09.1964 | M | Rash | 919 | 930 | Rash on soles of the feet & crack in between the toes | Terbinafine cream & Flucloxacillin | 5568 | |
| 22.07.2004 | 11.09.1924 | M | | 1305 | 1325 | He is not keen to go to MAU, SGH | | 5591 | Home visit. |
| 28.07.2004 | 17.08.1947 | F | | 1009 | 1024 | For MSU | | 56 | |
| 28.07.2004 | 17.04.1923 | M | RTI | 1006 | 1009 | Chesty cough | Ampicillin | 560 | |
| 23.07.2004 | 15.03.1967 | F | Rash | 1756 | 1804 | Itchy blisters on the soles of the feet | Fusidic Acid 2% + 1% Hydrocortisone cream | 5783 | |
| 30.07.2004 | 16.08.1950 | F | | 1631 | 1638 | To try regular OTC Lactulose for her constipation | | 583 | Penicillin allergy. |

Result of a query that lists all consultations from the 22nd to the end of July 2004 (ConsultationsSeenFrom22ndTillEndOfJul2004)

| SurgeryDate | DateOfBirth | Sex | Diagnosis | TimeIn | TimeOut | Complaints | Treatments | NumbersID | Notes |
|---|---|---|---|---|---|---|---|---|---|
| 30.07.2004 | 03.03.1946 | M | | 935 | 944 | Bilateral ankle oedema | For Open Access echocardiogram | 5845 | |
| 23.07.2004 | 24.09.1993 | M | | 940 | 943 | To continue with own Paracetamol for his resolving bad throat | | 5889 | |
| 23.07.2004 | 23.01.1989 | M | URTI | 937 | 940 | Ulcers in the throat & blisters | Amoxycillin | 5894 | |
| 23.07.2004 | 01.01.1953 | M | | 1658 | 1703 | Script for Viagra given - Private | | 5975 | |
| 26.07.2004 | 12.02.1938 | M | Hypertension | 1803 | 1820 | BP 179/130 | Nifedipine m/r capsules | 5997 | Script for Simvastatin given. |
| 30.07.2004 | 19.01.1964 | F | | 1003 | 1010 | She wants her period postponed whilst on holidays | Norethisterone | 6196 | |
| 30.07.2004 | 07.01.1987 | F | | 1010 | 1020 | Script for Microgynon-30 given | | 6197 | |
| 26.07.2004 | 18.10.1958 | M | | 1635 | 1642 | Reassured regarding his nagging abdominal pain | | 6245 | |
| 30.07.2004 | 05.03.1979 | F | | 1800 | 1808 | To get privately prescribed medication from Psychiatrist seen privately | | 6320 | Penicillin allergy. |
| 28.07.2004 | 31.07.1997 | F | | 1722 | 1728 | To observe small nodule on the (L) upper leg | | 6409 | |

Result of a query that lists all consultations from the 22nd to the end of July 2004 (ConsultationsSeenFrom22ndTillEndOfJul2004)

| SurgeryDate | DateOfBirth | Sex | Diagnosis | TimeIn | TimeOut | Complaints | Treatments | NumbersID | Notes |
|---|---|---|---|---|---|---|---|---|---|
| 28.07.2004 | 06.12.1962 | M | | 1728 | 1735 | He has stopped the Propranolol to see how he can do without them | | 6415 | |
| 30.07.2004 | 15.08.1999 | M | | 904 | 907 | Septic possible flea bites | Flucloxacillin | 6521 | |
| 29.07.2004 | 26.0101953 | M | | 918 | 925 | Abscess (R) lower gum | Amoxycillin | 6590 | |
| 29.07.2004 | 09.04.1944 | F | RTI | 934 | 946 | Cough | Amoxycillin | 6592 | Script for Injection MethylPrednisolone with Lidocaine given. |
| 27.07.2004 | 16.03.1929 | M | Pain | 1034 | 1041 | Gripping (L) upper abdominal pain | For CXR & upper abdominal USScan | 6647 | |
| 22.07.2004 | 04.05.1937 | F | | 1023 | 1040 | Script for Trimethoprim given | | 6723 | |
| 23.07.2004 | 16.01.1998 | F | | 1653 | 1658 | Script for Beclomethasone inhaler given | | 6809 | |
| 22.07.2004 | 30.04.1947 | M | Lump | 910 | 915 | Lump behind (R) ear | Referred to ENT Surgeon | 6968 | |
| 26.07.2004 | 17.09.1938 | M | | 1704 | 1712 | Script for Dihydrocodeine given | | 6997 | |
| 23.07.2004 | 20.04.1921 | F | | 1057 | 1109 | Constipation & vomiting | Macrogol compound npf oral powder 6.9g, Metoclopramide & Senna | 7017 | |

Result of a query that lists all consultations from the 22nd to the end of July 2004 (ConsultationsSeenFrom22ndTillEndOfJul2004)

| SurgeryDate | DateOfBirth | Sex | Diagnosis | TimeIn | TimeOut | Complaints | Treatments | NumbersID | Notes |
|---|---|---|---|---|---|---|---|---|---|
| 23.07.2004 | 28.03.1938 | M | Pain | 1013 | 1026 | Upper abdominal pain & discomfort | Omeprazole | 7065 | For FBC, ESR, U/Es, LFTs & USScan. |
| 26.07.2004 | 17.03.1940 | F | | 904 | 909 | Cholesterol 5.7 mmols/L | Simvastatin | 7213 | |
| 23.07.2004 | 15.03.1922 | F | RTI | 1007 | 1013 | Chesty cough | Erythromycin & Amoxycillin | 7229 | |
| 28.07.2004 | 09.06.1934 | M | | 1648 | 1655 | KUB USScan: Moderate hydronephrosis & difficulty passing urine | Referred to Urologist (Basildon Hospital) | 7277 | Penicillin allergy. |
| 30.07.2004 | 14.02.1952 | M | | 1738 | 1754 | For U/Es | | 7298 | |
| 27.07.2004 | 05.11.1924 | F | | 955 | 1014 | Script for Amoxycillin given | | 7301 | |
| 23.07.2004 | 03.07.1938 | M | | 1636 | 1644 | To take Colchicine for acute gout only | | 7305 | |
| 26.07.2004 | 08.10.1963 | M | | 1739 | 1758 | Script for Metformin given | | 7400 | |
| 22.07.2004 | 05.08.1936 | F | | 1008 | 1013 | Advised against taking Ibuprofen in view of her age | | 7424 | |
| 27.07.2004 | 25.08.1933 | F | | 910 | 916 | To increase the Atenolol to 50mg daily | | 7428 | |
| 23.07.2004 | 21.03.1949 | F | | 1734 | 1745 | Script for Loperamide given | | 7429 | |

Result of a query that lists all consultations from the 22nd to the end of July 2004 (ConsultationsSeenFrom22ndTillEndOfJul2004)

| SurgeryDate | DateOfBirth | Sex | Diagnosis | TimeIn | TimeOut | Complaints | Treatments | NumbersID | Notes |
|---|---|---|---|---|---|---|---|---|---|
| 30.07.2004 | 04.08.1936 | M | | 1717 | 1720 | Script for Dihydrocodeine given | | 7443 | |
| 22.07.2004 | 20.07.1989 | M | | 905 | 910 | He keeps choking | Referred to Paediatrician | 7557 | |
| 28.07.2004 | 07.03.1968 | F | URTI | 952 | 957 | Pain in the ears | Amoxycillin & Dexamethasone with neomycin ear spray | 7577 | |
| 23.07.2004 | 26.08.1938 | M | URTI | 917 | 923 | Sore throat | Erythromycin | 7670 | |
| 29.07.2004 | 07.02.1948 | M | Pain | 951 | 1000 | Pain (L) groin | Referred to General Surgeon | 7684 | |
| 27.07.2004 | 04.01.1950 | F | | 1041 | 1048 | X-Ray (L) foot showed un-united fracture of 2nd & 3rd MTs | Referred to Orthopaedic Surgeon | 7685 | |
| 30.07.2004 | 26.09.1937 | M | | 1724 | 1732 | Repeat prescriptions to be issued from the reception | | 7693 | |
| 22.07.2004 | 07.11.1968 | F | | 901 | 905 | Bad throat for 4 months | Referred to ENT Surgeon | 7739 | |
| 22.07.2004 | 23.12.1946 | M | | 1040 | 1056 | Script for Erythromycin given | | 7761 | |
| 23.07.2004 | 10.12.1971 | M | S/Leave | 901 | 904 | Injury (L) ankle | | 7776 | |
| 30.07.2004 | 10.12.1971 | M | S/Leave | 901 | 904 | Injury (L) ankle | | 7776 | |
| 27.07.2004 | 15.07.2002 | F | Rash | 916 | 922 | Wart in the (L) thumb | Salicylic acid topical solution 26% | 7833 | |
| 26.07.2004 | 06.10.1952 | M | RTI | 934 | 938 | Chesty cough | Amoxycillin | 7843 | |

## Result of a query that lists all consultations from the 22nd to the end of July 2004 (ConsultationsSeenFrom22ndTillEndOfJul2004)

| SurgeryDate | DateOfBirth | Sex | Diagnosis | TimeIn | TimeOut | Complaints | Treatments | NumbersID | Notes |
|---|---|---|---|---|---|---|---|---|---|
| 30.07.2004 | 01.12.1942 | M | | 1720 | 1724 | To get OTC Calms | | 7845 | |
| 29.07.2004 | 19.10.1938 | M | | 1033 | 1051 | 3rd PAR study visit | | 7847 | |
| 23.07.2004 | 13.02.1933 | F | Conjunctivitis | 910 | 914 | Sticky & itchy eyes | Chloramphenicol eye drops | 7850 | |
| 26.07.2004 | 02.08.2003 | F | Revisit | 1726 | 1730 | Still pulling at the ears | Referred to ENT Surgeon | 7917 | |
| 23.07.2004 | 30.10.1984 | F | Rash | 1703 | 1709 | Itchy rash on arms & legs | Loratadine | 980 | |
| 23.07.2004 | 06.09.1927 | F | | 1715 | 1724 | Script for Ipratropium with Salbutamol inhaler & Spacer/holding chamber device Type 2 given | | NP (DL) | |
| 28.07.2004 | 27.07.1979 | F | | 1715 | 1722 | Vaginal thrush | Fluconazole | NP (ER) | |
| 29.07.2004 | 16.09.1971 | M | S/Leave | 900 | 902 | Attending Counsellor | | NP (IMC) | |
| 29.07.2004 | 23.04.1923 | F | URTI | 1026 | 1033 | Sore throat | Amoxycillin | NP (JD) | Script for Co-codamol & Frusemide given. |
| 29.07.2004 | 13.09.1942 | F | RTI | 902 | 909 | Chesty cough | Erythromycin | NP (JH) | Penicillin allergy. |
| 23.07.2004 | 31.10.1986 | F | | 943 | 948 | To take own Paracetamol for her chest pain | | NP (JJ) | |
| 26.07.2004 | 22.06.1929 | M | Revisit | 1024 | 1030 | Still coughing | Erythromycin | NP (JL) | For CXR, FBC, ESR, PSA & U/Es. |
| 23.07.2004 | 19.11.1977 | F | | 1026 | 1034 | For Physiotherapy | | NP (KM) | |
| 26.07.2004 | 26.05.2004 | F | | 1758 | 1803 | Septic vaccination site | Fusidic Acid cream | NP (MH) | |

### Result of a query that lists all consultations from the 22nd to the end of July 2004 (ConsultationsSeenFrom22ndTillEndOfJul2004)

| SurgeryDate | DateOfBirth | Sex | Diagnosis | TimeIn | TimeOut | Complaints | Treatments | NumbersID | Notes |
|---|---|---|---|---|---|---|---|---|---|
| 30.07.2004 | 31.05.1930 | F | | 952 | 1003 | Mole/lesion above the upper lip, (L) side | Referred to Dermatologist (Basildon Hospital) | NP (SAW) | Script for Etodolac given. Penicillin & Paracetamol allergy. |
| 29.07.2004 | 14.08.1948 | F | Hypertension | 925 | 934 | BP 155/94 | Bendrofluazide | NP (SC) | |
| 26.07.2004 | 08.08.1995 | F | URTI | 1730 | 1734 | Sore throat | Amoxycillin | Temp | |
| 28.07.2004 | 11.02.1986 | F | | 1635 | 1644 | Gum abscess | Amoxycillin | Temp | Script for Ethinylestradiol with Levonorgestrel 30mcg + 150mcg given. |
| 28.07.2004 | 21.09.1983 | M | S/Leave | 1743 | 1754 | Headaches & dizziness - Private | | Temp | Script for Propranolol given. For FBC & Fasting Glucose. |

### Result of a query that lists all consultations from the 22nd to the end of July 2005 (ConsultationsSeenFrom22ndTillEndOfJul2005)

| SurgeryDate | DateOfBirth | Sex | Diagnosis | TimeIn | TimeOut | Complaints | Treatments | NumbersID | Notes |
|---|---|---|---|---|---|---|---|---|---|
| 27.07.2005 | 30.03.1923 | M | | 1812 | 1827 | Diarrhoea | Loperamide & oral rehydration salts oral | 1060 | |
| 27.07.2005 | 18.11.1946 | F | | 1635 | 1647 | She will take OTC Co-codamol for the arthritis in her knees | | 1307 | |
| 22.07.2005 | 06.01.1921 | M | Hypertension | 932 | 955 | BP 179/88 | Lisinopril | 1612 | Script for Allopurinol given. |

**Result of a query that lists all consultations from the 22nd to the end of July 2005 (ConsultationsSeenFrom22ndTillEndOfJul2005)**

| SurgeryDate | DateOfBirth | Sex | Diagnosis | TimeIn | TimeOut | Complaints | Treatments | NumbersID | Notes |
|---|---|---|---|---|---|---|---|---|---|
| 26.07.2005 | 02.10.1943 | M | Rash | 1815 | 1821 | Finger nail infections & of the feet | Terbinafine tablets | 1852 | |
| 29.07.2005 | 04.01.1962 | F | UTI | 1634 | 1642 | Dysuria | Amoxycillin | 1884 | For MSU. Trimethoprim allergy. |
| 29.07.2005 | 19.08.1926 | F | | 1646 | 1652 | Septic (L)GTN | Flucloxacillin | 1907 | |
| 29.07.2005 | 23.09.1931 | F | | 1028 | 1041 | Stool for C&S | | 1969 | |
| 25.07.2005 | 14.08.1927 | M | | 1727 | 1732 | Losing his nails on his (L) hand | Referred to Dermatologist (Basildon Hospital) | 2289 | |
| 25.07.2005 | 09.10.1949 | M | Rash | 950 | 1007 | Itchy rash on lower legs | Permethrin cream 5% w/w | 2326 | |
| 29.07.2005 | 20.06.1950 | M | Pain | 1642 | 1646 | Pain in (R) hip | For X-Ray | 2475 | |
| 28.07.2005 | 06.01.1955 | M | | 1658 | 1703 | Private script for Viagra given | | 2556 | |
| 27.07.2005 | 13.11.1970 | F | Pain | 1746 | 1754 | Burning sensation & pain on (L) side of pain | Referred to Neurologist | 2578 | |
| 22.07.2005 | 03.07.1989 | M | Rash | 905 | 908 | Mole on (R) shoulder | Referred to Dermatologist (Basildon Hospital) | 2625 | |
| 25.07.2005 | 06.01.1943 | F | | 1744 | 1750 | Vit. B12 - 110 ng/L, lowish | Referred to Haematologist | 2642 | |
| 27.07.2005 | 05.11.1965 | M | Pain | 1029 | 1042 | Lower abdominal pain | Referred to Surgical Dr. on call, SGH | 2663 | |
| 22.07.2005 | 08.06.1984 | M | S/Leave | 1044 | 1047 | Seizures - Med. 5 | | 2670 | |

## Result of a query that lists all consultations from the 22nd to the end of July 2005 (ConsultationsSeenFrom22ndTillEndOfJul2005)

| SurgeryDate | DateOfBirth | Sex | Diagnosis | TimeIn | TimeOut | Complaints | Treatments | NumbersID | Notes |
|---|---|---|---|---|---|---|---|---|---|
| 26.07.2005 | 24.03.1973 | M | Rash | 1011 | 1019 | Itchy rash spreading up the arms & onto the trunk | Referred to Dermatologist (Basildon Hospital) | 2787 | Cyst on the (L) fore-arm, referred to Orthopaedic Surgeon (Basildon Hospital). |
| 26.07.2005 | 21.09.1950 | F | | 1036 | 1047 | Script for Diclofenac e/c & Dihydrocodeine given | | 2796 | Letter to Whom it may concern. |
| 29.07.2005 | 01.02.1931 | M | RTI | 1724 | 1748 | Chesty cough | Amoxycillin | 2965 | Suspect glaucoma, referred to Ophthalmologist (BUPA). |
| 27.07.2005 | 11.02.1972 | M | | 1706 | 1716 | Script for Omeprazole given | | 3007 | For Direct Access Gastroscopy. |
| 22.07.2005 | 29.12.1954 | F | | 1635 | 1650 | Script for Metformin given | | 3128 | |
| 27.07.2005 | 06.12.1945 | M | S/Leave | 1647 | 1652 | Upper back pain | | 3198 | |
| 22.07.2005 | 08.10.1969 | F | | 1724 | 1747 | Script for 1% Hydrocortisone cream & ketoconazole shampoo given | | 3270 | |
| 25.07.2005 | 07.05.1974 | M | | 1712 | 1718 | Septic bitten lower lip | Amoxycillin | 3291 | |
| 28.07.2005 | 31.10.1915 | F | | 925 | 946 | Script for Hydrocortisone with nystatin & benzalkonium given | | 336 | |
| 25.07.2005 | 19.05.1992 | F | Lump | 905 | 914 | Lump (R) axilla | Erythromycin | 3581 | Penicillin allergy. |

Result of a query that lists all consultations from the 22nd to the end of July 2005 (ConsultationsSeenFrom22ndTillEndOFJul2005)

| SurgeryDate | DateOfBirth | Sex | Diagnosis | TimeIn | TimeOut | Complaints | Treatments | NumbersID | Notes |
|---|---|---|---|---|---|---|---|---|---|
| 22.07.2005 | 08.04.1971 | F | | 912 | 926 | She had MSU in the middle of her period | | 3633 | |
| 28.07.2005 | 24.04.1986 | M | | 946 | 953 | For FBC & ESR | | 3659 | |
| 28.07.2005 | 14.06.1957 | F | | 1648 | 1653 | Septic insect bite on abdomen | Erythromycin | 3661 | Septrin allergy. |
| 29.07.2005 | 18.05.1952 | F | Conjunctivitis | 951 | 1005 | Sticky eyes | Chloramphenicol eye drops | 3766 | Moles on back & face, referred to Dermatologist (Basildon Hospital). |
| 26.07.2005 | 07.07.1961 | F | | 904 | 911 | Script for Nicotine patch Clear 21mg given | | 3768 | |
| 26.07.2005 | 05.05.1924 | M | | 959 | 1006 | Script for Oxybutynin given | | 381 | For MSU. Penicillin allergy. |
| 25.07.2005 | 30.03.1949 | F | S/Leave | 923 | 933 | Swollen (L) foot | | 3824 | |
| 25.07.2005 | 06.03.1973 | F | S/Leave | 1709 | 1712 | Fractured distal phalanx (R) thumb | | 3896 | |
| 25.07.2005 | 21.05.1971 | F | | 1007 | 1025 | Script for Miconazole oral gel & Clotrimazole pessary given | | 39 | Penicillin allergy. |
| 27.07.2005 | 20.11.1938 | M | | 1220 | 1250 | Script for Co-codamol & Salbutamol inhaler given | | 4187 | Home visit. |

Result of a query that lists all consultations from the 22nd to the end of July 2005 (ConsultationsSeenFrom22ndTillEndOfJul2005)

| SurgeryDate | DateOfBirth | Sex | Diagnosis | TimeIn | TimeOut | Complaints | Treatments | NumbersID | Notes |
|---|---|---|---|---|---|---|---|---|---|
| 28.07.2005 | 25.07.1955 | F |  | 904 | 917 | Script for Estradiol vaginal tablets, Norgestrel and Conjugated (equine) tablets 150mcg + 625mcg & Flucloxacillin given |  | 4281 |  |
| 22.07.2005 | 30.10.1947 | M | S/Leave | 955 | 1000 | Waldenstrom's Macroglobulinemia |  | 431 |  |
| 25.07.2005 | 01.03.1967 | M | Pain | 914 | 923 | Injury (R) elbow | For X-Ray | 4390 | Script for Prednisolone e/c & Beclomethasone extrafine inhaler given. |
| 28.07.2005 | 31.07.1972 | F | URTI | 1023 | 1029 | (L) ear ache | Dexamethasone with neomycin ear spray | 4398 |  |
| 25.07.2005 | 26.12.1932 | F |  | 1330 | 1340 | Septic wound (R) hip | Flucloxacillin | 4437 |  |
| 26.07.2005 | 31.12.1922 | M |  | 1656 | 1703 | Bilateral pedal oedema | Frusemide | 4470 | Home visit. |
| 22.07.2005 | 29.05.1973 | M | S/Leave | 1800 | 1810 | Back Pain - Private |  | 4485 |  |
| 25.07.2005 | 09.10.1926 | M |  | 1025 | 1042 | Script for Paracetamol & Inj. MethylPrednisolone with Lidocaine given |  | 4567 |  |
| 27.07.2005 | 09.10.1926 | M |  | 1042 | 1102 | Injection Depo-Medrone with Lidocaine given to (L) shoulder |  | 4567 |  |

Result of a query that lists all consultations from the 22nd to the end of July 2005 (ConsultationsSeenFrom22ndTillEndOfJul2005)

| SurgeryDate | DateOfBirth | Sex | Diagnosis | TimeIn | TimeOut | Complaints | Treatments | NumbersID | Notes |
|---|---|---|---|---|---|---|---|---|---|
| 25.07.2005 | 21.02.1976 | F | S/Leave | 1705 | 1709 | Stress | | 4585 | |
| 27.07.2005 | 03.01.1914 | F | Pain | 1730 | 1737 | Neck Pain | Paracetamol | 4877 | |
| 26.07.2005 | 10.06.1921 | M | Pain | 916 | 932 | Painful & swollen (L) calf | Referred to DVT Clinic, SGH | 4972 | |
| 28.07.2005 | 10.06.1921 | M | | 1034 | 1052 | Injection Depo-Medrone with Lidocaine given to the (R) shoulder | | 4972 | |
| 27.07.2005 | 15.06.1988 | M | | 1754 | 1802 | To approach Orthopaedic Surgeon first regarding letter about his knee operation | | 5012 | |
| 26.07.2005 | 02.05.1985 | F | Rash | 1640 | 1647 | Itchy rash on body | Fexofenadine | 5114 | |
| 26.07.2005 | 20.06.1984 | M | | 1813 | 1815 | He will come back later regarding his RTA | | 5158 | |
| 26.07.2005 | 09.04.1926 | M | | 1019 | 1028 | He refuses to use Omeprazole | | 5248 | |
| 28.07.2005 | 01.02.1996 | M | | 953 | 1002 | For FBC | | 5336 | |
| 26.07.2005 | 30.03.1985 | M | Rash | 1727 | 1731 | Warts on hands | Salicylic acid topical solution 26% | 534 | |
| 29.07.2005 | 04.07.1986 | F | URTI | 1703 | 1724 | Sore throat | Amoxycillin | 5386 | |
| 26.07.2005 | 17.10.1965 | F | RTI | 1721 | 1727 | Chesty cough | Amoxycillin | 5571 | Itchy rash on elbows spreading, referred to Dermatologist (Basildon Hospital). |

Result of a query that lists all consultations from the 22nd to the end of July 2005 (ConsultationsSeenFrom22ndTillEndOfJul2005)

| SurgeryDate | DateOfBirth | Sex | Diagnosis | TimeIn | TimeOut | Complaints | Treatments | NumbersID | Notes |
|---|---|---|---|---|---|---|---|---|---|
| 26.07.2005 | 12.11.1968 | F | | 952 | 959 | Septic insect bite (R) leg | Flucloxacillin | 5590 | |
| 28.07.2005 | 24.04.1975 | F | | 1644 | 1648 | Late period | For Pregnancy test | 5635 | |
| 26.07.2005 | 27.01.1940 | F | | 932 | 944 | Script for Betamethasone scalp application given | | 588 | |
| 26.07.2005 | 29.05.1933 | M | | 1703 | 1714 | Script for Metformin given | | 591 | |
| 26.07.2005 | 23.03.1926 | M | | 1742 | 1813 | Advised to contact BVLA regarding reviewing his cognitive impairment | | 5954 | |
| 22.07.2005 | 07.01.1987 | F | | 1708 | 1715 | Vaginal thrush | Clotrimazole pessary | 6197 | |
| 29.07.2005 | 18.10.1958 | M | | 1005 | 1012 | Alternating constipation/ diarrhoea & pain (L) lower abdomen | Referred to Gastro-enterologist | 6245 | |
| 27.07.2005 | 18.06.1963 | F | | 1652 | 1706 | For repeat MSU in 8 weeks | | 6386 | |
| 25.07.2005 | 31.07.1997 | F | | 1718 | 1727 | Referred to Paediatrician regarding her Diabetes | | 6409 | |
| 26.07.2005 | 08.05.1939 | F | | 1731 | 1742 | Advised to contact BVLA regarding reviewing her driving Licence | | 6643 | |

Result of a query that lists all consultations from the 22nd to the end of July 2005 (ConsultationsSeenFrom22ndTillEndOfJul2005)

| SurgeryDate | DateOfBirth | Sex | Diagnosis | TimeIn | TimeOut | Complaints | Treatments | NumbersID | Notes |
|---|---|---|---|---|---|---|---|---|---|
| 26.07.2005 | 20.09.1965 | M | UTI | 911 | 916 | Dysuria & haematuria | Trimethoprim | 6725 | Referred to Urologist. For MSU. |
| 22.07.2005 | 31.01.1941 | F | | 1703 | 1708 | To remain on Atorvastatin all the time | | 673 | |
| 27.07.2005 | 19.12.1939 | F | | 938 | 959 | Script for Gliclazide & 1% Hydrocortisone cream given | | 6988 | |
| 22.07.2005 | 12.11.1950 | M | | 908 | 912 | Whitlow (R) thumb | Flucloxacillin | 7149 | Codeine allergy. |
| 26.07.2005 | 06.10.1944 | F | | 1647 | 1656 | For FBC, TFTs & Fasting Glucose | | 7262 | |
| 28.07.2005 | 19.06.1944 | F | | 917 | 925 | Script for Co-codamol & Diclofenac e/c given | | 7267 | |
| 28.07.2005 | 04.09.1949 | F | S/Leave | 1712 | 1722 | Chest pain | | 7285 | Script for Amoxycillin given. |
| 29.07.2005 | 26.04.1944 | F | | 1652 | 1703 | Script for Lisinopril & Peak Flow meter | | 7376 | |
| 22.07.2005 | 05.08.1936 | F | Pain | 1715 | 1724 | Injury (L) knee | For X-Ray | 7424 | |
| 26.07.2005 | 10.06.1921 | F | | 1225 | 1245 | (L) T4/5 shingles & vomiting | Famciclovir, Metoclopramide & Amitriptyline | 7442 | Home visit. |
| 25.07.2005 | 28.03.1960 | F | S/Leave | 1640 | 1651 | Depression - Med. 4 | | 7518 | |
| 27.07.2005 | 06.04.1938 | M | | 1716 | 1730 | Script for Allopurinol given | | 7626 | |
| 26.07.2005 | 01.10.1938 | F | | 944 | 952 | Script for Omeprazole & Ezetimibe given | | 7671 | |

## Result of a query that lists all consultations from the 22nd to the end of July 2005 (ConsultationsSeenFrom22ndTillEndOfJul2005)

| SurgeryDate | DateOfBirth | Sex | Diagnosis | TimeIn | TimeOut | Complaints | Treatments | NumbersID | Notes |
|---|---|---|---|---|---|---|---|---|---|
| 28.07.2005 | 07.02.1948 | M | | 1002 | 1018 | To persevere with the Metformin | | 7684 | |
| 27.07.2005 | 07.01.1944 | M | S/Leave | 916 | 931 | Pains in the knees - Med. 5 | | 7714 | For X-Ray. |
| 28.07.2005 | 04.09.1928 | M | | 1722 | 1732 | Script for Omeprazole given | | 7729 | Referred to Gastro-enterologist. |
| 25.07.2005 | 08.05.1962 | M | | 1737 | 1744 | Recurrent diarrhoea | Stool for C&S | 7777 | |
| 22.07.2005 | 08.12.1938 | F | Pain | 1655 | 1703 | Pain in (L) hip | Etodolac & Co-codamol | 7811 | Lump (R) breast, referred to Breast Surgeon (urgent). |
| 22.07.2005 | 29.11.1937 | F | | 1047 | 1054 | Septic insect bites on legs | Flucloxacillin | 7918 | |
| 22.07.2005 | 26.08.1987 | F | | 1650 | 1655 | Weepy discharge where the lump in (R) breast was removed | Flucloxacillin | 894 | |
| 27.07.2005 | 21.08.1979 | F | | 959 | 1005 | To put in self certificate for the first week for her whiplash injury | | NP (AA) | |
| 27.07.2005 | 26.03.1974 | F | | 1005 | 1015 | To put in self certificate for the first week for his whiplash injury | | NP (AA) | |
| 28.07.2005 | 18.06.1960 | F | | 1653 | 1658 | Back pain | Diclofenac e/c & Dihydrocodeine | NP (AF) | |
| 22.07.2005 | 03.06.1937 | M | | 1747 | 1800 | Tachycardia, known Woolf-Parkinson-White syndrome | Referred to Cardiologist | NP (AH) | |

Result of a query that lists all consultations from the 22nd to the end of July 2005 (ConsultationsSeenFrom22ndTillEndOfJul2005)

| SurgeryDate | DateOfBirth | Sex | Diagnosis | TimeIn | TimeOut | Complaints | Treatments | NumbersID | Notes |
|---|---|---|---|---|---|---|---|---|---|
| 26.07.2005 | 06.11.1961 | F | Lump | 1028 | 1036 | Something coming down, possible uterine prolapse | Referred to Gynaecologist (Basildon Hospital) | NP (BP) | |
| 26.07.2005 | 13.07.1987 | F | | 1006 | 1011 | Septic insect bite (R) foot | Flucloxacillin | NP (DI) | |
| 22.07.2005 | 28.09.1973 | F | URTI | 926 | 932 | Sore throat | Amoxycillin | NP (DS) | |
| 27.07.2005 | 03.03.1937 | M | | 906 | 916 | Script for Bendrofluazide & Chloramphenicol eye drops given | | NP (EJC) | |
| 27.07.2005 | 17.11.1937 | F | UTI | 1737 | 1746 | Frequency of micturition | Amoxycillin | NP (JC) | For MSU. |
| 22.07.2005 | 20.04.1945 | F | | 1024 | 1044 | Script for Simvastatin given | | NP (KY) | |
| 25.07.2005 | 05.06.1955 | M | | 1658 | 1705 | Referred to Dietician | | NP (MM) | |
| 25.07.2005 | 17.05.1943 | M | | 1651 | 1658 | For KUB USScan (urgent) | | NP (PC) | Penicillin allergy. |
| 25.07.2005 | 30.09.1942 | F | | 933 | 950 | Awaiting results of U/Es done on 19.07.05 | | NP (PLW) | |
| 29.07.2005 | 07.02.2005 | F | Rash | 923 | 931 | Impetigo-like rash on (R) arm & (L) leg | Fusidic Acid cream | NP (RH) | |
| 29.07.2005 | 23.06.1941 | M | UTI | 1012 | 1022 | Dysuria | Amoxycillin | NP (RS) | For MSU. |
| 25.07.2005 | 07.02.2004 | F | URTI | 1750 | 1755 | Infected rhinorrhoea | Amoxycillin | NP (SAW) | |
| 26.07.2005 | 14.10.1978 | F | S/Leave | 1714 | 1721 | Depression | | NP (TI) | |
| 27.07.2005 | 13.02.1985 | F | | 1802 | 1810 | Script for Femodene given | | Temp | |

Result of a query that lists all consultations from the 22nd to the end of July 2006 (ConsultationsSeenFrom22ndTillEndOfJul2006)

| SurgeryDate | DateOfBirth | Sex | Diagnosis | TimeIn | TimeOut | Complaints | Treatments | Initials | Notes |
|---|---|---|---|---|---|---|---|---|---|
| 24.07.2006 | 18.08.1957 | M | S/Leave | 945 | 957 | Back Pain - Private | | JA | Script for Diclofenac e/c & Dihydrocodeine given. |
| 24.07.2006 | 02.03.1948 | M | | 957 | 1015 | Referred to Gastroenterologist (BUPA) regarding his indigestion | | JHH | |
| 24.07.2006 | 26.09.1937 | M | | 1015 | 1038 | Script for Atenolol given | | DJD | |
| 24.07.2006 | 15.04.1927 | M | | 1038 | 1050 | Script for Co-codamol given | | JB | |
| 24.07.2006 | 20.05.1938 | F | | 1050 | 1058 | Script for Ezetimibe & Metformin given | | DSMS | |
| 24.07.2006 | 26.10.1943 | F | | 1058 | 1112 | Referred to Orthopaedic Surgeon regarding lump in (R) finger | | APM | |
| 24.07.2006 | 31.01.1938 | F | | 1112 | 1123 | Script for Ibuprofen & Omeprazole given | | JMS | |
| 24.07.2006 | 11.10.1938 | F | | 1123 | 1135 | To avoid salt-ladened foods | | JMS | |
| 24.07.2006 | 29.04.1935 | F | | 1135 | 1150 | Referred to Practice Counsellor regarding feeling low & being weepy | | CM | |

627

Result of a query that lists all consultations from the 22nd to the end of July 2006 (ConsultationsSeenFrom22ndTillEndOfJul2006)

| SurgeryDate | DateOfBirth | Sex | Diagnosis | TimeIn | TimeOut | Complaints | Treatments | Initials | Notes |
|---|---|---|---|---|---|---|---|---|---|
| 24.07.2006 | 30.05.1916 | M | | 1150 | 1200 | Referred to Colo-rectal Surgeon (cancer referral) regarding anal ulcer | | ER | |
| 24.07.2006 | 06.06.1958 | M | | 1645 | 1655 | To book appointment or stay till end of Surgery to have sutures removed | | SJC | |
| 24.07.2006 | 12.05.1936 | M | | 1653 | 1704 | Constipation | Macrogol npf oral powder 13.8g | AM | |
| 24.07.2006 | 02.03.2002 | F | URTI | 1704 | 1708 | Sore throat | Erythromycin | VSC | |
| 24.07.2006 | 28.03.1970 | F | | 1708 | 1712 | For X-Ray of 4th (L) toe | | LJ | |
| 24.07.2006 | 15.04.2003 | F | URTI | 1712 | 1717 | Sore throat | Erythromycin | LMC | |
| 24.07.2006 | 24.04.1966 | M | | 1717 | 1727 | For B12, Folate & Ferritin | | BSE | |
| 24.07.2006 | 17.12.1931 | M | | 1735 | 1742 | For TFTs in one month | | JGS | |
| 24.07.2006 | 22.07.1974 | F | | 1742 | 1750 | Trimethoprim | | KSR | For MSU. |
| 24.07.2006 | 06.04.1924 | F | | 1750 | 1800 | To see nurse for urinalysis | | EAS | |
| 24.07.2006 | 17.03.1968 | F | URTI | 1800 | 1810 | Sore throat | Erythromycin | NJB | Referred to Dermatologist regarding mole on back. |
| 24.07.2006 | 02.11.1977 | F | | 1810 | 1816 | Script for Ovranette | | CCW | |

Result of a query that lists all consultations from the 22nd to the end of July 2006 (ConsultationsSeenFrom22ndTillEndOfJul2006)

| SurgeryDate | DateOfBirth | Sex | Diagnosis | TimeIn | TimeOut | Complaints | Treatments | Initials | Notes |
|---|---|---|---|---|---|---|---|---|---|
| 24.07.2006 | 18.01.1950 | F | Conjunctivitis | 1826 | 1833 | Septic (L) stye with lower eye lid swelling | Chloramphenicol eye ointment & Amoxycillin | JS | |
| 25.07.2006 | 20.11.1945 | M | | 945 | 1002 | Red line on forehead which has now disappeared completely | | CJM | |
| 25.07.2006 | 11.02.1938 | M | | 1002 | 1028 | Dietary advice regarding high Triglycerides given | | RJH | |
| 25.07.2006 | 20.10.1983 | F | S/Leave | 1028 | 1104 | Chest infection & Asthma attack | | ARS | |
| 25.07.2006 | 21.09.1923 | M | | 1104 | 1115 | Referred to ENT Surgeon regarding his voice being gruff | | SAM | |
| 25.07.2006 | 12.08.1931 | F | | 1115 | 1124 | For MSU | | PRT | |
| 25.07.2006 | 16.12.1970 | F | | 1124 | 1132 | Script for Dihydrocodeine given | | KMB | |
| 25.07.2006 | 07.07.1983 | F | | 1132 | 1138 | Referred to Eye Dr. on call, SGH regarding sticky & sore (R) eye not improving with antibiotics | | AK | |
| 25.07.2006 | 12.05.1949 | F | | 1138 | 1154 | Script for Cinchocaine with hydrocortisone suppositories & ointment, Flucloxacillin & Dihydrocodeine given | | MK | |

Result of a query that lists all consultations from the 22nd to the end of July 2006 (ConsultationsSeenFrom22ndTillEndOfJul2006)

| SurgeryDate | DateOfBirth | Sex | Diagnosis | TimeIn | TimeOut | Complaints | Treatments | Initials | Notes |
|---|---|---|---|---|---|---|---|---|---|
| 26.07.2006 | 23.07.1919 | F | | 943 | 955 | Script for Lisinopril given | | KF | |
| 26.07.2006 | 04.09.1958 | F | S/Leave | 955 | 1004 | (R) foot operation | | LKW | |
| 26.07.2006 | 15.10.1937 | F | | 1004 | 1022 | Yearly Diabetic check | | GS | |
| 26.07.2006 | 27.04.1928 | M | | 1025 | 1044 | Script for Flucloxacillin given | | RFV | Referred to Orthopaedic Surgeon regarding (R) Olecranon bursa. |
| 26.07.2006 | 02.11.1984 | F | | 1047 | 1104 | Script for Ethinylestradiol with Levonorgestrel given | | TEG | |
| 26.07.2006 | 25.03.1946 | M | | 1104 | 1110 | Script for Ibuprofen given | | JE | |
| 26.07.2006 | 25.09.1961 | F | | 1110 | 1120 | Script for Ferrous Sulphate given | | SJB | |
| 26.07.2006 | 30.09.1941 | M | | 1120 | 1127 | Script for Penicillin V & Flucloxacillin given | | DGC | |
| 26.07.2006 | 18.04.1930 | F | | 1127 | 1144 | She will contact other chemists regarding availability of Tranxene | | IDB | |
| 26.07.2006 | 18.07.1978 | F | | 1144 | 1149 | Vaginal thrush | Clotrimazole pessary | TJS | |
| 26.07.2006 | 02.07.1924 | M | | 1149 | 1158 | Script for Co-codamol given | | TCC | |
| 26.07.2006 | 03.06.1977 | M | URTI | 1643 | 1653 | (L) ear ache | Amoxycillin & Otomize ear spray | SM | |

## Result of a query that lists all consultations from the 22nd to the end of July 2006 (ConsultationsSeenFrom22ndTillEndOfJul2006)

| SurgeryDate | DateOfBirth | Sex | Diagnosis | TimeIn | TimeOut | Complaints | Treatments | Initials | Notes |
|---|---|---|---|---|---|---|---|---|---|
| 26.07.2006 | 02.01.1933 | F | | 1656 | 1714 | Script for Atenolol given | | DLW | |
| 26.07.2006 | 21.06.1975 | F | | 1714 | 1725 | Referred to Practice Counsellor regarding being weepy & low | | AKE | |
| 26.07.2006 | 10.06.1969 | F | S/Leave | 1725 | 1739 | Caring for Son who had operation (Kardak's Procedure) | | JAT | |
| 26.07.2006 | 22.07.1968 | F | | 1739 | 1746 | Script for Flucloxacillin given | | RG | |
| 26.07.2006 | 30.03.1949 | F | | 1746 | 1809 | Referred to Orthopaedic Surgeon regarding (R) Carpal tunnel syndrome | | YAG | Script for Lisinopril given. |
| 26.07.2006 | 25.02.1986 | F | | 1809 | 1816 | Referred to Neurologist regarding her headaches | | SJH | |
| 26.07.2006 | 14.04.1970 | M | | 1816 | 1832 | Script for Diazepam given | | GB | |
| 26.07.2006 | 08.12.1978 | F | | 1832 | 1840 | Script for Alverine citrate given | | KW | For USScan of the abdomen. |
| 27.07.2006 | 09.12.1989 | F | | 941 | 954 | Script for Ciprofloxacin, Metoclopramide & Buscopan given | | Temp (DL) | |
| 27.07.2006 | 08.08.2003 | F | URTI | 954 | 1003 | Sore throat | Amoxycillin | SSSW | |
| 27.07.2006 | 18.10.1966 | F | | 1003 | 1014 | Yearly Diabetic check | | LAMW | |

631

Result of a query that lists all consultations from the 22nd to the end of July 2006 (ConsultationsSeenFrom22ndTillEndOfJul2006)

| SurgeryDate | DateOfBirth | Sex | Diagnosis | TimeIn | TimeOut | Complaints | Treatments | Initials | Notes |
|---|---|---|---|---|---|---|---|---|---|
| 27.07.2006 | 22.02.2004 | M | | 1014 | 1025 | Constipation | Glycerol suppositories & Lactulose | BJW | |
| 27.07.2006 | 22.06.1921 | F | | 1025 | 1035 | Script for Co-codamol & Flucloxacillin given | | FCH | |
| 27.07.2006 | 23.04.1958 | F | | 1035 | 1052 | Script for MethylPrednisolone tablets given | | LEB | |
| 27.07.2006 | 31.10.1915 | F | | 1052 | 1113 | Script for Bendrofluazide & Fusidic acid cream given | | MEC | |
| 27.07.2006 | 20.02.1930 | M | | 1113 | 1122 | For X-Ray (R) shoulder | | AL | |
| 27.07.2006 | 18.01.1977 | F | | 1122 | 1130 | For Pregnancy test (& TOP) | | MP | |
| 27.07.2006 | 26.06.2004 | F | | 1130 | 1136 | Dysuria | Amoxycillin | FGW | For MSU. |
| 27.07.2006 | 02.01.1926 | F | | 1310 | 1335 | Script for Electrolade, Buscopan & Lomotil given | | EG | Home visit. |
| 27.07.2006 | 27.08.1922 | M | | 1510 | 1535 | Referred to Surgical Dr. on call, SGH regarding his acute abdominal pain | | AC | Home visit. |
| 27.07.2006 | 06.02.1946 | F | | 1648 | 1659 | Script for Frovatriptan given | | KMT | |
| 27.07.2006 | 29.12.1982 | F | | 1659 | 1706 | Pregnancy test Positive | | HF | |

Result of a query that lists all consultations from the 22nd to the end of July 2006 (ConsultationsSeenFrom22ndTillEndOfJul2006)

| SurgeryDate | DateOfBirth | Sex | Diagnosis | TimeIn | TimeOut | Complaints | Treatments | Initials | Notes |
|---|---|---|---|---|---|---|---|---|---|
| 27.07.2006 | 28.08.1946 | F |  | 1706 | 1713 | Referred to Dermatologist regarding the contact dermatitis in his hands |  | VAG |  |
| 27.07.2006 | 25.09.1961 | F |  | 1716 | 1729 | Script for Lisinopril given |  | SJB |  |
| 27.07.2006 | 19.01.1954 | F |  | 1731 | 1747 | Referred to Dermatologist regarding moles on her body |  | DJD |  |
| 27.07.2006 | 03.09.1980 | F |  | 1747 | 1753 | Septic insect bite on (R) leg | Flucloxacillin | KCS |  |
| 27.07.2006 | 07.07.1980 | M |  | 1753 | 1805 | He will discuss about Clomipramine causing his body to heat up |  | DAC |  |
| 27.07.2006 | 01.09.1983 | F |  | 1805 | 1815 | Stool for C&S |  | KLM |  |
| 27.07.2006 | 02.12.1986 | M |  | 1815 | 1820 | Script for Flucloxacillin |  | SW |  |
| 28.07.2006 | 12.10.1948 | F |  | 941 | 952 | For repeat LFTs & Cholesterol |  | SRC |  |
| 28.07.2006 | 16.02.1931 | M |  | 952 | 1002 | Script for Ezetimibe given |  | CHH |  |
| 28.07.2006 | 23.01.1926 | F |  | 1002 | 1016 | Referred to Gastro-enterologist regarding recurrent anaemia |  | FN |  |

Result of a query that lists all consultations from the 22nd to the end of July 2006 (ConsultationsSeenFrom22ndTillEndOfJul2006)

| SurgeryDate | DateOfBirth | Sex | Diagnosis | TimeIn | TimeOut | Complaints | Treatments | Initials | Notes |
|---|---|---|---|---|---|---|---|---|---|
| 28.07.2006 | 05.07.1931 | F | | 1016 | 1033 | Script for Simvastatin given | | AVD | For B12, Folate & Ferritin. |
| 28.07.2006 | 11.03.2001 | F | | 1033 | 1040 | Script for Salbutamol inhaler given | | SJE | |
| 28.07.2006 | 08.03.1959 | F | | 1040 | 1047 | Script for Co-codamol & Diclofenac e/c given | | DM | For Cervical X-Ray. |
| 28.07.2006 | 15.05.1937 | M | | 1106 | 1128 | For Lumbar Spine X-Ray | | JHR | |
| 28.07.2006 | 10.12.1986 | F | S/Leave | 1128 | 1134 | Depression | | HEB | |
| 28.07.2006 | 05.02.1946 | F | | 1134 | 1142 | Referred to Orthopaedic Surgeon regarding (L) carpal tunnel syndrome | | ML | |
| 28.07.2006 | 18.11.1985 | M | | 1142 | 1150 | Script for Ibuprofen given | | Temp (KS) | |
| 28.07.2006 | 20.10.1929 | M | | 1300 | 1320 | For MSU | | PL | Home visit. |
| 28.07.2006 | 06.09.1984 | M | | 1647 | 1652 | Septic burn to (L) lower arm | Flucloxacillin & Fusidic acid cream | BJP | |
| 28.07.2006 | 26.05.1996 | M | RTI | 1652 | 1657 | (R) ear ache | Erythromycin | BF | |
| 28.07.2006 | 03.07.1950 | F | | 1721 | 1733 | Referred to Pain Management Specialist regarding pain in her (R) hand | | YC | |
| 28.07.2006 | 04.04.1953 | M | Pain | 1733 | 1741 | Pain (R) shoulder | Dihydrocodeine | GC | |
| 28.07.2006 | 10.05.2002 | M | RTI | 1741 | 1747 | Chesty cough | Erythromycin | KLC | |
| 28.07.2006 | 10.09.1997 | F | URTI | 1747 | 1754 | Sore throat | Amoxycillin | MJB | |

Result of a query that lists all consultations from the 22nd to the end of July 2006 (ConsultationsSeenFrom22ndTillEndOfJul2006)

| SurgeryDate | DateOfBirth | Sex | Diagnosis | TimeIn | TimeOut | Complaints | Treatments | Initials | Notes |
|---|---|---|---|---|---|---|---|---|---|
| 28.07.2006 | 01.06.1993 | M |  | 1758 | 1805 | Referred to Dermatologist (BUPA) regarding widespread body rash |  | DCE |  |
| 28.07.2006 | 04.08.1936 | M | URTI | 1805 | 1812 | Bilateral ear ache | Otomize ear spray & Amoxycillin | ECM |  |
| 28.07.2006 | 02.02.1951 | F |  | 1812 | 1822 | Script for Co-phenotrope & oral rehydration salts oral powder given |  | JMB | Stool for C&S. |
| 28.07.2006 | 18.01.1936 | M |  | 1822 | 1830 | For Fasting serum Cholesterol |  | PAP |  |

Result of a query that lists all consultations from the 22nd to the end of July 2007 (ConsultationsSeenFrom22ndTillEndOfJul2007)

| SurgeryDate | DateOfBirth | Sex | Diagnosis | TimeIn | TimeOut | Complaints | Treatments | Initials | Notes |
|---|---|---|---|---|---|---|---|---|---|
| 23.07.2007 | 01.10.1962 | F |  | 942 | 956 | Referred to Gynaecologist regarding being sterilized |  | CN |  |
| 23.07.2007 | 08.02.1939 | F |  | 956 | 1009 | Script for Quinine Sulphate given |  | IB |  |
| 23.07.2007 | 08.04.1945 | M |  | 1009 | 1019 | Referred to Gastroenterologist regarding persistent faecal leakage |  | GTW |  |

Result of a query that lists all consultations from the 22nd to the end of July 2007 (ConsultationsSeenFrom22ndTillEndOfJul2007)

| SurgeryDate | DateOfBirth | Sex | Diagnosis | TimeIn | TimeOut | Complaints | Treatments | Initials | Notes |
|---|---|---|---|---|---|---|---|---|---|
| 23.07.2007 | 20.06.1950 | M | | 1019 | 1029 | Referred to Rheumatologist regarding (L) shoulder & (L) arm pain | | PH | |
| 23.07.2007 | 05.04.1991 | F | | 1029 | 1038 | Referred to Gynaecologist regarding heavy periods with clots not improving with contraceptive pill | | LSR | |
| 23.07.2007 | 11.07.1956 | F | | 1038 | 1045 | Script for Nicotinell TTS patch 10 sq. cm given | | SAC | |
| 23.07.2007 | 17.07.1940 | F | | 1045 | 1105 | Referred to Orthopaedic Surgeon regarding swelling at the lower end of the (L) heel | | MPA | |
| 23.07.2007 | 12.11.1950 | M | | 1103 | 1110 | Referred to Dermatologist regarding multiple warts on his fore-head & neck | | MJP | |
| 23.07.2007 | 02.06.1955 | F | | 1110 | 1132 | Referred to Rheumatologist regarding multiple joints pain | | JPS | Script for Erythromycin given. |
| 23.07.2007 | 15.04.1956 | M | RTI | 1132 | 1140 | Chesty cough | Amoxycillin | MAO | |

636

Result of a query that lists all consultations from the 22nd to the end of July 2007 (ConsultationsSeenFrom22ndTillEndOfJul2007)

| SurgeryDate | DateOfBirth | Sex | Diagnosis | TimeIn | TimeOut | Complaints | Treatments | Initials | Notes |
|---|---|---|---|---|---|---|---|---|---|
| 23.07.2007 | 16.08.1992 | F | | 1140 | 1152 | Script for Co-codamol & Clindamycin with benzoyl peroxide gel given | | LMP | |
| 23.07.2007 | 20.12.1972 | F | | 1642 | 1648 | For FBC | | DEA | Her son came to Surgery. |
| 23.07.2007 | 18.09.1946 | F | | 1657 | 1706 | Script for Trimethoprim given | | SL | For MSU. |
| 23.07.2007 | 30.03.1949 | F | S/Leave | 1706 | 1715 | Chest infection & Depression | | YAG | |
| 23.07.2007 | 17.10.1989 | M | | 1715 | 1731 | Referred to Audiology Clinic regarding his worsening deafness | | JF | |
| 23.07.2007 | 21.09.1947 | M | | 1731 | 1738 | Referred to Orthopaedic Surgeon regarding pain in his (R) index finger | | DL | |
| 23.07.2007 | 10.05.1968 | F | | 1738 | 1744 | Referred to Physiotherapy regarding painful (R) leg | | AB | Script for Flucloxacillin given. |
| 23.07.2007 | 01.12.1967 | M | | 1744 | 1755 | To see the nurse regarding holidays vaccinations to Sri Lanka | | RAJ | |
| 23.07.2007 | 27.08.1983 | F | | 1755 | 1804 | Pregnancy test positive | | KLH | |

637

Result of a query that lists all consultations from the 22nd to the end of July 2007 (ConsultationsSeenFrom22ndTillEndOfJul2007)

| SurgeryDate | DateOfBirth | Sex | Diagnosis | TimeIn | TimeOut | Complaints | Treatments | Initials | Notes |
|---|---|---|---|---|---|---|---|---|---|
| 23.07.2007 | 16.08.1927 | F | | 1804 | 1814 | Script for Dihydrocodeine & Cefalexin given | | EFM | |
| 23.07.2007 | 29.01.1956 | M | | 1820 | 1832 | Script for Dihydrocodeine, Diclofenac e/c & Omeprazole given | | AJH | |
| 24.07.2007 | 13.05.1996 | F | RTI | 945 | 951 | Chesty cough | Amoxycillin | NMF | |
| 24.07.2007 | 11.12.1940 | M | | 951 | 1008 | Referred to Orthopaedic Surgeon regarding pain in both ankles | | FP | |
| 24.07.2007 | 26.11.1954 | M | | 1008 | 1017 | To continue with the same dose of Omeprazole for the next 2 months | | PHM | |
| 24.07.2007 | 23.03.1926 | M | | 1017 | 1034 | Script for Amitriptyline & GTN spray given | | JWH | |
| 24.07.2007 | 29.01.1941 | M | | 1034 | 1058 | Script for Citalopram & Trimethoprim given | | AD | |
| 24.07.2007 | 03.02.1946 | F | | 1058 | 1108 | Script for Conjugated Oestrogens equine tablets 300mcg given | | BKJ | |
| 24.07.2007 | 19.12.1945 | F | | 1108 | 1119 | Script for Omeprazole given | | JMB | |
| 24.07.2007 | 05.08.1936 | F | RTI | 1119 | 1124 | Chesty cough | Amoxycillin | SAMN | |
| 24.07.2007 | 15.01.2007 | F | RTI | 1124 | 1130 | Chesty cough | Amoxycillin | MRB | |

Result of a query that lists all consultations from the 22nd to the end of July 2007 (ConsultationsSeenFrom22ndTillEndOfJul2007)

| SurgeryDate | DateOfBirth | Sex | Diagnosis | TimeIn | TimeOut | Complaints | Treatments | Initials | Notes |
|---|---|---|---|---|---|---|---|---|---|
| 24.07.2007 | 10.09.1981 | F | | 1646 | 1658 | For Pregnancy test in one week | | HS | |
| 24.07.2007 | 15.05.1945 | M | | 1658 | 1703 | Script for Candesartan given | | VCC | |
| 24.07.2007 | 12.12.1948 | F | | 1703 | 1710 | Script for Amitriptyline & Amoxycillin given | | SMS | |
| 24.07.2007 | 05.10.1974 | M | | 1713 | 1730 | Script for Orlistat given | | SMG | |
| 24.07.2007 | 04.04.1953 | M | | 1730 | 1738 | Referred to Orthopaedic Surgeon regarding pain in his (L) ankle | | GC | Referred to Dermatologist regarding moles on his back. |
| 24.07.2007 | 25.03.1947 | F | | 1738 | 1751 | Script for Bendroflumethiazide given | | HER | |
| 24.07.2007 | 02.08.1948 | M | | 1751 | 1800 | To persevere with the Ikorel but at a lower dose | | KT | |
| 24.07.2007 | 20.05.1991 | F | | 1800 | 1807 | Script for Flucloxacillin given | | JS | |
| 24.07.2007 | 29.09.1932 | F | | 1807 | 1821 | Injection Depo-Medrone with Lidocaine given to the (L) knee | | SMD | |
| 24.07.2007 | 27.08.1948 | F | | 1826 | 1836 | Script for Amoxycillin & Clobetasol cream given | | BJH | |

Result of a query that lists all consultations from the 22$^{nd}$ to the end of July 2007 (ConsultationsSeenFrom22ndTillEndOfJul2007)

| SurgeryDate | DateOfBirth | Sex | Diagnosis | TimeIn | TimeOut | Complaints | Treatments | Initials | Notes |
|---|---|---|---|---|---|---|---|---|---|
| 24.07.2007 | 02.11.1938 | M | | 1836 | 1842 | Script for Bendroflumethiazide given | | MSH | |
| 25.07.2007 | 25.02.1988 | F | | 947 | 1002 | Script for Fluoxetine given | | MIG | |
| 25.07.2007 | 25.07.1984 | F | | 1002 | 1009 | Reassured regarding tingling in the (L) breast | | DDW | |
| 25.07.2007 | 04.01.1962 | F | | 1009 | 1020 | Script for Cefalexin given | | CEC | For MSU. Trimethoprim allergy. |
| 25.07.2007 | 17.02.1912 | F | | 1020 | 1032 | Script for Temazepam given | | IAA | Referred to Dermatologist regarding warty lesion on her face. |
| 25.07.2007 | 31.05.1997 | F | | 1032 | 1040 | Script for Erythromycin & Fusidic acid with hydrocortisone cream given | | SC | |
| 25.07.2007 | 02.06.1931 | M | | 1040 | 1055 | For Cervical & CXR as well as for TFTs & Fasting Glucose | | EWJE | |
| 25.07.2007 | 24.12.1975 | M | | 1055 | 1106 | For USScan of testicles (urgent) | | DWDS | |
| 25.07.2007 | 25.08.1934 | M | | 1106 | 1122 | To get details of the Parkinson's Society from the reception | | NTRR | |

Result of a query that lists all consultations from the 22nd to the end of July 2007 (ConsultationsSeenFrom22ndTillEndOfJul2007)

| SurgeryDate | DateOfBirth | Sex | Diagnosis | TimeIn | TimeOut | Complaints | Treatments | Initials | Notes |
|---|---|---|---|---|---|---|---|---|---|
| 25.07.2007 | 25.09.1960 | M | | 1122 | 1136 | Referred to Neurologist regarding his epilepsy | | JM | |
| 25.07.2007 | 06.01.1955 | M | | 1647 | 1654 | Script for Prochlorperazine & Private script for Viagra given | | MAS | |
| 25.07.2007 | 17.08.1961 | F | | 1654 | 1702 | Referred to Podiatrist regarding bilateral bunions | | JT | |
| 25.07.2007 | 29.03.1974 | F | | 1706 | 1715 | Late Period | For urine pregnancy test | GJP | |
| 25.07.2007 | 15.07.1956 | F | | 1715 | 1729 | Referred to General Surgeon regarding lump just inferior to the (R) Clavicle | | DHC | |
| 25.07.2007 | 02.06.1974 | F | | 1729 | 1755 | Referred to Breast Surgeon regarding (R) nipple discharge. | | MEG | Script for Flucloxacillin given |
| 25.07.2007 | 16.03.1978 | M | S/Leave | 1755 | 1804 | Depression following Heroin withdrawal - Med. 5 | | JWPS | Script for Diazepam given |
| 25.07.2007 | 23.11.1960 | M | | 1804 | 1819 | Referred to ENT Surgeon regarding cyst in the (R) ear lobe | | DNT | Referred to Dermatologist regarding lesion behind the (R) ear. |

## Result of a query that lists all consultations from the 22nd to the end of July 2007 (ConsultationsSeenFrom22ndTillEndOfJul2007)

| SurgeryDate | DateOfBirth | Sex | Diagnosis | TimeIn | TimeOut | Complaints | Treatments | Initials | Notes |
|---|---|---|---|---|---|---|---|---|---|
| 25.07.2007 | 18.03.1987 | F | | 1819 | 1836 | Letter to Whom it may concern that she cannot attend gymnasium | | LP | Referred to Physiotherapy privately regarding whiplash injury. |
| 25.07.2007 | 30.03.1943 | M | | 946 | 953 | For MSU | | BWF | |
| 25.07.2007 | 03.07.1938 | M | | 953 | 1002 | For repeat FBC in 3 to 6 months with the nurse | | DBW | |
| 25.07.2007 | 08.11.1921 | F | | 1002 | 1020 | Script for Oxybutynin given | | JW | Referred to the Incontinence nurse regarding her urgency of micturition. |
| 25.07.2007 | 19.02.1947 | M | | 1020 | 1042 | Script for Gliclazide given | | SMB | |
| 25.07.2007 | 23.10.1932 | F | | 1042 | 1058 | Script for Vitamin bpc given | | CFAB | |
| 25.07.2007 | 16.08.1927 | F | | 1058 | 1109 | Script for Erythromycin & Furosemide given | | EFM | |
| 25.07.2007 | 06.04.1937 | M | | 1109 | 1126 | Script for Bendroflumethiazide given | | GWH | |
| 25.07.2007 | 25.04.1943 | F | | 1126 | 1139 | For FBC, U/Es & TFTs | | SJH | |
| 25.07.2007 | 19.08.1917 | F | | 1139 | 1149 | Script for Ferrous Sulphate given | | VL | |

Result of a query that lists all consultations from the 22nd to the end of July 2007 (ConsultationsSeenFrom22ndTillEndOfJul2007)

| SurgeryDate | DateOfBirth | Sex | Diagnosis | TimeIn | TimeOut | Complaints | Treatments | Initials | Notes |
|---|---|---|---|---|---|---|---|---|---|
| 25.07.2007 | 09.04.1938 | M | | 1149 | 1158 | Script for Candesartan given | | NWH | |
| 25.07.2007 | 09.10.1926 | M | | 1158 | 1206 | Script for Fexofenadine given | | RAC | |
| 25.07.2007 | 25.06.1921 | M | | 1206 | 1218 | Chemotherapy appointment re-arranged for him | | HRP | |
| 25.07.2007 | 21.09.1947 | M | | 1645 | 1655 | Script for Bendroflumethiazide & Metformin given | | DL | |
| 25.07.2007 | 11.06.1968 | F | | 1655 | 1705 | For repeat U/Es in 3 months | | TR | |
| 25.07.2007 | 28.07.1961 | F | | 1705 | 1720 | Referred to Psychiatrist regarding manic depression | | KTN | |
| 25.07.2007 | 19.05.1988 | F | | 1720 | 1725 | Human bite to lower lip | Co-Amoxiclav | DRC | |
| 25.07.2007 | 23.06.1978 | F | | 1725 | 1739 | Referred to Gynaecologist regarding hormonal imbalance | | NPS | Referred to Practice Counsellor regarding inability to deal with her miscarriage. |
| 25.07.2007 | 15.11.1972 | M | | 1739 | 1749 | To see me in one month for BP check | | SIH | |
| 25.07.2007 | 14.08.1947 | F | S/Leave | 1749 | 1759 | pain in (L) leg & Back - Med. 5 | | PJH | |
| 25.07.2007 | 22.01.1932 | M | | 1808 | 1818 | He will observe his mild constipation for now | | JBW | |

643

Result of a query that lists all consultations from the 22$^{nd}$ to the end of July 2007 (ConsultationsSeenFrom22ndTillEndOfJul2007)

| SurgeryDate | DateOfBirth | Sex | Diagnosis | TimeIn | TimeOut | Complaints | Treatments | Initials | Notes |
|---|---|---|---|---|---|---|---|---|---|
| 25.07.2007 | 22.02.1971 | M | | 1818 | 1827 | Awaiting letter from Basildon Hospital | | SB | |
| 25.07.2007 | 23.02.1940 | M | | 1831 | 1912 | Nationwide Insurance Medical done | | BWH | |
| 27.07.2007 | 05.06.1998 | F | | 945 | 1006 | Script for Trimethoprim given | | PG | Referred to Paediatrician regarding recurrent back pains & headaches. For USScan of the kidneys. |
| 27.07.2007 | 28.03.1999 | M | | 1006 | 1019 | Referred to Paediatrician regarding lacking concentration & being inattentive | | TAH | |
| 27.07.2007 | 03.12.1989 | F | | 1019 | 1034 | Referred to Neurologist regarding her migraine attacks | | EDB | Script for Erythromycin given. Penicillin allergy. |
| 27.07.2007 | 28.10.1930 | F | | 1034 | 1049 | Script for Lisinopril & Prochlorperazine given | | KBC | |
| 27.07.2007 | 18.01.1950 | F | | 1049 | 1110 | Script for Levothyroxine given | | JS | Referred to ENT Surgeon regarding persistent itchy spot on the ear lobe. |

Result of a query that lists all consultations from the 22nd to the end of July 2007 (ConsultationsSeenFrom22ndTillEndOfJul2007)

| SurgeryDate | DateOfBirth | Sex | Diagnosis | TimeIn | TimeOut | Complaints | Treatments | Initials | Notes |
|---|---|---|---|---|---|---|---|---|---|
| 27.07.2007 | 07.12.1968 | M | | 1110 | 1124 | Script for Diazepam given | | SKF | |
| 27.07.2007 | 07.04.1971 | F | URTI | 1124 | 1131 | Sore throat | Amoxycillin | TM | Script for Sibutramine given. |
| 27.07.2007 | 21.08.1934 | M | | 1131 | 1137 | To see the nurse in 6 months for repeat U/Es | | KW | |
| 27.07.2007 | 17.07.1983 | F | S/Leave | 1137 | 1147 | Pain in the (R) arm - Med. 5 | | DLR | Script for Dihydrocodeine given. |
| 27.07.2007 | 14.10.1949 | F | | 1147 | 1156 | Referred to Fracture Clinic regarding her fractured (L) Humerus | | SW | |
| 27.07.2007 | 27.04.1925 | M | | 1158 | 1208 | To see me if he is ballooning up or his urine output is significantly falling | | RWF | |
| 30.07.2007 | 18.06.1963 | M | | 940 | 957 | Script for Co-codamol & Diclofenac e/c given | | RR | Referred to Physiotherapist regarding pain down back of his leg with numbness. For X-Ray Lumbar Spine, hips & Pelvis. |
| 30.07.2007 | 24.05.1959 | M | S/Leave | 957 | 1004 | Excess Alcohol Intake | | KMH | |

Result of a query that lists all consultations from the 22nd to the end of July 2007 (ConsultationsSeenFrom22ndTillEndOfJul2007)

| SurgeryDate | DateOfBirth | Sex | Diagnosis | TimeIn | TimeOut | Complaints | Treatments | Initials | Notes |
|---|---|---|---|---|---|---|---|---|---|
| 30.07.2007 | 13.03.1944 | F | | 1004 | 1011 | Script for Simvastatin given | | BCO | For FBC, U/Es, Cholesterol & LFTs. |
| 30.07.2007 | 29.01.1956 | M | S/Leave | 1011 | 1021 | Injury to back - Med. 5 | | AJH | Referred to Orthopaedic Surgeon (BUPA) regarding his back injury. |
| 30.07.2007 | 20.04.1947 | F | S/Leave | 1025 | 1032 | Stress & (R) leg pain | | PA | For FBC. Penicillin allergy. |
| 30.07.2007 | 04.02.1963 | F | S/Leave | 1108 | 1119 | Shingles - Med. 5 | | SAL | Script for Acyclovir given. |
| 30.07.2007 | 27.10.1960 | F | S/Leave | 1119 | 1126 | Back Pain - Med. 4 | | DLK | |
| 30.07.2007 | 01.09.1983 | F | | 1126 | 1138 | Script for Acyclovir tablets given | | KLM | Co-trimoxazole allergy. |
| 30.07.2007 | 31.08.1906 | F | Conjunctivitis | 1325 | 1337 | (L) eye is red & sore | Chloramphenicol eye drops | EM | Home visit. |
| 30.07.2007 | 25.02.1912 | F | | 1345 | 1355 | Bilateral pedal oedema | Furosemide | AK | Home visit. |
| 30.07.2007 | 16.07.1936 | F | | 1644 | 1649 | Script for Simvastatin given | | EG | |
| 30.07.2007 | 24.07.1956 | M | | 1655 | 1710 | Script for Bendroflumethiazide given | | SS | Referred to Physiotherapist regarding pain in both shoulders. |
| 30.07.2007 | 28.06.1959 | M | | 1710 | 1727 | Script for Lisinopril & Doxazosin given | | SCU | |

Result of a query that lists all consultations from the 22<sup>nd</sup> to the end of July 2007 (ConsultationsSeenFrom22ndTillEndOfJul2007)

| SurgeryDate | DateOfBirth | Sex | Diagnosis | TimeIn | TimeOut | Complaints | Treatments | Initials | Notes |
|---|---|---|---|---|---|---|---|---|---|
| 30.07.2007 | 19.05.1956 | F |  | 1727 | 1733 | Script for Sodium bicarbonate ear drops given |  | VJM |  |
| 30.07.2007 | 10.03.2004 | M |  | 1733 | 1741 | Script for Diprobase given |  | DFJB | Referred to Dermatologist regarding eczema & spots on his back. |
| 30.07.2007 | 11.06.1980 | M |  | 1741 | 1748 | Script for Diprobase & Flucloxacillin given |  | MLP |  |
| 30.07.2007 | 22.07.1982 | F | S/Leave | 1748 | 1756 | Urinary Tract Infection - Private |  | USK |  |
| 30.07.2007 | 25.01.1939 | F |  | 1756 | 1812 | Her bilateral pedal oedema is probably due to the Verapamil |  | PMC |  |
| 30.07.2007 | 10.08.1962 | M |  | 1812 | 1521 | For serum Uric acid & Rheumatoid Factor |  | DPS |  |
| 30.07.2007 | 18.11.1979 | M |  | 1821 | 1828 | Script for Co-codamol & Diclofenac e/c given |  | JAS |  |
| 30.07.2007 | 15.04.1956 | M |  | 1828 | 1843 | Script for Salbutamol nebulising fluid given |  | MAO |  |

Result of a query that lists all consultations from the 22$^{nd}$ to the end of July 2008 (ConsultationsSeenFrom22ndTillEndOfJul2008)

| SurgeryDate | DateOfBirth | Sex | Diagnosis | TimeIn | TimeOut | Complaints | Treatments | Initials | Notes |
|---|---|---|---|---|---|---|---|---|---|
| 22.07.2008 | 08.08.1940 | F | | 944 | 952 | Referred to Ophthalmologist for glaucoma check | | WAW | |
| 22.07.2008 | 13.09.1918 | M | | 952 | 1024 | To take own Paracetamol for the arthritis in his hands | | EJG | |
| 22.07.2008 | 23.03.1926 | M | | 1024 | 1032 | Referred to Physiotherapist regarding weakness of the (L) leg | | JWH | |
| 22.07.2008 | 03.03.1937 | M | | 1032 | 1035 | Script for Co-codamol given | | EJC | |
| 22.07.2008 | 23.02.1969 | M | S/Leave | 1035 | 1040 | Shoulder pain - Med. 5 | | DJP | |
| 22.07.2008 | 20.04.1938 | M | RTI | 1040 | 1045 | Chesty cough | Amoxycillin | DAD | |
| 22.07.2008 | 22.12.1936 | F | | 1045 | 1052 | Medication Review Done | | VMG | |
| 22.07.2008 | 04.05.1937 | F | | 1052 | 1111 | Script for Ferrous Sulphate given | | DMB | Stool for C&S. |
| 22.07.2008 | 29.04.1935 | F | | 1111 | 1117 | Medication Review Done | | CM | |
| 22.07.2008 | 17.03.1967 | M | | 1117 | 1123 | Referred to Dermatologist regarding scaly skin & possible fungal nails infection | | TCS | |
| 22.07.2008 | 25.09.1960 | M | | 1123 | 1128 | For X-Rays of the (L) shoulder | | JM | |

Result of a query that lists all consultations from the 22nd to the end of July 2008 (ConsultationsSeenFrom22ndTillEndOfJul2008)

| SurgeryDate | DateOfBirth | Sex | Diagnosis | TimeIn | TimeOut | Complaints | Treatments | Initials | Notes |
|---|---|---|---|---|---|---|---|---|---|
| 22.07.2008 | 29.08.1915 | F |  | 1320 | 1327 | Script for Co-codamol given |  | FJ | Home visit. |
| 22.07.2008 | 23.10.1932 | F |  | 1340 | 1355 | Letter to expedite appointment to see the Neurologist |  | CFAB | Home visit. |
| 22.07.2008 | 10.09.1919 | F |  | 1400 | 1425 | Script for Buccastem & Salivix pastilles given |  | ALG | Home visit. |
| 22.07.2008 | 25.07.1939 | F | S/Leave | 1646 | 1700 | Diarrhoea & Vomiting - Med. 5 |  | JLB |  |
| 22.07.2008 | 02.12.1992 | M |  | 1700 | 1710 | Script for Amoxycillin given |  | TJN | For FBC. |
| 22.07.2008 | 27.04.1944 | M |  | 1710 | 1717 | Script for Bendroflumethiazide & Simvastatin given |  | JN |  |
| 22.07.2008 | 26.06.1990 | M | Rash | 1717 | 1721 | Itchy rash all over | Loratadine | KSH |  |
| 22.07.2008 | 15.01.1962 | M |  | 1721 | 1725 | Script for Erythromycin given |  | PWL |  |
| 22.07.2008 | 27.05.1959 | F |  | 1725 | 1728 | Script for Fusidic acid cream given |  | SM |  |
| 22.07.2008 | 03.07.1950 | F |  | 1728 | 1732 | For X-Rays (L) elbow |  | YC |  |
| 22.07.2008 | 04.04.1953 | M |  | 1732 | 1736 | Script for Co-codamol given |  | GC |  |
| 22.07.2008 | 01.09.1983 | F |  | 1740 | 1746 | No evidence of infection at the injection site |  | KLM |  |

Result of a query that lists all consultations from the 22nd to the end of July 2008 (ConsultationsSeenFrom22ndTillEndOfJul2008)

| SurgeryDate | DateOfBirth | Sex | Diagnosis | TimeIn | TimeOut | Complaints | Treatments | Initials | Notes |
|---|---|---|---|---|---|---|---|---|---|
| 22.07.2008 | 03.05.1951 | F | | 1746 | 1756 | Patient to come & see me regarding possible vaginal prolapse when she comes back from Dorset | | GAG | Husband came to the Surgery. |
| 22.07.2008 | 19.07.1960 | F | | 1811 | 1818 | Script for Amoxycillin given | | CLP | |
| 23.07.2008 | 16.09.1936 | M | | 941 | 945 | Private script for Viagra given | | LPCE | |
| 23.07.2008 | 09.04.1938 | M | | 945 | 950 | Medication Review Done | | NWH | |
| 23.07.2008 | 25.08.1936 | M | | 950 | 957 | Script for Furosemide & Prochlorperazine given | | CAJ | |
| 23.07.2008 | 23.10.1947 | F | | 957 | 1004 | Script for Omeprazole & Hyoscine butyl bromide given | | EEV | For USScan of the upper abdomen. |
| 23.07.2008 | 17.07.1940 | F | | 1004 | 1016 | Script for Simvastatin given | | MPA | |
| 23.07.2008 | 26.06.1955 | F | | 1022 | 1030 | Script for Amitriptyline & Clotrimazole with hydrocortisone cream given | | TAP | |
| 23.07.2008 | 21.02.1916 | F | | 1030 | 1040 | Script for Aspirin dispersible, Fusidic acid eye drops & Paracetamol given | | EFH | |

Result of a query that lists all consultations from the 22nd to the end of July 2008 (ConsultationsSeenFrom22ndTillEndOfJul2008)

| SurgeryDate | DateOfBirth | Sex | Diagnosis | TimeIn | TimeOut | Complaints | Treatments | Initials | Notes |
|---|---|---|---|---|---|---|---|---|---|
| 23.07.2008 | 22.05.1920 | F | | 1040 | 1049 | Medication Review Done | | VHC | |
| 23.07.2008 | 07.03.1941 | F | | 1049 | 1056 | For X-Rays of the (R) knee | | PJE | |
| 23.07.2008 | 21.01.1949 | M | | 1103 | 1113 | To see the nurse for ear syringing after getting OTC Sodium bicarbonate ear drops | | PH | |
| 23.07.2008 | 20.03.1987 | M | | 1113 | 1122 | Referred to Practice Counsellor regarding being unable to manage his anger & inability to cope | | CRS | |
| 23.07.2008 | 01.04.1945 | F | | 1648 | 1654 | Script for Co-codamol given | | IPB | |
| 23.07.2008 | 31.10.1951 | F | | 1654 | 1700 | Script for Diclofenac e/c & Furosemide given | | BAL | |
| 23.07.2008 | 01.04.1988 | F | | 1700 | 1703 | For FBC & U/Es | | KRW | |
| 23.07.2008 | 29.12.2000 | F | | 1706 | 1715 | Referred to Dermatologist regarding her eczema | | MMS | Referred to the ENT Surgeon regarding her worsening nasal speech. |
| 23.07.2008 | 07.07.1961 | F | RTI | 1715 | 1720 | Chesty cough | Erythromycin | SSA | Penicillin allergy. |
| 23.07.2008 | 13.03.1932 | M | UTI | 1720 | 1727 | Dysuria | Trimethoprim | RJW | For MSU. |
| 23.07.2008 | 09.06.1993 | F | URTI | 1742 | 1747 | Sore throat | Amoxycillin | AL | |
| 23.07.2008 | 29.11.1929 | F | | 1747 | 1757 | Medication Review Done | | JMB | Her daughter came to the Surgery. |

Result of a query that lists all consultations from the 22nd to the end of July 2008 (ConsultationsSeenFrom22ndTillEndOfJul2008)

| SurgeryDate | DateOfBirth | Sex | Diagnosis | TimeIn | TimeOut | Complaints | Treatments | Initials | Notes |
|---|---|---|---|---|---|---|---|---|---|
| 23.07.2008 | 24.01.2005 | M | Rash | 1757 | 1802 | Cradle cap | Fusidic acid with hydrocortisone cream | CRRD | |
| 23.07.2008 | 08.03.1959 | F | | 1802 | 1809 | To get OTC 1% Hydrocortisone cream for her itchy rash | | DM | |
| 23.07.2008 | 02.01.1926 | F | | 1840 | 1850 | Script for Trimethoprim given | | EAG | For MSU. |
| 24.07.2008 | 08.06.1952 | F | S/Leave | 945 | 954 | Back Pain | | PMA | |
| 24.07.2008 | 17.04.1923 | M | | 954 | 1003 | Medication Review Done | | JWD | |
| 24.07.2008 | 06.01.1994 | F | | 1003 | 1016 | She will like her period postponed | Norethisterone | GW | |
| 24.07.2008 | 30.08.1995 | F | | 1016 | 1032 | She will like her period postponed | Norethisterone | LW | Referred to Dermatologist regarding rash on her upper arms. |
| 24.07.2008 | 31.07.1927 | F | | 1032 | 1038 | Referred to Orthopaedic Surgeon regarding persistent pain in the (L) foot | | SMM | |
| 24.07.2008 | 30.01.1989 | M | S/Leave | 1046 | 1051 | Chesty Pain - Med. 5 | | CDB | |
| 24.07.2008 | 14.04.1964 | F | RTI | 1056 | 1104 | Chesty cough | Amoxycillin | JV | |
| 24.07.2008 | 10.02.1947 | F | | 1108 | 1116 | For MSU | | CAM | |
| 24.07.2008 | 14.09.1947 | F | URTI | 1120 | 1129 | (L) ear ache | Amoxycillin | CEJY | |
| 24.07.2008 | 23.06.1994 | M | | 1706 | 1713 | Script for Erythromycin given | | KCDA | Penicillin allergy. |
| 24.07.2008 | 20.11.1923 | M | | 1713 | 1723 | Script for Furosemide given | | WEG | |

Result of a query that lists all consultations from the 22nd to the end of July 2008 (ConsultationsSeenFrom22ndTillEndOfJul2008)

| SurgeryDate | DateOfBirth | Sex | Diagnosis | TimeIn | TimeOut | Complaints | Treatments | Initials | Notes |
|---|---|---|---|---|---|---|---|---|---|
| 24.07.2008 | 21.05.1949 | M | | 1728 | 1751 | Script for Omeprazole given | | JJH | For Chest X-Rays. For USScan of the abdomen. |
| 24.07.2008 | 08.12.1962 | F | | 1751 | 1804 | Script for Diclofenac e/c & Co-codamol given | | BJM | Referred to Rheumatologist regarding (L) elbow pain. Referred to Gynaecologist regarding menorrhagia. |
| 24.07.2008 | 06.08.1941 | M | | 1804 | 1813 | To see the nurse in 3 months for repeat HbA1c | | AJM | |
| 24.07.2008 | 24.02.2007 | M | | 1804 | 1813 | Script for Salbutamol inhaler given | | ASMP | |
| 24.07.2008 | 29.11.1969 | M | S/Leave | 1820 | 1830 | Rectal Bleeding - Private | | CW | |
| 25.07.2008 | 25.03.1947 | F | | 925 | 945 | Referred to Endocrinologist regarding getting heat intolerance | | HER | |
| 25.07.2008 | 04.06.1958 | F | | 945 | 955 | Script for Lactulose given | | JDC | |
| 25.07.2008 | 23.01.1926 | F | | 955 | 1000 | for serum BNP | | FGN | |
| 25.07.2008 | 05.06.1930 | F | | 1000 | 1008 | Referred to Chest Physician regarding getting HRCT to exclude (R) lung base bronchiectasis | | JMF | |

Result of a query that lists all consultations from the 22nd to the end of July 2008 (ConsultationsSeenFrom22ndTillEndOfJul2008)

| SurgeryDate | DateOfBirth | Sex | Diagnosis | TimeIn | TimeOut | Complaints | Treatments | Initials | Notes |
|---|---|---|---|---|---|---|---|---|---|
| 25.07.2008 | 07.02.1948 | M | | 1008 | 1019 | Referred to ENT Surgeon regarding wanting to clear his throat all the time | | GRC | Referred to Gastroenterologist regarding passing dark stools & anaemia. |
| 25.07.2008 | 13.11.1970 | F | | 1019 | 1028 | Referred to ENT Surgeon regarding persistent (L) ear discomfort | | SD | |
| 25.07.2008 | 23.05.1971 | F | | 1028 | 1038 | (L) eye infection | Chloramphenicol eye drops | BCR | |
| 25.07.2008 | 04.07.1961 | F | | 1038 | 1046 | Script for Amoxycillin given | | JB | For MSU & for USScan of the abdomen. |
| 25.07.2008 | 04.04.1992 | F | | 1046 | 1053 | Referred to Dermatologist regarding itchy dry skin under the eyes & brown patches on the back | | SAG | |
| 25.07.2008 | 30.08.1950 | F | | 1053 | 1100 | Referred to Dermatologist regarding small brownish lesion on the (L) temple | | AB | |
| 25.07.2008 | 15.10.1923 | F | | 1100 | 1108 | Script for Flucloxacillin & Salbutamol inhaler given | | DWB | |

654

Result of a query that lists all consultations from the 22nd to the end of July 2008 (ConsultationsSeenFrom22ndTillEndOfJul2008)

| SurgeryDate | DateOfBirth | Sex | Diagnosis | TimeIn | TimeOut | Complaints | Treatments | Initials | Notes |
|---|---|---|---|---|---|---|---|---|---|
| 25.07.2008 | 17.07.1983 | F | URTI | 1115 | 1120 | Sore throat | Amoxycillin | DLR | |
| 25.07.2008 | 24.08.1918 | F | | 1130 | 1153 | Script for Doxazosin & Naftidrofuryl given | | GPE | |
| 25.07.2008 | 08.11.2007 | F | | 1203 | 1213 | Script for Amoxycillin, Lactulose & Maxolon Paediatric given | | OTA | |
| 25.07.2008 | 20.11.1938 | M | | 1651 | 1705 | Script for Chloramphenicol eye drops & Ciprofloxacin given | | GL | Home visit. |
| 28.07.2008 | 27.04.1939 | F | | 944 | 948 | For serum BNP | | DBS | |
| 28.07.2008 | 25.01.1944 | F | | 958 | 1004 | For Chest X-Rays | | HPS | Script for Co-codamol given. |
| 28.07.2008 | 15.03.1934 | F | | 1004 | 1011 | Script for Ciprofloxacin given | | PJB | |
| 28.07.2008 | 03.07.1989 | M | | 1011 | 1016 | Infected (R) In growing toe nail | Flucloxacillin | WDH | |
| 28.07.2008 | 30.11.1945 | F | | 1016 | 1026 | Referred to General Surgeon regarding big lipoma in the * axilla | | JBJ | |
| 28.07.2008 | 13.12.1940 | F | | 1026 | 1031 | Results of Coeliac screen test is not yet back | | JAL | |

Result of a query that lists all consultations from the 22nd to the end of July 2008 (ConsultationsSeenFrom22ndTillEndOfJul2008)

| SurgeryDate | DateOfBirth | Sex | Diagnosis | TimeIn | TimeOut | Complaints | Treatments | Initials | Notes |
|---|---|---|---|---|---|---|---|---|---|
| 28.07.2008 | 12.05.1949 | F | RTI | 1035 | 1041 | Chesty cough | Amoxycillin | MK | Script for Co-codamol given. For letter to whom it may concern that she is taking Co-codamol for back pain. |
| 28.07.2008 | 02.07.1926 | M | RTI | 1046 | 1052 | Chesty cough | | BLB | |
| 28.07.2008 | 07.04.1950 | M | S/Leave | 1055 | 1104 | Chest Infection - Private | Ciprofloxacin | DML | Script for Ciprofloxacin given. |
| 28.07.2008 | 07.05.1974 | M | | 1104 | 1116 | Private script for Viagra given | | SBK | |
| 28.07.2008 | 30.11.1936 | M | | 1116 | 1124 | To use OTC Sodium bicarbonate ear drops & get his ears syringed | | GEE | |
| 28.07.2008 | 28.06.1959 | F | | 1124 | 1129 | Script for Flucloxacillin given | | PIS | For FBC & Fasting Glucose. |
| 28.07.2008 | 29.11.1929 | F | | 1350 | 1410 | Script for Trimethoprim given | | JMB | Home visit. For MSU. |
| 28.07.2008 | 20.05.1921 | F | | 1419 | 1450 | To contact DAU, SGH to review her | | CMB | Home visit. |
| 28.07.2008 | 03.05.1951 | F | | 1651 | 1658 | Referred to Gynaecologist (Benenden) regarding vaginal prolapse | | GAG | |

Result of a query that lists all consultations from the 22nd to the end of July 2008 (ConsultationsSeenFrom22ndTillEndOfJul2008)

| SurgeryDate | DateOfBirth | Sex | Diagnosis | TimeIn | TimeOut | Complaints | Treatments | Initials | Notes |
|---|---|---|---|---|---|---|---|---|---|
| 28.07.2008 | 06.09.1924 | M | | 1658 | 1703 | Medication Review Done | | FE | |
| 28.07.2008 | 28.06.1959 | M | | 1703 | 1707 | For FBC & serum Ferritin | | SCU | |
| 28.07.2008 | 06.07.1968 | F | | 1709 | 1718 | For FSH | | TEM | |
| 28.07.2008 | 30.09.1970 | F | | 1718 | 1723 | Referred to Ophthalmologist regarding recurrent blurred visions & temporary losses of sight | | LJL | |
| 28.07.2008 | 24.12.1962 | F | | 1732 | 1738 | Medication Review Done | | CAW | |
| 28.07.2008 | 16.05.1967 | M | | 1755 | 1801 | Script for Fluoxetine given | | JPZ | |
| 28.07.2008 | 20.07.1956 | M | | 1801 | 1809 | Referred to Physiotherapy regarding locking (R) knee | | MDJ | |
| 28.07.2008 | 11.11.1961 | M | RTI | 1809 | 1816 | Chesty cough | Ciprofloxacin | AMP | For Chest X-Rays. |
| 29.07.2008 | 31.12.1960 | F | | 944 | 1001 | Script for Diclofenac e/c, Fusidic acid with Hydrocortisone cream & Levothyroxine given | | SAS | |
| 29.07.2008 | 26.10.1943 | F | | 1001 | 1010 | Script for Metformin given | | APM | |
| 29.07.2008 | 28.03.1926 | F | | 1010 | 1019 | Medication Review Done | | JD | |

Result of a query that lists all consultations from the 22nd to the end of July 2008 (ConsultationsSeenFrom22ndTillEndOfJul2008)

| SurgeryDate | DateOfBirth | Sex | Diagnosis | TimeIn | TimeOut | Complaints | Treatments | Initials | Notes |
|---|---|---|---|---|---|---|---|---|---|
| 29.07.2008 | 24.09.1937 | M | S/Leave | 1019 | 1027 | Bereavement - Med. 5 | | DA | |
| 29.07.2008 | 23.04.1923 | F | | 1027 | 1039 | For MSU | | JD | |
| 29.07.2008 | 23.02.1969 | M | S/Leave | 1045 | 1054 | (R) shoulder pain | | DJP | |
| 29.07.2008 | 10.02.1947 | F | | 1054 | 1100 | For repeat MSU in 2 weeks | | CAM | |
| 29.07.2008 | 15.10.1969 | F | | 1100 | 1108 | Script for Qvar inhaler given | | MAC | |
| 29.07.2008 | 29.08.1939 | M | | 1108 | 1121 | Script for Fusidic acid with Hydrocortisone cream given | | JFP | |
| 29.07.2008 | 30.10.1958 | M | | 1121 | 1133 | Script for Ciprofloxacin, Co-phenotrope & Hyoscine butyl bromide given | | MSE | |
| 29.07.2008 | 20.09.2006 | F | | 1648 | 1654 | Referred to Paediatrician regarding unequal legs length | | IEHG | |
| 29.07.2008 | 18.05.1975 | F | S/Leave | 1654 | 1700 | Non-epileptic seizure & Depression - Med. 5 | | EGHG | |
| 29.07.2008 | 06.05.1971 | M | | 1700 | 1710 | Referred to Orthopaedic Surgeon regarding recurrent medial dislocation of the (L) knee | | RHG | Script for Omeprazole given. |

658

Result of a query that lists all consultations from the 22nd to the end of July 2008 (ConsultationsSeenFrom22ndTillEndOfJul2008)

| SurgeryDate | DateOfBirth | Sex | Diagnosis | TimeIn | TimeOut | Complaints | Treatments | Initials | Notes |
|---|---|---|---|---|---|---|---|---|---|
| 29.07.2008 | 23.01.1991 | F | | 1710 | 1716 | Script for Citalopram & Microgynon 30 given | | DSLB | |
| 29.07.2008 | 02.07.1937 | M | RTI | 1716 | 1719 | Chesty cough | Erythromycin | GG | Penicillin allergy. |
| 29.07.2008 | 31.10.1943 | M | RTI | 1719 | 1724 | Chesty cough | Amoxycillin | NFH | |
| 29.07.2008 | 01.10.1976 | F | | 1731 | 1740 | Medication Review Done | | AEC | |
| 29.07.2008 | 14.02.1952 | M | | 1740 | 1745 | For X-Rays of the Lumbar Spine | | BHCH | |
| 29.07.2008 | 06.03.1969 | F | | 1757 | 1811 | To keep her next dermatological appointment regarding the melanoma | | KSLC | |
| 29.07.2008 | 01.02.1980 | F | | 1811 | 1819 | Script for Amoxycillin & Otomize ear spray given | | LTK | |
| 29.07.2008 | 03.03.1984 | M | | 1819 | 1826 | Script for Amoxycillin & Qvar inhaler given | | PWK | |
| 30.07.2008 | 20.04.1927 | F | | 945 | 950 | Medication Review Done | | MW | |
| 30.07.2008 | 05.03.1973 | F | | 950 | 955 | Late period | For Pregnancy test | HAF | |
| 30.07.2008 | 12.04.1932 | F | | 958 | 1011 | Script for Co-codamol & Simvastatin given | | JMA | |

Result of a query that lists all consultations from the 22nd to the end of July 2008 (ConsultationsSeenFrom22ndTillEndOfJul2008)

| SurgeryDate | DateOfBirth | Sex | Diagnosis | TimeIn | TimeOut | Complaints | Treatments | Initials | Notes |
|---|---|---|---|---|---|---|---|---|---|
| 30.07.2008 | 08.12.1938 | F | | 1018 | 1024 | Script for Flucloxacillin & Fusidic acid cream given | | EVB | |
| 30.07.2008 | 02.07.1924 | M | | 1024 | 1036 | Referred to Dermatologist regarding crumbling (L) big toe nail | | TCC | |
| 30.07.2008 | 01.04.1945 | F | | 1036 | 1045 | Referred to General Surgeon regarding (R) Inguinal hernia | | IPB | |
| 30.07.2008 | 10.04.1986 | M | S/Leave | 1045 | 1055 | Injury to the (R) hand | | BML | For X-Rays of the (R) hand. |
| 30.07.2008 | 25.01.1957 | M | | 1055 | 1102 | Referred to Physiotherapist regarding (R) sided back pain | | GWC | For FBC, U/Es & LFTs. |
| 30.07.2008 | 21.08.1934 | F | | 1106 | 1116 | Script for Gliclazide given | | IEW | |
| 30.07.2008 | 23.05.1932 | M | | 1116 | 1125 | The Parking Badge Scheme for Disabled People Medical Practitioner Report, form ESS208B, completed with the patient (& his daughter) | | EB | |
| 30.07.2008 | 14.04.2007 | M | URTI | 1125 | 1131 | Smelly ears | Amoxycillin | JJH | |

Result of a query that lists all consultations from the 22nd to the end of July 2008 (ConsultationsSeenFrom22ndTillEndOfJul2008)

| SurgeryDate | DateOfBirth | Sex | Diagnosis | TimeIn | TimeOut | Complaints | Treatments | Initials | Notes |
|---|---|---|---|---|---|---|---|---|---|
| 30.07.2008 | 25.09.1996 | F | URTI | 1131 | 1137 | Fever & poking her ears | Erythromycin | JLN | |
| 30.07.2008 | 07.12.1940 | F | | 1412 | 1425 | Script for Ciprofloxacin & Co-codamol given | | MWC | Home visit. |
| 30.07.2008 | 25.07.1939 | F | | 1643 | 1655 | For B12, Folate & serum Ferritin | | JLB | |
| 30.07.2008 | 07.03.1955 | F | | 1655 | 1701 | Script for Lisinopril given | | DN | |
| 30.07.2008 | 03.04.1920 | F | | 1701 | 1708 | Script for Prochlorperazine given | | JA | |
| 30.07.2008 | 25.08.1961 | F | | 1708 | 1716 | To come back later for her sick leave | | MFD | |
| 30.07.2008 | 15.07.1971 | F | | 1716 | 1720 | Script for Microgynon 30 given | | KZ | |
| 30.07.2008 | 07.04.1971 | F | RTI | 1720 | 1724 | Chesty cough | Ciprofloxacin | TJB | |
| 30.07.2008 | 11.09.1947 | M | | 1801 | 1814 | Referred to Dermatologist (BUPA) regarding itchy lesion under (R) nipple, possibly an accessory nipple | | TSN | |
| 30.07.2008 | 04.06.1958 | F | RTI | 1814 | 1821 | Chesty cough | Amoxycillin | JDC | |
| 30.07.2008 | 11.04.1982 | F | | 1821 | 1826 | Late period | For pregnancy test | JLS | |
| 30.07.2008 | 02.01.1944 | M | | 1857 | 1920 | Script for Electrolade & Ciprofloxacin given | | JKC | Home visit. |

661

Result of a query that lists all consultations from the 22nd to the end of July 2009 (ConsultationsSeenFrom22ndTillEndOfJul2009)

| SurgeryDate | DateOfBirth | Sex | Diagnosis | TimeIn | TimeOut | Complaints | Treatments | Initials | Notes |
|---|---|---|---|---|---|---|---|---|---|
| 22.07.2009 | 22.03.1936 | F | | 952 | 959 | Medication Review Done | | MEE | |
| 22.07.2009 | 18.11.1946 | F | | 959 | 1006 | Referred to Podiatrist regarding (L) foot pain on plantar-flexing the toes | | JML | |
| 22.07.2009 | 21.02.1959 | F | | 1006 | 1014 | For KUB USScan | | GT | |
| 22.07.2009 | 07.03.1968 | F | | 1017 | 1026 | Referred to Physiotherapist regarding pain in the (L) knee | | AMR | |
| 22.07.2009 | 07.04.1933 | M | | 1026 | 1047 | Medication Review Done | | JM | |
| 22.07.2009 | 24.01.1958 | F | Rash | 1048 | 1054 | Itchy rash on the upper eye lids | 0.5% Hydrocortisone cream | JDB | |
| 22.07.2009 | 16.08.1927 | F | | 1054 | 1103 | The results of the TFTs & echocardiogram which were normal were explained to the patient | | GC | |
| 22.07.2009 | 22.01.2006 | F | | 1103 | 1110 | Parents will observe her enlarged tonsils for now | | KEGM | |

662

Result of a query that lists all consultations from the 22nd to the end of July 2009 (ConsultationsSeenFrom22ndTillEndOfJul2009)

| SurgeryDate | DateOfBirth | Sex | Diagnosis | TimeIn | TimeOut | Complaints | Treatments | Initials | Notes |
|---|---|---|---|---|---|---|---|---|---|
| 22.07.2009 | 10.01.1958 | M | | 1646 | 1700 | Script for Beconase Aqueous nasal spray given | | ARH | Referred to Dermatologist regarding largish area of depigmentation on the (R) fore-arm. |
| 22.07.2009 | 17.04.1930 | M | | 1700 | 1710 | Medication Review Done | | FL | |
| 22.07.2009 | 16.09.1936 | M | | 1710 | 1714 | Private script for Viagra given | | LPCE | |
| 22.07.2009 | 07.07.1991 | M | | 1714 | 1721 | To take own analgesia for his painful (R) knee | | DW | |
| 22.07.2009 | 30.05.1964 | M | | 1721 | 1731 | Script for Omeprazole given | | ED | |
| 22.07.2009 | 13.07.2008 | M | | 1731 | 1742 | Script for Dicycloverine & Oral rehydration salts oral powder given | | MJD | Stool for C&S. |
| 22.07.2009 | 16.07.2006 | F | URTI | 1742 | 1748 | Sore throat | Amoxycillin | LB | |
| 22.07.2009 | 12.01.1992 | F | | 1748 | 1758 | Advised to attend the Family Planning clinic to get her Minipill (name not known) where she has been getting it | | SAL | |
| 22.07.2009 | 06.08.1941 | M | | 1758 | 1808 | Script for Prochlorperazine given | | AJM | |

Result of a query that lists all consultations from the 22nd to the end of July 2009 (ConsultationsSeenFrom22ndTillEndOfJul2009)

| SurgeryDate | DateOfBirth | Sex | Diagnosis | TimeIn | TimeOut | Complaints | Treatments | Initials | Notes |
|---|---|---|---|---|---|---|---|---|---|
| 23.07.2009 | 08.07.1952 | F | S/Leave | 943 | 952 | Back Pain | | PMA | |
| 23.07.2009 | 01.10.1954 | M | | 952 | 1005 | Referred to Cardiologist regarding ache in the chest on exertion and palpitations | | PJL | |
| 23.07.2009 | 07.12.1986 | F | | 1005 | 1017 | She is happy to continue with the dose of Propranolol that the Neurologist commenced her on | | SDB | |
| 23.07.2009 | 21.11.1954 | M | | 1020 | 1034 | For fasting lipids | | GLS | |
| 23.07.2009 | 08.06.1989 | M | | 1034 | 1046 | Referred to Physiotherapist regarding back pain | | AJS | |
| 23.07.2009 | 03.04.1997 | M | | 1046 | 1052 | Script for Chloramphenicol eye drops given | | LAJ | |
| 23.07.2009 | 03.10.1939 | M | | 1052 | 1107 | Script for Quinine Sulphate given | | NS | |
| 23.07.2009 | 30.04.1986 | F | | 1107 | 1134 | Script for Daktarin gel & Noriday given | | SJ | Routine 6 weeks post-natal check done. |
| 23.07.2009 | 23.08.1925 | F | | 1134 | 1140 | Medication Review Done | | REP | |
| 23.07.2009 | 13.09.1918 | M | | 1645 | 1706 | Medication Review Done | | EJG | |

Result of a query that lists all consultations from the 22nd to the end of July 2009 (ConsultationsSeenFrom22ndTillEndOfJul2009)

| SurgeryDate | DateOfBirth | Sex | Diagnosis | TimeIn | TimeOut | Complaints | Treatments | Initials | Notes |
|---|---|---|---|---|---|---|---|---|---|
| 23.07.2009 | 11.01.1964 | F | S/Leave | 1706 | 1721 | Flu Symptoms - Med. 5 | | KW | Referred to Neurologist regarding persistent headaches. |
| 23.07.2009 | 26.09.1973 | F | | 1721 | 1726 | Script for Flucloxacillin & Fusidic acid cream given | | SJS | |
| 23.07.2009 | 03.07.1940 | F | | 1726 | 1740 | Medication Review Done | | JMM | |
| 23.07.2009 | 10.08.1931 | M | | 1740 | 1756 | Constipation | Liquid paraffin/ Magnesium hydroxide oral emulsion | REW | |
| 23.07.2009 | 02.03.1948 | M | | 1756 | 1810 | Script for Prochlorperazine given | | JHH | Referred to Dermatologist (BUPA) regarding the warty lesion on the bridge of the nose close to the (L) eye. |
| 23.07.2009 | 18.03.1987 | F | | 1810 | 1819 | Script for Prochlorperazine given | | LP | |
| 23.07.2009 | 11.05.1959 | F | | 1819 | 1830 | Script for Cinchocaine with Hydrocortisone cream & suppositories given | | LJE | |

Result of a query that lists all consultations from the 22nd to the end of July 2009 (ConsultationsSeenFrom22ndTillEndOfJul2009)

| SurgeryDate | DateOfBirth | Sex | Diagnosis | TimeIn | TimeOut | Complaints | Treatments | Initials | Notes |
|---|---|---|---|---|---|---|---|---|---|
| 24.07.2009 | 12.11.1950 | M | S/Leave | 928 | 942 | Flu Symptoms - Med. 5 | | MJP | |
| 24.07.2009 | 09.03.1966 | M | | 942 | 949 | Script for Dihydrocodeine given | | MS | Referred to Physiotherapist regarding his back pain. |
| 24.07.2009 | 06.10.1952 | M | | 949 | 959 | For Cervical spine X-Rays | | CJG | Referred to Rheumatologist regarding neck pain & feeling hot. |
| 24.07.2009 | 15.06.1974 | F | URTI | 959 | 1004 | Sore throat | Amoxycillin | SAH | |
| 24.07.2009 | 03.07.1950 | F | RTI | 1004 | 1025 | Chesty cough | Amoxycillin | YC | Script for Dixarit & Sertraline given. |
| 24.07.2009 | 27.05.1968 | M | S/Leave | 1025 | 1033 | Back Pain - Med. 5 | | LJH | |
| 24.07.2009 | 24.02.2007 | M | | 1033 | 1039 | Script for Erythromycin & Fusidic acid cream given | | ASMP | |
| 24.07.2009 | 03.05.2009 | M | | 1039 | 1044 | His mum re-assured about lower abdomen that goes hard when he cries | | HAP | |
| 24.07.2009 | 26.06.1959 | M | | 1044 | 1058 | Script for Erythromycin & Fusidic acid with Hydrocortisone cream given | | SCU | Penicillin allergy. |

666

Result of a query that lists all consultations from the 22nd to the end of July 2009 (ConsultationsSeenFrom22ndTillEndOfJul2009)

| SurgeryDate | DateOfBirth | Sex | Diagnosis | TimeIn | TimeOut | Complaints | Treatments | Initials | Notes |
|---|---|---|---|---|---|---|---|---|---|
| 24.07.2009 | 01.07.1927 | F | | 1058 | 1113 | Referred to Urologist regarding large residual bladder volume post micturition | | DMSG | Script for Lisinopril given. |
| 24.07.2009 | 07.05.1974 | M | | 1113 | 1136 | Script for Amoxycillin & Ibuprofen given | | SC | |
| 24.07.2009 | 27.09.1988 | M | RTI | 1136 | 1142 | Chesty cough | Amoxycillin | SJA | |
| 24.07.2009 | 31.05.1930 | F | | 1535 | 1555 | Script for Stemetil & Ciprofloxacin given | | SAW | Penicillin & Paracetamol allergy. Home visit. |
| 27.07.2009 | 26.01.1953 | M | | 945 | 958 | Medication Review Done | | BGN | |
| 27.07.2009 | 16.04.1949 | M | | 958 | 1004 | Medication Review Done | | DRT | |
| 27.07.2009 | 11.09.1978 | M | | 1009 | 1017 | Referred to ENT Surgeon regarding recurrent discharge from the (L) ear | | CPB | |
| 27.07.2009 | 24.01.1944 | M | | 1017 | 1025 | Referred to ENT Surgeon regarding poor hearing | | PDS | |
| 27.07.2009 | 26.03.1965 | F | | 1031 | 1037 | For X-Rays of the (R) foot | | CP | |
| 27.07.2009 | 24.10.1989 | F | | 1037 | 1047 | Mat B1 from completed for the patient | | MC | |

Result of a query that lists all consultations from the 22nd to the end of July 2009 (ConsultationsSeenFrom22ndTillEndOfJul2009)

| SurgeryDate | DateOfBirth | Sex | Diagnosis | TimeIn | TimeOut | Complaints | Treatments | Initials | Notes |
|---|---|---|---|---|---|---|---|---|---|
| 27.07.2009 | 27.05.1959 | F | RTI | 1047 | 1054 | Chesty cough | Amoxycillin | SM | Script for Easyhaler Salbutamol inhaler given. |
| 27.07.2009 | 06.11.1935 | F |  | 1057 | 1114 | Script for Co-codamol & Quinine Sulphate given |  | SRB | Referred to Orthopaedic Surgeon regarding pain in the (L) hip. |
| 27.07.2009 | 20.10.1929 | M |  | 1439 | 1452 | Script for Fucidin cream & Flucloxacillin given |  | PL | Home visit. |
| 27.07.2009 | 14.01.1934 | F |  | 1458 | 1507 | Script for Haloperidol given |  | MRP | Home visit. |
| 27.07.2009 | 29.12.1954 | F |  | 1651 | 1702 | Script for Citalopram & Doxazosin given |  | PAK |  |
| 27.07.2009 | 31.01.1964 | F |  | 1702 | 1712 | For FBC, U/Es, FSH, CRP & Rheumatoid Factor |  | DH |  |
| 27.07.2009 | 01.02.1996 | M |  | 1712 | 1723 | Referred to Paediatrician regarding his bilateral gynaecomastia |  | CTH |  |
| 27.07.2009 | 18.06.1981 | M |  | 1723 | 1733 | Referred to General Surgeon regarding his para-umbilical hernia |  | SCJ |  |
| 27.07.2009 | 02.10.1992 | M |  | 1733 | 1748 | For KUB USScan, MSU, U/Es & FBC |  | LF |  |

Result of a query that lists all consultations from the 22nd to the end of July 2009 (ConsultationsSeenFrom22ndTillEndOfJul2009)

| SurgeryDate | DateOfBirth | Sex | Diagnosis | TimeIn | TimeOut | Complaints | Treatments | Initials | Notes |
|---|---|---|---|---|---|---|---|---|---|
| 27.07.2009 | 07.03.1968 | F | | 1748 | 1800 | Patient informed that if she needs to have OPD gynae. procedure done, then it ought to be done under General anaesthesia | | AMR | |
| 27.07.2009 | 01.04.2009 | M | | 1800 | 1805 | Medication Review Done | | OPAW | |
| 27.07.2009 | 24.02.1992 | F | | 1805 | 1828 | Script for Citalopram given | | ELP | |
| 27.07.2009 | 14.01.1951 | F | | 1828 | 1834 | Referred to Colorectal Surgeon regarding her recurrent piles | | RD | |
| 28.07.2009 | 04.11.1984 | M | | 944 | 957 | Patient informed that his clotting screen was normal | | CJRK | |
| 28.07.2009 | 07.02.1948 | M | | 1004 | 1014 | We will look into him being referred for gastric banding | | GRC | |
| 28.07.2009 | 06.02.1946 | F | | 1014 | 1022 | Referred to Rheumatologist regarding pain in the (L) heel | | KMT | |
| 28.07.2009 | 22.04.1951 | M | S/Leave | 1022 | 1040 | Injury to the (R) knee - Private & Med. 5 | | PJT | |
| 28.07.2009 | 10.09.1981 | F | | 1040 | 1053 | Script for Ferrous Sulphate | | HAS | |

669

Result of a query that lists all consultations from the 22nd to the end of July 2009 (ConsultationsSeenFrom22ndTillEndOfJul2009)

| SurgeryDate | DateOfBirth | Sex | Diagnosis | TimeIn | TimeOut | Complaints | Treatments | Initials | Notes |
|---|---|---|---|---|---|---|---|---|---|
| 28.07.2009 | 10.01.1924 | M | | 1053 | 1105 | For FBC, TFTs, Fasting Glucose, B12, Folate & Ferritin | | HAJB | |
| 28.07.2009 | 01.08.1951 | F | | 1105 | 1116 | Referred to ENT Surgeon regarding feeling of wanting to clear her throat all the time | | JM | |
| 28.07.2009 | 15.10.1923 | F | | 1116 | 1145 | Referred to Rheumatologist regarding her worsening neck pain | | DWR | |
| 28.07.2009 | 27.11.1992 | F | | 1145 | 1154 | Burst condom | Levonorgestrel | CJK | |
| 28.07.2009 | 28.09.1924 | F | | 1415 | 1435 | Script for Flucloxacillin given | | VMG | Referred to DAU, SGH, regarding her bad bilateral pedal oedema. Home visit. Macrodantin allergy. |
| 28.07.2009 | 09.05.1937 | F | | 1643 | 1658 | Script for Levothyroxine given | | KMN | Referred to Vascular Surgeon regarding her Varicose veins causing eczema. |
| 28.07.2009 | 02.02.1928 | M | | 1658 | 1706 | For B12, Folate & Ferritin | | DH | |

Result of a query that lists all consultations from the 22nd to the end of July 2009 (ConsultationsSeenFrom22ndTillEndOfJul2009)

| SurgeryDate | DateOfBirth | Sex | Diagnosis | TimeIn | TimeOut | Complaints | Treatments | Initials | Notes |
|---|---|---|---|---|---|---|---|---|---|
| 28.07.2009 | 26.09.1973 | F | | 1706 | 1713 | Script for Loratadine given | | SJS | Referred to Gynaecologist regarding heavy prolonged periods with clots. |
| 28.07.2009 | 21.09.1947 | M | | 1713 | 1730 | Referred to Endocrinologist regarding his Addison's disease & Diabetes Mellitus | | DL | |
| 28.07.2009 | 26.03.1988 | M | S/Leave | 1730 | 1747 | Sore Rash - Private | | SL | Script for Acyclovir tablets & Flucloxacillin given. |
| 28.07.2009 | 05.04.1964 | F | | 1747 | 1812 | For FBC, U/Es, serum Cholesterol, TFTs, HbA1c, BNP, CRP & Chest X-Rays | | JL | |
| 28.07.2009 | 09.08.1961 | M | | 1812 | 1823 | Referred to Colorectal Surgeon (urgent) regarding his persistent constipation | | SRC | |
| 28.07.2009 | 15.01.1962 | M | | 1823 | 1833 | Referred to Neurologist regarding puns & needles with numbness down both arms | | PWL | |

Result of a query that lists all consultations from the 22nd to the end of July 2009 (ConsultationsSeenFrom22ndTillEndOfJul2009)

| SurgeryDate | DateOfBirth | Sex | Diagnosis | TimeIn | TimeOut | Complaints | Treatments | Initials | Notes |
|---|---|---|---|---|---|---|---|---|---|
| 28.07.2009 | 10.04.1984 | M | | 1833 | 1849 | Referred to ENT Surgeon regarding difficulty swallowing & a feeling of something getting stuck | | BM | |
| 28.07.2009 | 18.06.1993 | F | | 1849 | 1904 | Script for Fexofenadine given | | LT | Referred to Podiatrist regarding tender lump on the sole of her (L) foot. |
| 29.07.2009 | 29.06.1934 | M | | 946 | 1000 | Script for Omeprazole given | | PM | |
| 29.07.2009 | 01.10.1920 | M | | 1000 | 1015 | Medication Review Done | | JM | Wife came to the Surgery. |
| 29.07.2009 | 09.04.1944 | F | | 1015 | 1024 | Medication Review Done | | JN | |
| 29.07.2009 | 15.07.1955 | F | | 1024 | 1037 | Script for Frovatriptan given | | JDU | |
| 29.07.2009 | 13.05.1982 | F | | 1037 | 1049 | Script for Amoxycillin, Calamine lotion & Chlorphenamine given | | DMB | |
| 29.07.2009 | 13.11.1918 | M | | 1049 | 1057 | Referred to Dermatologist (urgent) regarding darkish scab on the (R) temple | | DTM | |

Result of a query that lists all consultations from the 22nd to the end of July 2009 (ConsultationsSeenFrom22ndTillEndOfJul2009)

| SurgeryDate | DateOfBirth | Sex | Diagnosis | TimeIn | TimeOut | Complaints | Treatments | Initials | Notes |
|---|---|---|---|---|---|---|---|---|---|
| 29.07.2009 | 29.10.1981 | F | | 1057 | 1109 | Referred to Dermatologist regarding discolouration of the toe nails | | ACM | |
| 29.07.2009 | 08.03.1946 | F | | 1109 | 1114 | Referred to Dermatologist regarding mole on the inner aspect of the (R) thigh | | GRC | |
| 29.07.2009 | 08.02.1939 | F | URTI | 1114 | 1122 | Sore throat | Amoxycillin | IB | Script for Codeine & Omeprazole given. |
| 29.07.2009 | 13.11.1974 | F | | 1122 | 1128 | Script for Cefalexin given | | LEM | |
| 29.07.2009 | 19.12.1954 | F | | 1645 | 1655 | Medication Review Done | | SAH | |
| 29.07.2009 | 13.06.1997 | F | Rash | 1655 | 1701 | Impetigo rash on chin | Flucloxacillin & Fusidic acid cream | EZN | |
| 29.07.2009 | 25.06.1996 | F | | 1713 | 1728 | Referred to Paediatrician regarding her functional dyspepsia & low Hb | | ERY | |
| 29.07.2009 | 04.04.1938 | M | | 1728 | 1736 | Script for Amoxycillin & Fusidic acid eye drops given | | DB | |

Result of a query that lists all consultations from the 22nd to the end of July 2009 (ConsultationsSeenFrom22ndTillEndOfJul2009)

| SurgeryDate | DateOfBirth | Sex | Diagnosis | TimeIn | TimeOut | Complaints | Treatments | Initials | Notes |
|---|---|---|---|---|---|---|---|---|---|
| 29.07.2009 | 16.07.1952 | F | | 1736 | 1747 | Script for Simvastatin given | | KAM | |
| 29.07.2009 | 11.02.1972 | M | | 1747 | 1753 | Referred to Physiotherapist regarding whiplash injury post RTA | | DJB | |
| 29.07.2009 | 02.05.1991 | M | | 1753 | 1758 | Pinworms | Mebendazole | PDC | |
| 29.07.2009 | 18.02.1968 | F | | 1758 | 1808 | Referred to Dermatologist regarding her hairs falling off | | PAC | Script for Orlistat given. |
| 29.07.2009 | 27.07.1967 | F | | 1808 | 1818 | Script for Co-codamol & Noriday given | | JTR | |
| 30.07.2009 | 21.11.1923 | M | RTI | 1006 | 1020 | Chesty cough | Amoxycillin | RU | Script for Prochlorperazine & Otomize ear spray given. |
| 30.07.2009 | 06.03.1925 | F | | 1020 | 1033 | Script for Prochlorperazine given | | MHT | For Cervical Spine X-Rays. |
| 30.07.2009 | 26.10.1960 | F | | 1033 | 1046 | Script for Flucloxacillin & Fusidic acid with Hydrocortisone cream given | | DME | For FBC, U/Es, FSH & Fasting Glucose. |
| 30.07.2009 | 06.05.1971 | M | | 1046 | 1052 | Script for Amoxycillin, Erythromycin & Co-codamol given | | RHG | |

Result of a query that lists all consultations from the 22$^{nd}$ to the end of July 2009 (ConsultationsSeenFrom22ndTillEndOfJul2009)

| SurgeryDate | DateOfBirth | Sex | Diagnosis | TimeIn | TimeOut | Complaints | Treatments | Initials | Notes |
|---|---|---|---|---|---|---|---|---|---|
| 30.07.2009 | 19.11.1969 | F | RTI | 1052 | 1100 | Chesty cough | Amoxycillin | LMG | For Chest X-Rays. |
| 30.07.2009 | 12.12.1959 | M | | 1100 | 1105 | He will come back later for the extension of his sick leave | | RJW | |
| 30.07.2009 | 13.04.1985 | F | RTI | 1105 | 1115 | Chesty cough | Amoxycillin | CLA | Script for Sertraline given. |
| 30.07.2009 | 30.09.1925 | M | | 1115 | 1122 | For X-Rays of the (R) thigh to exclude/ locate foreign body (war shrapnel) | | JCA | |
| 30.07.2009 | 25.11.1943 | M | | 1646 | 1707 | Script for Fusidic acid with Hydrocortisone cream given | | AES | |
| 30.07.2009 | 05.02.1960 | F | | 1707 | 1713 | Script for Co-codamol given | | SJW | For X-Rays of the hips |
| 30.07.2009 | 15.08.1943 | M | | 1713 | 1721 | Script for Clotrimazole cream given | | LCAH | Referred to Dermatologist regarding the rash on the (L) little finger. |
| 30.07.2009 | 09.04.1938 | M | | 1721 | 1737 | To discuss with DVT clinic regarding (R) swollen calf | | NWH | |
| 30.07.2009 | 25.05.1939 | F | | 1737 | 1748 | Referred to Ophthalmologist regarding problems with her eyes post cataract operations | | DET | |

### Result of a query that lists all consultations from the 22nd to the end of July 2009 (ConsultationsSeenFrom22ndTillEndOfJul2009)

| SurgeryDate | DateOfBirth | Sex | Diagnosis | TimeIn | TimeOut | Complaints | Treatments | Initials | Notes |
|---|---|---|---|---|---|---|---|---|---|
| 30.07.2009 | 17.07.1985 | F | | 1748 | 1756 | Script for Fusidic acid with Hydrocortisone cream given | | ZB | |
| 30.07.2009 | 16.07.2006 | F | | 1756 | 1800 | Referred to ENT Surgeon regarding persistently inflamed & enlarged tonsils | | LB | |
| 30.07.2009 | 02.08.1956 | M | | 1803 | 1813 | Medication Review Done | | KRC | |
| 30.07.2009 | 11.01.1964 | F | URTI | 1813 | 1821 | Sore throat | Amoxycillin | TJR | |
| 30.07.2009 | 25.09.1961 | F | | 1821 | 1838 | Script for Omeprazole given | | SJB | |

### Result of a query that lists all consultations from the 22nd to the end of July 2010 (ConsultationsSeenFrom22ndTillEndOfJul2010)

| SurgeryDate | DateOfBirth | Sex | Diagnosis | TimeIn | TimeOut | Complaints | Treatments | Initials | Notes |
|---|---|---|---|---|---|---|---|---|---|
| 22.07.2010 | 09.04.1930 | M | | 946 | 1006 | Script for Bendroflumethiazide & Perindopril given | | NWH | |
| 22.07.2010 | 01.02.1931 | M | | 1006 | 1024 | Referred to the Care of the Elderly regarding his possible collapse in Portugal | | MDS | For FBC, Fasting Glucose, LFTs, TFTs & U/Es. |
| 22.07.2010 | 06.10.1933 | M | | 1024 | 1030 | Medication Review Done | | RJK | |

Result of a query that lists all consultations from the 22nd to the end of July 2010 (ConsultationsSeenFrom22ndTillEndOfJul2010)

| SurgeryDate | DateOfBirth | Sex | Diagnosis | TimeIn | TimeOut | Complaints | Treatments | Initials | Notes |
|---|---|---|---|---|---|---|---|---|---|
| 22.07.2010 | 16.09.1936 | M | | 1030 | 1033 | Private script for Viagra given | | LPCE | |
| 22.07.2010 | 06.06.1961 | M | S/Leave | 1033 | 1039 | Med. 3 04/10 given for Stress for one month from 21.07.10 | | LG | Script for Citalopram given. |
| 22.07.2010 | 31.12.1953 | F | | 1039 | 1058 | Script for Citalopram given | | JWH | |
| 22.07.2010 | 18.02.1968 | F | | 1103 | 1127 | Script for Omeprazole given | | PAC | |
| 22.07.2010 | 27.01.1934 | F | | 1645 | 1658 | Script for Ferrous Sulphate given | | JWC | |
| 22.07.2010 | 27.02.1934 | M | | 1658 | 1709 | Medication Review Done | | RAC | |
| 22.07.2010 | 05.06.2004 | M | | 1709 | 1714 | To see Health Visitor regarding his hearing problems picked up at school | | JMT | |
| 22.07.2010 | 23.01.1950 | F | | 1714 | 1727 | Script for Co-codamol, Diclofenac e/c & Omeprazole given | | SM | For X-Rays of the (L) knee. |
| 22.07.2010 | 23.05.1932 | M | | 1727 | 1733 | Daughter came in regarding lasting power of Attorney which I declined to sign | | EB | |
| 22.07.2010 | 24.10.1959 | M | | 1733 | 1742 | Referred for Gastroscopy (urgent) | | BRH | |

Result of a query that lists all consultations from the 22nd to the end of July 2010 (ConsultationsSeenFrom22ndTillEndOfJul2010)

| SurgeryDate | DateOfBirth | Sex | Diagnosis | TimeIn | TimeOut | Complaints | Treatments | Initials | Notes |
|---|---|---|---|---|---|---|---|---|---|
| 22.07.2010 | 07.07.1961 | F | | 1742 | 1748 | Referred to Orthopaedic Surgeon regarding her grating neck which is painful | | SSA | |
| 22.07.2010 | 10.08.1962 | M | | 1749 | 1758 | Private script for Viagra given | | DPS | |
| 22.07.2010 | 04.07.1953 | M | S/Leave | 1758 | 1805 | Med. 3 04/10 given for (R) Fibular Fracture from 10.07.10 for 2 months | | VWH | |
| 23.07.2010 | 05.02.1946 | F | | 932 | 938 | Medication Review Done | | ML | |
| 23.07.2010 | 09.08.1939 | M | | 938 | 944 | Script for Co-codamol given | | JL | |
| 23.07.2010 | 17.09.1965 | F | | 944 | 954 | Referred to Cardiologist regarding her central chest pain going down the (L) arm | | PAE | |
| 23.07.2010 | 27.10.1950 | F | | 1005 | 1014 | Medication Review Done | | KB | |
| 23.07.2010 | 14.11.1963 | F | | 1014 | 1024 | Referred to Oncology Dr. on call, SGH regarding her persistent vomiting | | SJK | |
| 23.07.2010 | 28.03.1945 | M | | 1024 | 1032 | Medication Review Done | | APD | |

678

Result of a query that lists all consultations from the 22nd to the end of July 2010 (ConsultationsSeenFrom22ndTillEndOfJul2010)

| SurgeryDate | DateOfBirth | Sex | Diagnosis | TimeIn | TimeOut | Complaints | Treatments | Initials | Notes |
|---|---|---|---|---|---|---|---|---|---|
| 23.07.2010 | 07.10.1933 | M | | 1032 | 1037 | Script for Ferrous Sulphate given | | FDF | |
| 23.07.2010 | 11.10.1942 | M | | 1037 | 1059 | Medication Review Done | | RWA | |
| 23.07.2010 | 25.02.1934 | M | | 1059 | 1116 | Medication Review Done | | BAC | |
| 23.07.2010 | 11.03.1968 | F | | 1116 | 1125 | Script for Ciprofloxacin, Co-phenotrope & oral rehydration salts oral powder given | | EJA | Stool for C&S. |
| 23.07.2010 | 24.01.1958 | F | Pain | 1125 | 1133 | Back Pain | Co-codamol | JDB | |
| 26.07.2010 | 26.01.1955 | F | | 942 | 950 | For Cervical Spine X-Rays | | CYR | For MSU. |
| 26.07.2010 | 17.04.1945 | F | | 950 | 1000 | To persevere with the Ferrous Sulphate tablets | | MC | |
| 26.07.2010 | 29.12.2000 | F | | 1000 | 1014 | Script for Clenil Modulite inhaler given | | MMS | |
| 26.07.2010 | 20.06.1974 | F | | 1014 | 1018 | Script for Salicylic acid 26% solution given | | SLS | |
| 26.07.2010 | 19.01.1964 | F | | 1028 | 1037 | Referred to Oral Surgeon regarding pain around her excised (L) Parotid gland | | NAB | |

Result of a query that lists all consultations from the 22nd to the end of July 2010 (ConsultationsSeenFrom22ndTillEndOfJul2010)

| SurgeryDate | DateOfBirth | Sex | Diagnosis | TimeIn | TimeOut | Complaints | Treatments | Initials | Notes |
|---|---|---|---|---|---|---|---|---|---|
| 26.07.2010 | 03.01.2004 | F |  | 1037 | 1046 | Referred to Ophthalmologist regarding her (R) eye squint |  | RLT |  |
| 26.07.2010 | 29.12.1954 | F |  | 1046 | 1054 | To try taking the Bisoprolol in the evening to see if the daytime tiredness improves |  | PAK |  |
| 26.07.2010 | 05.12.1973 | F |  | 1056 | 1105 | Script for Amoxycillin & Macrogol compound half-strength oral powder sachets npf given |  | VNB |  |
| 26.07.2010 | 27.03.1931 | F |  | 1105 | 1112 | Referred to Dermatologist regarding welts on the under surface of both breasts |  | MMA |  |
| 26.07.2010 | 10.03.2004 | M |  | 1112 | 1121 | Script for Amoxycillin given |  | CJCB |  |
| 26.07.2010 | 10.08.1950 | M |  | 1121 | 1130 | Script for Flucloxacillin & Clotrimazole with Hydrocortisone cream given |  | JD |  |
| 26.07.2010 | 27.04.1928 | M |  | 1417 | 1440 | BP 120/80 |  | RFV | Home visit. Aspirin allergy. |

Result of a query that lists all consultations from the 22nd to the end of July 2010 (ConsultationsSeenFrom22ndTillEndOfJul2010)

| SurgeryDate | DateOfBirth | Sex | Diagnosis | TimeIn | TimeOut | Complaints | Treatments | Initials | Notes |
|---|---|---|---|---|---|---|---|---|---|
| 26.07.2010 | 01.01.1953 | M | | 1645 | 1652 | Medication Review Done | | TPH | |
| 26.07.2010 | 28.07.1939 | F | | 1652 | 1713 | Script for Amitriptyline, Ezetimibe, Benzydamine mouth wash & MST continus tablets given | | RMM | |
| 26.07.2010 | 16.07.2009 | M | | 1713 | 1721 | Referred to Paediatrician regarding runny stools, worse with cow's milk | | CLB | |
| 26.07.2010 | 18.02.1968 | F | S/Leave | 1721 | 1729 | Med. 3 04/10 given for Abdominal Wound Infection from 22.07.10 for one month | | PAC | |
| 26.07.2010 | 25.01.1944 | F | | 1729 | 1734 | Script for Diclofenac e/c & Omeprazole given | | HPS | For X-Rays of the (L) knee. |
| 26.07.2010 | 30.09.1991 | M | S/Leave | 1734 | 1740 | Med. 3 04/10 given for Back Pain from 25.07.10 for one week | | MNDDR | |
| 26.07.2010 | 21.09.1947 | M | | 1740 | 1746 | To increase his intake of tomato, tomato juice & bananas to improve his hypokalaemia | | DL | |

Result of a query that lists all consultations from the 22nd to the end of July 2010 (ConsultationsSeenFrom22ndTillEndOfJul2010)

| SurgeryDate | DateOfBirth | Sex | Diagnosis | TimeIn | TimeOut | Complaints | Treatments | Initials | Notes |
|---|---|---|---|---|---|---|---|---|---|
| 26.07.2010 | 23.04.2007 | M | | 1746 | 1754 | To continue with Calpol for his night fevers & come back in 4 weeks if still present | | HB | |
| 26.07.2010 | 08.06.1974 | M | S/Leave | 1802 | 1810 | Med. 3 04/10 given for Diarrhoea & Vomiting from 26.07.10 until 27.07.10 | | SWM | |
| 26.07.2010 | 15.11.1969 | M | | 1815 | 1829 | Referred to Neurologist regarding his recurrent headaches with numbness of one side of the face | | DWK | |
| 27.07.2010 | 12.05.1949 | F | | 944 | 957 | Script for Citalopram given | | MK | |
| 27.07.2010 | 01.07.1948 | M | | 957 | 1004 | Script for Furosemide given | | JFE | |
| 27.07.2010 | 24.08.1946 | M | | 1004 | 1009 | Medication Review Done | | RL | |
| 27.07.2010 | 03.03.1937 | M | | 1009 | 1034 | Referred to Ophthalmologist regarding the chalazion/stye in his (L) upper eye lid | | EJC | |
| 27.07.2010 | 09.03.1937 | F | | 1034 | 1043 | Script for Co-codamol & Gliclazide given | | HGE | |

Result of a query that lists all consultations from the 22nd to the end of July 2010 (ConsultationsSeenFrom22ndTillEndOfJul2010)

| SurgeryDate | DateOfBirth | Sex | Diagnosis | TimeIn | TimeOut | Complaints | Treatments | Initials | Notes |
|---|---|---|---|---|---|---|---|---|---|
| 27.07.2010 | 15.04.1927 | M | | 1043 | 1054 | Medication Review Done | | JB | |
| 27.07.2010 | 25.08.1983 | M | | 1054 | 1103 | Referred to ENT Surgeon regarding being only able to breathe from the (L) nostril | | SCW | |
| 27.07.2010 | 23.07.1953 | M | | 1103 | 1113 | For Cervical spine X-Rays, Ferritin, B12 & Folate | | THM | |
| 27.07.2010 | 07.04.1950 | M | | 1644 | 1649 | Script for Co-codamol given | | DML | |
| 27.07.2010 | 14.01.1951 | F | | 1646 | 1653 | Referred to Physiotherapist regarding pain in the (L) hip | | RD | |
| 27.07.2010 | 20.11.1936 | M | | 1704 | 1712 | Medication Review Done | | NN | |
| 27.07.2010 | 18.05.1949 | M | | 1712 | 1729 | Script for Amoxycillin, Metformin, Levothyroxine & Simvastatin given | | JJ | |
| 27.07.2010 | 14.08.1935 | M | | 1729 | 1745 | Script for Gliclazide given | | RAT | For serum Ferritin & Folate. |
| 27.07.2010 | 29.02.1944 | F | | 1745 | 1750 | Referred to ENT Surgeon regarding lesion on the (R) side of her nose | | CFC | |

Result of a query that lists all consultations from the 22nd to the end of July 2010 (ConsultationsSeenFrom22ndTillEndOfJul2010)

| SurgeryDate | DateOfBirth | Sex | Diagnosis | TimeIn | TimeOut | Complaints | Treatments | Initials | Notes |
|---|---|---|---|---|---|---|---|---|---|
| 27.07.2010 | 03.02.1971 | F | | 1759 | 1804 | Script for Otomize ear spray given | | MT | |
| 27.07.2010 | 30.03.1943 | M | | 1804 | 1813 | Script for Amoxycillin given | | BWF | |
| 27.07.2010 | 15.04.1973 | F | | 1813 | 1824 | Script for Amoxycillin given | | LJB | For Urine Pregnancy test. |
| 27.07.2010 | 21.07.1959 | F | | 1824 | 1829 | Script for Amoxycillin given | | GT | For MSU. |
| 27.07.2010 | 02.01.2010 | M | | 1829 | 1837 | Script for Erythromycin given | | BLS | Penicillin allergy. |
| 28.07.2010 | 31.08.1964 | M | | 945 | 954 | Script for Serrtraline given | | CJW | |
| 28.07.2010 | 06.12.1940 | F | | 954 | 1002 | Referred to Physiotherapist regarding the pain in her (R) hip | | MC | |
| 28.07.2010 | 20.07.1956 | M | | 1002 | 1016 | Medication Review Done | | MDJ | |
| 28.07.2010 | 23.01.1994 | F | | 1017 | 1024 | Script for Driclor 20% solution given | | WMS | |
| 28.07.2010 | 12.05.1983 | M | | 1024 | 1029 | Script for Hydrocortisone with Fusidic acid cream & Loratadine given | | NDM | |
| 28.07.2010 | 15.04.1951 | F | | 1034 | 1052 | Script for Trimethoprim given | | MM | |
| 28.07.2010 | 01.01.1976 | M | | 1052 | 1058 | Script for Co-Amoxiclav given | | JJH | |

Result of a query that lists all consultations from the 22nd to the end of July 2010 (ConsultationsSeenFrom22ndTillEndOfJul2010)

| SurgeryDate | DateOfBirth | Sex | Diagnosis | TimeIn | TimeOut | Complaints | Treatments | Initials | Notes |
|---|---|---|---|---|---|---|---|---|---|
| 28.07.2010 | 24.10.1929 | F | | 1058 | 1112 | Script for Aspirin dispersible, Diclofenac e/c & Omeprazole given | | LL | |
| 28.07.2010 | 26.04.1943 | M | | 1112 | 1122 | Script for Erythromycin & Hyoscine butylbromide given | | WWH | |
| 28.07.2010 | 16.12.1970 | F | | 1648 | 1653 | Script for Co-codamol given | | KMB | |
| 28.07.2010 | 09.07.1959 | F | | 1653 | 1722 | Medication Review Done | | LH | |
| 28.07.2010 | 02.01.1955 | M | S/Leave | 1722 | 1731 | Med. 3 04/10 given for (L) sided Bell's Palsy from 27.07.10 for 2 weeks | | TRE | |
| 28.07.2010 | 01.06.1937 | M | | 1731 | 1748 | For serum Ferritin & TFTs | | JNN | |
| 28.07.2010 | 01.11.1939 | M | | 1748 | 1755 | Referred to ENT Surgeon regarding wax in his ears & perforated ear drum | | JN | |
| 28.07.2010 | 01.01.1951 | F | | 1755 | 1806 | Medication Review Done | | CR | |
| 28.07.2010 | 04.04.1938 | M | | 1806 | 1816 | Script for Bendroflumethiazide given | | DB | |

685

Result of a query that lists all consultations from the 22nd to the end of July 2010 (ConsultationsSeenFrom22ndTillEndOfJul2010)

| SurgeryDate | DateOfBirth | Sex | Diagnosis | TimeIn | TimeOut | Complaints | Treatments | Initials | Notes |
|---|---|---|---|---|---|---|---|---|---|
| 28.07.2010 | 19.12.1949 | M | | 1816 | 1820 | For GTT | | DJB | Referred to Physiotherapist regarding painful (L) knee. For X-Rays of the (L) knee. |
| 28.07.2010 | 01.03.1947 | M | | 1820 | 1827 | Script for Metformin given | | JRW | |
| 29.07.2010 | 03.05.2009 | M | RTI | 955 | 959 | Cough | Amoxycillin | HAP | |
| 29.07.2010 | 24.02.2007 | M | RTI | 959 | 1003 | Cough | Amoxycillin | ASMP | |
| 29.07.2010 | 16.08.1927 | F | | 1003 | 1009 | Medication Review Done | | GC | |
| 29.07.2010 | 02.04.1988 | F | | 1026 | 1030 | Script for Logynon ED given | | JB | |
| 29.07.2010 | 22.02.1936 | F | | 1030 | 1050 | Script for Furosemide given | | RPM | For serum BNP. |
| 29.07.2010 | 19.04.1996 | M | Rash | 1050 | 1054 | Acne rash on face | Benzoyl Peroxide with Clindamycin gel | SAM | |
| 29.07.2010 | 29.07.1951 | F | | 1054 | 1103 | Script for Salicylic acid 26% solution given | | CF | |
| 29.07.2010 | 08.02.1939 | F | | 1103 | 1123 | Script for Morphine tablets given | | IB | |
| 29.07.2010 | 03.12.1955 | F | | 1123 | 1132 | Referred to Counsellor regarding feeling low & depressed since losing her grand daughter | | CAD | For FBC, TFTs, Fasting Glucose & U/Es. |

## Result of a query that lists all consultations from the 22nd to the end of July 2010 (ConsultationsSeenFrom22ndTillEndOfJul2010)

| SurgeryDate | DateOfBirth | Sex | Diagnosis | TimeIn | TimeOut | Complaints | Treatments | Initials | Notes |
|---|---|---|---|---|---|---|---|---|---|
| 29.07.2010 | 20.04.1947 | F | S/Leave | 1646 | 1705 | Med. 3 04/10 given for Vaginal Carcinoma from 29.07.10 until 02.08.10 | | PA | |
| 29.07.2010 | 31.01.1964 | F | | 1705 | 1730 | Script for Lisinopril & Prochlorperazine given | | DH | |
| 29.07.2010 | 15.02.1929 | F | | 1730 | 1737 | Script for Dihydrocodeine given | | NLA | |
| 29.07.2010 | 17.03.2008 | M | URTI | 1737 | 1742 | Sore throat | Amoxycillin | JLP | |
| 29.07.2010 | 15.07.1955 | F | | 1742 | 1751 | Script for Metformin given | | JDU | |
| 29.07.2010 | 27.05.2000 | M | | 1751 | 1755 | Script for Amoxycillin & Dicycloverine given | | NCB | |
| 29.07.2010 | 21.09.1983 | M | | 1755 | 1801 | Script for Lansoprazole given | | JH | |
| 29.07.2010 | 31.05.1997 | F | URTI | 1801 | 1805 | Sore throat | Erythromycin | SC | Penicillin allergy |
| 29.07.2010 | 17.06.1968 | M | | 1805 | 1816 | Script for Lisinopril given | | SOY | |
| 30.07.2010 | 24.10.1954 | M | S/Leave | 929 | 939 | Med. 3 04/10 given for Closure of Wound (R) shin for one week from 30.07.10 | | PW | |
| 30.07.2010 | 29.07.1947 | F | | 939 | 950 | Script for Furosemide given | | KM | For serum BNP, U/E, FBC & TFTs. |

687

Result of a query that lists all consultations from the 22nd to the end of July 2010 (ConsultationsSeenFrom22ndTillEndOfJul2010)

| SurgeryDate | DateOfBirth | Sex | Diagnosis | TimeIn | TimeOut | Complaints | Treatments | Initials | Notes |
|---|---|---|---|---|---|---|---|---|---|
| 30.07.2010 | 06.01.1969 | F | S/Leave | 950 | 1005 | Med. 3 04/10 given for Stress for one month from 30.07.10 | | KEL | Referred to Counsellor regarding being stressed about what is going on in her home & family. |
| 30.07.2010 | 11.11.1969 | F | | 1005 | 1010 | To see the nurse for yearly TFTs | | TLP | |
| 30.07.2010 | 15.09.1946 | F | | 1010 | 1017 | Medication Review Done | | IP | |
| 30.07.2010 | 23.03.1926 | M | | 1017 | 1026 | Referred to Physiotherapist regarding his shoulder pains | | JWH | Script for BuTrans patches given. |
| 30.07.2010 | 08.05.1939 | F | | 1026 | 1035 | Script for Trimethoprim given | | JCH | For MSU. |
| 30.07.2010 | 22.01.1937 | M | | 1035 | 1046 | Constipation | Glycerol suppositories & Macrogol compound half-strength oral powder sachets NPF | AM | |
| 30.07.2010 | 04.01.1967 | F | S/Leave | 1046 | 1055 | Med. 3 04/10 given for Headaches for 2 weeks from 30.07.10 | | MC | |

Result of a query that lists all consultations from the 22nd to the end of July 2011 (ConsultationsSeenFrom22ndTillEndOfJul2011)

| SurgeryDate | DateOfBirth | Sex | Diagnosis | TimeIn | TimeOut | Complaints | Treatments | Initials | Notes |
|---|---|---|---|---|---|---|---|---|---|
| 22.07.2011 | 17.06.1965 | F | | 933 | 940 | Script for MST Continus given | | JLP | |
| 22.07.2011 | 06.08.1941 | M | | 940 | 954 | Medication Review Done | | AJM | |
| 22.07.2011 | 25.12.1942 | M | | 954 | 1008 | Script for Depo-Medrone with Lidocaine injection given | | RFL. | For X-Rays of the (R) shoulder. |
| 22.07.2011 | 30.04.1941 | F | | 1008 | 1018 | To see the nurse in 3 t 6 months for repeat LFTs | | VRG | |
| 22.07.2011 | 22.05.1931 | F | URTI | 1018 | 1026 | (L) ear ache | Amoxycillin | DK | |
| 22.07.2011 | 05.06.2010 | M | | 1026 | 1033 | To see the Optician & to contact the Health visitor regarding the frequent blinking of the eyes over the past few days | | EM | |
| 22.07.2011 | 07.12.1937 | M | | 1033 | 1039 | Referred to Dermatologist regarding the BCC-like lesion on his cheeks | | AS | |
| 22.07.2011 | 20.10.2010 | F | | 1039 | 1047 | Referred to Paediatrician regarding unequal legs skin creases & the apparent shortening of the (L) leg | | GEA | Script for Chloromycetin eye drops given. |

Result of a query that lists all consultations from the 22nd to the end of July 2011 (ConsultationsSeenFrom22ndTillEndOFJul2011)

| SurgeryDate | DateOfBirth | Sex | Diagnosis | TimeIn | TimeOut | Complaints | Treatments | Initials | Notes |
|---|---|---|---|---|---|---|---|---|---|
| 22.07.2011 | 30.07.1989 | F | URTI | 1047 | 1050 | Sore throat | Amoxycillin | CJB | |
| 22.07.2011 | 05.02.1946 | F | RTI | 1054 | 1104 | Chesty cough | Erythromycin | ML | |
| 25.07.2011 | 23.05.1927 | M | | 944 | 1003 | Script for Buprenorphine patch and Paracetamol given | | JM | |
| 25.07.2011 | 25.08.1989 | F | | 1003 | 1014 | Urine Pregnancy test positive | | LMD | |
| 25.07.2011 | 25.04.1935 | M | | 1014 | 1020 | Referred to ENT Surgeon regarding foods getting stuck in the throat intermittently | | FCW | Script for Lansoprazole given. |
| 25.07.2011 | 19.09.1962 | M | S/Leave | 1020 | 1030 | Med. 3 04/10 given for Pain in the (R) leg for 1 day from 21.07.11 | | KPW | That he may be fit for work from amended duties as arranged with his employer. |
| 25.07.2011 | 13.03.1934 | M | | 1030 | 1046 | Script for Diltiazem & Nafudrofuryl given | | KRF | For FBC, U/Es, Fasting Glucose, Fasting Lipids, TFTs & LFTs. |
| 25.07.2011 | 15.03.1940 | F | | 1046 | 1056 | Medication Review Done | | BRS | |
| 25.07.2011 | 08.04.1942 | M | | 1100 | 1108 | Script for Simvastatin given | | GFT | |
| 25.07.2011 | 15.01.1934 | F | | 1651 | 1701 | Script for Loratadine & Co-Amoxiclav given | | SMC | |

Result of a query that lists all consultations from the 22nd to the end of July 2011 (ConsultationsSeenFrom22ndTillEndOfJul2011)

| SurgeryDate | DateOfBirth | Sex | Diagnosis | TimeIn | TimeOut | Complaints | Treatments | Initials | Notes |
|---|---|---|---|---|---|---|---|---|---|
| 25.07.2011 | 10.01.1958 | M | | 1702 | 1720 | Referred to Colorectal Surgeon (urgent) regarding rectal bleeding | | ARH | For FBC & U/Es. |
| 25.07.2011 | 06.07.1948 | M | | 1720 | 1727 | To use olive oil & then to use Sodium bicarbonate ear drop for the wax in his ears and then to see the nurse to have the ears syringed | | DRS | |
| 25.07.2011 | 15.01.1962 | M | | 1748 | 1804 | Referred to Dermatologist regarding the mole on the (R) side of his neck | | PWL | Referred to General Surgeon regarding the pain in his (L) groin region. |
| 26.07.2011 | 10.04.1969 | F | S/Leave | 945 | 1010 | Med. 3 04/10 given for Depression and Heavy bleeding for 3 months from 26.07.11 | | LAJ | Script for Ferrous Fumarate given. Referred to One stop Breast Clinic regarding her (R) breast feeling heavy. |
| 26.07.2011 | 29.07.1969 | M | | 1010 | 1016 | Referred for Colonoscopy regarding alternating diarrhoea & constipation with bloated abdomen | | AKL | |

Result of a query that lists all consultations from the 22nd to the end of July 2011 (ConsultationsSeenFrom22ndTillEndOfJul2011)

| SurgeryDate | DateOfBirth | Sex | Diagnosis | TimeIn | TimeOut | Complaints | Treatments | Initials | Notes |
|---|---|---|---|---|---|---|---|---|---|
| 26.07.2011 | 15.01.1935 | F | | 1016 | 1025 | Script for Trimethoprim & Co-codamol given | | JRS | For MSU. |
| 26.07.2011 | 06.06.1947 | M | | 1025 | 1030 | Patient informed that he has got Diabetes Mellitus | | TLS | |
| 26.07.2011 | 31.05.1967 | M | | 1049 | 1055 | For USScan of the neck | | GKP | |
| 26.07.2011 | 08.02.1939 | F | | 1205 | 1220 | Script for Buprenorphine patch given | | IB | |
| 26.07.2011 | 25.02.1912 | F | | 1325 | 1340 | She is in Valentine's Lodge Nursing Home for TLC | | AEK | Home visit. |
| 26.07.2011 | 08.12.1962 | F | URTI | 1645 | 1650 | Sore throat | Erythromycin | BJM | Penicillin allergy. |
| 26.07.2011 | 15.01.1948 | F | | 1650 | 1659 | Script for Qvar inhaler & Salbutamol inhaler given | | EAW | Husband came to Surgery. |
| 26.07.2011 | 16.09.1936 | M | | 1700 | 1706 | Private script for Viagra given | | LPCE | |
| 26.07.2011 | 17.05.1955 | M | | 1706 | 1720 | Script for Dihydrocodeine & Orlistat given | | SJM | |
| 26.07.2011 | 08.09.1981 | M | | 1722 | 1727 | Script for Hydrocortisone/ Miconazole cream given | | SK | |

Result of a query that lists all consultations from the 22nd to the end of July 2011 (ConsultationsSeenFrom22ndTillEndOfJul2011)

| SurgeryDate | DateOfBirth | Sex | Diagnosis | TimeIn | TimeOut | Complaints | Treatments | Initials | Notes |
|---|---|---|---|---|---|---|---|---|---|
| 26.07.2011 | 10.09.1981 | F | | 1727 | 1740 | Script for Microgynon 30 given | | HAS | Referred to Rheumatologist with view to being investigated for Lupus. |
| 26.07.2011 | 14.04.1946 | F | | 1741 | 1749 | Script for Ibuprofen given | | VBB | |
| 27.07.2011 | 11.11.1934 | M | | 949 | 1003 | Script for Prednisolone, Salbutamol inhaler & Tiotropium inhalers given | | VRB | |
| 27.07.2011 | 21.11.1993 | M | | 1003 | 1020 | Script for Lactulose given | | JHR | For FBC, U/Es, MSU & Fasting Glucose. |
| 27.07.2011 | 09.06.1934 | M | | 1020 | 1037 | Referred to Colorectal Surgeon (urgent0 regarding his rectal bleeding | | MKC | |
| 27.07.2011 | 07.10.1933 | M | | 1037 | 1041 | Script for Olanzapine given | | FDF | |
| 27.07.2011 | 17.10.1978 | F | | 1041 | 1049 | She has anal skin tags & will see me later today with the nurse about them | | NHB | |
| 27.07.2011 | 10.08.1963 | M | S/Leave | 1049 | 1100 | Med. 3 04/10 given for (R) Cataract operation for 3 months from 26.07.11 | | FN | Script for Carmellose & Loteprednol eye drops given. |

Result of a query that lists all consultations from the 22nd to the end of July 2011 (ConsultationsSeenFrom22ndTillEndOfJul2011)

| SurgeryDate | DateOfBirth | Sex | Diagnosis | TimeIn | TimeOut | Complaints | Treatments | Initials | Notes |
|---|---|---|---|---|---|---|---|---|---|
| 27.07.2011 | 06.06.1936 | F | | 1100 | 1111 | Medication Review Done | | AJW | |
| 27.07.2011 | 17.10.1978 | F | | 1111 | 1124 | Referred to Colorectal Surgeon regarding anal skin tags that she will like removed | | NHB | |
| 27.07.2011 | 25.12.1942 | M | | 1124 | 1138 | Injection Depo-Medrone with Lidocaine given to the (R) shoulder | | RFL | |
| 27.07.2011 | 12.07.1967 | M | | 1645 | 1655 | Script for Amitripyline given | | KRG | |
| 27.07.2011 | 18.05.1952 | F | | 1655 | 1700 | Script for Amoxycillin given | | JN | |
| 27.07.2011 | 09.08.1971 | M | | 1701 | 1705 | Script for Erythromycin & Fusidic acid cream given | | JCW | Penicillin allergy. |
| 27.07.2011 | 14.08.1935 | M | | 1705 | 1714 | To see the nurse in 3 months for FBC, U/Es, B12, Folate & Ferritin | | RAT | |
| 27.07.2011 | 10.04.1969 | F | | 1716 | 1721 | Sick leave amended to read Depression and Heavy bleeding | | LAJ | |
| 27.07.2011 | 30.09.1961 | M | | 1730 | 1736 | Script for Erythromycin/Zinc lotion given | | IMB | |

Result of a query that lists all consultations from the 22nd to the end of July 2011 (ConsultationsSeenFrom22ndTillEndOfJul2011)

| SurgeryDate | DateOfBirth | Sex | Diagnosis | TimeIn | TimeOut | Complaints | Treatments | Initials | Notes |
|---|---|---|---|---|---|---|---|---|---|
| 27.07.2011 | 23.02.1969 | M | | 1736 | 1750 | Script for Flucloxacillin & Simvastatin given | | DJP | |
| 27.07.2011 | 02.05.1949 | M | | 1754 | 1807 | Script for Salbutamol inhaler given | | RB | |
| 27.07.2011 | 03.05.1951 | F | | 1807 | 1819 | Script for Tramadol given | | GAG | |
| 28.07.2011 | 15.10.1937 | F | | 946 | 952 | Script for Ferrous Fumarate given | | GS | |
| 28.07.2011 | 15.10.1925 | F | | 952 | 1008 | Script for Diltiazem & Simvastatin given | | RAA | For Ferritin, Folate & B12. |
| 28.07.2011 | 26.12.1951 | F | | 1008 | 1012 | Script for Hydrocortisone/ Miconazole given | | DCP | |
| 28.07.2011 | 02.09.1941 | F | | 1012 | 1022 | Script for Pizotifen given | | MS | |
| 28.07.2011 | 29.07.1947 | F | | 1022 | 1035 | Script for Amoxicillin, Prednisolone & Salbutamol inhaler given | | KM | For Chest X-Rays. |
| 28.07.2011 | 06.03.1991 | M | | 1035 | 1041 | Script for Clobetasol scalp application given | | DRA | For FBC, Fasting Glucose & U/Es. |
| 28.07.2011 | 20.04.1929 | F | | 1041 | 1052 | Referred to Pain Management specialist regarding her multiple joints pains | | JMG | |

695

## Result of a query that lists all consultations from the 22nd to the end of July 2011 (ConsultationsSeenFrom22ndTillEndOfJul2011)

| SurgeryDate | DateOfBirth | Sex | Diagnosis | TimeIn | TimeOut | Complaints | Treatments | Initials | Notes |
|---|---|---|---|---|---|---|---|---|---|
| 28.07.2011 | 31.05.1967 | M | | 1058 | 1112 | Referred to Counsellor regarding his depression & mood swings | | GKP | |
| 28.07.2011 | 16.06.1967 | M | | 1645 | 1659 | Script for Diprobase cream, Flucloxacillin & Fusidic acid cream given | | PBK | |
| 28.07.2011 | 01.07.1976 | M | | 1704 | 1719 | Script for Fexofenadine, Lansoprazole & Otomize ear spray given | | LJM | Referred to Physiotherapist regarding his back pain. |
| 28.07.2011 | 18.09.1946 | F | | 1719 | 1726 | Script for Loratadine given | | SL | |
| 28.07.2011 | 24.06.2001 | M | | 1726 | 1731 | Referred to Paediatrician regarding his chest pains | | JSB | |
| 28.07.2011 | 02.03.1948 | M | | 1731 | 1735 | Referred to Dermatologist regarding the whitish spot/area on his upper lip | | JHH | |
| 28.07.2011 | 26.05.1936 | M | | 1735 | 1741 | Script for Furosemide given | | TC | |
| 29.07.2011 | 15.07.1956 | M | | 928 | 942 | For FBC, U/Es, ESR, CRP & USScan of the (R) axilla | | DHH | |

Result of a query that lists all consultations from the 22nd to the end of July 2011 (ConsultationsSeenFrom22ndTillEndOfJul2011)

| SurgeryDate | DateOfBirth | Sex | Diagnosis | TimeIn | TimeOut | Complaints | Treatments | Initials | Notes |
|---|---|---|---|---|---|---|---|---|---|
| 29.07.2011 | 21.09.1947 | M |  | 942 | 951 | For X-Rays of the Pelvis & hips |  | DL |  |
| 29.07.2011 | 25.03.1911 | M |  | 951 | 1000 | Referred to Paediatrician regarding his persistent cough & wheezing |  | JAB | Script for Salbutamol inhaler & Volumatic with Paediatric mask given. |
| 29.07.2011 | 15.04.1973 | F | URTI | 1000 | 1010 | Sore throat | Amoxycillin | LJB |  |
| 29.07.2011 | 26.04.1944 | F |  | 1015 | 1025 | Script for Flucloxacillin & Fusidic acid cream given |  | AW |  |
| 29.07.2011 | 25.07.1938 | F |  | 1025 | 1035 | Medication Review Done |  | MR |  |
| 29.07.2011 | 08.01.1998 | F |  | 1035 | 1043 | Script for Erythromycin given |  | ELB |  |
| 29.07.2011 | 11.06.1932 | M |  | 1043 | 1050 | Script for Enoxaparin injection given |  | DHC |  |

Result of a query that lists all consultations from the 22nd to the end of July 2012 (ConsultationsSeenFrom22ndTillEndOfJul2012)

| SurgeryDate | DateOfBirth | Sex | Diagnosis | TimeIn | TimeOut | Complaints | Treatments | Initials | Notes |
|---|---|---|---|---|---|---|---|---|---|
| 23.07.2012 | 20.06.1974 | F |  | 945 | 950 | Script for Amitriptyline given |  | SLS |  |
| 23.07.2012 | 07.04.1950 | M |  | 1000 | 1012 | Script for Tramadol given |  | DML |  |

Result of a query that lists all consultations from the 22nd to the end of July 2012 (ConsultationsSeenFrom22ndTillEndOfJul2012)

| SurgeryDate | DateOfBirth | Sex | Diagnosis | TimeIn | TimeOut | Complaints | Treatments | Initials | Notes |
|---|---|---|---|---|---|---|---|---|---|
| 23.07.2012 | 23.10.1941 | M | | 1012 | 1017 | Medication Review Done | | RJH | |
| 23.07.2012 | 04.07.1929 | M | | 1017 | 1025 | For USScan of the abdomen | | RMC | |
| 23.07.2012 | 09.10.1967 | M | | 1025 | 1032 | Script for Salbutamol inhaler given | | KDL | |
| 23.07.2012 | 05.02.1960 | F | | 1032 | 1050 | Script for Amoxycillin, Prednisolone & Simvastatin given | | SJW | |
| 23.07.2012 | 06.12.1947 | M | | 1050 | 1059 | Script for Codeine Linctus given | | BSK | For Spirometry & for Chest X-Rays. |
| 23.07.2012 | 26.11.1964 | F | | 1059 | 1111 | Script for Fluoxetine given | | DN | |
| 23.07.2012 | 11.10.1938 | F | | 1115 | 1132 | Script for Chloramphenicol eye ointment given | | JMS | |
| 23.07.2012 | 16.09.1936 | M | | 1645 | 1649 | Private script for Viagra given | | LPCE | |
| 23.07.2012 | 24.08.2010 | M | | 1652 | 1702 | Script for Hydrocortisone/ Fusidic acid cream given | | JIS | |
| 23.07.2012 | 18.07.1956 | F | S/Leave | 1707 | 1716 | Med. 3 04/10 given for Multiple joint pains & injury to (R) foot from 23.07.12. for 3 months | | MTC | Referred to Physiotherapist regarding pain in her (R) hip & wrist. |

698

Result of a query that lists all consultations from the 22nd to the end of July 2012 (ConsultationsSeenFrom22ndTillEndOfJul2012)

| SurgeryDate | DateOfBirth | Sex | Diagnosis | TimeIn | TimeOut | Complaints | Treatments | Initials | Notes |
|---|---|---|---|---|---|---|---|---|---|
| 23.07.2012 | 03.11.1971 | F | | 1726 | 1740 | Advised to check with Mr. Lee via his secretary about blood test for Estrogen level | | KDM | |
| 23.07.2012 | 05.09.1998 | F | | 1740 | 1757 | She changed her mind about going on medication delay her period | | EVW | |
| 23.07.2012 | 09.12.1964 | M | | 1757 | 1803 | Script for Amoxycillin given | | ST | |
| 23.07.2012 | 08.04.1971 | F | | 1803 | 1811 | Script for Ferrous Fumarate given | | JRB | |
| 23.07.2012 | 24.09.1930 | F | | 1811 | 1818 | Script for Paracetamol & Trimethoprim given | | JMC | |
| 23.07.2012 | 25.07.1964 | M | | 1818 | 1824 | Script for Chloramphenicol eye drops given | | SJP | |
| 24.07.2012 | 25.07.1934 | M | | 945 | 955 | Script for Lisinopril given | | SCC | For serum Ferritin, Folate and B12. |
| 24.07.2012 | 02.09.1951 | F | | 955 | 1008 | BP 105/66 | | CMS | |
| 24.07.2012 | 31.07.1956 | M | | 1008 | 1014 | Script for Co-codamol & Colofac MR given | | RVGH | |
| 24.07.2012 | 12.04.1938 | M | | 1014 | 1021 | Medication Review Done | | MAF | |
| 24.07.2012 | 05.06.1924 | M | | 1023 | 1031 | Script for Omeprazole given | | DAC | |

Result of a query that lists all consultations from the 22nd to the end of July 2012 (ConsultationsSeenFrom22ndTillEndOfJul2012)

| SurgeryDate | DateOfBirth | Sex | Diagnosis | TimeIn | TimeOut | Complaints | Treatments | Initials | Notes |
|---|---|---|---|---|---|---|---|---|---|
| 24.07.2012 | 21.04.1949 | M | | 1031 | 1047 | Script for Carbimazole given | | RL | Referred to Endocrinologist regarding his hyperthyroidism. Referred to General Surgeon regarding the possible lipoma on the back of his neck. |
| 24.07.2012 | 27.01.1934 | F | | 1047 | 1058 | To stop the Indapamide & to see me in one month for review | | JWC | |
| 24.07.2012 | 17.02.1957 | F | | 1058 | 1114 | Referred to Physiotherapist regarding pain in the feet | | VMC | For X-Rays of the (L) foot. |
| 24.07.2012 | 20.10.1929 | M | | 1318 | 1324 | To continue with TLC | | PL | Home visit. |
| 24.07.2012 | 24.08.1918 | F | | 1345 | 1400 | Script for Movicol Half strength & Trimethoprim given | | GPE | Home visit. |
| 24.07.2012 | 31.07.1923 | M | | 1646 | 1654 | Script for Canesten HC cream & Capasal shampoo given | | HO | |
| 24.07.2012 | 08.04.1945 | M | | 1654 | 1703 | Cryotherapy blasts applied to fingers warts | | GTW | |

Result of a query that lists all consultations from the 22nd to the end of July 2012 (ConsultationsSeenFrom22ndTillEndOfJul2012)

| SurgeryDate | DateOfBirth | Sex | Diagnosis | TimeIn | TimeOut | Complaints | Treatments | Initials | Notes |
|---|---|---|---|---|---|---|---|---|---|
| 24.07.2012 | 18.03.1987 | F | S/Leave | 1741 | 1748 | Med. 3 04/10 given for Back Pain from 24.07.12 to 25.07.12, phased return | | LP | |
| 24.07.2012 | 27.05.1968 | M | S/Leave | 1748 | 1752 | Med. 3 04/10 given for Back Pain from 23.07.12. for 2 weeks | | LJH | |
| 24.07.2012 | 21.09.1947 | M | | 1751 | 1755 | Patient came in for DVLA examination but we have no form for him, he will contact DVLA to get the form | | DL | |
| 24.07.2012 | 08.01.1998 | F | | 1807 | 1813 | Script for Duac gel given | | ELB | |
| 25.07.2012 | 23.12.1952 | F | | 944 | 957 | Script for Atorvastatin given | | GCB | |
| 25.07.2012 | 26.02.1934 | F | | 957 | 1003 | BP 127/88 | | DIM | |
| 25.07.2012 | 10.04.1969 | F | S/Leave | 1003 | 1018 | Med. 3 04/10 given for Depression and Heavy Bleeding from 25.07.12 for 6 months | | LAJ | |
| 25.07.2012 | 04.11.1924 | F | | 1018 | 1026 | Referred to Physiotherapist regarding her painful back due to her curvature | | OJR | |
| 25.07.2012 | 23.05.1971 | F | | 1026 | 1036 | Script for Cetirizine given | | JW | |

701

Result of a query that lists all consultations from the 22nd to the end of July 2012 (ConsultationsSeenFrom22ndTillEndOfJul2012)

| SurgeryDate | DateOfBirth | Sex | Diagnosis | TimeIn | TimeOut | Complaints | Treatments | Initials | Notes |
|---|---|---|---|---|---|---|---|---|---|
| 25.07.2012 | 17.09.1965 | F | URTI | 1036 | 1041 | Sore throat | Amoxycillin | PAE | |
| 25.07.2012 | 15.09.1925 | F | | 1041 | 1056 | Script for Amoxycillin & Fucidin H cream given | | DFS | |
| 25.07.2012 | 14.03.1936 | F | | 1056 | 1107 | General discussion with the patient about the bad effects of high cholesterol | | ST | |
| 25.07.2012 | 26.06.1997 | F | | 1107 | 1137 | Referred to Paediatric Dr. on call regarding her very high fasting Glucose & very abnormal TFTs | | EBF | |
| 25.07.2012 | 17.03.1968 | F | | 1644 | 1702 | Referred to Dr. Gil for removal of the mole on the (R) shoulder | | NJB | |
| 25.07.2012 | 03.10.1991 | F | | 1702 | 1709 | Script for Erythromycin & Otosporin ear drops given | | ARC | |
| 25.07.2012 | 08.04.1948 | M | | 1709 | 1713 | Script for Flucloxacillin given | | WRT | |
| 25.07.2012 | 02.08.1948 | M | | 1713 | 1723 | Script for Bisoprolol given | | KT | |
| 25.07.2012 | 02.05.1949 | M | | 1723 | 1730 | Script for Canesten HC cream given | | RB | |
| 25.07.2012 | 24.01.2001 | F | | 1730 | 1734 | Script for Calamine lotion given | | NKJ | |

## Result of a query that lists all consultations from the 22nd to the end of July 2012 (ConsultationsSeenFrom22ndTillEndOfJul2012)

| SurgeryDate | DateOfBirth | Sex | Diagnosis | TimeIn | TimeOut | Complaints | Treatments | Initials | Notes |
|---|---|---|---|---|---|---|---|---|---|
| 25.07.2012 | 14.08.1927 | M | | 1734 | 1740 | Script for Flucloxacillin given | | RJW | For serum Uric acid. |
| 25.07.2012 | 03.02.2008 | F | | 1740 | 1748 | Script for Salbutamol inhaler given | | AAL | |
| 25.07.2012 | 25.09.1961 | F | S/Leave | 1753 | 1810 | Med. 3 04/10 given for (R) Elbow Injury from 25.07.12 for 3 months | | SJB | |
| 26.07.2012 | 09.11.1972 | F | | 944 | 957 | Script for Flucloxacillin given | | LSS | |
| 26.07.2012 | 21.11.1994 | F | | 957 | 1003 | Script for Beconase Aqueous nasal spray & Salbutamol inhaler given | | HJA | |
| 26.07.2012 | 19.06.1927 | F | | 1003 | 1010 | Medication Review Done | | GEG | |
| 26.07.2012 | 29.11.1998 | F | | 1010 | 1022 | For MSU | | MLYG | |
| 26.07.2012 | 27.07.1995 | F | | 1022 | 1028 | Script for Cetirizine solution, Diprobase & Salbutamol inhaler given | | BM | |
| 26.07.2012 | 18.04.1965 | M | S/Leave | 1032 | 1041 | Med. 3 04/10 given for Stress from 23.07.12 for 2 weeks | | MGF | |
| 26.07.2012 | 17.08.1947 | F | | 1041 | 1053 | Script for Flucloxacillin & Tramadol m/r capsule given | | SAA | |

Result of a query that lists all consultations from the 22nd to the end of July 2012 (ConsultationsSeenFrom22ndTillEndOfJul2012)

| SurgeryDate | DateOfBirth | Sex | Diagnosis | TimeIn | TimeOut | Complaints | Treatments | Initials | Notes |
|---|---|---|---|---|---|---|---|---|---|
| 26.07.2012 | 16.08.1943 | M | | 1053 | 1108 | Script for Codeine, Gliclazide & Naproxen given | | MJG | |
| 26.07.2012 | 24.10.1959 | M | | 1108 | 1124 | Script for Metoclopramide given | | BRH | For FBC, TFTs, U/Es, Chest X-Rays (urgent) & USScan of the Abdomen (urgent). |
| 26.07.2012 | 06.12.1962 | M | | 1124 | 1134 | Referred to ENT Surgeon regarding pressure in his (L) ear persistently | | DAB | |
| 26.07.2012 | 06.12.2006 | F | | 1134 | 1140 | Script for Cetirizine solution & Flucloxacillin given | | ALS | |
| 26.07.2012 | 09.04.1938 | M | | 1644 | 1654 | Referred for Colonoscopy (urgent) regarding his diarrhoea & abdominal pain with poor appetite & weight loss | | NWH | |
| 26.07.2012 | 16.03.1956 | F | | 1654 | 1659 | Script for Qvar 50 inhaler given | | SPD | |
| 26.07.2012 | 15.12.1935 | F | | 1659 | 1709 | Referred to Dermatologist regarding the BCC-like lesion on her face | | DL | |

Result of a query that lists all consultations from the 22nd to the end of July 2012 (ConsultationsSeenFrom22ndTillEndOfJul2012)

| SurgeryDate | DateOfBirth | Sex | Diagnosis | TimeIn | TimeOut | Complaints | Treatments | Initials | Notes |
|---|---|---|---|---|---|---|---|---|---|
| 26.07.2012 | 09.12.1964 | M | S/Leave | 1709 | 1712 | Med. 3 04/10 given for Throat infection from 23.07.12 for 1 week | | ST | |
| 26.07.2012 | 24.09.1995 | F | | 1713 | 1726 | Script for Rigevidon tablets given | | GEM | |
| 26.07.2012 | 02.09.1934 | M | | 1726 | 1730 | Script for Aqueous cream & Otosporin ear drops given | | DBM | |
| 26.07.2012 | 15.03.1930 | M | | 1730 | 1749 | Script for Paracetamol given | | JLC | |
| 27.07.2012 | 06.01.1969 | F | S/Leave | 951 | 1000 | Med. 3 04/10 given for (R) Knee arthroscopy from 27.07.12 for 1 month | | KEL | |
| 27.07.2012 | 20.02.1954 | F | | 1000 | 1011 | For Thyroid antibodies | | VB | |
| 27.07.2012 | 18.05.1952 | F | | 1011 | 1020 | Script for Fluoxetine given | | JN | |
| 27.07.2012 | 11.11.1981 | F | | 1020 | 1029 | Referred to Gynaecologist regarding her primary infertility | | SC | |
| 27.07.2012 | 31.12.1965 | F | | 1029 | 1039 | Script for Ferrous Fumarate given | | BV | |
| 27.07.2012 | 25.08.1989 | F | S/Leave | 1039 | 1047 | Med. 3 04/10 given for Dehydration and Vomiting in Pregnancy from 28.05.12 to 02.07.12 | | LMD | |

Result of a query that lists all consultations from the 22nd to the end of July 2012 (ConsultationsSeenFrom22ndTillEndOfJul2012)

| SurgeryDate | DateOfBirth | Sex | Diagnosis | TimeIn | TimeOut | Complaints | Treatments | Initials | Notes |
|---|---|---|---|---|---|---|---|---|---|
| 27.07.2012 | 09.08.1971 | M | | 1047 | 1057 | Script for Candesartan given | | JCW | Referred to Physiotherapist regarding his painful (L) knee. |
| 27.07.2012 | 18.10.1974 | F | RTI | 1057 | 1101 | Chesty cough | Amoxycillin | HAW | |
| 27.07.2012 | 25.02.1975 | M | | 1101 | 1111 | Referred to Dermatologist regarding bleeding scrotal spots | | GHD | Referred to Ophthalmologist (Dr. Idre) regarding pain in the (R) eye after getting grit into the eye. |
| 30.07.2012 | 27.03.1948 | M | | 945 | 951 | He has CKD stage 3A | | BAG | |
| 30.07.2012 | 22.05.1988 | M | S/Leave | 951 | 957 | Med. 3 04/10 given for Depression from 23.07.12 for 3 months | | MCC | |
| 30.07.2012 | 06.09.1974 | M | | 958 | 1010 | Script for Metformin given | | DGH | |
| 30.07.2012 | 02.05.1965 | M | | 1010 | 1019 | Script for Fexofenadine, Flucloxacillin, Naseptin cream & Tacrolimus given | | GJB | |
| 30.07.2012 | 25.06.1934 | F | | 1029 | 1041 | Script for Driclor solution given | | EW | |
| 30.07.2012 | 10.11.2000 | M | | 1041 | 1046 | Script for Salbutamol inhaler given | | CJM | |

Result of a query that lists all consultations from the 22nd to the end of July 2012 (ConsultationsSeenFrom22ndTillEndOfJul2012)

| SurgeryDate | DateOfBirth | Sex | Diagnosis | TimeIn | TimeOut | Complaints | Treatments | Initials | Notes |
|---|---|---|---|---|---|---|---|---|---|
| 30.07.2012 | 15.09.2011 | M | | 1046 | 1050 | To continue to use own Oilatum cream | | SKC | |
| 30.07.2012 | 04.07.1959 | F | | 1050 | 1100 | Script for Simvastatin given | | SAB | For FBC & TFTs. |
| 30.07.2012 | 02.06.1994 | F | | 1100 | 1105 | To see the Practice nurse in 6 months for repeat FBC & serum Ferritin | | EPB | |
| 30.07.2012 | 24.02.1921 | F | | 1314 | 1326 | Script for Amoxycillin & Furosemide given | | EIW | Home visit. |
| 30.07.2012 | 05.02.1943 | M | | 1645 | 1653 | Referred to General Surgeon regarding lumps on his back | | MJV | |
| 30.07.2012 | 03.03.1951 | M | | 1653 | 1703 | For FBC, U/Es, TFTs, Fasting lipids, Fasting Glucose & TFTs | | SWP | |
| 30.07.2012 | 16.03.1963 | F | S/Leave | 1703 | 1712 | Med. 3 04/10 given for Depression from 23.07.12 for 6 months | | TJC | Script for Duac gel given. |
| 30.07.2012 | 09.09.1962 | F | | 1712 | 1719 | Medication Review Done | | MLF | |
| 30.07.2012 | 11.03.1968 | F | | 1719 | 1728 | Script for Hydroxocobalamin injection given | | EJA | |
| 30.07.2012 | 16.06.1967 | M | | 1728 | 1735 | Script for Canesten HC cream & Furosemide given | | PBK | |

## Result of a query that lists all consultations from the 22nd to the end of July 2012 (ConsultationsSeenFrom22ndTillEndOfJul2012)

| SurgeryDate | DateOfBirth | Sex | Diagnosis | TimeIn | TimeOut | Complaints | Treatments | Initials | Notes |
|---|---|---|---|---|---|---|---|---|---|
| 30.07.2012 | 28.07.1939 | F | | 1750 | 1830 | She is unable to come to terms with the reversal of the diagnosis of her MS | | RMM | |
| 30.07.2012 | 07.03.1973 | F | | 1830 | 1835 | Script for Levonelle 1500mcg tablet given | | MJC | |

## Result of a query that lists all consultations from the 22nd to the end of July 2013 (ConsultationsSeenFrom22ndTillEndOfJul2013)

| SurgeryDate | DateOfBirth | Sex | Diagnosis | TimeIn | TimeOut | Complaints | Treatments | Initials | Notes |
|---|---|---|---|---|---|---|---|---|---|
| 22.07.2013 | 10.04.1969 | F | S/Leave | 944 | 950 | Med. 3 04/10 given for Depression and Heavy Bleeding for 6 months from 22.07.13 | | LAJ | |
| 22.07.2013 | 25.11.1946 | M | | 952 | 1000 | For X-Rays of the (R) knee | | DBY | |
| 22.07.2013 | 07.06.1955 | F | S/Leave | 1000 | 1011 | Med. 3 04/10 given for Pain in the Back & (L) Hip for 3 months from 19.07.13 | | JM | For MSU. |
| 22.07.2013 | 03.08.1935 | M | | 1011 | 1026 | For serum Ferritin, B12 & Folate | | RH | |
| 22.07.2013 | 04.06.1988 | F | | 1026 | 1032 | To attend FP clinic regarding the specific progesterone only pill that she is after | | ALB | |

Result of a query that lists all consultations from the 22nd to the end of July 2013 (ConsultationsSeenFrom22ndTillEndOfJul2013)

| SurgeryDate | DateOfBirth | Sex | Diagnosis | TimeIn | TimeOut | Complaints | Treatments | Initials | Notes |
|---|---|---|---|---|---|---|---|---|---|
| 22.07.2013 | 16.03.1956 | F | | 1032 | 1041 | For MSU | | SPD | |
| 22.07.2013 | 26.06.1955 | F | | 1041 | 1048 | Referred to Orthopaedic Surgeon regarding the lump on the volar aspect of her (L) wrist | | TAP | |
| 22.07.2013 | 15.10.1937 | F | | 1048 | 1054 | Medications Review Done | | GS | |
| 22.07.2013 | 23.04.1963 | F | | 1054 | 1107 | Referred to General Surgeon regarding the lipoma-like lesion on her upper back | | FN | |
| 22.07.2013 | 18.07.1978 | F | | 1107 | 1120 | For Pelvic USScan | | TJS | |
| 22.07.2013 | 15.04.1927 | M | | 1324 | 1342 | Script for Loperamide & Dioralyte given | | JB | Home visit. |
| 22.07.2013 | 06.03.1957 | F | | 1643 | 1652 | Referred to Audiology clinic regarding her bilateral deafness | | CMT | |
| 22.07.2013 | 31.01.1969 | F | | 1652 | 1700 | Script for Amoxycillin & Co-codamol given | | JP | |
| 22.07.2013 | 06.03.1966 | F | | 1700 | 1712 | Script for Norethisterone given | | JLL | Referred to Vascular Surgeon (BUPA) regarding her painful & aching varicose veins in the (L) leg. |
| 22.07.2013 | 05.11.2006 | F | URTI | 1712 | 1719 | Sore throat | Amoxycillin | ALA | |

709

Result of a query that lists all consultations from the 22nd to the end of July 2013 (ConsultationsSeenFrom22ndTillEndOfJul2013)

| SurgeryDate | DateOfBirth | Sex | Diagnosis | TimeIn | TimeOut | Complaints | Treatments | Initials | Notes |
|---|---|---|---|---|---|---|---|---|---|
| 22.07.2013 | 23.09.1944 | M | | 1719 | 1729 | Script for Prochlorperazine given | | VRE | For FBC, TFT, LFTs, serum cholesterol, U/Es & Fasting Glucose. |
| 22.07.2013 | 31.01.1969 | M | | 1729 | 1736 | Advised to put in a self-certificate for the first week | | DRA | |
| 22.07.2013 | 30.07.1983 | F | RTI | 1736 | 1745 | Chesty cough | Amoxycillin | YP | |
| 22.07.2013 | 05.12.2007 | F | URTI | 1745 | 1752 | (R) ear ache | Amoxycillin | ABH | |
| 22.07.2013 | 08.11.1941 | F | | 1752 | 1800 | Toothache | Amoxycillin & Metronidazole | PET | |
| 23.07.2013 | 08.01.1942 | F | | 941 | 954 | Script for BuTrans patch given | | SM | |
| 23.07.2013 | 21.08.1934 | M | | 954 | 1008 | Script for Codeine tablets & Oramorph given | | KW | |
| 23.07.2013 | 28.02.1960 | F | | 1008 | 1025 | Script for Lansoprazole given | | JS | Referred to General Surgeon regarding diffuse goitre shown on the USScan of the neck. |
| 23.07.2013 | 24.03.1935 | F | | 1025 | 1033 | Script for Hirudoid cream, Lansoprazole & Co-codamol given | | PW | Referred to Orthopaedic Surgeon regarding her right sided carpal tunnel syndrome. |

710

Result of a query that lists all consultations from the 22nd to the end of July 2013 (ConsultationsSeenFrom22ndTillEndOfJul2013)

| SurgeryDate | DateOfBirth | Sex | Diagnosis | TimeIn | TimeOut | Complaints | Treatments | Initials | Notes |
|---|---|---|---|---|---|---|---|---|---|
| 23.07.2013 | 23.09.1936 | M | | 1033 | 1045 | Script for Codeine tablets given | | TH | For X-Rays of the (R) knee. |
| 23.07.2013 | 17.05.1943 | M | | 1045 | 1054 | For Chest X-Rays | | PJC | |
| 23.07.2013 | 02.05.1962 | F | | 1054 | 1102 | For MSU in 2 to 3 months, form given to the patient | | DP | |
| 23.07.2013 | 03.03.1946 | M | RTI | 1102 | 1111 | Chesty cough | Amoxycillin | SP | For Chest X-Rays. |
| 23.07.2013 | 01.09.1958 | F | S/Leave | 1111 | 1118 | Med. 3 04/10 given for (R) Inguinal hernia repair for 2 weeks from 17.07.13 | | RM | |
| 23.07.2013 | 15.12.1939 | M | | 1645 | 1651 | Cryotherapy blasts x2 applied to warts on (R) hand | | ERC | |
| 23.07.2013 | 18.07.1956 | F | S/Leave | 1651 | 1656 | Med. 3 04/10 given for Multiple joint pains & injury to (R) foot for 3 months from 23.07.13 | | MTC | |
| 23.07.2013 | 04.07.1929 | M | | 1656 | 1703 | Cryotherapy blasts x2 applied to warts on the back | | RMC | |
| 23.07.2013 | 23.02.1991 | M | | 1716 | 1725 | Script for Fucibet cream given | | MSK | |
| 23.07.2013 | 26.03.1974 | M | | 1725 | 1731 | Script for Flucloxacillin & Clenil Modulite inhaler given | | MPF | |

Result of a query that lists all consultations from the 22nd to the end of July 2013 (ConsultationsSeenFrom22ndTillEndOfJul2013)

| SurgeryDate | DateOfBirth | Sex | Diagnosis | TimeIn | TimeOut | Complaints | Treatments | Initials | Notes |
|---|---|---|---|---|---|---|---|---|---|
| 23.07.2013 | 03.02.1964 | F | | 1731 | 1736 | Script for Erythromycin given | | SB | |
| 23.07.2013 | 13.11.1949 | M | | 1736 | 1742 | Referred for Colonoscopy (urgent) regarding his rectal bleeding | | BEP | |
| 23.07.2013 | 26.10.1987 | M | S/Leave | 1742 | 1749 | Med. 3 04/10 given for (R) ear infection for 1 week from 22.07.13 | | RML | |
| 23.07.2013 | 08.11.1941 | F | | 1749 | 1801 | Script for Naproxen & Omeprazole given | | PET | |
| 23.07.2013 | 20.10.1953 | M | | 1819 | 1826 | BP 130/80 | | PJH | |
| 24.07.2013 | 08.03.1946 | F | | 944 | 950 | She will observe her (L) ankle swelling which happens on & off for now | | GRC | |
| 24.07.2013 | 18.02.1968 | F | | 950 | 957 | For serum BNP | | PAC | |
| 24.07.2013 | 06.12.1947 | M | | 957 | 1007 | Script for Tobradex eye drops given | | BSK | |
| 24.07.2013 | 17.11.1937 | F | | 1007 | 1017 | Script for Hyoscine butylbromide given | | JTC | For FBC, U/Es, serum Ferritin, fasting Glucose, Folate, B12. |
| 24.07.2013 | 23.01.1947 | F | | 1017 | 1024 | Script for Co-codamol given | | BW | |
| 24.07.2013 | 30.04.1941 | F | | 1024 | 1029 | For FBC, U/Es, serum cholesterol & LFTs | | VRG | |

Result of a query that lists all consultations from the 22nd to the end of July 2013 (ConsultationsSeenFrom22ndTillEndOfJul2013)

| SurgeryDate | DateOfBirth | Sex | Diagnosis | TimeIn | TimeOut | Complaints | Treatments | Initials | Notes |
|---|---|---|---|---|---|---|---|---|---|
| 24.07.2013 | 23.09.1951 | F | | 1029 | 1037 | Script for Fucidin 2% cream given | | DJS | |
| 24.07.2013 | 07.02.1952 | M | | 1325 | 1335 | No obvious evidence of hernia or groin swelling, although patient was difficult to examine | | GAH | Home visit. |
| 24.07.2013 | 05.07.1990 | F | | 1646 | 1656 | For MSU | | RLS | |
| 24.07.2013 | 21.08.1946 | F | | 1656 | 1703 | Medications Review Done | | JK | |
| 24.07.2013 | 06.01.1955 | M | | 1703 | 1707 | Private script for Viagra given | | MAS | |
| 24.07.2013 | 31.01.1969 | M | S/Leave | 1715 | 1724 | Med. 3 04/10 given for Migraine & Depression for 6 months from 05.04.13 | | DRA | |
| 24.07.2013 | 25.10.1966 | M | | 1724 | 1731 | Script for Omeprazole given | | WBG | |
| 24.07.2013 | 13.10.1983 | M | S/Leave | 1733 | 1742 | Med. 3 04/10 given for Injury to (R) wrist for 2 months from 22.07.13 | | RGW | |
| 24.07.2013 | 16.05.1944 | F | | 1742 | 1747 | To use OTC Sodium bicarbonate ear drops for a couple of weeks & to see the nurse for ear syringing | | JRL | |

Result of a query that lists all consultations from the 22nd to the end of July 2013 (ConsultationsSeenFrom22ndTillEndOfJul2013)

| SurgeryDate | DateOfBirth | Sex | Diagnosis | TimeIn | TimeOut | Complaints | Treatments | Initials | Notes |
|---|---|---|---|---|---|---|---|---|---|
| 24.07.2013 | 17.02.1987 | F | | 1747 | 1801 | Script for Laxido Orange oral powder sachets given | | KMT | |
| 24.07.2013 | 05.04.1964 | F | | 1801 | 1810 | Referred to Orthopaedic Surgeon regarding pain in her (R) knee | | JL | |
| 25.07.2013 | 09.04.1938 | M | | 945 | 952 | BP 145/81 | | MWH | |
| 25.07.2013 | 21.04.1949 | M | | 952 | 958 | He will observe the painful arthritic (R) shoulder for now | | RL | |
| 25.07.2013 | 14.06.1945 | M | | 958 | 1005 | BP 139/76 | | BL | |
| 25.07.2013 | 22.05.1931 | F | | 1041 | 1055 | Script for Allopurinol, Flucloxacillin, Naproxen & Omeprazole given | | DK | For serum uric acid, U/Es, serum cholesterol & LFTs. |
| 25.07.2013 | 19.08.1917 | F | | 1248 | 1308 | Referred to Neurologist regarding her unsteadiness & confusion since hitting her head a few months ago | | VL | Referred to Audiology clinic regarding her deafness. Home visit. |
| 25.07.2013 | 19.08.1939 | F | | 1644 | 1706 | Script for Citalopram & Levothyroxine given | | JEN | |
| 25.07.2013 | 18.10.1949 | M | | 1706 | 1723 | Script for Sildenafil given | | BJG | |

Result of a query that lists all consultations from the 22nd to the end of July 2013 (ConsultationsSeenFrom22ndTillEndOfJul2013)

| SurgeryDate | DateOfBirth | Sex | Diagnosis | TimeIn | TimeOut | Complaints | Treatments | Initials | Notes |
|---|---|---|---|---|---|---|---|---|---|
| 25.07.2013 | 20.11.1936 | M | | 1723 | 1731 | Script for Co-codamol, Naproxen & Omeprazole given | | NN | |
| 25.07.2013 | 15.12.1939 | M | URTI | 1731 | 1736 | Sore throat | Amoxycillin | ERC | |
| 25.07.2013 | 20.05.1991 | F | | 1736 | 1745 | Script for Microgynon 30 given | | JS | |
| 25.07.2013 | 19.10.1944 | F | | 1745 | 1752 | Script for Flucloxacillin given | | IS | |
| 26.07.2013 | 17.03.1961 | M | | 942 | 951 | Script for Sertraline & Sumatriptan given | | LDM | |
| 26.07.2013 | 07.10.1933 | M | | 951 | 1000 | For TFTs & FBC | | FDF | |
| 26.07.2013 | 27.02.2008 | F | | 1000 | 1005 | Script for Erythromycin given | | SCAB | |
| 26.07.2013 | 11.12.1968 | F | | 1017 | 1027 | Infected insect bites | Flucloxacillin | ALH | |
| 26.07.2013 | 23.09.1933 | M | | 1027 | 1032 | Script for Paracetamol & Naproxen given | | JFRB | |
| 26.07.2013 | 20.09.1934 | M | | 1032 | 1046 | For U/Es | | EWM | |
| 26.07.2013 | 11.08.1983 | F | | 1102 | 1112 | Script for Noriday & Propranolol given | | RJN | |
| 26.07.2013 | 29.04.1937 | M | | 1112 | 1123 | Script for Pinexel PR & Trimethoprim given | | PGS | For MSU, U/Es, FBC, serum cholesterol & LFTs. |
| 29.07.2013 | 11.09.1947 | M | | 942 | 948 | Medications Review Done | | TSN | |
| 29.07.2013 | 15.01.1959 | M | S/Leave | 948 | 959 | Med. 3 04/10 given for Back Pain for 2 weeks from 28.07.13 | | ROW | |

715

Result of a query that lists all consultations from the 22nd to the end of July 2013 (ConsultationsSeenFrom22ndTillEndOfJul2013)

| SurgeryDate | DateOfBirth | Sex | Diagnosis | TimeIn | TimeOut | Complaints | Treatments | Initials | Notes |
|---|---|---|---|---|---|---|---|---|---|
| 29.07.2013 | 09.10.1926 | M | | 959 | 1012 | Script for BuTrans transdermal patches given | | RAC | |
| 29.07.2013 | 01.01.1951 | F | | 1012 | 1018 | Script for Trimethoprim given | | CR | For MSU. |
| 29.07.2013 | 08.01.1966 | F | | 1020 | 1030 | For X-Rays of the (R) knee | | AJK | |
| 29.07.2013 | 12.08.1993 | M | | 1037 | 1050 | Referred to Occupational therapist regarding him getting new pairs of in-soles for his flat feet | | DTA | |
| 29.07.2013 | 19.06.1944 | F | | 1050 | 1101 | For TFT's | | PJL | |
| 29.07.2013 | 24.02.1962 | M | | 1101 | 1110 | Medications Review Done | | SAB | |
| 29.07.2013 | 11.10.1938 | F | | 1110 | 1120 | Medications Review Done | | JMS | |
| 29.07.2013 | 08.06.1961 | M | | 1647 | 1701 | To leave the holiday cancellation form at the Reception to be completed | | MPB | |
| 29.07.2013 | 18.03.1967 | F | | 1701 | 1711 | For X-Rays of the (L) hand | | SO | |
| 29.07.2013 | 04.03.1982 | F | | 1711 | 1716 | Referred to Colorectal Surgeon regarding her rectal bleeding on & off | | GV | |

Result of a query that lists all consultations from the 22nd to the end of July 2013 (ConsultationsSeenFrom22ndTillEndOfJul2013)

| SurgeryDate | DateOfBirth | Sex | Diagnosis | TimeIn | TimeOut | Complaints | Treatments | Initials | Notes |
|---|---|---|---|---|---|---|---|---|---|
| 29.07.2013 | 05.06.1947 | M | | 1716 | 1723 | Script for Solaraze 3% gel given | | DTR | |
| 29.07.2013 | 27.11.1967 | M | | 1723 | 1732 | Script for Codeine tablets given | | DMS | |
| 29.07.2013 | 05.08.1942 | M | | 1732 | 1736 | BP 130/81 | | RP | |
| 29.07.2013 | 25.06.1938 | F | | 1736 | 1749 | Script for Furosemide given | | JEL | Referred to Dermatologist regarding her multiple seborrheic dermatoses |
| 29.07.2013 | 04.09.1966 | M | | 1754 | 1803 | Script for Amoxycillin given | | PLM | |
| 30.07.2013 | 01.09.1958 | F | S/Leave | 943 | 958 | Med. 3 04/10 given for (R) Inguinal hernia repair from 30.07.13 to 02.08.13 | | RM | Script for Fucidin H cream given. |
| 30.07.2013 | 19.10.1971 | M | | 958 | 1004 | Script for DHC Continus & Naproxen given | | PSSC | |
| 30.07.2013 | 31.12.1965 | F | | 1004 | 1009 | Referred to Podiatrist regarding bunion on the (R) foot | | BV | |
| 30.07.2013 | 15.04.1927 | M | | 1009 | 1019 | For FBC & U/Es | | JB | |
| 30.07.2013 | 28.07.1946 | M | | 1019 | 1036 | Script for Timolol 0.25% eye drops given | | PWD | |
| 30.07.2013 | 05.06.1930 | F | | 1036 | 1046 | Script for Seebri Breezhaler given | | JMF | Her son came to the Surgery. |

Result of a query that lists all consultations from the 22nd to the end of July 2013 (ConsultationsSeenFrom22ndTillEndOfJul2013)

| SurgeryDate | DateOfBirth | Sex | Diagnosis | TimeIn | TimeOut | Complaints | Treatments | Initials | Notes |
|---|---|---|---|---|---|---|---|---|---|
| 30.07.2013 | 11.07.1962 | M | | 1046 | 1053 | Script for Bendroflumethiazide & Lisinopril given | | JEG | |
| 30.07.2013 | 25.12.1948 | M | | 1053 | 1100 | To continue with the present doses of his medications | | CGB | |
| 30.07.2013 | 19.01.1940 | F | | 1110 | 1136 | Script for Doxazosin given | | VS | |
| 30.07.2013 | 31.10.1927 | F | | 1338 | 1355 | Script for Laxido, Co-codamol, BuTrans patches & Trimethoprim given | | VFL | Home visit. |
| 30.07.2013 | 27.08.1933 | M | | 1645 | 1653 | Script for Trimethoprim given | | HGH | For MSU. |
| 30.07.2013 | 19.08.1939 | F | | 1653 | 1709 | For Chest X-Rays | | JEN | |
| 30.07.2013 | 10.09.1989 | F | | 1709 | 1717 | Script for Citalopram & Erythromycin given | | SED | For Pelvic USScan (urgent). |
| 30.07.2013 | 02.10.1943 | M | | 1717 | 1724 | Script for Gabapentin given | | SHS | |
| 30.07.2013 | 21.04.1949 | M | | 1724 | 1730 | Medications Review Done | | RL | |
| 30.07.2013 | 09.03.2012 | F | | 1740 | 1748 | Script for Amoxycillin given | | LRP | |
| 30.07.2013 | 28.09.1978 | F | | 1748 | 1756 | Referred to Orthopaedic Surgeon regarding her persistent back pain | | TLJ | |

718

## Result of a query that lists all consultations from the 22nd to the end of July 2013 (ConsultationsSeenFrom22ndTillEndOfJul2013)

| SurgeryDate | DateOfBirth | Sex | Diagnosis | TimeIn | TimeOut | Complaints | Treatments | Initials | Notes |
|---|---|---|---|---|---|---|---|---|---|
| 30.07.2013 | 17.07.1983 | M | | 1756 | 1802 | Script for Flucloxacillin given | | JRC | |
| 30.07.2013 | 14.08.1946 | M | | 1802 | 1840 | Routine Taxi Medical Examination done | | RBG | |

## Result of a query that lists all consultations from the 22nd to the end of July 2014 (ConsultationsSeenFrom22ndTillEndOfJul2014)

| SurgeryDate | DateOfBirth | Sex | Diagnosis | TimeIn | TimeOut | Complaints | Treatments | Initials | Notes |
|---|---|---|---|---|---|---|---|---|---|
| 22.07.2014 | 11.07.1962 | M | | 944 | 958 | Script for Amlodipine given | | JEG | For FBC, Fasting Glucose, TFTs, U/Es, LFTs & Cholesterol. |
| 22.07.2014 | 28.06.1956 | M | | 958 | 1003 | Medications Review Done | | TLP | |
| 22.07.2014 | 01.12.1942 | M | | 1003 | 1016 | Script for Doxycycline & Chloramphenicol eye drops given | | MP | For FBC, U/Es, Cholesterol, LFTs. |
| 22.07.2014 | 23.12.1942 | F | | 1016 | 1024 | Script for Loratadine given | | JASP | For FBC, U/Es, HbA1c, Cholesterol, LFTs & urine microalbumin screen. |
| 22.07.2014 | 22.05.1931 | F | | 1024 | 1043 | She may come back for us to refer her back to Dr. Won, Rheumatologist | | DK | |

Result of a query that lists all consultations from the 22nd to the end of July 2014 (ConsultationsSeenFrom22ndTillEndOfJul2014)

| SurgeryDate | DateOfBirth | Sex | Diagnosis | TimeIn | TimeOut | Complaints | Treatments | Initials | Notes |
|---|---|---|---|---|---|---|---|---|---|
| 22.07.2014 | 31.10.1943 | M | | 1043 | 1050 | Script for Transvasin Heat Rub cream given | | NFH | |
| 22.07.2014 | 22.02.1936 | F | | 1050 | 1114 | Script for Aymes given | | RPM | She may need letter to Gastroenterologist to expedite her appointment. |
| 22.07.2014 | 20.06.1974 | F | S/Leave | 1114 | 1121 | Med. 3 04/10 given for Dizziness & Vomiting for 2 weeks from 22.07.14 | | SLS | Script for Amitriptyline given. |
| 22.07.2014 | 03.07.1940 | F | | 1121 | 1130 | Script for Co-codamol given | | JMM | |
| 22.07.2014 | 11.08.1943 | F | | 1645 | 1656 | Medications Review Done | | JMEH | |
| 22.07.2014 | 02.05.1987 | F | | 1652 | 1702 | For FBC, U/Es, Fasting Glucose & TFTs | | JT | |
| 22.07.2014 | 07.02.1948 | M | | 1702 | 1725 | Script for Orlistat given | | GRC | |
| 22.07.2014 | 06.07.1948 | M | | 1725 | 1736 | Referred for Colonoscopy regarding his recurrent diarrhoea | | DRS | For LFTs, Clotting screen & USScan of the abdomen. |
| 22.07.2014 | 17.03.1958 | M | | 1736 | 1747 | Script for Permethrin 5% cream & Tears Naturale eye drops given | | KEW | Referred to Ophthalmologist (Dr. Idre) regarding his weepy & sore eyes. |

Result of a query that lists all consultations from the 22nd to the end of July 2014 (ConsultationsSeenFrom22ndTillEndOfJul2014)

| SurgeryDate | DateOfBirth | Sex | Diagnosis | TimeIn | TimeOut | Complaints | Treatments | Initials | Notes |
|---|---|---|---|---|---|---|---|---|---|
| 22.07.2014 | 07.05.1974 | M | | 1747 | 1757 | Script for Ventolin evohaler given | | SC | Referred to Dermatologist regarding the mole in his perineal area. |
| 22.07.2014 | 16.09.1980 | F | | 1757 | 1801 | For Urine Pregnancy test | | LCY | |
| 22.07.2014 | 13.01.1966 | M | | 1801 | 1814 | Referred to Orthopaedic Surgeon (Knee Surgeon) privately regarding injury to the (R) knee | | PJB | |
| 22.07.2014 | 06.08.1941 | M | | 1814 | 1827 | Script for Forxiga given | | AJM | |
| 23.07.2014 | 23.09.1951 | F | | 942 | 956 | For Rheumatoid Factor & Bone profile | | DJS | |
| 23.07.2014 | 02.05.1990 | F | | 956 | 1004 | Script for Citalopram given | | MTG | |
| 23.07.2014 | 08.01.2009 | M | RTI | 1004 | 1010 | Chesty cough | Amoxycillin | CNC | |
| 23.07.2014 | 17.04.1945 | F | | 1010 | 1018 | Script for Lansoprazole given | | MC | |
| 23.07.2014 | 20.05.1987 | F | | 1021 | 1030 | Referred to Counsellor regarding feeling low & unable to cope | | DADS | |
| 23.07.2014 | 09.12.1945 | F | | 1030 | 1037 | Script for Canesten HC cream given | | AML | |

Result of a query that lists all consultations from the 22nd to the end of July 2014 (ConsultationsSeenFrom22ndTillEndOfJul2014)

| SurgeryDate | DateOfBirth | Sex | Diagnosis | TimeIn | TimeOut | Complaints | Treatments | Initials | Notes |
|---|---|---|---|---|---|---|---|---|---|
| 23.07.2014 | 18.02.1968 | F | | 1041 | 1052 | I explained to her that I am not happy to be prescribing her 2 litres of Gaviscon monthly regularly | | PAC | |
| 23.07.2014 | 23.05.1952 | F | | 1052 | 1104 | Script for Cetirizine given | | MEH | For DEXA scan. |
| 23.07.2014 | 01.02.1931 | M | | 1235 | 1250 | Clinically he does not appear to be in any pain or discomfort | | MDS | Home visit. |
| 23.07.2014 | 05.09.1963 | M | | 1645 | 1652 | Script for Simvastatin given | | RJW | |
| 23.07.2014 | 21.08.1934 | F | | 1652 | 1701 | Stool for C&S | | IEW | |
| 23.07.2014 | 09.04.1971 | M | | 1701 | 1710 | Script for Paracetamol given | | MH | |
| 23.07.2014 | 18.11.1982 | F | | 1710 | 1720 | Script for Metronidazole & Erythromycin given | | VAB | Penicillin allergy. |
| 23.07.2014 | 22.04.1942 | F | | 1720 | 1725 | Medications Review Done | | JS | |
| 23.07.2014 | 15.09.1939 | M | | 1725 | 1732 | For serum Ferritin, Folate & B12 | | WJS | |
| 23.07.2014 | 12.11.1944 | F | | 1741 | 1753 | Referred to Neurosurgeon (Mr. Pollock) to expedite her clinic appointment | | PM | |
| 23.07.2014 | 01.12.1934 | F | | 1753 | 1803 | Script for Isotard XL given | | LFM | |

Result of a query that lists all consultations from the 22nd to the end of July 2014 (ConsultationsSeenFrom22ndTillEndOfJul2014)

| SurgeryDate | DateOfBirth | Sex | Diagnosis | TimeIn | TimeOut | Complaints | Treatments | Initials | Notes |
|---|---|---|---|---|---|---|---|---|---|
| 23.07.2014 | 14.12.1971 | M | | 1803 | 1814 | Script for Mirtazapine given | | SPH | |
| 23.07.2014 | 05.04.1964 | F | | 1814 | 1824 | Script for Canesten HC cream & Doxycycline given | | JL | |
| 24.07.2014 | 28.06.1959 | M | | 946 | 959 | BP 144/90 | | SCU | |
| 24.07.2014 | 23.07.1953 | M | | 959 | 1011 | Referred to ENT Surgeon regarding pain & blockage in the (R) ear, to be deferred for now | | THM | |
| 24.07.2014 | 19.06.1944 | F | | 1011 | 1018 | Script for Co-codamol & Docusate capsules given | | PJL | |
| 24.07.2014 | 03.09.1951 | M | | 1018 | 1025 | Script for Trimethoprim given | | GLF | For MSU. |
| 24.07.2014 | 02.12.1973 | F | | 1025 | 1042 | Referred to Gynaecologist regarding her persistent heavy persistent prolonged periods | | MC | |
| 24.07.2014 | 20.02.1930 | M | | 1042 | 1056 | Referred to Gastroenterologist regarding his dark stools & anaemia | | AL | |
| 24.07.2014 | 22.05.1931 | F | | 1056 | 1106 | Referred to DVT clinic to exclude DVT (L) leg | | DK | |

Result of a query that lists all consultations from the 22nd to the end of July 2014 (ConsultationsSeenFrom22ndTillEndOfJul2014)

| SurgeryDate | DateOfBirth | Sex | Diagnosis | TimeIn | TimeOut | Complaints | Treatments | Initials | Notes |
|---|---|---|---|---|---|---|---|---|---|
| 24.07.2014 | 31.06.1975 | F | | 1106 | 1115 | Script for Co-Amoxiclav oral suspension given | | AKE | |
| 24.07.2014 | 04.08.1936 | M | | 1115 | 1139 | Script for Doxycycline given | | ECM | |
| 24.07.2014 | 06.01.1955 | M | | 1640 | 1647 | Private script for Sildenafil given | | MAS | |
| 24.07.2014 | 14.10.1938 | F | | 1649 | 1715 | Referred to Vascular Surgeon regarding pain in both legs on walking short distances | | DT | For FBC, U/Es, HbA1c, urine microalbumin screen, LFTs & Cholesterol. |
| 24.07.2014 | 08.01.1942 | F | | 1715 | 1722 | Script for Fucidin H cream & Doxycycline given | | SM | |
| 24.07.2014 | 03.03.1946 | M | | 1722 | 1734 | Referred to Dermatologist (Community) regarding fungal nail infection & fluid coming from under the nail bed | | SP | |
| 24.07.2014 | 27.07.1999 | M | | 1734 | 1740 | Script for Canesten HC cream given | | JJB | |
| 24.07.2014 | 05.10.1974 | M | | 1740 | 1748 | Referred to Orthopaedic Surgeon (knee surgeon) regarding persistent pain & swelling in the (L) knee following a fall | | SMG | |

724

Result of a query that lists all consultations from the 22nd to the end of July 2014 (ConsultationsSeenFrom22ndTillEndOfJul2014)

| SurgeryDate | DateOfBirth | Sex | Diagnosis | TimeIn | TimeOut | Complaints | Treatments | Initials | Notes |
|---|---|---|---|---|---|---|---|---|---|
| 24.07.2014 | 21.05.1958 | F | | 1754 | 1802 | For MSU | | SB | |
| 24.07.2014 | 03.07.2001 | M | | 1802 | 1816 | Script for Co-Amoxiclav & Terbinafine cream given | | TLM | For FBC, U/Es & Fasting Glucose. |
| 25.07.2014 | 07.06.1955 | F | S/Leave | 943 | 1004 | Med. 3 04/10 given for Pain in the Back & (L) Hip for 6 months from 25.07.14 | | JM | Script for Ferrous Fumarate & Forxiga given. |
| 25.07.2014 | 13.11.1952 | F | | 1004 | 1010 | Script for Fucidin H cream given | | LH | |
| 25.07.2014 | 14.07.1982 | F | | 1010 | 1016 | Script for Anugesic-HC cream & Uniroid HC suppositories given | | SMR | |
| 25.07.2014 | 11.07.2014 | M | | 1016 | 1019 | To try Gripe water for his infantile colic | | JISL | |
| 25.07.2014 | 09.03.2012 | F | | 1019 | 1026 | Script for Oilatum Junior cream given | | LRP | |
| 25.07.2014 | 21.10.1929 | F | | 1026 | 1034 | Script for Mepore dressings & Clarithromycin given | | PMJ | |
| 25.07.2014 | 02.07.1924 | M | | 1037 | 1056 | His daughter came to discuss his placement for respite care in a Kent home to collect the paper work, fee 1.00 pound | | TCC | |

725

Result of a query that lists all consultations from the 22nd to the end of July 2014 (ConsultationsSeenFrom22ndTillEndOfJul2014)

| SurgeryDate | DateOfBirth | Sex | Diagnosis | TimeIn | TimeOut | Complaints | Treatments | Initials | Notes |
|---|---|---|---|---|---|---|---|---|---|
| 25.07.2014 | 04.07.1929 | M |  | 1056 | 1105 | Eprex 2000iu/0.5ml given in (R) Deltoid |  | RMC |  |
| 28.07.2014 | 13.03.1938 | F |  | 945 | 955 | Script for Prochlorperazine given |  | DGP |  |
| 28.07.2014 | 27.03.1987 | F | S/Leave | 955 | 1005 | Med. 3 04/10 given for Possible Urticarial Rash for 1 month from 25.07.14 |  | MMW | Script for Hydroxychloroquine & Microgynon 30 given. |
| 28.07.2014 | 09.07.1940 | M |  | 1005 | 1022 | Script for Amoxycillin given |  | WW | For Fasting Glucose, HbA1c & TFTs. |
| 28.07.2014 | 04.10.1968 | F |  | 1022 | 1030 | She is due to be seen in Eye clinic in Southend hospital on 30.07.14 |  | AW |  |
| 28.07.2014 | 13.04.1944 | M |  | 1030 | 1039 | Script for Furosemide given |  | RAP | For serum BNP. |
| 28.07.2014 | 29.11.1937 | F |  | 1043 | 1102 | Script for Fenbid 5% gel & Quinine Sulphate given |  | MRS |  |
| 28.07.2014 | 04.07.1929 | M |  | 1102 | 1110 | Eprex 2000iu/0.5ml given in (R) Deltoid |  | RMC |  |
| 28.07.2014 | 06.10.2013 | F |  | 1110 | 1120 | Script for Amoxycillin & Paracetamol given |  | MJJR |  |
| 28.07.2014 | 03.02.1957 | M |  | 1649 | 1659 | Awaiting response from Podiatrist to find out what type of consultant they want him referred to |  | ER |  |

Result of a query that lists all consultations from the 22nd to the end of July 2014 (ConsultationsSeenFrom22ndTillEndOfJul2014)

| SurgeryDate | DateOfBirth | Sex | Diagnosis | TimeIn | TimeOut | Complaints | Treatments | Initials | Notes |
|---|---|---|---|---|---|---|---|---|---|
| 28.07.2014 | 31.01.1969 | F | | 1659 | 1706 | To remain on Levothyroxine permanently | | JP | |
| 28.07.2014 | 10.10.1964 | F | | 1706 | 1715 | For DEXA scan | | KF | |
| 28.07.2014 | 03.07.1939 | M | | 1715 | 1724 | For B12, Folate & Ferritin | | RFL | |
| 28.07.2014 | 06.09.1984 | M | | 1724 | 1737 | Script for Flucloxacillin given | | BJP | |
| 28.07.2014 | 16.07.1968 | F | S/Leave | 1737 | 1747 | Med. 3 04/10 given for Breathlessness for 1 month from 28.07.14 | | JLF | Script for Ventolin Evohaler & Qvar inhaler given. For Chest X-Rays. |
| 28.07.2014 | 29.12.1975 | F | | 1747 | 1757 | For MSU & Pelvic USScan | | JC | |
| 28.07.2014 | 29.04.1984 | M | | 1759 | 1806 | Script for Ibuprofen & Co-codamol given | | RJB | |
| 29.07.2014 | 17.08.1912 | F | | 942 | 958 | Script for Clarithromycin & Simple Linctus given | | IAA | For Chest X-Rays. |
| 29.07.2014 | 09.03.1937 | F | | 958 | 1006 | For Ferritin, Folate, B12, TFTs & urine microalbumin screen | | HGE | |
| 29.07.2014 | 28.02.1960 | F | | 1006 | 1017 | She will like to see the pain management specialist before starting on Gabapentin | | JS | |

727

Result of a query that lists all consultations from the 22nd to the end of July 2014 (ConsultationsSeenFrom22ndTillEndOfJul2014)

| SurgeryDate | DateOfBirth | Sex | Diagnosis | TimeIn | TimeOut | Complaints | Treatments | Initials | Notes |
|---|---|---|---|---|---|---|---|---|---|
| 29.07.2014 | 14.07.1932 | F | | 1017 | 1029 | Script for Furosemide & Doxycycline given | | JB | For FBC, U/Es, TFTs & BNP. |
| 29.07.2014 | 18.03.1967 | F | | 1029 | 1036 | Script for Amoxycillin, Cetraben cream & Loratadine given | | SO | |
| 29.07.2014 | 23.06.1962 | M | | 1036 | 1042 | For repeat FBC in one month, form given to the patient | | RJE | |
| 29.07.2014 | 23.05.1927 | M | | 1042 | 1100 | Script for Fenbid 5% gel, Clarithromycin & Permethrin 5% cream given | | JM | |
| 29.07.2014 | 13.03.1932 | M | | 1100 | 1112 | Medications Review Done | | BJC | |
| 29.07.2014 | 19.06.1943 | M | | 1338 | 1350 | Script for Oramorph given | | BFS | Home visit. |
| 29.07.2014 | 10.03.2004 | M | | 1651 | 1659 | Script for Clonidine given | | CJCB | |
| 29.07.2014 | 16.12.1987 | M | | 1659 | 1705 | Script for Duac gel given | | NM | |
| 29.07.2014 | 18.07.1965 | F | | 1705 | 1721 | For repeat TFTs in 2 months, form given to the patient | | LSC | |
| 29.07.2014 | 08.01.1972 | M | | 1722 | 1730 | Referred to Rheumatologist regarding pains in both arms, worse on the (L) side | | EM | |

Result of a query that lists all consultations from the 22nd to the end of July 2014 (ConsultationsSeenFrom22ndTillEndOFJul2014)

| SurgeryDate | DateOfBirth | Sex | Diagnosis | TimeIn | TimeOut | Complaints | Treatments | Initials | Notes |
|---|---|---|---|---|---|---|---|---|---|
| 29.07.2014 | 19.10.1978 | M | | 1740 | 1753 | Script for Flucloxacillin given | | JDS | |
| 29.07.2014 | 21.06.1975 | F | | 1753 | 1840 | Taxi Medical Examination Done | | AKE | |
| 30.07.2014 | 12.08.1936 | M | | 946 | 952 | For repeat MSU in one month, form given to the patient | | RHP | |
| 30.07.2014 | 28.06.1959 | M | | 952 | 1002 | To see the nurse monthly for BP checks | | SCU | |
| 30.07.2014 | 03.09.1951 | M | | 1002 | 1013 | For FBC, U/Es, PSA & repeat MSU in one month | | GLH | |
| 30.07.2014 | 28.06.1959 | F | | 1013 | 1022 | Referred back to ENT Surgeon regarding her painful (L) ear | | PIS | |
| 30.07.2014 | 05.12.2007 | F | | 1022 | 1027 | For MSU | | ABH | |
| 30.07.2014 | 31.07.1961 | F | | 1027 | 1040 | Script for Citalopram given | | CMW | |
| 30.07.2014 | 22.05.1931 | F | | 1051 | 1058 | Script for Furosemide given | | DK | |
| 30.07.2014 | 26.10.1943 | F | | 1103 | 1109 | Script for Janumet given | | APM | |
| 30.07.2014 | 05.04.1937 | M | | 1230 | 1245 | BP 98/50 | | JM | Home visit. |
| 30.07.2014 | 25.03.1944 | M | | 1644 | 1653 | For X-Rays of the (L) knee | | RFB | |

Result of a query that lists all consultations from the 22nd to the end of July 2014 (ConsultationsSeenFrom22ndTillEndOfJul2014)

| SurgeryDate | DateOfBirth | Sex | Diagnosis | TimeIn | TimeOut | Complaints | Treatments | Initials | Notes |
|---|---|---|---|---|---|---|---|---|---|
| 30.07.2014 | 04.01.1932 | F | | 1653 | 1700 | To stop the Loperamide & to take own Dioralyte if necessary | | EAC | |
| 30.07.2014 | 09.05.1955 | M | | 1700 | 1708 | For KUB USScan | | SL | |
| 30.07.2014 | 28.09.1937 | F | | 1708 | 1715 | To try OTC OroCalm spray | | MR | |
| 30.07.2014 | 15.01.1935 | F | | 1715 | 1722 | Script for Doxycycline given | | JRS | |
| 30.07.2014 | 22.10.2009 | F | | 1724 | 1732 | Hygiene measures discussed including Savlon & salt baths | | CMGM | |
| 30.07.2014 | 14.01.1994 | F | | 1753 | 1818 | Travel Claims Medical Certificate completed | | GJG | |

Result of a query that lists all consultations from the 22nd to the end of July 2015 (ConsultationsSeenFrom22ndTillEndOfJul2015)

| SurgeryDate | DateOfBirth | Sex | Diagnosis | TimeIn | TimeOut | Complaints | Treatments | Initials | Notes |
|---|---|---|---|---|---|---|---|---|---|
| 22.07.2015 | 20.07.1961 | M | | 947 | 1013 | For FBC, U/Es, LFTs, Cholesterol, Testosterone & Fasting Glucose | | DIC | |
| 22.07.2015 | 20.11.1944 | M | | 1003 | 1010 | Medications Review Done | | JE | |
| 22.07.2015 | 26.12.1951 | F | | 1010 | 1017 | Script for Acyclovir tablets given | | DCP | |

Result of a query that lists all consultations from the 22nd to the end of July 2015 (ConsultationsSeenFrom22ndTillEndOfJul2015)

| SurgeryDate | DateOfBirth | Sex | Diagnosis | TimeIn | TimeOut | Complaints | Treatments | Initials | Notes |
|---|---|---|---|---|---|---|---|---|---|
| 22.07.2015 | 17.05.1939 | M | | 1017 | 1025 | He is happy to take Paracetamol for his (R) shoulder & (R) knee pain | | JTN | |
| 22.07.2015 | 16.05.1938 | M | | 1025 | 1034 | Referred to Dermatologist (Private - Benenden) regarding BCC lesion on his (R) cheek | | CJW | |
| 22.07.2015 | 08.07.1940 | F | | 1034 | 1042 | Script for Voltarol Emugel given | | MTB | |
| 22.07.2015 | 18.04.1930 | F | | 1045 | 1114 | Script for Doxycycline, Qvar inhaler, Scholl softgrip class 2 below knee stocking given | | IDB | For Chest X-Rays, FBC, U/Es, LFTs, Cholesterol. |
| 22.07.2015 | 22.06.1979 | M | | 1114 | 1122 | Script for Fucibet cream & Prednisolone tablets given | | DC | |
| 22.07.2015 | 08.11.1929 | M | | 1300 | 1316 | Referred to Occupational Therapist regarding his knee which keeps giving way & for assessment for wearable support | | FAD | For X-Rays of the (L) knee. Home visit. |

Result of a query that lists all consultations from the 22nd to the end of July 2015 (ConsultationsSeenFrom22ndTillEndOfJul2015)

| SurgeryDate | DateOfBirth | Sex | Diagnosis | TimeIn | TimeOut | Complaints | Treatments | Initials | Notes |
|---|---|---|---|---|---|---|---|---|---|
| 22.07.2015 | 29.11.1946 | F | | 1645 | 1655 | Script for Doxycycline, Prednisolone & Ventolin Evohaler given | | PW | |
| 22.07.2015 | 24.10.1954 | M | | 1655 | 1707 | Referred to Physiotherapist regarding persistent pain in the the (R) knee as requested by Physiotherapist | | PW | |
| 22.07.2015 | 08.07.1998 | F | | 1707 | 1714 | Medications Review Done | | COSP | |
| 22.07.2015 | 30.03.1960 | F | | 1722 | 1734 | Script for Co-Amoxiclav given | | MTP | |
| 22.07.2015 | 29.09.1995 | M | | 1734 | 1743 | Script for Erythromycin given | | JSC | |
| 22.07.2015 | 01.09.1985 | F | | 1745 | 1843 | Referred to Gynaecologist regarding her recurrent offensive yellow vaginal discharge | | SS | |
| 22.07.2015 | 09.05.1991 | F | | 1803 | 1813 | Script for Erythromycin given | | CEB | Penicillin allergy. |
| 23.07.2015 | 23.06.1994 | M | | 944 | 954 | BP 133/78 | | KCDA | |
| 23.07.2015 | 22.02.1944 | M | | 954 | 1000 | Medications Review Done | | AS | |

Result of a query that lists all consultations from the 22nd to the end of July 2015 (ConsultationsSeenFrom22ndTillEndOfJul2015)

| SurgeryDate | DateOfBirth | Sex | Diagnosis | TimeIn | TimeOut | Complaints | Treatments | Initials | Notes |
|---|---|---|---|---|---|---|---|---|---|
| 23.07.2015 | 12.09.1994 | F | | 1009 | 1024 | For FBC, U/Es, TFTs, Fasting Glucose, Bone profile, LFTs & Fasting Lipids | | TS | |
| 23.07.2015 | 22.03.1931 | F | | 1024 | 1039 | Script for Carmellose eye drops, Fostair inhaler & Fucidin H cream | | HH | |
| 23.07.2015 | 07.08.1996 | F | | 1039 | 1048 | Referred to Haematologist regarding her bruises as advised by the Haematologist | | NP | |
| 23.07.2015 | 10.06.2002 | F | | 1048 | 1058 | Script for Erythromycin, Paracetamol & Ibuprofen given | | PCC | For FBC, U/Es & Fasting Glucose. Penicillin allergy. |
| 23.07.2015 | 30.04.1941 | F | | 1058 | 1106 | Script for Flucloxacillin given | | VRG | |
| 23.07.2015 | 08.05.1974 | M | S/Leave | 1106 | 1124 | Med. 3 04/10 given for Back Pain for 3 months from 09.07.15 | | TW | Referred to Orthopaedic Surgeon regarding his persistent (L) dislocated index finger. |
| 23.07.2015 | 15.10.1925 | F | | 1248 | 1310 | Script for Trimethoprim & Paracetamol given | | RAA | Home visit. |

733

Result of a query that lists all consultations from the 22nd to the end of July 2015 (ConsultationsSeenFrom22ndTillEndOfJul2015)

| SurgeryDate | DateOfBirth | Sex | Diagnosis | TimeIn | TimeOut | Complaints | Treatments | Initials | Notes |
|---|---|---|---|---|---|---|---|---|---|
| 23.07.2015 | 25.06.1938 | F | | 1649 | 1702 | Referred to Orthopaedic Surgeon regarding pain in the (R) hip | | JEL | |
| 23.07.2015 | 09.07.1940 | M | | 1702 | 1717 | Referred to Cardiologist regarding his palpitations & dizziness attacks | | WW | |
| 23.07.2015 | 06.07.1936 | F | | 1717 | 1732 | Script for Clarithromycin & Lansoprazole given | | MLW | For FBC, U/Es, HbA1c, Cholesterol & LFTs. Penicillin & Doxazosin allergy. |
| 23.07.2015 | 16.03.1956 | F | | 1732 | 1742 | For Chest X-Rays & MSU | | SPD | |
| 23.07.2015 | 08.06.1957 | F | | 1742 | 1752 | She will continue with the anti-epileptic medication & does not want to go back to see the Neurologist yet | | JAR | |
| 23.07.2015 | 15.09.1957 | M | S/Leave | 1752 | 1758 | Med. 3 04/10 given for Injury to the (R) knee for 3 months from 23.07.15 | | PSB | |
| 23.07.2015 | 23.10.1996 | F | | 1758 | 1804 | Urine Pregnancy test is positive | | JAS | |

Result of a query that lists all consultations from the 22nd to the end of July 2015 (ConsultationsSeenFrom22ndTillEndOfJul2015)

| SurgeryDate | DateOfBirth | Sex | Diagnosis | TimeIn | TimeOut | Complaints | Treatments | Initials | Notes |
|---|---|---|---|---|---|---|---|---|---|
| 23.07.2015 | 11.08.1983 | F | | 1804 | 1820 | Script for Co-Amoxiclav given | | RJN | For MSU, Ferritin, FBC, U/Es, Folate & USScan of the kidneys. |
| 24.07.2015 | 20.04.1938 | M | | 944 | 957 | To see me in 3 months for repeat FBC, U/Es & PSA | | DAD | |
| 24.07.2015 | 02.03.1957 | F | | 957 | 1005 | Script for Doxycycline & Otomize ear spray given | | EPS | |
| 24.07.2015 | 06.04.1937 | M | | 1005 | 1016 | BP 142/70 | | GWH | |
| 24.07.2015 | 21.06.1942 | M | | 1016 | 1025 | BP 138/85 | | WJB | |
| 24.07.2015 | 25.11.1987 | F | | 1025 | 1035 | Script for Ferrous Sulphate & Dermovate scalp application | | KMB | |
| 24.07.2015 | 06.10.1933 | M | | 1035 | 1049 | Script for Nasacort Allergy nasal spray given | | FJK | For PSA, Cholesterol, FBC, U/Es, LFTs & for X-Rays of the (R) hip. |
| 24.07.2015 | 04.07.1929 | M | | 1049 | 1059 | To see what the Haematologist say about his anaemia when he sees them next month | | RMC | |

Result of a query that lists all consultations from the 22nd to the end of July 2015 (ConsultationsSeenFrom22ndTillEndOfJul2015)

| SurgeryDate | DateOfBirth | Sex | Diagnosis | TimeIn | TimeOut | Complaints | Treatments | Initials | Notes |
|---|---|---|---|---|---|---|---|---|---|
| 24.07.2015 | 04.08.1936 | M | | 1059 | 1107 | He does not want to use the Praxilene any more as he has not found them particularly useful | | ECM | |
| 27.07.2015 | 04.04.1953 | M | S/Leave | 944 | 954 | Med. 3 04/10 given for (L) ankle revision for 1 month from 25.07.15 | | GC | |
| 27.07.2015 | 23.04.1950 | F | | 954 | 1003 | Script for Premarin 0.3mg tablets given | | PEH | |
| 27.07.2015 | 24.04.1939 | M | | 1003 | 1013 | Script for Allopurinol & Colchicine given | | JC | |
| 27.07.2015 | 24.04.1948 | F | | 103 | 1028 | Script for Lisinopril given | | CSP | For FBC, U/Es, Cholesterol, LFTs, TFTs & Fasting Lipids. |
| 27.07.2015 | 23.09.1951 | F | S/Leave | 1032 | 1042 | Med. 3 04/10 given for (L) ankle revision for 1 month from 25.07.15 | | DJS | |
| 27.07.2015 | 23.12.1952 | F | | 1051 | 1102 | For LFTs | | GCB | Drinks diary given to the patient to be completed. |
| 27.07.2015 | 15.10.1925 | F | | 1220 | 1240 | Script for Oramorph given | | RAA | Home visit. |
| 27.07.2015 | 27.08.1935 | M | | 1243 | 1300 | Script for Flagyl & Doxycycline given | | AAS | Home visit. |

Result of a query that lists all consultations from the 22nd to the end of July 2015 (ConsultationsSeenFrom22ndTillEndOfJul2015)

| SurgeryDate | DateOfBirth | Sex | Diagnosis | TimeIn | TimeOut | Complaints | Treatments | Initials | Notes |
|---|---|---|---|---|---|---|---|---|---|
| 27.07.2015 | 29.10.1949 | F | | 1704 | 1717 | Script for Indapamide given | | DT | For FBC, U/Es, Cholesterol & LFTs. |
| 27.07.2015 | 04.07.1961 | F | | 1717 | 1727 | Script for Amoxycillin given | | JB | |
| 27.07.2015 | 24.12.1930 | M | | 1727 | 1756 | Nitromin sublingual spray & Indapamide give | | DJJ | For FBC, U/Es, LFTs, TFTs, Fasting Glucose, Fasting Lipids & Chest X-Rays. |
| 27.07.2015 | 02.01.1955 | M | | 1756 | 1808 | Advised to inform the DVLA about his sleep apnoea | | TRE | |
| 27.07.2015 | 19.09.1984 | M | | 1808 | 1820 | Referred for Vasectomy | | RLWL | |
| 28.07.2015 | 06.04.1937 | M | | 944 | 954 | BP 144/78 | | GWH | |
| 28.07.2015 | 02.04.1963 | M | S/Leave | 954 | 1000 | Med. 3 04/10 given for Bereavement for 1 month from 28.07.15 | | AIM | |
| 28.07.2015 | 18.09.1974 | M | | 1000 | 1008 | Script for Lansoprazole given | | RVM | |
| 28.07.2015 | 14.08.1935 | M | | 1008 | 1030 | For FBC, U/Es, HbA1c, Cholesterol, LFTs, TFTs & Urine microalbumin screen | | RAT | |

Result of a query that lists all consultations from the 22nd to the end of July 2015 (ConsultationsSeenFrom22ndTillEndOfJul2015)

| SurgeryDate | DateOfBirth | Sex | Diagnosis | TimeIn | TimeOut | Complaints | Treatments | Initials | Notes |
|---|---|---|---|---|---|---|---|---|---|
| 28.07.2015 | 24.07.1956 | M | | 1030 | 1040 | Script for Dermovate 0.05% scalp application, Fexofenadine & Prednisolone tablets given | | SS | |
| 28.07.2015 | 03.07.1940 | F | | 1040 | 1111 | Script for BuTrans patches & Tramulief SR given | | JMM | |
| 28.07.2015 | 25.11.1949 | M | | 1111 | 1116 | For PSA | | GJD | |
| 28.07.2015 | 11.05.2015 | F | | 1116 | 1123 | Script for Chloramphenicol eye drops given | | SAK | |
| 28.07.2015 | 01.07.1948 | M | | 1645 | 1708 | Script for Citalopram given | | JFE | For FBC, U/Es, HbA1c, LFTs, Cholesterol, TFTs & urine microalbumin screen. |
| 28.07.2015 | 23.01.2015 | F | | 1708 | 1713 | Script for Nystan oral suspension & Paracetamol given | | MAPL | |
| 28.07.2015 | 30.03.1943 | M | | 1713 | 1721 | Script for Doxycycline & Prednisolone given | | BWF | |
| 28.07.2015 | 07.06.1955 | F | | 1721 | 1730 | Script for Co-Amoxiclav given | | JM | |
| 28.07.2015 | 06.04.1960 | M | | 1734 | 1744 | Script for Tramadol & Citalopram given | | AMB | |

Result of a query that lists all consultations from the 22nd to the end of July 2015 (ConsultationsSeenFrom22ndTillEndOfJul2015)

| SurgeryDate | DateOfBirth | Sex | Diagnosis | TimeIn | TimeOut | Complaints | Treatments | Initials | Notes |
|---|---|---|---|---|---|---|---|---|---|
| 28.07.2015 | 09.06.1993 | F | | 1744 | 1750 | For Urine Pregnancy test | | AL | |
| 28.07.2015 | 17.09.1961 | F | | 1750 | 1800 | Script for Amoxycillin & Laxido orange given | | TJB | |
| 28.07.2015 | 06.08.1981 | M | | 1800 | 1812 | To see me in 4 to 6 weeks to review the mole on his (R) fore-arm | | REH | |
| 29.07.2015 | 28.12.1962 | M | | 946 | 1001 | Script for Allopurinol & Diclofenac given | | KF | For X-Rays of the (R) foot, U/Es, Cholesterol, LFTs, Uric acid & Fasting Glucose. |
| 29.07.2015 | 18.10.1974 | F | | 1001 | 1010 | Script for Doxycycline given | | HAW | For Chest X-Rays, FBC, U/Es, Cholesterol & LFTs. |
| 29.07.2015 | 27.02.1938 | F | | 1010 | 1022 | To continue to leave off the Co-Tenidone and to see the nurse in 3 months for BP check | | REH | |
| 29.07.2015 | 12.08.1993 | M | | 1027 | 1042 | Script for Balneum Plus bath oil, Balneum Plus cream & Fexofenadine given | | DTA | Referred to Dermatologist regarding his severe eczema. |

Result of a query that lists all consultations from the 22nd to the end of July 2015 (ConsultationsSeenFrom22ndTillEndOfJul2015)

| SurgeryDate | DateOfBirth | Sex | Diagnosis | TimeIn | TimeOut | Complaints | Treatments | Initials | Notes |
|---|---|---|---|---|---|---|---|---|---|
| 29.07.2015 | 05.03.1965 | F | | 1042 | 1051 | Referred to Dermatologist (Community) regarding her multiple dermatological problems (skin thickenings, Vitiligo & Psoriasis | | ALG | |
| 29.07.2015 | 31.05.1946 | F | | 1051 | 1101 | Referred to Orthopaedic Surgeon (knee Surgeon) regarding Baker's cyst on the (L) knee | | VIL | For X-Rays of the (L) knee. |
| 29.07.2015 | 22.07.1961 | M | | 1101 | 1111 | Script for Codeine tablets, Diazepam & Naproxen given | | PWL | |
| 29.07.2015 | 01.07.2014 | M | | 1111 | 1118 | Referred to Paediatrician regarding his constipation | | KRMF | Script for Laxido Paediatric Plain oral powder given |
| 29.07.2015 | 03.01.1939 | M | | 1303 | 1316 | Script for Amoxycillin given | | GJS | Home visit. |
| 29.07.2015 | 16.12.1956 | M | | 1647 | 1657 | Referred Gastroscopy regarding his Barrett's oesophagus | | PGT | |
| 29.07.2015 | 03.05.1938 | F | | 1657 | 1706 | For Ferritin, Folate & B12 | | MFB | |

740

Result of a query that lists all consultations from the 22nd to the end of July 2015 (ConsultationsSeenFrom22ndTillEndOfJul2015)

| SurgeryDate | DateOfBirth | Sex | Diagnosis | TimeIn | TimeOut | Complaints | Treatments | Initials | Notes |
|---|---|---|---|---|---|---|---|---|---|
| 29.07.2015 | 22.09.1967 | F | S/Leave | 1706 | 1730 | Med. 3 04/10 given for Myasthenia Gravis for 2 months from 20.07.15 | | SG | |
| 29.07.2015 | 12.10.1973 | F | | 1730 | 1745 | Script for Fluoxetine, Ibuprofen, Omeprazole & Quetiapine given | | DMB | |
| 29.07.2015 | 21.11.1954 | M | | 1745 | 1757 | Script for Ramipril given | | GLS | |
| 29.07.2015 | 01.09.1983 | F | | 1757 | 1807 | Script for Erythromycin & Otomize ear spray given | | KLH | Penicillin allergy. |
| 30.07.2015 | 24.09.1995 | F | S/Leave | 945 | 958 | Med. 3 04/10 given for Sepsis for 1 week from 30.07.15 | | GEM | |
| 30.07.2015 | 06.01.1965 | F | | 958 | 1021 | Script for Citalopram, Co-Amoxiclav & Fenbid forte 10% gel given | | LAR | |
| 30.07.2015 | 27.08.1996 | F | | 1021 | 1041 | Referred to Counsellor regarding her depression & being unable to cope | | CRMW | |
| 30.07.2015 | 25.02.1948 | M | | 1041 | 1055 | Referred to General Surgeon regarding probable ventral hernia | | TPB | |

Result of a query that lists all consultations from the 22nd to the end of July 2015 (ConsultationsSeenFrom22ndTillEndOfJul2015)

| SurgeryDate | DateOfBirth | Sex | Diagnosis | TimeIn | TimeOut | Complaints | Treatments | Initials | Notes |
|---|---|---|---|---|---|---|---|---|---|
| 30.07.2015 | 14.05.1971 | M | | 1055 | 1108 | Script for Co-Amoxiclav & Fucidin 2% cream given | | NJF | |
| 30.07.2015 | 15.05.1962 | F | | 1108 | 1128 | Script for Citalopram given | | JMD | |
| 30.07.2015 | 09.12.1945 | F | | 1128 | 1142 | Script for Daktacort cream & Dermovate scalp application given | | AML | |
| 30.07.2015 | 02.02.1951 | F | | 1640 | 1648 | Script for Clarithromycin given | | CAT | Penicillin allergy. |
| 30.07.2015 | 27.09.1931 | F | | 1648 | 1658 | Script for Amoxycillin & Fucidin H cream given | | JJ | |
| 30.07.2015 | 14.09.1947 | F | | 1658 | 1718 | Referred to Orthopaedic Surgeon regarding painful (L) knee | | CEJY | |
| 30.07.2015 | 23.08.1963 | F | | 1718 | 1726 | Reassured regarding her slightly reduced Prothrombin Time | | GPB | |
| 30.07.2015 | 13.02.1950 | M | | 1726 | 1738 | Script for Aspirin & Atorvastatin given | | DCF | For FBC, U/Es, LFTs, Fasting Glucose, Fasting Lipids & Cortisol. |
| 30.07.2015 | 20.03.1652 | F | | 1738 | 1748 | Script for Dermovate scalp application given | | LJF | Referred to Rheumatologist regarding her multiple joints pain. |

742

Result of a query that lists all consultations from the 22nd to the end of July 2015 (ConsultationsSeenFrom22ndTillEndOfJul2015)

| SurgeryDate | DateOfBirth | Sex | Diagnosis | TimeIn | TimeOut | Complaints | Treatments | Initials | Notes |
|---|---|---|---|---|---|---|---|---|---|
| 30.07.2015 | 18.06.1981 | M | | 1748 | 1756 | Script for Allopurinol given | | SCJ | |
| 30.07.2015 | 08.12.1962 | F | | 1756 | 1807 | Script for Codeine tablets & Lisinopril | | BJM | |
| 30.07.2015 | 26.06.2015 | F | | 1807 | 1818 | Referred to Paediatrician regarding the recurrent red rash on her face & neck when she is feeding | | LRA | |
| 30.07.2015 | 24.07.2015 | M | | 1818 | 1828 | Script for Chloramphenicol eye drops given | | CB | |

# RESULTS OF QUERIES THAT LIST ALL CONSULTATIONS FROM THE 22ND TO THE END OF AUGUST 1997 TO AUGUST 2014

Result of a query that lists all consultations from the 22nd to the end of August 1997 (ConsultationsSeenFrom22ndTillEndOfAug1997)

| SurgeryDate | DateOfBirth | Sex | Diagnosis | TimeIn | TimeOut | Complaints | Treatments | NumbersID | Notes |
|---|---|---|---|---|---|---|---|---|---|
| 22.08.97 | 29.05.84 | F | URTI | 1820 | 1825 | Sore throat & (L) ear ache | Erymax | 2337 | Penicillin allergy. |
| 22.08.97 | 02.12.34 | F | | 1714 | 1718 | Feels tired all the time | For FBC | 2436 | |
| 22.08.97 | 26.10.84 | F | | 1644 | 1647 | (L) ear ache | Orosporin | 2827 | |
| 22.08.97 | 05.07.90 | F | | 1706 | 1713 | Frequent nose bleeds | Flixonase | 2912 | |
| 22.08.97 | 06.10.24 | F | RTI | 1340 | 1415 | Cough | Amoxycillin & Salbutamol inhaler | 312 | Home visit. Ensure plus & Enlive also prescribed. |
| 23.08.97 | 23.08.91 | M | Revisit | 1027 | 1031 | Still coughing | To continue Amoxycillin | 3358 | If he is no better in 3 to 4 days, to come back. |
| 22.08.97 | 07.05.83 | M | URTI | 1801 | 1808 | Sore throat & (L) ear ache | Amoxycillin & Orosporin | 3390 | |
| 22.08.97 | 29.06.85 | M | Lump | 1648 | 1651 | Infected lump (L) breast | Amoxycillin & Flucloxacillin | 3769 | |
| 23.08.97 | 04.09.85 | M | RTI | 1008 | 1018 | Cough | Co-Amoxiclav & Stemetil | 3959 | He also has vomiting. |
| 23.08.97 | 21.01.29 | F | Revisit | 1019 | 1026 | Eyes still feel sore & gritty | Amoxycillin & Fucithalmic | 4116 | Patient requested Amoxycillin. |
| 22.08.97 | 08.12.25 | M | | 1726 | 1734 | Uric acid high | Allopurinol | 4296 | |
| 22.08.97 | 27.03.66 | M | | 1738 | 1741 | Bilateral athletes foot | Lamisil cream | 4516 | |
| 23.08.97 | 07.06.66 | F | | 1033 | 1038 | Vaginal thrush | Diflucan | 46 | |
| 22.08.97 | 06.10.94 | M | | 1735 | 1738 | Dad feels he has in grown toe nail | To see a Chiropodist | 4617 | |
| 23.08.97 | 05.06.26 | F | Rash | 1003 | 1007 | Spot on (R) cheek | Trimovate cream | 4719 | |
| 22.08.97 | 04.07.96 | M | | 931 | 948 | Child keeps falling, going blue & eyes rolling | Referred to Paediatrician, Rapid access clinic | 5312 | |

Result of a query that lists all consultations from the 22nd to the end of August 1997 (ConsultationsSeenFrom22ndTillEndOfAug1997)

| SurgeryDate | DateOfBirth | Sex | Diagnosis | TimeIn | TimeOut | Complaints | Treatments | NumbersID | Notes |
|---|---|---|---|---|---|---|---|---|---|
| 22.08.97 | 07.05.63 | M | | 1005 | 1015 | Infected insect bite on shoulder | Co-Amoxiclav | 5327 | He has frequent skin infection & tender cervical gland. For FBC & Glucose. He also has skin tag on his upper eye brow, for excision. |
| 22.08.97 | 25.01.23 | M | Rash | 1635 | 1643 | Feet peeling off | Canesten cream | 5370 | He also complained of dizziness & nausea, Rx. Stemetil. Ears itchy & buzzing, Rx. Otosporin. |
| 22.08.97 | 12.10.45 | F | S/Leave | 956 | 1004 | Asthma & Diabetes | | 5457 | Movelat script also given. |
| 22.08.97 | 07.04.19 | F | | 1719 | 1725 | Indigestion | Lansoprazole | 5558 | Referred to Gastroenterologist. |
| 23.08.97 | 27.07.83 | F | | 1104 | 1108 | Glandular fever positive | | 5588 | |
| 22.08.97 | 18.02.52 | M | | 1754 | 1758 | Cholesterol 5.3 mmols/L | For repeat Cholesterol in 6 months | 5690 | |
| 22.08.97 | 24.03.60 | M | | 900 | 916 | Infra patella bursitis | Diclofenac | 640 | ?Foreign body present, for X-Ray (R) Knee. |
| 22.08.97 | 08.01.86 | F | Revisit | 1830 | 1834 | Sore throat still | Augmentin-Duo | 794 | |

747

Result of a query that lists all consultations from the 22nd to the end of August 1997 (ConsultationsSeenFrom22ndTillEndOfAug1997)

| SurgeryDate | DateOfBirth | Sex | Diagnosis | TimeIn | TimeOut | Complaints | Treatments | NumbersID | Notes |
|---|---|---|---|---|---|---|---|---|---|
| 22.08.97 | 20.09.45 | M | S/Leave | 919 | 930 | Salmonella infection | | 89 | |
| 23.08.97 | 01.08.46 | M | | 1055 | 1103 | Diarrhoea | Rehidrat & Loperamide | Temp | He also has abdominal pain, Rx. Buscopan. |

Result of a query that lists all consultations from the 22nd to the end of August 1998 (ConsultationsSeenFrom22ndTillEndOfAug1998)

| SurgeryDate | DateOfBirth | Sex | Diagnosis | TimeIn | TimeOut | Complaints | Treatments | NumbersID | Notes |
|---|---|---|---|---|---|---|---|---|---|
| 25.08.98 | 04.06.81 | F | URTI | 1014 | 1017 | Sore throat | Amoxycillin | 1104 | |
| 25.08.98 | 11.08.27 | M | | 1100 | 1117 | Taxi Medical Examination done. £58.50 paid | | 1214 | |
| 26.08.98 | 11.08.65 | M | | 1705 | 1714 | Tooth abscess | Amoxycillin & Metronidazole | 1368 | New Patient check done. He also has diarrhoea, Rx. Loperamide. |
| 28.08.98 | 21.09.24 | F | | 1632 | 1643 | Clinistix script given | | 1419 | |
| 26.08.98 | 17.01.26 | F | | 1325 | 1335 | Fever & dyspnoea | Ciprofloxacin | 1537 | New Patient check done. Home visit. Penicillin allergy. Pacemaker in-situ. |
| 25.08.98 | 27.06.44 | M | URTI | 931 | 936 | Sore throat | Co-Amoxiclav | 1673 | |
| 24.08.98 | 26.06.53 | M | S/Leave | 1647 | 1652 | (L) knee operation | | 1681 | He also has cellulitis (L) knee wound, Rx. Co-Amoxiclav. |

748

Result of a query that lists all consultations from the 22nd to the end of August 1998 (ConsultationsSeenFrom22ndTillEndOfAug1998)

| SurgeryDate | DateOfBirth | Sex | Diagnosis | TimeIn | TimeOut | Complaints | Treatments | NumbersID | Notes |
|---|---|---|---|---|---|---|---|---|---|
| 27.08.98 | 05.02.35 | M | | 953 | 956 | Infected insect bite (R) arm | Flucloxacillin | 1834 | |
| 27.08.98 | 18.02.30 | M | RTI | 1652 | 1701 | Dry throat & wheezy | Amoxycillin, Salbutamol & Bendrofluazide | 1926 | |
| 28.08.98 | 14.12.48 | M | | 1043 | 1050 | (R) Otitis ext. | Flucloxacillin & Sofradex ear drops | 1964 | New Patient check done. |
| 26.08.98 | 11.02.75 | M | URTI | 1725 | 1728 | Sore throat | Amoxycillin | 2039 | |
| 24.08.98 | 04.04.40 | M | | 1654 | 1704 | (L) kidney pain again | Diclofenac enteric coated | 21 | For USScan of the kidneys. |
| 24.08.98 | 23.09.68 | M | URTI | 1751 | 1756 | Sore throat | Amoxycillin | 2136 | New Patient check done. |
| 27.08.98 | 19.12.57 | M | S/Leave | 922 | 934 | Fractured (R) index finger | | 2267 | |
| 25.08.98 | 17.02.22 | F | | 1632 | 1640 | Frusemide script given | | 2285 | For U/Es. |
| 28.08.98 | 24.09.37 | M | | 1754 | 1800 | Bendrofluazide script given | | 2329 | |
| 24.08.98 | 23.04.50 | F | Rash | 950 | 958 | Red stinging rash on neck | Flucloxacillin & Fucidin-H cream | 2369 | New Patient check done. |
| 28.08.39 | 28.03.70 | F | Depressed | 1800 | 1807 | Stressed at work | Efexor XL | 2375 | |
| 26.08.98 | 19.07.61 | F | | 946 | 952 | Late period | For Pregnancy test | 2505 | |
| 25.08.98 | 17.09.70 | M | | 1807 | 1812 | X-Ray (R) knee - Normal | | 2555 | |
| 28.08.98 | 03.09.88 | F | | 1705 | 1710 | Ventolin inhaler | | 2565 | |

Result of a query that lists all consultations from the 22nd to the end of August 1998 (ConsultationsSeenFrom22ndTillEndOfAug1998)

| SurgeryDate | DateOfBirth | Sex | Diagnosis | TimeIn | TimeOut | Complaints | Treatments | NumbersID | Notes |
|---|---|---|---|---|---|---|---|---|---|
| 28.08.98 | 30.10.60 | F | | 1657 | 1705 | Seeing a solicitor regarding a claim for injury | | 2572 | |
| 26.08.98 | 05.03.49 | M | Lump | 1747 | 1804 | Olecranon bursitis | Flucloxacillin | 2726 | He also has hypertension, Rx. Atenolol. |
| 24.08.98 | 23.05.32 | M | Pain | 1638 | 1647 | Pain in the perineum | Co-dydramol | 274 | |
| 26.08.98 | 11.12.54 | M | | 1728 | 1733 | Indigestion still quite bad | Referred to Gastro-enterologist | 295 | New Patient check done. |
| 29.08.98 | 14.03.83 | F | | 1055 | 1101 | (R) ear sore | Amoxycillin & Otosporin | 296 | |
| 25.08.98 | 07.04.65 | F | Revisit | 950 | 956 | Abdominal pain still bad | Referred to Gastro-enterologist | 2962 | |
| 26.08.98 | 01.08.48 | F | | 920 | 925 | Abdominal distension & constipation | Lactulose & Spasmonal | 3009 | |
| 28.08.98 | 23.08.63 | F | | 1037 | 1043 | Wax in (R) ear | Cerumol ear drops | 3038 | For syringing. |
| 24.08.98 | 16.12.59 | F | | 1026 | 1045 | Private cervical smear abnormal | For smear asap | 311 | New Patient check done. |
| 26.08.98 | 01.02.80 | F | | 1824 | 1827 | Pruritus vulvae, ?thrush | Diflucan | 3118 | New Patient check done. |
| 24.08.98 | 13.11.53 | M | | 1747 | 1751 | (R) ear ache | Amoxycillin | 3119 | |
| 24.08.98 | 06.10.24 | F | | 1056 | 1101 | Atenolol script given | | 312 | |
| 27.08.98 | 17.11.61 | F | Pain | 1716 | 1729 | Headaches, ?migraine | Imigran | 319 | New Patient check done. Referred to Neurologist (Basildon hospital). |

Result of a query that lists all consultations from the 22nd to the end of August 1998 (ConsultationsSeenFrom22ndTillEndOfAug1998)

| SurgeryDate | DateOfBirth | Sex | Diagnosis | TimeIn | TimeOut | Complaints | Treatments | NumbersID | Notes |
|---|---|---|---|---|---|---|---|---|---|
| 26.08.98 | 07.07.62 | M | Pain | 1835 | 1840 | Hit in the perineum, sore | Co-dydramol & Diclofenac SR | 3240 | New Patient check done. |
| 26.08.98 | 16.03.25 | M | | 1634 | 1645 | Sinus problems for years | Rhinocort Aqua nasal spray | 3245 | |
| 25.08.98 | 06.06.91 | F | URTI | 939 | 945 | Sore throat | Amoxycillin & Paracetamol | 3259 | New Patient check done. |
| 26.08.98 | 12.08.32 | M | Pain | 1030 | 1035 | Epigastric discomfort | Omeprazole | 3344 | New Patient check done. |
| 27.08.98 | 14.08.35 | M | Hypertension | 1729 | 1802 | BP 170/110 | Referred to Cardiologist | 3353 | |
| 27.08.98 | 31.10.15 | F | | 934 | 937 | (L) bloodshot eye | Chloramphenicol eye drops | 336 | |
| 27.08.98 | 11.06.56 | F | Lump | 1701 | 1715 | Lump (L) breast | Referred to Surgeon | 3371 | She had radical vulvectomy for vulval carcinoma. New Patient check done. |
| 27.08.98 | 02.05.91 | M | | 943 | 953 | Warts on middle finger & under lower lip | Cuplex gel | 3411 | New Patient check done. |
| 27.08.98 | 20.07.61 | M | | 1816 | 1824 | He will consider about having vasectomy | | 3412 | New Patient check done. |
| 25.08.98 | 06.05.64 | F | Pain | 1649 | 1702 | (R) sided chest pain | For CXR | 3474 | |
| 27.08.98 | 12.08.39 | M | | 905 | 922 | Restandol script given | | 3475 | |
| 25.08.98 | 27.02.92 | M | URTI | 1720 | 1724 | (L) ear ache | Erythromycin | 3589 | |
| 26.08.98 | 30.09.81 | M | URTI | 1714 | 1718 | Sore throat | Erythromycin | 371 | New Patient check done. Penicillin allergy. |

Result of a query that lists all consultations from the 22nd to the end of August 1998 (ConsultationsSeenFrom22ndTillEndOfAug1998)

| SurgeryDate | DateOfBirth | Sex | Diagnosis | TimeIn | TimeOut | Complaints | Treatments | NumbersID | Notes |
|---|---|---|---|---|---|---|---|---|---|
| 27.08.98 | 23.05.27 | M | | 1025 | 1035 | Diabetic on diet, urine negative | | 3716 | |
| 24.08.98 | 01.10.23 | F | | 905 | 915 | Co-dydramol script given | | 3750 | |
| 26.08.98 | 29.09.37 | F | RTI | 1025 | 1030 | Chesty cough | Ciprofloxacin | 3835 | |
| 25.08.98 | 11.03.30 | F | | 1032 | 1100 | Wants Prednisolone withdrawn | To gradually withdraw by 1 mg every 2 weeks | 3887 | New Patient check done. For ESR every 6 weeks. |
| 28.08.98 | 16.10.59 | F | | 1006 | 1014 | Hb 10.20 g/dl | Ferrous Sulphate | 3929 | |
| 28.08.98 | 25.01.83 | F | URTI | 1643 | 1654 | Sore throat | Amoxycillin & Paracetamol | 3930 | New Patient check done. |
| 25.08.98 | 11.01.91 | F | Rash | 1702 | 1710 | Rash (L) axilla | Referred to Dermatologist | 3945 | |
| 25.08.98 | 02.11.78 | M | Rash | 1812 | 1817 | Itchy viral rash all over | Co-dydramol & Loratadine | 404 | |
| 26.08.98 | 25.09.58 | M | | 1827 | 1830 | Due to do a parachute jump. He wants to know who gives the form of fitness | To check with the club | 405 | New Patient check done. |
| 26.08.98 | 29.01.73 | F | Rash | 1004 | 1014 | Red, weepy & itchy rash on face | Erythromycin & Fucidin-H cream | 4063 | |
| 25.08.98 | 21.08.41 | M | Pain | 1756 | 1807 | Epigastric pain | Omeprazole | 4229 | New Patient check done. |
| 24.08.98 | 06.08.64 | F | UTI | 1807 | 1812 | Dysuria | Trimethoprim | 425 | New Patient check done. |

Result of a query that lists all consultations from the 22nd to the end of August 1998 (ConsultationsSeenFrom22ndTillEndOfAug1998)

| SurgeryDate | DateOfBirth | Sex | Diagnosis | TimeIn | TimeOut | Complaints | Treatments | NumbersID | Notes |
|---|---|---|---|---|---|---|---|---|---|
| 27.08.98 | 29.08.73 | F | | 1802 | 1816 | Unwell & feverish | Amoxycillin | 4262 | She also has nausea, Rx. Metoclopramide. Mefenamic acid script also given. |
| 25.08.98 | 26.11.75 | M | S/Leave | 921 | 926 | Back pain - Private | | 4410 | New Patient check done. |
| 27.08.98 | 22.03.18 | F | Pain | 1226 | 1242 | Pain (L) shoulder | Ibuprofen | 4411 | Home visit. She also has ear infection, Rx. Ciprofloxacin. |
| 27.08.98 | 17.09.38 | M | RTI | 1824 | 1829 | Cough | Amoxycillin | 4448 | New Patient check done. |
| 29.08.98 | 18.11.91 | M | Pain | 1016 | 1020 | Headaches | Paracetamol | 4475 | New Patient check done. |
| 24.08.98 | 08.04.93 | M | RTI | 1020 | 1026 | Cough | Amoxycillin | 4476 | New Patient check done. |
| 29.08.98 | 24.05.66 | M | | 1002 | 1016 | Peptic ulcer symptoms | Lansoprazole | 4487 | New Patient check done. He is also tired all the time, for FBC. |
| 25.08.98 | 03.04.69 | F | Pain | 1731 | 1738 | Abdominal pain | Referred to Gynaecologist | 4508 | She was seen by Gastro-enterologist who suggested that she is referred to Gynaecologist. |

753

Result of a query that lists all consultations from the 22nd to the end of August 1998 (ConsultationsSeenFrom22ndTillEndOfAug1998)

| SurgeryDate | DateOfBirth | Sex | Diagnosis | TimeIn | TimeOut | Complaints | Treatments | NumbersID | Notes |
|---|---|---|---|---|---|---|---|---|---|
| 26.08.98 | 07.06.66 | F | RTI | 1830 | 1835 | Cough | Amoxycillin | 46 | New Patient check done. She is also tired all the time, for FBC & TFTs. FP1001 (GMS4) form signed. |
| 29.08.98 | 07.06.66 | F | Revisit | 1101 | 1125 | Quite wheezy | Nebulizer given | 46 | Erythromycin, Ventolin & Flixotide inhalers also given. |
| 27.08.98 | 30.01.68 | F | | 937 | 943 | Vaginal thrush | Canesten cream | 461 | She is 13 weeks gestation. Gaviscon script also given. |
| 24.08.98 | 03.09.86 | F | | 1812 | 1818 | (L) buttock abscess | Flucloxacillin | 4623 | New Patient check done. |
| 26.08.98 | 06.04.78 | F | | 1816 | 1824 | Infected TB vaccination site | Fucidin cream & Erythromycin | 4647 | FP1001 (GMS4) form signed. |
| 26.08.98 | 07.08.42 | F | | 1718 | 1725 | Lungs feel congested | Amoxycillin | 4695 | |
| 26.08.98 | 27.04.62 | F | Pain | 1043 | 1049 | Neck pain | Diclofenac enteric coated | 4724 | Involved in RTA yesterday. |
| 26.08.98 | 09.03.75 | M | Rash | 1653 | 1705 | Itchy rash all over, ?Scabies | Lyclear Dermal cream | 4771 | New Patient check done. |
| 26.08.98 | 22.04.62 | F | | 937 | 946 | Itchy mole in front of (L) ear lobe | Fucidin-H cream | 4831 | |
| 25.08.98 | 17.03.95 | F | Pain | 1724 | 1731 | Abdominal pain | Merbentyl & Lactulose | 4844 | |
| 25.08.98 | 17.03.67 | M | S/Leave | 1710 | 1714 | Tenosynovitis (R) wrist | | 4854 | |

## Result of a query that lists all consultations from the 22nd to the end of August 1998 (ConsultationsSeenFrom22ndTillEndOfAug1998)

| SurgeryDate | DateOfBirth | Sex | Diagnosis | TimeIn | TimeOut | Complaints | Treatments | NumbersID | Notes |
|---|---|---|---|---|---|---|---|---|---|
| 24.08.98 | 13.08.15 | M | | 1235 | 1300 | Unwell, ?CCF | Referred to Medical Dr. on call, SGH | 4865 | Home visit. |
| 25.08.98 | 13.08.15 | M | | 1305 | 1309 | Told that a Domiciliary visit has been arranged for him & to get his new telephone number | | 4865 | |
| 26.08.98 | 14.02.76 | F | Rash | 1804 | 1811 | Itchy rash all over, ?Scabies | Lyclear Dermal cream & Loratadine | 4868 | New Patient check done. Dianette script also given. |
| 26.08.98 | 20.06.93 | M | Rash | 1811 | 1816 | Itchy rash all over, ?Scabies | Lyclear Dermal cream & Loratadine | 4869 | Mum came to Surgery. |
| 27.08.98 | 27.02.47 | M | Pain | 1829 | 1835 | Back pain | Arthrotec 50 | 488 | New Patient check done. |
| 24.08.98 | 09.04.55 | F | | 1012 | 1020 | Unhappy about private Psychiatrist report | | 491 | |
| 24.08.98 | 19.06.85 | F | Rash | 958 | 1012 | Folliculitis on scalp & face | Referred to Dermatologist | 494 | New Patient check done. Retinova cream has not helped. |
| 28.08.98 | 25.01.61 | F | Depressed | 1745 | 1754 | Feels vacant | Referred to CPN | 4991 | |
| 24.08.98 | 25.06.38 | F | Revisit | 1704 | 1710 | Rash worse with Fucidin-H cream | Lamisil cream | 5 | |
| 27.08.98 | 30.03.17 | M | | 1008 | 1018 | (L) thumb infected | Erythromycin | 5005 | New Patient check done. Penicillin allergy. |

Result of a query that lists all consultations from the 22nd to the end of August 1998 (ConsultationsSeenFrom22ndTillEndOfAug1998)

| SurgeryDate | DateOfBirth | Sex | Diagnosis | TimeIn | TimeOut | Complaints | Treatments | NumbersID | Notes |
|---|---|---|---|---|---|---|---|---|---|
| 26.08.98 | 23.04.21 | F | RTI | 1645 | 1653 | Cough | Amoxycillin & Sudafed Plus | 5108 | New Patient check done. Tetanus toxoid Booster given. |
| 25.08.98 | 11.01.81 | M | | 926 | 931 | Cystic Lump on fore-skin | Referred to Surgeon | 5250 | |
| 28.08.98 | 12.08.44 | M | S/Leave | 1824 | 1830 | Abdominal pain | | 5364 | He is still passing mucus PR & abdominal pain, referred to Gastro-enterologist. |
| 27.08.98 | 25.01.23 | M | Rash | 1003 | 1008 | Rash on chest | To observe | 5370 | Vit. B Co. script also given. |
| 27.08.98 | 13.03.25 | F | RTI | 956 | 1003 | Cough | Amoxycillin | 5371 | New Patient check done. |
| 24.08.98 | 19.12.81 | F | Rash | 1730 | 1738 | Itchy rash on the arms & legs | Loratadine | 5384 | |
| 28.08.98 | 03.11.22 | M | UTI | 1030 | 1037 | Dysuria | Trimethoprim | 5444 | |
| 28.08.98 | 08.12.82 | F | Pain | 934 | 946 | Pain (L) shoulder | Ibuprofen & Cuplex gel | 545 | New Patient check done. |
| 24.08.98 | 25.06.21 | M | | 1756 | 1801 | Pavacol-D & Omeprazole script given | | 5474 | |
| 24.08.98 | 28.01.60 | M | | 1052 | 1056 | Tylex script given | | 5500 | |
| 25.08.98 | 23.05.79 | F | | 1017 | 1024 | Late period | For pregnancy test | 5522 | |
| 28.08.98 | 23.05.79 | F | | 1729 | 1737 | Pregnancy test positive. Requests TOP | | 5522 | |

Result of a query that lists all consultations from the 22nd to the end of August 1998 (ConsultationsSeenFrom22ndTillEndOfAug1998)

| SurgeryDate | DateOfBirth | Sex | Diagnosis | TimeIn | TimeOut | Complaints | Treatments | NumbersID | Notes |
|---|---|---|---|---|---|---|---|---|---|
| 25.08.98 | 21.09.69 | F | | 1024 | 1032 | Husband has reversal of vasectomy, he wants semen analysis | Husband needs to come in | 5524 | |
| 24.08.98 | 18.03.91 | M | | 1801 | 1807 | Balanitis | Augmentin-Duo | 5535 | |
| 28.08.98 | 28.10.36 | M | Revisit | 930 | 934 | Pain (L) heel persists | Referred to Orthopaedic Surgeon | 554 | X-Ray: Os calcis - NAD. |
| 28.08.98 | 06.07.42 | F | | 946 | 955 | Hb 11.6 g/dl | Ferrous Sulphate | 556 | New Patient check done. Gaviscon script also given. |
| 28.08.98 | 26.08.25 | M | | 1807 | 1824 | Prostatism, enlarged prostate | Referred to Urologist | 5581 | For MSU. |
| 25.08.98 | 06.05.97 | M | URTI | 1714 | 1720 | Pulling (R) ear | Erythromycin | 5645 | Penicillin allergy. |
| 24.08.98 | 25.09.17 | F | | 1220 | 1227 | Dizziness | Prochlorperazine | 5665 | Home visit. |
| 27.08.98 | 25.09.17 | F | Revisit | 1200 | 1220 | Still unwell | Amoxycillin | 5665 | For FBC, U/Es, LFTs & Glucose. Home visit. |
| 25.08.98 | 02.04.57 | F | | 915 | 921 | Nail infection | Lamisil | 5685 | Chlorpromazine script also given. |
| 24.08.98 | 19.07.39 | F | | 935 | 950 | H. pylori positive | Amoxycillin, Clarithromycin & Lansoprazole | 5727 | Stemetil script also given. |
| 28.08.98 | 19.07.39 | F | | 910 | 924 | Lansoprazole script given | | 5727 | |
| 24.08.98 | 09.11.52 | M | | 1045 | 1050 | Diarrhoea again | Stool for C&S | 582 | |
| 26.08.98 | 30.10.97 | M | Rash | 1733 | 1747 | Loose nappy & nappy rash | Electrolade & Timodine cream | 5847 | |

Result of a query that lists all consultations from the 22nd to the end of August 1998 (ConsultationsSeenFrom22ndTillEndOfAug1998)

| SurgeryDate | DateOfBirth | Sex | Diagnosis | TimeIn | TimeOut | Complaints | Treatments | NumbersID | Notes |
|---|---|---|---|---|---|---|---|---|---|
| 24.08.98 | 270.9.21 | F | Revisit | 1710 | 1730 | Still rubbing the epigastric region | Referred to the care of the elderly specialist | 5856 | For FBC, U/Es & USScan of the abdomen. |
| 28.08.98 | 06.01.35 | M | | 1024 | 1030 | 0.5% Malathion liquid | | 5872 | |
| 25.08.98 | 04.02.33 | F | | 1007 | 1014 | Infected mole has fallen off her chest | Flucloxacillin | 5880 | She also has pain (L) shoulder, Rx. Co-dydramol. |
| 28.08.98 | 08.06.50 | M | | 1654 | 1657 | Adalat 60 script | | 5939 | |
| 26.08.98 | 24.01.91 | F | | 1014 | 1025 | Warts on fingers | Cuplex gel | 6026 | |
| 26.08.98 | 20.08.59 | M | S/Leave | 1035 | 1043 | Laceration (L) wrist (Ulnar nerve involved) - Med 5 | | 6029 | |
| 29.08.98 | 23.06.45 | F | Revisit | 1038 | 1055 | (L) knee is still painful | For Physiotherapy | 6040 | Flucloxacillin & Diclofenac e/c script also given. |
| 27.08.98 | 06.08.55 | F | S/Leave | 1018 | 1025 | (R) Breast cancer | | 6048 | |
| 25.08.98 | 01.08.68 | M | Pain | 1750 | 1756 | Pain (R) hip | To use own Nurofen | 6068 | |
| 26.08.98 | 27.11.58 | M | | 958 | 1004 | Infected hair follicle | Fucidin cream | 6107 | |
| 25.08.98 | 30.05.98 | M | | 1640 | 1649 | Rash on face | To continue Aqueous cream | 6127 | |
| 28.08.98 | 08.11.73 | F | | 955 | 1006 | 15 weeks gestation. Per vagina bleeding has stopped | | 6138 | |
| 29.08.98 | 21.03.73 | M | | 1031 | 1038 | Tender glands & fever | Amoxycillin | 6142 | |

758

## Result of a query that lists all consultations from the 22nd to the end of August 1998 (ConsultationsSeenFrom22ndTillEndOfAug1998)

| SurgeryDate | DateOfBirth | Sex | Diagnosis | TimeIn | TimeOut | Complaints | Treatments | NumbersID | Notes |
|---|---|---|---|---|---|---|---|---|---|
| 24.08.98 | 21.07.98 | F | | 1830 | 1845 | Unwell, crying | Paracetamol & Amoxycillin | 6160 | |
| 26.08.98 | 16.01.70 | F | | 925 | 927 | Mole on back | To observe | 6172 | |
| 26.08.98 | 22.11.91 | F | Revisit | 927 | 931 | Still coughing | Erythromycin & Simple Linctus | 6173 | |
| 26.08.98 | 22.07.17 | F | | 907 | 920 | Lyclear Dermal cream script given | | 6182 | |
| 28.08.98 | 22.01.44 | M | | 1710 | 1720 | Betaloc script given | | 6183 | |
| 28.08.98 | 09.06.44 | F | URTI | 1720 | 1729 | Sore throat | Amoxycillin | 6184 | Her husband came to Surgery. |
| 24.08.98 | 20.09.28 | F | | 915 | 924 | Referred to Physiotherapist, SGH | | 663 | |
| 29.08.98 | 27.02.41 | M | RTI | 1025 | 1031 | Cough | Tavanic | 675 | |
| 27.08.98 | 30.07.64 | F | | 1835 | 1840 | Wants her period delayed for holidays | Norethisterone | 707 | New Patient check done. |
| 28.08.98 | 13.12.25 | M | | 1014 | 1024 | Bendrofluazide script given | | 736 | New Patient check done. For FBC, U/Es & Cholesterol. |
| 25.08.98 | 20.09.14 | F | | 1738 | 1743 | Ears normal | | 746 | |
| 28.08.98 | 04.09.85 | F | Pain | 1737 | 1745 | Back pain | Referred to Physiotherapist | 811 | Her mum came to Surgery. |
| 27.08.98 | 17.04.40 | F | | 1641 | 1652 | Heart missing a beat | For FBC, TFTs, LH & FSH | 86 | New Patient check done. |
| 26.08.98 | 14.08.60 | M | | 935 | 937 | Wife has thrush | Diflucan | 881 | His wife came to Surgery. |
| 26.08.98 | 05.09.61 | F | | 931 | 935 | Vaginal thrush | Diflucan | 882 | |

Result of a query that lists all consultations from the 22nd to the end of August 1998 (ConsultationsSeenFrom22ndTillEndOfAug1998)

| SurgeryDate | DateOfBirth | Sex | Diagnosis | TimeIn | TimeOut | Complaints | Treatments | NumbersID | Notes |
|---|---|---|---|---|---|---|---|---|---|
| 24.08.98 | 05.10.76 | M | | 1738 | 1747 | Came to Surgery regarding his girlfriend who is pregnant, a patient registered elsewhere | | 913 | |
| 25.08.98 | 25.05.97 | M | URTI | 956 | 1007 | Infected rhinorrhoea | Amoxycillin | NP | He also has rash on his (L) leg, Rx. Unguentum Merck cream. Script for Paracetamol, Bonjela teething gel & Conotrane cream given. |
| 25.08.98 | 12.06.74 | M | RTI | 945 | 950 | Cough | Amoxycillin | Temp | |
| 27.08.98 | 18.09.90 | M | Rash | 1635 | 1641 | Itchy rash all over | Loratadine & Calamine lotion | Temp | |
| 27.08.98 | 28.11.97 | F | Rash | 1840 | 1845 | Rash & unwell | Amoxycillin | Temp | |
| 29.08.98 | 18.12.69 | M | URTI | 1020 | 1025 | Sore throat | Amoxycillin & Co-dydramol | Temp | |

Result of a query that lists all consultations from the 22nd to the end of August 1999 (ConsultationsSeenFrom22ndTillEndOfAug1999)

| SurgeryDate | DateOfBirth | Sex | Diagnosis | TimeIn | TimeOut | Complaints | Treatments | NumbersID | Notes |
|---|---|---|---|---|---|---|---|---|---|
| 24.08.99 | 16.10.78 | F | | 1721 | 1736 | Late period | For Pregnancy test | Temp | |
| 26.08.99 | 17.05.85 | M | | 952 | 957 | Diarrhoea | Electrolade | Temp | |

760

## Result of a query that lists all consultations from the 22$^{nd}$ to the end of August 1999 (ConsultationsSeenFrom22ndTillEndOfAug1999)

| SurgeryDate | DateOfBirth | Sex | Diagnosis | TimeIn | TimeOut | Complaints | Treatments | NumbersID | Notes |
|---|---|---|---|---|---|---|---|---|---|
| 26.08.99 | 02.07.87 | F | URTI | 957 | 1000 | Sore throat | Amoxycillin | Temp | |
| 26.08.99 | 09.05.68 | F | URTI | 1717 | 1722 | Sore throat | Amoxycillin | Temp | Script for Bricanyl inhaler & Flixotide inhaler given. |
| 27.08.99 | 25.05.97 | F | | 1648 | 1652 | Script for Alpha Keri bath & Keri lotion given | | Temp | |
| 31.08.99 | 30.10.29 | M | | 1006 | 1016 | Script for Glipizide & Metformin given | | NP | |
| 27.08.99 | 05.01.71 | F | | 958 | 1006 | Sneezing & snuffling | She will observe | 1003 | |
| 26.08.99 | 03.10.69 | F | | 1009 | 1012 | Script for Trinovum given | | 1206 | |
| 24.08.99 | 10.07.43 | F | URTI | 923 | 931 | (L) ear ache | Amoxycillin & Otomize ear spray | 1232 | Script for Spasmonal given. |
| 24.08.99 | 08.04.64 | F | RTI | 931 | 936 | Cough | Amoxycillin | 1362 | |
| 27.08.99 | 13.04.43 | F | Rash | 1716 | 1722 | Vitiligo rash (R) shoulder | Referred to Dermatologist | 1377 | |
| 24.08.99 | 06.08.41 | M | Pain | 1808 | 1818 | Pain (R) Achilles tendon | Diclofenac enteric coated | 1425 | He also has rash on his back, ?infected/?shingles, Rx. Flucloxacillin. |
| 23.08.99 | 05.04.72 | M | | 1642 | 1645 | Advised to continue finger mobilization exercises | | 1427 | |
| 25.08.99 | 11.09.47 | M | | 1812 | 1823 | He had tooth extraction & on Penicillin V | | 1503 | |
| 31.08.99 | 20.07.21 | F | Pain | 1330 | 1348 | Abdominal pain | Buscopan | 1517 | Home visit. |

Result of a query that lists all consultations from the 22nd to the end of August 1999 (ConsultationsSeenFrom22ndTillEndOfAug1999)

| SurgeryDate | DateOfBirth | Sex | Diagnosis | TimeIn | TimeOut | Complaints | Treatments | NumbersID | Notes |
|---|---|---|---|---|---|---|---|---|---|
| 31.08.99 | 08.08.24 | F |  | 1709 | 1724 | Script for Multivitamin & Glandosane given |  | 1559 |  |
| 25.08.99 | 22.12.59 | M |  | 926 | 932 | (L) ear is fuzzy & painful | Amoxycillin & Otomize ear spray | 1595 |  |
| 25.08.99 | 17.10.67 | F | Pain | 1734 | 1740 | Colicky abdominal pain & dysuria | Buscopan | 1646 | For MSU. |
| 25.08.99 | 08.05.66 | M | Conjunctivitis | 1640 | 1643 | Sticky & sore (L) eye | Chloramphenicol eye drops | 1745 |  |
| 31.08.99 | 11.10.38 | F | Pain | 1637 | 1641 | Pain (R) leg | Co-dydramol & Ibuprofen | 1832 |  |
| 26.08.99 | 17.10.53 | F | Pain | 1012 | 1030 | Severe abdominal pain | Referred to Surgical Dr. on call, SGH | 2020 |  |
| 27.08.99 | 21.02.76 | M |  | 1748 | 1756 | Sepsis (R) big toe | Flucloxacillin | 2031 | Tetanus toxoid Booster given. Script for Diclomax was also given. |
| 23.08.99 | 22.12.36 | F | Revisit | 903 | 919 | She still gets lumpy feeling in her throat | Referred to ENT Surgeon | 208 | USScan of the neck - normal. |
| 27.08.99 | 09.07.40 | M | S/Leave | 1055 | 1106 | Pain (L) shoulder |  | 2152 | Script for Atorvastatin & Kapake also given. |
| 31.08.99 | 03.11.57 | F |  | 1748 | 1752 | PER VAGINA bleeding over past 3 weeks | For pregnancy test | 2210 |  |

Result of a query that lists all consultations from the 22nd to the end of August 1999 (ConsultationsSeenFrom22ndTillEndOfAug1999)

| SurgeryDate | DateOfBirth | Sex | Diagnosis | TimeIn | TimeOut | Complaints | Treatments | NumbersID | Notes |
|---|---|---|---|---|---|---|---|---|---|
| 23.08.99 | 06.11.15 | M | | 1650 | 1657 | For LFTs, gamma-GT, TFTs & Reticulocyte count | | 229 | |
| 31.08.99 | 06.11.15 | M | Pain | 1033 | 1046 | Epigastric pain | Omeprazole | 229 | He was also referred to Gastro-enterologist. He also has unexplained macrocytosis, referred to Haematologist. |
| 24.08.99 | 28.05.85 | F | Revisit | 1001 | 1009 | Eye lump has got bigger | Referred to eye Dr. on call, Eye clinic SGH | 2387 | |
| 31.08.99 | 26.03.87 | M | URTI | 1821 | 1825 | Ear infections bilaterally | Sofradex ear drops & Co-Amoxiclav | 2439 | |
| 24.08.99 | 16.06.15 | M | Pain | 1042 | 1053 | (L) shoulder pain | Inj. Depo-Medrone with Lidocaine | 245 | |
| 27.08.99 | 07.11.88 | F | Pain | 941 | 946 | Pain in her head | Referred to Paediatrician | 2451 | She has a strong family history of berry aneurysm. |
| 31.08.99 | 01.10.20 | M | | 1019 | 1033 | Infected abrasion (R) fore-arm | Flucloxacillin | 2463 | |
| 23.08.99 | 21.11.88 | F | URTI | 1638 | 1642 | Sore throat | Amoxycillin | 2507 | |
| 27.08.99 | 09.01.38 | F | Revisit | 1702 | 1708 | X-Ray neck: moderate narrowing of the disc space between C5-C6 | Referred to Orthopaedic Surgeon | 2508 | |

Result of a query that lists all consultations from the 22nd to the end of August 1999 (ConsultationsSeenFrom22ndTillEndOfAug1999)

| SurgeryDate | DateOfBirth | Sex | Diagnosis | TimeIn | TimeOut | Complaints | Treatments | NumbersID | Notes |
|---|---|---|---|---|---|---|---|---|---|
| 23.08.99 | 06.01.43 | F | S/Leave | 900 | 903 | Abdominal pain | | 2642 | |
| 26.08.99 | 08.11.86 | M | | 1648 | 1655 | To use ear plugs when he is swimming | | 2649 | |
| 25.08.99 | 15.02.46 | F | S/Leave | 944 | 949 | Sinusitis | | 2792 | Script for Amoxycillin was also given. She also has sticky eyes, Rx. Chloramphenicol eye drops. |
| 26.08.99 | 10.09.36 | M | Pain | 1710 | 1717 | Skin tingles after shingles | Diclofenac enteric coated & Co-dydramol | 284 | |
| 23.08.99 | 24.09.70 | F | URTI | 1030 | 1034 | (R) ear ache | Otomize ear spray & Flucloxacillin | 2935 | |
| 25.08.99 | 20.03.19 | F | Revisit | 1643 | 1646 | Cough is still better but she is still wheezy | Clarithromycin | 2943 | |
| 23.08.99 | 08.03.40 | M | | 1750 | 1753 | He got screw driver into his (L) hand | Flucloxacillin | 2977 | |
| 31.08.99 | 08.01.44 | F | | 1703 | 1709 | Phlebitis (L) shin | Erythromycin & Ibuprofen | 2996 | Penicillin allergy. |
| 25.08.99 | 16.12.39 | F | | 932 | 940 | Script for Tramadol given | | 3003 | |
| 26.08.99 | 01.08.48 | F | URTI | 1730 | 1739 | Both ears sore | Flucloxacillin & Otomize ear spray | 3009 | |
| 26.08.99 | 22.02.91 | M | RTI | 1812 | 1817 | Fever & cough | Amoxycillin | 3196 | |
| 23.08.99 | 22.02.44 | M | S/Leave | 1730 | 1744 | Backache, Osteo-arthritis multiple joints & cervical laminectomy - Med 4 | | 3203 | |

Result of a query that lists all consultations from the 22nd to the end of August 1999 (ConsultationsSeenFrom22ndTillEndOfAug1999)

| SurgeryDate | DateOfBirth | Sex | Diagnosis | TimeIn | TimeOut | Complaints | Treatments | NumbersID | Notes |
|---|---|---|---|---|---|---|---|---|---|
| 27.08.99 | 09.08.61 | M | Rash | 1652 | 1656 | Itchy rash on chest | Balneum Plus bath oil, Diprobase cream & Fucidin-H cream | 3217 | |
| 31.08.99 | 15.04.53 | F | Revisit | 1800 | 1805 | (L) shoulder is still painful | Referred to Orthopaedic Surgeon (BUPA) | 3228 | |
| 24.08.99 | 17.07.42 | M | Pain | 1652 | 1657 | Joint pains | Ibuprofen | 3244 | CXR - normal. |
| 25.08.99 | 25.07.66 | F | Revisit | 910 | 920 | Back pain persists | Referred to Orthopaedic Surgeon | 3261 | |
| 25.08.99 | 23.08.91 | M | Rash | 920 | 926 | Red itchy rash on arms & groin | Lyclear Dermal cream | 3358 | |
| 25.08.99 | 17.01.61 | M | RTI | 1823 | 1829 | Cough & wheezy | Co-Amoxiclav & Prednisolone | 3410 | New Patient check done. Nebulizer given. |
| 27.08.99 | 18.03.69 | M | RTI | 1708 | 1711 | Cough | Amoxycillin | 3435 | |
| 26.08.99 | 14.01.72 | M | Rash | 1752 | 1801 | Dry skin patches on face | Fucidin-H cream | 346 | New Patient check done. Tetanus toxoid Booster given. |
| 25.08.99 | 02.03.48 | M | Conjunctivitis | 1759 | 1812 | Sticky eyes | Chloramphenicol eye drops | 3473 | |
| 31.08.99 | 10.01.92 | M | | 1659 | 1703 | Infected insect bite (L) upper eye lid | Cetirizine & Erythromycin | 3492 | Penicillin allergy. |

765

## Result of a query that lists all consultations from the 22nd to the end of August 1999 (ConsultationsSeenFrom22ndTillEndOfAug1999)

| SurgeryDate | DateOfBirth | Sex | Diagnosis | TimeIn | TimeOut | Complaints | Treatments | NumbersID | Notes |
|---|---|---|---|---|---|---|---|---|---|
| 26.08.99 | 03.12.44 | F | | 1704 | 1710 | She feels depressed | | 3509 | Her daughter came to Surgery. She is to persuade her mother to come to the Surgery. |
| 27.08.99 | 03.12.44 | F | | 1801 | 1816 | Panicky, ?menopausal | Premique | 3509 | |
| 26.08.99 | 19.05.92 | F | RTI | 938 | 942 | Cough | Amoxycillin | 3581 | |
| 26.08.99 | 02.05.92 | M | RTI | 949 | 952 | Cough | Amoxycillin | 3606 | |
| 24.08.99 | 05.12.39 | M | Pain | 1015 | 1207 | Back pain | Co-dydramol, Lactulose & Co-danthramer | 3646 | |
| 27.08.99 | 05.12.37 | M | Revisit | 946 | 954 | Back pain worse | Tramadol | 3646 | |
| 27.08.99 | 09.05.91 | F | URTI | 1820 | 1823 | Sore throat | Erythromycin & Paracetamol | 3651 | Penicillin allergy. |
| 23.08.99 | 31.12.19 | F | | 919 | 926 | Difficulty breathing & pitting ankle oedema | Bumetanide | 3704 | |
| 27.08.99 | 18.03.48 | M | | 1830 | 1837 | He is applying for Orange badge | | 3712 | |
| 24.08.99 | 26.01.91 | M | Rash | 1814 | 1823 | Urticarial type rash | Clarityn & Calamine | 3724 | |
| 23.08.99 | 29.08.34 | F | | 1710 | 1715 | Script for Prochlorperazine given | | 3729 | |
| 24.08.99 | 24.09.41 | F | RTI | 1756 | 1808 | Cough & wheezy | Amoxycillin, Clarithromycin & Prednisolone | 3760 | Nebulizer was also given. |

Result of a query that lists all consultations from the 22nd to the end of August 1999 (ConsultationsSeenFrom22ndTillEndOfAug1999)

| SurgeryDate | DateOfBirth | Sex | Diagnosis | TimeIn | TimeOut | Complaints | Treatments | NumbersID | Notes |
|---|---|---|---|---|---|---|---|---|---|
| 27.08.99 | 29.09.41 | F | Revisit | 1041 | 1055 | Acute asthmatic attack | Referred to Medical Dr. on call, SGH | 3760 | |
| 27.08.99 | 26.10.61 | M | | 1012 | 1019 | For Creatinine clearance test & MSU | | 3820 | |
| 25.08.99 | 02.12.92 | M | Rash | 1646 | 1652 | Bald patch on head & itchy rash on feet | Nizoral shampoo & Fucidin-H cream | 3826 | |
| 27.08.99 | 29.09.37 | F | RTI | 1816 | 1820 | Cough | Amoxycillin | 3835 | |
| 31.08.99 | 31.05.86 | M | Lump | 1742 | 1748 | (L) cervical node palpable | Advised to come to surgery in 3-6 months | 3881 | |
| 31.08.99 | 31.05.86 | M | URTI | 1738 | 1742 | Bilateral ear infection | Otomize ear spray | 3882 | |
| 31.08.99 | 23.04.84 | M | | 1724 | 1727 | Verrucae both feet | Cuplex gel | 3883 | |
| 25.08.99 | 19.09.51 | F | S/Leave | 940 | 944 | Back pain | | 3910 | Script for Frusemide was also given. |
| 31.08.99 | 29.01.56 | M | S/Leave | 1727 | 1732 | Back pain - private | | 3935 | Script for Co-Proxamol & Ibuprofen given. |
| 24.08.99 | 04.09.85 | M | RTI | 1645 | 1652 | Cough | Clarithromycin | 3959 | |
| 27.08.99 | 01.08.47 | F | | 1635 | 1644 | Advised to continue her own Gaviscon | | 398 | |
| 26.08.99 | 03.02.71 | F | UTI | 1739 | 1745 | Dysuria & Haematuria | Cefadroxil | 4003 | FP1001 (GMS4) form signed. For MSU. |
| 25.08.99 | 27.06.72 | M | | 1722 | 1728 | Redness & swelling (L) hand | Flucloxacillin, Ibuprofen & Clarityn | 4012 | |

Result of a query that lists all consultations from the 22nd to the end of August 1999 (ConsultationsSeenFrom22ndTillEndOfAug1999)

| SurgeryDate | DateOfBirth | Sex | Diagnosis | TimeIn | TimeOut | Complaints | Treatments | NumbersID | Notes |
|---|---|---|---|---|---|---|---|---|---|
| 23.08.99 | 18.06.93 | F | Revisit | 933 | 936 | She still snores quite a lot | Referred to ENT Surgeon | 4038 | |
| 27.08.99 | 07.10.33 | M | | 954 | 958 | Script for Haloperidol & Procyclidine given | | 4055 | |
| 24.08.99 | 30.04.84 | M | URTI | 1736 | 1742 | (L) ear ache | Flucloxacillin & Sofradex ear drops | 4131 | |
| 31.08.99 | 21.02.16 | F | Pain | 1641 | 1646 | Pain (R) ear | Co-Proxamol & Otomize ear spray | 4178 | Penicillin allergy. |
| 31.08.99 | 20.11.38 | M | | 1910 | 1935 | Patient fell in front of his house, no obvious injury | | 4187 | Home visit. |
| 25.08.99 | 03.07.40 | F | | 949 | 956 | Numbness (L) thigh & back pain | Referred to Orthopaedic Surgeon | 4223 | Penicillin allergy. |
| 26.08.99 | 19.05.89 | M | URTI | 1659 | 1704 | Sore throat | Amoxycillin | 4257 | |
| 26.08.99 | 19.11.24 | M | | 1030 | 1039 | Giddy & insomnia | Prochlorperazine & Zolpidem | 4264 | For FBC & Cholesterol. |
| 27.08.99 | 02.10.53 | M | Pain | 914 | 921 | Abdominal pain | Spasmonal | 4266 | |
| 23.08.99 | 30.10.69 | F | Pain | 944 | 959 | Persistent chest pain | Referred to Cardiologist | 4275 | For CXR & serum Cholesterol. |
| 31.08.99 | 30.12.28 | F | Lump | 1651 | 1659 | Painful prolapsed pile | Co-Amoxiclav, Scheriproct suppositories & Scheriproct ointment | 430 | New Patient check done. |
| 31.08.99 | 09.03.63 | F | RTI | 951 | 955 | Cough | Amoxycillin | 4368 | Script for Paroxetine was also given. |

Result of a query that lists all consultations from the 22nd to the end of August 1999 (ConsultationsSeenFrom22ndTillEndOfAug1999)

| SurgeryDate | DateOfBirth | Sex | Diagnosis | TimeIn | TimeOut | Complaints | Treatments | NumbersID | Notes |
|---|---|---|---|---|---|---|---|---|---|
| 27.08.99 | 31.12.22 | M | | 1106 | 1120 | Script for Co-Proxamol, Lactulose & Co-danthrusate given | | 4470 | |
| 31.08.99 | 31.12.22 | M | | 1315 | 1328 | Pedal oedema & dysuria | Trimethoprim & Bumetanide | 4470 | Home visit. |
| 26.08.99 | 03.05.46 | F | | 925 | 938 | Hot flushes | Estraderm MX | 4483 | Her sister has Crohn's disease & her bowels are very loose. Referred to Gastro-enterologist. |
| 23.08.99 | 10.04.89 | M | Conjunctivitis | 959 | 1002 | Sticky red eyes | Fucithalmic eye drops | 4524 | |
| 23.08.99 | 04.06.61 | F | | 1034 | 1101 | Her husband is physically & mentally assaulting her | | 4605 | Her mum came to the Surgery. |
| 26.08.99 | 31.03.42 | F | | 942 | 949 | Script for Dienoestrol cream given | | 4609 | |
| 24.08.99 | 27.08.22 | M | Pain | 936 | 940 | Injury (L) shoulder | X-Ray (L) shoulder | 4624 | |
| 25.08.99 | 13.01.29 | F | Conjunctivitis | 1023 | 1026 | Sticky (L) eye | Chloramphenicol eye drops | 4627 | |
| 24.08.99 | 22.04.59 | F | Revisit | 1718 | 1721 | Breasts still itchy & congested | Advised to make appointment with P/Nurse for breasts examination | 463 | |
| 31.08.99 | 22.04.59 | F | Revisit | 1646 | 1651 | (R) breast lump | Referred to Surgeon | 463 | |

769

Result of a query that lists all consultations from the 22nd to the end of August 1999 (ConsultationsSeenFrom22ndTillEndOfAug1999)

| SurgeryDate | DateOfBirth | Sex | Diagnosis | TimeIn | TimeOut | Complaints | Treatments | NumbersID | Notes |
|---|---|---|---|---|---|---|---|---|---|
| 24.08.99 | 20.11.83 | F | Pain | 1715 | 1718 | Headaches | Ibuprofen & Paracetamol | 464 | |
| 27.08.99 | 14.02.37 | F | | 935 | 941 | Script for Glucobay, Metformin, Paracetamol & Medisense test strips given | | 4672 | |
| 26.08.99 | 07.08.42 | F | | 1635 | 1648 | USScan of neck: Nodular masses in (R) & (L) Thyroid lobes | Referred to neck Surgeon | 4695 | |
| 24.08.99 | 10.06.20 | F | | 903 | 907 | Script for Isosorbide Mononitrate & Fru-Co given | | 4699 | |
| 25.08.99 | 19.01.24 | F | Revisit | 956 | 1002 | Red itchy rash on neck worse | Referred to Dermatologist (urgent) | 4708 | |
| 27.08.99 | 13.02.74 | M | | 1734 | 1741 | His hearing on (R) side is worse | Referred to ENT Surgeon | 4731 | His hear is also throbbing, Rx. Otosporin ear drops. He also has darkish ring around his eyes, referred to Dermatologist. |
| 31.08.99 | 21.04.85 | M | | 936 | 945 | Infected BCG site | Flucloxacillin & Fucidin cream | 4768 | He also has verruca (L) foot, Rx. Cuplex gel. |
| 31.08.99 | 28.08.84 | M | Rash | 1732 | 1738 | Acne spots on his face & upper trunk | Topicycline lotion | 4862 | |
| 24.08.99 | 23.06.83 | M | | 1710 | 1715 | Fell on glass, ?foreign body present in arm | | 4888 | For X-Ray (L) arm. |

770

Result of a query that lists all consultations from the 22nd to the end of August 1999 (ConsultationsSeenFrom22ndTillEndOfAug1999)

| SurgeryDate | DateOfBirth | Sex | Diagnosis | TimeIn | TimeOut | Complaints | Treatments | NumbersID | Notes |
|---|---|---|---|---|---|---|---|---|---|
| 31.08.99 | 27.02.74 | F | | 1354 | 1405 | Routine P/Natal check | | 4977 | Home visit. |
| 27.08.99 | 25.02.62 | M | S/Leave | 1826 | 1830 | Depression | | 5034 | Script for Citalopram given. |
| 27.08.99 | 10.12.43 | M | S/Leave | 1644 | 1648 | Dizziness & chest pain | | 5054 | |
| 23.08.99 | 03.03.77 | M | | 1804 | 1809 | Spots on the penile shaft | Metronidazole & Clarithromycin | 5104 | |
| 24.08.99 | 11.01.57 | F | | 1639 | 1645 | Script for Multivitamin given | | 5113 | |
| 25.08.99 | 06.11.26 | F | | 1031 | 1039 | Script for Paracetamol given | | 5181 | |
| 31.08.99 | 18.02.43 | M | Pain | 945 | 951 | Epigastric pain & discomfort | Referred to Gastro-enterologist | 519 | |
| 31.08.99 | 17.04.45 | F | | 1016 | 1019 | On Tizanidine | For LFTs | 5207 | |
| 31.08.99 | 15.10.69 | F | | 903 | 914 | Pregnancy test positive | | 5239 | |
| 25.08.99 | 30.05.37 | M | | 1002 | 1007 | Buzzing both ears | Otomize ear spray | 5299 | |
| 27.08.99 | 04.07.96 | M | RTI | 1823 | 1826 | Cough | Amoxycillin & Paracetamol | 5312 | |
| 27.08.99 | 01.02.96 | M | | 1026 | 1041 | Excessive weight gain & tiredness | Referred to Paediatrician | 5336 | For FBC, U/Es, MSU & Glucose. |
| 26.08.99 | 29.12.37 | F | | 1042 | 1047 | Hot flushes & night cramps | Premarin & Quinine Bisulphate | 5395 | |

Result of a query that lists all consultations from the 22nd to the end of August 1999 (ConsultationsSeenFrom22ndTillEndOfAug1999)

| SurgeryDate | DateOfBirth | Sex | Diagnosis | TimeIn | TimeOut | Complaints | Treatments | NumbersID | Notes |
|---|---|---|---|---|---|---|---|---|---|
| 23.08.99 | 16.10.96 | F | Rash | 1715 | 1723 | Impetigo rash on face | Penicillin V, Flucloxacillin, Aveeno oil & Bactroban ointment | 5409 | |
| 25.08.99 | 03.02.96 | M | RTI | 1728 | 1734 | Cough | Clarithromycin | 5421 | |
| 23.08.99 | 07.02.53 | M | S/Leave | 1726 | 1730 | Oesophagus tumour | | 5425 | |
| 27.08.99 | 31.05.67 | F | S/Leave | 905 | 909 | Stress & anxiety | | 5565 | |
| 23.08.99 | 27.07.83 | F | Rash | 1657 | 1705 | Rash on arms, ?viral | Advised to observe | 5588 | |
| 31.08.99 | 08.01.73 | F | | 1052 | 1101 | She was seen in A/E 3 days ago with bilateral ear ache | | 5592 | |
| 24.08.99 | 30.03.84 | F | URTI | 1704 | 1710 | Sore throat | Amoxycillin & Paracetamol | 5608 | |
| 24.08.99 | 24.12.59 | F | URTI | 1700 | 1704 | Tender glands & sore throat | Cephalexin | 5609 | Penicillin allergy. |
| 26.08.99 | 28.10.70 | M | | 1801 | 1812 | He requests a letter to whom it may concern regarding application to get his driving banning from drinking revoked | | 5661 | |
| 23.08.99 | 26.06.94 | F | URTI | 1705 | 1710 | Sore throat & fever | Amoxycillin & Ibuprofen | 5711 | |
| 31.08.99 | 21.04.85 | F | Pain | 926 | 936 | Abdominal pain & lump | For USScan of the abdomen | 5798 | Script for Hydroxyzine was given. |

Result of a query that lists all consultations from the 22nd to the end of August 1999 (ConsultationsSeenFrom22ndTillEndOfAug1999)

| SurgeryDate | DateOfBirth | Sex | Diagnosis | TimeIn | TimeOut | Complaints | Treatments | NumbersID | Notes |
|---|---|---|---|---|---|---|---|---|---|
| 25.08.99 | 16.08.50 | F | | 1652 | 1659 | Hot flushes & angina | For FSH, LH & serum Cholesterol | 583 | |
| 31.08.99 | 18.06.74 | M | Pain | 1046 | 1050 | Back pain | Co-dydramol & Ibuprofen | 5830 | |
| 23.08.99 | 03.03.46 | M | | 1002 | 1015 | He wants a letter that was written to me by his employer | I explained to him that I need to get their permission first | 5845 | |
| 31.08.99 | 04.02.33 | F | Revisit | 1805 | 1817 | Increasing dyspnoea | For CXR | 5880 | |
| 31.08.99 | 24.04.67 | F | | 1817 | 1821 | She had a nasty fire in her house & she wants s/Lcave | Advised to put in a self-certificate | 5903 | |
| 27.08.99 | 10.08.94 | M | Rash | 1019 | 1026 | Impetigo rash all over | Bactroban ointment & Flucloxacillin | 5905 | |
| 24.08.99 | 08.10.97 | F | URTI | 1258 | 1306 | Infected rhinorrhoea | Amoxycillin & Ibuprofen | 5906 | |
| 25.08.99 | 02.12.86 | F | URTI | 1755 | 1759 | Sore throat | Co-Amoxiclav | 5908 | |
| 26.08.99 | 14.08.56 | M | Conjunctivitis | 1039 | 1042 | Sore & sticky eyes | Chloramphenicol eye drops | 5936 | |
| 26.08.99 | 14.05.71 | M | RTI | 1745 | 1749 | Cough & (R) ear ache | Co-Amoxiclav & Sofradex ear drops | 6017 | |
| 26.08.99 | 23.06.45 | F | Pain | 1817 | 1824 | Red, painful & swollen (L) knee | Co-dydramol & Flucloxacillin | 6040 | |
| 23.08.99 | 20.10.77 | F | | 1809 | 1816 | USScan of pelvis - normal | | 611 | Her abdominal pain also persists, Rx. Colofac. |

Result of a query that lists all consultations from the 22nd to the end of August 1999 (ConsultationsSeenFrom22ndTillEndOfAug1999)

| SurgeryDate | DateOfBirth | Sex | Diagnosis | TimeIn | TimeOut | Complaints | Treatments | NumbersID | Notes |
|---|---|---|---|---|---|---|---|---|---|
| 26.08.99 | 08.11.73 | F | URTI | 1047 | 1052 | Sore throat | Amoxycillin | 6138 | |
| 26.08.99 | 28.09.39 | F | | 903 | 916 | She is on waiting list for operation on her toes | | 6176 | |
| 23.08.99 | 22.07.17 | F | | 1744 | 1750 | Abscess (L) anterior abdominal wall | Ciprofloxacin & Fucidin cream | 6182 | Penicillin allergy. |
| 24.08.99 | 20.12.53 | M | Pain | 911 | 916 | Neck pain | Tylex & Transvasin cream | 6201 | |
| 24.08.99 | 13.05.82 | F | RTI | 1742 | 1747 | Cough | Amoxycillin | 6210 | |
| 27.08.99 | 04.12.54 | F | RTI | 931 | 935 | Cough | Amoxycillin | 6220 | |
| 26.08.99 | 21.11.24 | M | Pain | 1000 | 1009 | Pain (R) calf | Naftidrofuryl | 6221 | Script for Exorex lotion & Co-codamol was also given. |
| 26.08.99 | 20.02.77 | M | | 1722 | 1730 | Advised to see P/ Nurse for proper strapping of his broken fingers | | 6254 | Penicillin allergy. |
| 27.08.99 | 20.02.77 | M | S/Leave | 1656 | 1702 | Fracture 5th MC bone (L) hand | | 6254 | He also has verruca (R) foot, Rx. Cuplex gel. Script for Co-dydramol was also given. |
| 31.08.99 | 27.01.80 | F | | 955 | 1006 | Pregnancy test positive | | 6283 | |
| 25.08.99 | 07.12.98 | F | Rash | 1740 | 1755 | Nappy rash | Timodine cream | 6313 | |
| 26.08.99 | 12.12.98 | M | | 1655 | 1659 | Croaky voice | Amoxycillin | 6314 | |

Result of a query that lists all consultations from the 22nd to the end of August 1999 (ConsultationsSeenFrom22ndTillEndOfAug1999)

| SurgeryDate | DateOfBirth | Sex | Diagnosis | TimeIn | TimeOut | Complaints | Treatments | NumbersID | Notes |
|---|---|---|---|---|---|---|---|---|---|
| 24.08.99 | 05.06.98 | F | Conjunctivitis | 1013 | 1015 | (L) eye is red | Chloramphenicol eye drops | 6318 | |
| 24.08.99 | 13.10.69 | F | Conjunctivitis | 1009 | 1013 | Sore, watery & red (R) eye | Chloramphenicol eye ointment | 6327 | |
| 25.08.99 | 14.04.46 | F | | 1711 | 1722 | Per vagina bleeding since starting Premique cycle | She will observe | 6333 | |
| 27.08.99 | 11.05.76 | M | URTI | 921 | 931 | Sore throat | Amoxycillin | 6334 | |
| 23.08.99 | 04.03.86 | M | RTI | 1632 | 1638 | Cough & vomiting | Amoxycillin & Metoclopramide | 641 | New Patient check done. |
| 27.08.99 | 09.11.41 | F | | 1711 | 1716 | Dizziness | Prochlorperazine | 6442 | For FBC & Glucose. |
| 26.08.99 | 09.12.45 | F | | 916 | 925 | She feels tired after taking Tidiem LA | | 6467 | |
| 24.08.99 | 17.07.99 | F | | 1027 | 1042 | The baby is restless & doesn't pass urine well | Referred to Paediatric Dr. on call, SGH | 6488 | |
| 24.08.99 | 05.06.25 | F | | 1747 | 1756 | Swollen & painful gums | Metronidazole & Co-Amoxiclav | 6493 | Script for Ranitidine was also given. |
| 23.08.99 | 05.11.58 | F | Revisit | 1753 | 1804 | Itchy rash spreading | Referred to Dermatologist | 6517 | |
| 27.08.99 | 14.02.76 | M | S/Leave | 1756 | 1801 | Vomiting - private | | 778 | |
| 31.08.99 | 20.09.62 | F | | 923 | 926 | USScan of the abdomen - normal | | 808 | |
| 31.08.99 | 07.03.64 | M | | 914 | 923 | Script for Thioridazine given | | 810 | |

## Result of a query that lists all consultations from the 22nd to the end of August 1999 (ConsultationsSeenFrom22ndTillEndOfAug1999)

| SurgeryDate | DateOfBirth | Sex | Diagnosis | TimeIn | TimeOut | Complaints | Treatments | NumbersID | Notes |
|---|---|---|---|---|---|---|---|---|---|
| 24.08.99 | 16.12.33 | M | Conjunctivitis | 940 | 943 | (L) eye is blood shot | Chloramphenicol eye drops | 863 | |
| 24.08.99 | 02.09.76 | M | S/Leave | 916 | 923 | Fractured (L) Lateral malleolus - Med 5 | | 929 | |
| 23.08.99 | 08.12.62 | F | URTI | 1723 | 1726 | Sore throat | Erythromycin | 981 | Penicillin allergy. |

## Result of a query that lists all consultations from the 22nd to the end of August 2000 (ConsultationsSeenFrom22ndTillEndOfAug2000)

| SurgeryDate | DateOfBirth | Sex | Diagnosis | TimeIn | TimeOut | Complaints | Treatments | NumbersID | Notes |
|---|---|---|---|---|---|---|---|---|---|
| 22.08.2000 | 02.05.1998 | F | URTI | 1833 | 1841 | Infected rhinorrhoea & itchy rash | Calamine lotion, Amoxycillin, Paracetamol & Chlorpheniramine | Temp | |
| 23.08.2000 | 07.08.1991 | F | | 929 | 933 | Septic wound (R) wrist | Augmentin-Duo & Fucidin cream | Temp | |
| 25.08.2000 | 31.07.1945 | M | Pain | 1755 | 1800 | Pain (L) knee | For X-Ray (L) knee | NP | Penicillin allergy. |
| 25.08.2000 | 27.09.1944 | F | Conjunctivitis | 1800 | 1806 | Infection (L) upper eye lid | Chloramphenicol eye ointment | Temp | Script for Kliofem given. |
| 30.08.2000 | 30.07.1970 | F | Depression | 930 | 938 | Weepy & unable to cope | Sertraline | Temp | |
| 23.08.2000 | 31.10.1969 | F | Revisit | 1809 | 1826 | (R) vaginal area is still quite lumpy & sore | Referred to Gynaecologist | 1029 | |
| 29.08.2000 | 13.03.1954 | F | | 912 | 919 | Script for Minocin MR given | | 1172 | |

Result of a query that lists all consultations from the 22nd to the end of August 2000 (ConsultationsSeenFrom22ndTillEndOfAug2000)

| SurgeryDate | DateOfBirth | Sex | Diagnosis | TimeIn | TimeOut | Complaints | Treatments | NumbersID | Notes |
|---|---|---|---|---|---|---|---|---|---|
| 22.08.2000 | 04.07.1916 | F | | 940 | 944 | Blood tests results are not yet available | | 1199 | |
| 24.08.2000 | 04.07.1916 | F | | 1647 | 1653 | Hb 10.9 g/dl | For Ferritin, B12 & Folate | 1199 | |
| 30.08.2000 | 04.07.1916 | F | | 1641 | 1702 | Pitting ankle oedema & jaundiced | Frusemide | 1199 | For LFTs, clotting screen, U/Es, fasting Glucose & USS of upper abdomen. |
| 25.08.2000 | 13.09.1938 | F | Hypertension | 1640 | 1647 | BP 150/100 | Atenolol | 1215 | Script for Simvastatin given. For LFTs. |
| 23.08.2000 | 20.02.1930 | M | Rash | 900 | 909 | Allergic rash to Erythromycin | | 1254 | |
| 25.08.2000 | 05.08.1946 | F | | 1746 | 1755 | Script for Vioxx given | | 1268 | |
| 30.08.2000 | 18.05.1980 | M | | 1747 | 1754 | Pain (R) side of abdomen & haematuria, now settled | For MSU | 1473 | |
| 30.08.2000 | 17.12.1938 | F | Lump | 1230 | 1240 | Warry lump on (R) thigh | Referred to Surgeon | 154 | Home visit. |
| 25.08.2000 | 18.01.1936 | M | | 1653 | 1659 | (R) gum is swollen | Amoxycillin & Co-dydramol | 1620 | |
| 24.08.2000 | 04.04.1936 | F | | 939 | 952 | Orthopaedic Surgeon will contact her regarding follow-up for Colle's fracture | | 1999 | |
| 24.08.2000 | 12.02.1917 | M | RTI | 952 | 955 | Cough | Amoxycillin | 2006 | |

Result of a query that lists all consultations from the 22nd to the end of August 2000 (ConsultationsSeenFrom22ndTillEndOfAug2000)

| SurgeryDate | DateOfBirth | Sex | Diagnosis | TimeIn | TimeOut | Complaints | Treatments | NumbersID | Notes |
|---|---|---|---|---|---|---|---|---|---|
| 25.08.2000 | 09.01.1983 | M | Pain | 912 | 918 | Lower back pain | Ibuprofen & Co-dydramol | 2021 | |
| 24.08.2000 | 28.11.1980 | F | RTI | 1728 | 1735 | cough | Amoxycillin | 2393 | Whitish skin scales, Rx. 1% Hydrocortisone cream. |
| 25.08.2000 | 05.11.1941 | M | | 1740 | 1746 | Script for Allopurinol given | | 251 | For Serum Uric Acid. |
| 30.08.2000 | 24.06.1932 | F | | 1021 | 1029 | Advised to continue her present medication | | 2629 | |
| 30.08.2000 | 01.09.1989 | M | | 1016 | 1021 | Fore-skin is tight & painful to pull back | Referred to Surgeon | 2657 | |
| 30.08.2000 | 21.09.1950 | F | | 916 | 930 | Script for Kapake, Bactroban & Norethisterone given | | 2796 | |
| 24.08.2000 | 16.11.1973 | F | URTI | 1038 | 1042 | Sore throat | Co-Amoxiclav | 2836 | |
| 30.08.2000 | 24.02.1932 | F | URTI | 950 | 1005 | Pain (R) ear & congested | Amoxycillin & Otomize ear spray | 2853 | Script for Paracetamol & Amitriptyline given. |
| 25.08.2000 | 02.08.1988 | F | Revisit | 900 | 912 | Recurrent dysuria | Trimethoprim | 2919 | |
| 22.08.2000 | 31.01.1938 | M | | 1002 | 1015 | Dizziness & nausea | Prochlorperazine | 3001 | |
| 22.08.2000 | 29.01.1956 | F | | 1700 | 1703 | Flucloxacillin makes her feel sick | Co-Amoxiclav | 3034 | |
| 29.08.2000 | 15.06.1988 | M | Pain | 1746 | 1751 | Septic pierced (L) eye brow | Erythromycin | 3149 | Penicillin allergy. |

Result of a query that lists all consultations from the 22nd to the end of August 2000 (ConsultationsSeenFrom22ndTillEndOfAug2000)

| SurgeryDate | DateOfBirth | Sex | Diagnosis | TimeIn | TimeOut | Complaints | Treatments | NumbersID | Notes |
|---|---|---|---|---|---|---|---|---|---|
| 22.08.2000 | 05.11.1988 | F | | 1746 | 1755 | HVS: Beta-haemolytic streptococci Lancefield group A sensitive to Penicillin | Penicillin V | 3297 | |
| 30.08.2000 | 12.08.1932 | M | | 938 | 941 | Abdominal pain now improving | | 3344 | |
| 23.08.2000 | 02.03.1948 | M | Revisit | 1720 | 1734 | Ranula cystic lump is still present under the tongue | Referred to Oral Surgeon | 3473 | |
| 30.08.2000 | 10.08.1910 | F | Pain | 1220 | 1230 | Body pains | Co-codamol soluble | 3485 | Home visit. General condition poor. |
| 25.08.2000 | 03.12.1944 | F | Rash | 1716 | 1724 | Spotty infected rash on back | Flucloxacillin | 3509 | Body pains, Rx. Co-dydramol. |
| 30.08.2000 | 09.12.1933 | F | Rash | 1005 | 1016 | Itchy, scaly & reddish rash around the nose | Fucidin-H cream | 3583 | Tetracycline allergy. |
| 29.08.2000 | 04.05.1992 | F | | 1033 | 1037 | Verrucae both feet | Cuplex gel | 3700 | |
| 29.08.2000 | 02.12.1992 | M | | 1014 | 1019 | Itchy white spots on the tongue | Daktarin oral gel | 3810 | |
| 22.08.2000 | 11.03.1930 | F | | 1155 | 1210 | Script for Frusemide given | | 3887 | Home visit. |
| 29.08.2000 | 29.01.1956 | M | | 1000 | 1014 | Panic attacks | Citalopram | 3935 | Neck pain & headaches, for Cervical X-Ray. |
| 24.08.2000 | 04.09.1985 | M | URTI | 1805 | 1810 | Sore throat | Amoxycillin & Paracetamol | 3959 | Nuts allergy. |

Result of a query that lists all consultations from the 22nd to the end of August 2000 (ConsultationsSeenFrom22ndTillEndOfAug2000)

| SurgeryDate | DateOfBirth | Sex | Diagnosis | TimeIn | TimeOut | Complaints | Treatments | NumbersID | Notes |
|---|---|---|---|---|---|---|---|---|---|
| 30.08.2000 | 19.05.1964 | M | | 1633 | 1641 | He wants to have vasectomy reversal under BUPA | | 3995 | |
| 23.08.2000 | 07.10.1933 | M | | 1017 | 1021 | Script for Haloperidol & Procyclidine given | | 4055 | |
| 22.08.2000 | 04.09.1952 | M | Pain | 934 | 940 | Pain (R) kidney area | For MSU | 4128 | |
| 25.08.2000 | 25.07.1931 | F | Pain | 955 | 1004 | Pain from her Gall bladder stones is quite bad | Kapake & Buscopan | 4156 | |
| 24.08.2000 | 21.02.1916 | F | Revisit | 1653 | 1659 | Leg wound is still sore | Clarithromycin | 4178 | Penicillin allergy. |
| 30.08.2000 | 21.02.1916 | F | Revisit | 1034 | 1040 | Leg wound is still septic | Erythromycin | 4178 | Penicillin allergy. |
| 30.08.2000 | 20.11.1938 | M | | 1240 | 1315 | Wife wants a mobile aid for her husband | To be arranged | 4187 | Home visit. |
| 22.08.2000 | 27.03.1943 | F | | 1029 | 1033 | Recurrent chest infections | For CXR | 4203 | |
| 30.08.2000 | 10.03.1936 | M | | 1732 | 1740 | Script for Chloramphenicol eye drops given | | 425 | Private script for Viagra was also given. |
| 23.08.2000 | 14.10.1958 | M | Rash | 1643 | 1652 | Allergic rash to Metronidazole & Voltarol | Loratadine | 4250 | |
| 24.08.2000 | 23.06.1972 | F | | 1027 | 1038 | Script for Dianette given | | 4336 | FP1001 (GMS4) form signed. |
| 25.08.2000 | 31.05.1986 | F | Rash | 1724 | 1729 | Impetigo-like rash on the ears | Flucloxacillin & Bactroban | 4369 | |
| 23.08.2000 | 29.05.1973 | M | | 1744 | 1749 | Script for Flixonase nasal spray given | | 4485 | |

Result of a query that lists all consultations from the 22nd to the end of August 2000 (ConsultationsSeenFrom22ndTillEndOfAug2000)

| SurgeryDate | DateOfBirth | Sex | Diagnosis | TimeIn | TimeOut | Complaints | Treatments | NumbersID | Notes |
|---|---|---|---|---|---|---|---|---|---|
| 25.08.2000 | 01.03.1930 | F | RTI | 1635 | 1640 | Cough | Ciprofloxacin | 4652 | |
| 25.08.2000 | 16.11.1962 | F | | 1004 | 1030 | I explained to her that I cannot give further Zopiclone without adequately monitoring the previous Zopiclone doses | | 4655 | |
| 29.08.2000 | 16.11.1962 | F | | 1754 | 1834 | Script for Zopiclone given | | 4655 | |
| 24.08.2000 | 02.07.1943 | M | Pain | 930 | 939 | Pain (R) elbow | Inj. Depo-Medrone with Lidocaine | 4667 | |
| 25.08.2000 | 02.07.1943 | M | | 1049 | 1100 | Inj. Depo-Medrone with Lidocaine given to (R) elbow | | 4667 | |
| 22.08.2000 | 06.03.1913 | F | URTI | 900 | 921 | (R) Otitis ext. | Flucloxacillin & Otosporin ear drops | 4919 | |
| 30.08.2000 | 25.07.1978 | M | | 1706 | 1712 | Tender lump (L) axilla | Flucloxacillin | 5015 | ?Foreign body (R) thumb, for X-Ray (R) thumb. |
| 22.08.2000 | 27.02.1931 | F | RTI | 1640 | 1645 | Cough | Amoxycillin | 5036 | |
| 25.08.2000 | 19.06.1961 | F | | 918 | 929 | Script for Fluconazole given | | 5131 | |
| 30.08.2000 | 22.04.1983 | F | Pain | 1205 | 1220 | Pains in her joints | Kapake & Amitripyline | 5228 | Script for Senna tablets given. Home visit. |
| 25.08.2000 | 21.03.1996 | F | RTI | 1647 | 1653 | Cough | Amoxicillin | 5233 | |

Result of a query that lists all consultations from the 22nd to the end of August 2000 (ConsultationsSeenFrom22ndTillEndOfAug2000)

| SurgeryDate | DateOfBirth | Sex | Diagnosis | TimeIn | TimeOut | Complaints | Treatments | NumbersID | Notes |
|---|---|---|---|---|---|---|---|---|---|
| 22.08.2000 | 11.11.1930 | F | | 921 | 931 | Bruising of (R) leg following angioplasty | Advised to stop Clopidogrel for now | 5275 | |
| 25.08.2000 | 17.02.1972 | F | | 1039 | 1043 | Cervical Spine X-Ray: No bony injury seen. Probable muscle spasm | | 5279 | Penicillin allergy. |
| 30.08.2000 | 08.12.1978 | F | Rash | 1044 | 1101 | Urticaria rash | Fexofenadine | 5293 | Referred to Dermatologist (BUPA). |
| 24.08.2000 | 11.11.1969 | F | | 1704 | 1718 | Hb 10.9 g/dl | Ferrograd-Folic | 5363 | 28 weeks gestation. |
| 25.08.2000 | 17.10.1929 | M | | 931 | 938 | Script for Bendrofluazide & Simvastatin given | | 5469 | |
| 24.08.2000 | 24.02.1918 | M | | 1635 | 1647 | X-Ray Pelvis/Hips: Mild OA changes both hips | | 5490 | |
| 29.08.2000 | 08.02.1945 | M | Rash | 1720 | 1727 | Red spotty rash | Flucloxacillin & Fucidin cream | 5516 | |
| 23.08.2000 | 08.10.1967 | M | Revisit | 1633 | 1640 | He still has pain in both shoulders | Referred to Rheumatologist (BUPA) | 5525 | |
| 30.08.2000 | 05.08.1976 | F | | 1723 | 1732 | Script for Microgynon-30, Capasal shampoo & Betacap lotion given | | 5702 | |
| 30.08.2000 | 21.08.1997 | M | Rash | 1712 | 1717 | Chicken Pox rash | Chlorpheniramine & Paracetamol | 5768 | |

Result of a query that lists all consultations from the 22nd to the end of August 2000 (ConsultationsSeenFrom22ndTillEndOfAug2000)

| SurgeryDate | DateOfBirth | Sex | Diagnosis | TimeIn | TimeOut | Complaints | Treatments | NumbersID | Notes |
|---|---|---|---|---|---|---|---|---|---|
| 30.08.2000 | 17.01.1956 | F | Rash | 941 | 950 | Infected spots (R) upper arm | Tetracycline & Bactroban | 5796 | |
| 23.08.2000 | 16.08.1950 | M | | 953 | 1008 | ?Anaemia | For FBC | 583 | |
| 30.08.2000 | 16.08.1950 | F | Anaemia | 1024 | 1034 | Hb 11.3 g/dl | For B12, Folate & Ferritin | 583 | |
| 23.08.2000 | 02.06.1977 | M | | 944 | 953 | Weakness & palpitations | For FBC & TFTs | 585 | |
| 22.08.2000 | 25.03.1963 | M | RTI | 1645 | 1651 | Cough | Ciprofloxacin & Simple Linctus | 5853 | |
| 29.08.2000 | 25.03.1963 | M | Revisit | 919 | 926 | He still has chesty cough | For CXR | 5853 | |
| 23.08.2000 | 13.12.1982 | M | Pain | 1652 | 1715 | Back & chest pain | Ibuprofen & Co-dydramol | 586 | Penicillin allergy. |
| 22.08.2000 | 19.01.1983 | F | Revisit | 1651 | 1700 | Still chesty | For CXR | 5907 | Penicillin allergy. |
| 29.08.2000 | 19.01.1983 | F | S/Leave | 1700 | 1708 | Persistent cough | | 5907 | Penicillin allergy. |
| 23.08.2000 | 02.12.1986 | F | Rash | 1749 | 1752 | Acne rash on face | Zineryt lotion | 5908 | |
| 29.08.2000 | 22.12.1997 | F | RTI | 926 | 930 | Cough | Amoxycillin | 5919 | |
| 24.08.2000 | 28.11.1980 | F | URTI | 1718 | 1728 | Sore throat | Amoxycillin | 5938 | Script for Dalacin-T lotion given. |
| 29.08.2000 | 26.10.1997 | F | RTI | 1656 | 1700 | Cough | Amoxycillin | 6084 | Script for Prednisolone given. |
| 24.08.2000 | 22.02.1924 | M | Pain | 919 | 930 | Pain (R) shoulder | For X-Ray (R) shoulder | 6094 | |
| 22.08.2000 | 22.02.1966 | F | | 1716 | 1730 | Pregnancy test positive | | 6106 | |
| 25.08.2000 | 04.06.1969 | F | | 1729 | 1734 | Strange sensation in both ears & giddiness | EarCalm & Prochlorperazine | 6130 | Penicillin & Sulphur allergy. |

783

## Result of a query that lists all consultations from the 22nd to the end of August 2000 (ConsultationsSeenFrom22ndTillEndOfAug2000)

| SurgeryDate | DateOfBirth | Sex | Diagnosis | TimeIn | TimeOut | Complaints | Treatments | NumbersID | Notes |
|---|---|---|---|---|---|---|---|---|---|
| 23.08.2000 | 03.12.1955 | F | | 1734 | 1744 | Script for Citalopram & Colpermin given | | 614 | |
| 25.08.2000 | 22.07.1917 | F | | 1659 | 1710 | Pins & needles both feet | Hirudoid cream | 6182 | Penicillin & Vallergan allergy. |
| 22.08.2000 | 09.06.1944 | F | URTI | 1708 | 1716 | Sinuses congested | Amoxycillin | 6184 | Script for Constipated, Lactulose & Senna given. |
| 23.08.2000 | 21.05.1958 | F | Revisit | 933 | 944 | Back pain has persisted | For Physiotherapy | 6209 | |
| 23.08.2000 | 09.11.1910 | F | | 912 | 919 | Dyspnoea again | For CXR | 626 | |
| 22.08.2000 | 07.04.1981 | F | | 931 | 934 | Diarrhoea with Flucloxacillin | To try & take the antibiotics for at least 5 days | 6275 | |
| 29.08.2000 | 28.03.1945 | M | Revisit | 1834 | 1842 | Pain (R) knee is still present | Vioxx & Zacin cream | 6357 | Script for Tetracycline given. |
| 25.08.2000 | 03.03.1999 | F | | 1030 | 1039 | Septic wound & blister on (L) foot | Flucloxacillin & Fucidin cream | 6376 | |
| 29.08.2000 | 07.01.1980 | F | | 950 | 1000 | PER VAGINA bleeding | Referred to Gynaecology Dr. on call, SGH | 6397 | 8 weeks gestation. |
| 25.08.2000 | 18.07.1936 | F | | 938 | 944 | Her NatWest's Premium has been increased because of hypertension | | 6444 | |
| 24.08.2000 | 24.19.1924 | M | | 1742 | 1747 | Septic (R) cheek lump | Clarithromycin | 6492 | Penicillin allergy. |

## Result of a query that lists all consultations from the 22<sup>nd</sup> to the end of August 2000 (ConsultationsSeenFrom22ndTillEndOfAug2000)

| SurgeryDate | DateOfBirth | Sex | Diagnosis | TimeIn | TimeOut | Complaints | Treatments | NumbersID | Notes |
|---|---|---|---|---|---|---|---|---|---|
| 23.08.2000 | 27.08.1948 | F | | 1752 | 1809 | Script for Estraderm MX & Dydrogesterone given | | 6538 | |
| 24.08.2000 | 03.07.1974 | M | Pain | 1205 | 1225 | Chest pain | GTN spray | 6546 | Home visit. Referred to Care of the elderly Physician. Penicillin allergy. |
| 23.08.2000 | 03.09.1926 | M | Lump | 1008 | 1017 | Lipoma (R) fore-head | Referred to Plastic Surgeon (Basildon hospital) | 6568 | Script for ROC cream. |
| 24.08.2000 | 13.11.1943 | F | URTI | 958 | 1007 | Sore throat, (R) ear ache, dizziness & nausea | Amoxycillin, Prochlorperazine & Otomize ear spray | 6601 | Itchy rash on (R) leg, Rx. 1% Hydrocortisone cream. |
| 22.08.2000 | 22.04.1954 | M | S/Leave | 944 | 951 | Chest pain - Private | | 6614 | |
| 29.08.2000 | 09.11.1978 | F | | 1400 | 1428 | Diarrhoea & vomiting | Ciprofloxacin & Loperamide | 6622 | PR bleeding. Home visit. |
| 24.08.2000 | 20.02.1953 | F | | 1659 | 1704 | Septic insect bites on face | Flucloxacillin & Loratadine | 6633 | |
| 29.08.2000 | 16.03.1929 | M | Pain | 1708 | 1720 | (L) chest pain | GTN spray & Imdur | 6647 | |
| 24.08.2000 | 02.09.1994 | F | | 1013 | 1017 | Diarrhoea | Electrolade | 6719 | Cough, Rx. Simple Linctus. Head lice. Rx. 0.5% Malathion. |

Result of a query that lists all consultations from the 22nd to the end of August 2000 (ConsultationsSeenFrom22ndTillEndOfAug2000)

| SurgeryDate | DateOfBirth | Sex | Diagnosis | TimeIn | TimeOut | Complaints | Treatments | NumbersID | Notes |
|---|---|---|---|---|---|---|---|---|---|
| 30.08.2000 | 11.01.1951 | F | | 1717 | 1723 | Script for Zafirlukast given | | 6735 | |
| 29.08.2000 | 16.07.1969 | F | | 1643 | 1656 | Routine ante-natal check | | 6747 | 38+4 weeks gestation. |
| 24.08.2000 | 27.02.1941 | M | S/Leave | 1735 | 1742 | Emphysema - Private | | 675 | He would like to be referred back to chest Physician, referred to Chest Physician (Basildon hospital). |
| 22.08.2000 | 23.08.1971 | F | | 1755 | 1825 | 1st Accolate safety study test | | 6762 | |
| 24.08.2000 | 18.05.2000 | M | | 1007 | 1013 | Diarrhoea | Dioralyte | 6787 | |
| 30.08.2000 | 13.12.1970 | F | | 1040 | 1044 | For repeat FBC in 6 months | | 6792 | |
| 22.08.2000 | 10.03.1951 | F | | 951 | 955 | Pain at site of laceration | Advised to use own analgesia | 683 | |
| 25.08.2000 | 22.06.1999 | F | | 1043 | 1049 | Vomiting | Paracetamol & Metoclopramide | 6837 | |
| 24.08.2000 | 10.11.1976 | F | | 909 | 919 | She keeps feeling faint | For FBC & MSU | 6838 | 13 weeks gestation. |
| 24.08.2000 | 16.10.1979 | M | Lump | 902 | 909 | Mole on chest | For excision | 6859 | |
| 22.08.2000 | 12.05.1982 | F | Pain | 1015 | 1029 | Fell on her back | Paracetamol soluble | 6860 | She is 6 months pregnant. For MSU. |
| 24.08.2000 | 17.09.1956 | M | | 1810 | 1822 | Script for Simvastatin given | | 793 | |
| 23.08.2000 | 01.09.1961 | M | | 1715 | 1720 | Spots on the penis | Daktarin cream | 832 | |

| \multicolumn{8}{c}{Result of a query that lists all consultations from the 22$^{nd}$ to the end of August 2000 (ConsultationsSeenFrom22ndTillEndOfAug2000)} |
| SurgeryDate | DateOfBirth | Sex | Diagnosis | TimeIn | TimeOut | Complaints | Treatments | NumbersID | Notes |
| --- | --- | --- | --- | --- | --- | --- | --- | --- | --- |
| 30.08.2000 | 05.10.1974 | M | S/Leave | 858 | 903 | Pain (R) shoulder | | 918 | |
| 29.08.2000 | 26.06.1945 | M | | 1727 | 1746 | Hay fever | Fexofenadine | 939 | Script for Fexofenadine given. For FSH & LH. |

| \multicolumn{8}{c}{Result of a query that lists all consultations from the 22$^{nd}$ to the end of August 2001 (ConsultationsSeenFrom22ndTillEndOfAug2001)} |
| SurgeryDate | DateOfBirth | Sex | Diagnosis | TimeIn | TimeOut | Complaints | Treatments | NumbersID | Notes |
| --- | --- | --- | --- | --- | --- | --- | --- | --- | --- |
| 22.08.2001 | 09.03.1922 | M | | 1010 | 1015 | Bilateral pedal oedema | Frusemide | NP | For U/Es & FBC. |
| 22.08.2001 | 09.04.1953 | F | S/Leave | 1743 | 1750 | Pain (R) lower chest | | Temp | Script for Thyroxine given. |
| 22.08.2001 | 19.07.1934 | F | | 1818 | 1827 | (L) arm went numb & heavy | Aspirin Dispersible | Temp | |
| 23.08.2001 | 19.07.1934 | F | | 1718 | 1735 | Advised to go to Smoking Cessation clinic | | Temp | |
| 23.08.2001 | 21.12.2000 | F | Rash | 1808 | 1812 | Red rash both cheeks, ?slapped cheek syndrome | Fucidin cream & Flucloxacillin | Temp | |
| 24.08.2001 | 10.12.1978 | F | | 1035 | 1044 | She will come later for her anti-eczema rash medication | | Temp | |
| 28.08.2001 | 12.09.1983 | F | | 1826 | 1833 | Burst condom | Levonelle-2 | Temp | |
| 30.08.2001 | 19.05.1943 | F | Pain | 1711 | 1717 | Abdominal pain | Buscopan | Temp | |

Result of a query that lists all consultations from the 22nd to the end of August 2001 (ConsultationsSeenFrom22ndTillEndOfAug2001)

| SurgeryDate | DateOfBirth | Sex | Diagnosis | TimeIn | TimeOut | Complaints | Treatments | NumbersID | Notes |
|---|---|---|---|---|---|---|---|---|---|
| 30.08.2001 | 25.05.1997 | F | | 1803 | 1808 | Script for Diprobase cream & Fucidin cream given | | Temp | |
| 24.08.2001 | 31.10.1969 | F | | 1800 | 1804 | Persistent per vagina bleeding | Norethisterone | 1022 | FP1001 (GMS4) form signed. |
| 22.08.2001 | 11.08.1943 | F | | 904 | 933 | Advised to continue Dosulepin | | 1024 | Husband came to Surgery. |
| 28.08.2001 | 11.08.1943 | F | | 1707 | 1719 | Vaginal irritation | Clotrimazole cream | 1024 | Script for Dosulepin given. For Fasting Cholesterol. |
| 28.08.2001 | 08.02.1939 | F | | 1757 | 1801 | Whitlow (R) middle finger | Flucloxacillin & Fucidin cream | 113 | Trimethoprim allergy. |
| 29.08.2001 | 19.06.1959 | M | Deafness | 956 | 959 | Wax in the ears | Waxsol ear drops | 1191 | |
| 22.08.2001 | 24.10.1929 | F | | 1716 | 1721 | Script for Pravastatin given | | 1255 | Script for Cerivastatin given. |
| 23.08.2001 | 05.02.1946 | F | | 922 | 930 | Phlebitis (L) leg | Flucloxacillin & 0.3% Heparinoid cream | 1268 | |
| 30.08.2001 | 10.08.1985 | F | Pain | 1724 | 1729 | Back pain | Naprosyn | 1268 | For X-Ray Lumbar Spine. |
| 23.08.2001 | 13.08.1935 | M | | 938 | 946 | Foods get stuck in the throat | Referred to Gastro-enterologist | 1269 | |
| 22.08.2001 | 28.04.1981 | F | | 933 | 939 | Constipation | Lactulose & Senna | 1287 | |
| 30.08.2001 | 15.07.1936 | F | | 944 | 955 | Script for Premique given | | 1309 | Letter to whom it may concern. |

Result of a query that lists all consultations from the 22nd to the end of August 2001 (ConsultationsSeenFrom22ndTillEndOfAug2001)

| SurgeryDate | DateOfBirth | Sex | Diagnosis | TimeIn | TimeOut | Complaints | Treatments | NumbersID | Notes |
|---|---|---|---|---|---|---|---|---|---|
| 30.08.2001 | 06.07.1948 | M | URTI | 931 | 937 | (R) ear is reddish | Amoxycillin | 1356 | |
| 24.08.2001 | 06.12.1939 | M | | 1758 | 1800 | Script for Simvastatin & Bendrofluazide given | | 1414 | Advised to stop Cerivastatin. |
| 28.08.2001 | 02.05.1959 | M | | 1748 | 1757 | He trod on a nail, (R) foot | Flucloxacillin | 1451 | For Fasting Cholesterol. Tetanus Toxoid Booster given. |
| 28.08.2001 | 09.01.1991 | M | | 1815 | 1819 | Wants his sutures removed | Advised to go to A/E | 1470 | Mum was unhappy. |
| 28.08.2001 | 17.09.1916 | F | | 906 | 918 | She came in regarding her failing hearing aid | | 1531 | |
| 28.08.2001 | 14.12.1924 | M | | 1225 | 1245 | Bilateral pedal oedema | Metolazone & Frusemide | 1586 | Home visit. Script for Multivitamins given. |
| 29.08.2001 | 11.11.1940 | M | Revisit | 1718 | 1722 | Wound (R) thumb is healing slowly | Flucloxacillin & Fucidin cream | 1611 | |
| 30.08.2001 | 18.01.1936 | M | Pain | 1011 | 1018 | Pain (R) heel | Ibuprofen & Co-dydramol | 1620 | |
| 23.08.2001 | 17.08.1984 | F | URTI | 1006 | 1010 | Pain in (R) ear | Otosporin ear drops | 2001 | |
| 28.08.2001 | 22.03.1933 | F | | 1725 | 1729 | Sore mouth & swollen gums | Amoxycillin | 2179 | |
| 29.08.2001 | 21.10.1982 | M | | 1036 | 1042 | Letter to expedite Dermatology clinic appointment | | 2196 | |

Result of a query that lists all consultations from the 22nd to the end of August 2001 (ConsultationsSeenFrom22ndTillEndOfAug2001)

| SurgeryDate | DateOfBirth | Sex | Diagnosis | TimeIn | TimeOut | Complaints | Treatments | NumbersID | Notes |
|---|---|---|---|---|---|---|---|---|---|
| 23.08.2001 | 11.06.1968 | F | Pain | 1748 | 1758 | Lower abdominal pain has got worse despite taking Trimethoprim | Referred to Surgical Dr. on call, SGH | 2261 | |
| 23.08.2001 | 06.11.1915 | M | Revisit | 903 | 922 | Persistent sweating & (R) sided back pain | Referred to Dr. on duty, MAU, SGH | 229 | |
| 29.08.2001 | 22.08.1980 | F | | 1702 | 1710 | Script for Dianette given | | 2300 | FP1001 (GMS4) form signed. |
| 28.08.2001 | 23.08.1937 | F | | 1801 | 1815 | (R) upper abdominal pain & heartburn | Lansoprazole | 2304 | For USScan of the upper abdomen. |
| 22.08.2001 | 24.09.1937 | M | | 1703 | 1708 | He may need modified GTT now or later after a repeat fasting Glucose | | 2329 | |
| 22.08.2001 | 01.10.1920 | M | Pain | 1750 | 1802 | Painful (R) big toe & red | Flucloxacillin & Ibuprofen | 2463 | For Uric Acid. For X-Ray (R) big toe (& (R) foot). |
| 28.08.2001 | 11.12.1987 | M | Rash | 944 | 950 | Impetigo rash on (R) arm & (R) leg | Mupirocin cream & Flucloxacillin | 2473 | |
| 30.08.2001 | 03.09.1988 | F | URTI | 937 | 944 | (L) ear ache | Erythromycin | 2565 | Penicillin allergy. |
| 30.08.2001 | 12.06.1983 | M | S/Leave | 929 | 931 | Sore throat - Private | | 2719 | Script for Amoxycillin given. |
| 28.08.2001 | 25.05.1976 | F | | 1732 | 1743 | Script for Microgynon-30 given | | 2797 | Cefaclor allergy. For MSU |
| 29.08.2001 | 25.02.1966 | M | | 1744 | 1754 | Palpitations & tachycardia | Atenolol | 2856 | |
| 23.08.2001 | 22.05.1983 | F | | 1635 | 1639 | Late Period | For Pregnancy test | 3142 | |

790

Result of a query that lists all consultations from the 22nd to the end of August 2001 (ConsultationsSeenFrom22ndTillEndOfAug2001)

| SurgeryDate | DateOfBirth | Sex | Diagnosis | TimeIn | TimeOut | Complaints | Treatments | NumbersID | Notes |
|---|---|---|---|---|---|---|---|---|---|
| 29.08.2001 | 22.05.1983 | F | | 1636 | 1643 | Pregnancy test positive | | 3142 | |
| 24.08.2001 | 20.03.1959 | F | | 1750 | 1758 | She wants her period delayed whilst on holidays | Norethisterone | 3166 | Septrin allergy. |
| 22.08.2001 | 02.11.1953 | F | Revisit | 1028 | 1033 | Pain (R) leg is worse | Referred to Physician (BUPA) | 3182 | Penicillin allergy. |
| 29.08.2001 | 04.07.1929 | M | | 907 | 913 | Due to be seen in Urology OPD in 2/52 | | 322 | |
| 24.08.2001 | 23.07.1971 | F | S/Leave | 1642 | 1651 | Pain (R) Achilles | | 3465 | Script for Ibuprofen & Co-dydramol given. FP1001 (GMS4) form signed. |
| 23.08.2001 | 19.11.1967 | F | Pain | 1812 | 1816 | Painful swelling (L) ankle | Ibuprofen | 3484 | Penicillin allergy. |
| 30.08.2001 | 13.12.1966 | M | S/Leave | 922 | 929 | Abscess (L) side of face – Private | | 3512 | Sebaceous cyst on face, referred to Surgeon. |
| 24.08.2001 | 09.12.1933 | F | | 1011 | 1016 | Oral thrush again | Miconazole oral gel | 3583 | Oxytetracycline allergy. |
| 22.08.2001 | 14.04.1930 | M | | 1015 | 1028 | Advised to continue Cedocard & Isotard XL | | 3584 | |
| 29.08.2001 | 21.02.1992 | F | RTI | 920 | 929 | Cough | Erythromycin | 3586 | Penicillin allergy. |
| 22.08.2001 | 24.01.1932 | F | Rash | 958 | 1001 | Itchy rash on (R) sole | Daktacort | 3609 | |

Result of a query that lists all consultations from the 22nd to the end of August 2001 (ConsultationsSeenFrom22ndTillEndOfAug2001)

| SurgeryDate | DateOfBirth | Sex | Diagnosis | TimeIn | TimeOut | Complaints | Treatments | NumbersID | Notes |
|---|---|---|---|---|---|---|---|---|---|
| 22.08.2001 | 16.08.1927 | F | URTI | 943 | 949 | Sinus problems & (L) ear discharge | Amoxycillin & Otosporin ear drops | 3717 | |
| 30.08.2001 | 17.11.1919 | M | URTI | 1742 | 1803 | Discharging (L) ear | Otosporin | 3825 | Script for Potassium Bicarbonate given. |
| 29.08.2001 | 20.04.1936 | M | | 1754 | 1805 | Lump (L) thigh has changed in size recenly | Referred to Orthopaedic Surgeon | 3840 | Script for Co-dydramol given. |
| 28.08.2001 | 02.11.1973 | F | URTI | 1702 | 1707 | (L) ear ache | Otosporin ear drops | 3864 | |
| 23.08.2001 | 24.12.1981 | M | RTI | 1804 | 1808 | Cough | Amoxycillin | 3871 | |
| 24.08.2001 | 16.10.1959 | F | Lump | 1651 | 1701 | USScan of Thyroid: mild diffuse goitre | | 3929 | |
| 28.08.2001 | 04.09.1985 | M | | 1719 | 1725 | Ear ache & cough | Amoxycillin & Otosporin ear drops | 3959 | Nuts allergy. |
| 29.08.2001 | 16.07.1967 | F | | 1805 | 1808 | Vaginal thrush | Fluconazole | 3993 | |
| 24.08.2001 | 03.02.1971 | F | | 1804 | 1810 | Bleeding piles | Glyceryl Trinitrate ointment 0.2% w/w | 4003 | |
| 30.08.2001 | 07.10.1933 | M | | 955 | 957 | Script for Olanzapine given | | 4055 | |
| 29.08.2001 | 21.02.1916 | F | | 959 | 1008 | Script for Inj. Depo-Medrone with Lidocaine given | | 4178 | Penicillin allergy. |
| 30.08.2001 | 21.02.1916 | F | | 1031 | 1042 | Inj. Depo-Medrone with Lidocaine given to (R) knee | | 4178 | Penicillin allergy. |

Result of a query that lists all consultations from the 22nd to the end of August 2001 (ConsultationsSeenFrom22ndTillEndOfAug2001)

| SurgeryDate | DateOfBirth | Sex | Diagnosis | TimeIn | TimeOut | Complaints | Treatments | NumbersID | Notes |
|---|---|---|---|---|---|---|---|---|---|
| 28.08.2001 | 03.06.1974 | F | | 1202 | 1215 | Routine P/Natal visit | | 4219 | Home visit. |
| 28.08.2001 | 15.04.1951 | F | | 1819 | 1826 | Inside of mouth is sore, ?oral thrush | Nystatin pastilles | 4258 | |
| 29.08.2001 | 13.09.1992 | F | URTI | 1821 | 1826 | (R) ear ache & bunged up | Amoxycillin, Paracetamol & Ibuprofen | 4259 | |
| 29.08.2001 | 24.06.1928 | M | Pain | 1012 | 1018 | Pain (L) kidney region | Tramadol | 4312 | Penicillin allergy. For MSU. |
| 24.08.2001 | 16.04.1993 | F | Revisit | 1735 | 1747 | Facial rash is worse with Fucidin-H | Loratadine & Calamine lotion | 4327 | |
| 22.08.2001 | 04.10.1928 | F | | 955 | 958 | She lost her son recently | Diazepam | 4403 | Husband came to Surgery. |
| 22.08.2001 | 14.08.1929 | M | | 949 | 955 | He lost his son recently | Diazepam | 4404 | |
| 23.08.2001 | 26.11.1975 | M | Pain | 1758 | 1804 | Stiff & painful neck | Ibuprofen & Co-dydramol | 4410 | |
| 30.08.2001 | 10.08.1985 | F | URTI | 1738 | 1742 | Sore throat | Amoxycillin | 4429 | |
| 28.08.2001 | 26.12.1932 | F | Revisit | 927 | 931 | Mole on arm is tender & looks septic | Flucloxacillin & Fucidin cream | 4437 | |
| 28.08.2001 | 02.09.1948 | F | Pain | 1145 | 1152 | Abdominal pain | Buscopan | 4444 | Penicillin allergy. Home visit. |
| 28.08.2001 | 06.11.1968 | F | | 1654 | 1702 | Script for Citalopram given | | 4479 | |
| 29.08.2001 | 03.04.1969 | F | URTI | 1714 | 1718 | Sore throat & ear ache | Erythromycin | 4508 | Penicillin allergy. |
| 29.08.2001 | 22.04.1959 | F | | 1808 | 1815 | CXR: Possible calcification due to past chicken Pox pneumonia | | 463 | |

793

Result of a query that lists all consultations from the 22nd to the end of August 2001 (ConsultationsSeenFrom22ndTillEndOfAug2001)

| SurgeryDate | DateOfBirth | Sex | Diagnosis | TimeIn | TimeOut | Complaints | Treatments | NumbersID | Notes |
|---|---|---|---|---|---|---|---|---|---|
| 23.08.2001 | 22.11.1983 | F | URTI | 1648 | 1718 | (R) ear is red & sore | Amoxycillin & Otomize ear spray | 464 | Pain in hips & knees, Rx. Co-dydramol. Referred to Orthopaedic Surgeon. |
| 29.08.2001 | 23.05.1987 | F | Rash | 931 | 941 | Impetigo-like rash on (R) arm & back | Erythromycin, Mupirocin cream & Paracetamol | 4653 | Penicillin allergy. |
| 23.08.2001 | 03.07.1967 | F | | 1029 | 1040 | Script for Microgynon-30 given | | 4657 | FP1001 (GMS4) form given. |
| 24.08.2001 | 09.10.1926 | M | Revisit | 954 | 1006 | Penile thrush | Fluconazole | 4657 | |
| 24.08.2001 | 17.08.1935 | F | | 946 | 954 | Script for Simvastatin given | | 4670 | |
| 30.08.2001 | 05.02.1946 | F | URTI | 1720 | 1724 | Sore throat | Amoxycillin | 4691 | |
| 28.08.2001 | 13.12.1974 | M | URTI | 1637 | 1654 | (R) ear ache | Otosporin | 4731 | Persistent (R) ear ache, referred to ENT Surgeon. |
| 30.08.2001 | 13.02.1974 | M | | 1813 | 1841 | HGV medical done | | 4731 | |
| 24.08.2001 | 10.12.1944 | M | | 902 | 907 | Advised to stop Lansoprazole until he sees the Gastro-enterologist | | 4780 | |
| 24.08.2001 | 11.07.1953 | M | | 918 | 939 | Advised to stop Ibuprofen | | 4968 | |
| 24.08.2001 | 07.04.1949 | F | Hypertension | 1704 | 1712 | BP 140/96 | Bendrofluazide | 513 | |
| 30.08.2001 | 23.05.1978 | F | | 1637 | 1707 | She had epileptic fit 5 days ago after taking excess alcohol | | 5204 | |
| 22.08.2001 | 11.11.1932 | F | ?UTI | 1816 | 1818 | Pain in the groins | For MSU | 5290 | |

794

## Result of a query that lists all consultations from the 22nd to the end of August 2001 (ConsultationsSeenFrom22ndTillEndOfAug2001)

| SurgeryDate | DateOfBirth | Sex | Diagnosis | TimeIn | TimeOut | Complaints | Treatments | NumbersID | Notes |
|---|---|---|---|---|---|---|---|---|---|
| 28.08.2001 | 10.08.1996 | M | | 918 | 927 | Advised to continue eye drops & Erythromycin as prescribed by Health call Dr. | | 5353 | |
| 28.08.2001 | 17.10.1929 | M | | 1729 | 1732 | On Simvastatin | | 5469 | Worried about Cerivastatin. |
| 22.08.2001 | 09.02.1963 | F | Anaemia | 1802 | 1808 | Hb 10.8 g/dl | Ferrous Sulphate | 5567 | |
| 23.08.2001 | 17.08.1947 | F | | 1735 | 1748 | Night cramps | Quinine Sulphate | 56 | |
| 22.08.2001 | 25.09.1917 | F | | 1033 | 1040 | Script for Dihydrocodeine given | | 5665 | Tetanus Toxoid allergy. |
| 24.08.2001 | 18.04.1969 | M | Depression | 1016 | 1028 | Weepy, unable to cope & suicidal | Referred to Psychiatric Dr. on call, SGH | 5736 | |
| 29.08.2001 | 18.04.1969 | M | | 949 | 956 | Advised to contact Council regarding his housing application | | 5736 | |
| 30.08.2001 | 21.06.1933 | M | Pain | 1002 | 1006 | Pain (L) shoulder | Inj. Depo-Medrone with Lidocaine | 5771 | |
| 28.08.2001 | 21.11.1939 | M | | 1000 | 1010 | Script for Citalopram given | | 5777 | |
| 23.08.2001 | 12.05.1939 | F | | 946 | 956 | Panicky, palpations & tearful | Atenolol | 5782 | |
| 29.08.2001 | 25.03.1963 | M | Rash | 1710 | 1714 | Mole on (R) shoulder | Referred to Dermatologist (BUPA) | 5853 | |
| 24.08.2001 | 15.07.1936 | M | Anaemia | 1028 | 1035 | Hb 10.7 g/dl | Ferrous Sulphate | 5881 | |

| SurgeryDate | DateOfBirth | Sex | Diagnosis | TimeIn | TimeOut | Complaints | Treatments | NumbersID | Notes |
|---|---|---|---|---|---|---|---|---|---|
| 28.08.2001 | 21.11.1997 | M | URTI | 1018 | 1026 | Sore throat, fever & vomiting | Amoxycillin & Metoclopramide | 5898 | |
| 24.08.2001 | 23.02.1952 | M | URTI | 1701 | 1704 | Sore throat | Amoxycillin | 594 | |
| 29.08.2001 | 23.07.1929 | M | RTI | 1008 | 1012 | Cough | Amoxycillin | 6057 | |
| 29.08.2001 | 28.03.1969 | M | Pain | 913 | 920 | Back Pain | Co-dydramol & Ibuprofen | 6074 | |
| 30.08.2001 | 20.04.1933 | F | Rash | 957 | 1002 | Eczema-like rash on finger | 1% Hydrocortisone cream | 6110 | |
| 24.08.2001 | 11.11.1934 | M | | 1724 | 1735 | Advised to contact smoking cessation clinic | | 6121 | |
| 28.08.2001 | 03.12.1955 | F | | 1743 | 1748 | Script for Citalopram given | | 614 | |
| 29.08.2001 | 26.04.1918 | M | | 1815 | 1821 | Bruising (L) fore-arm | 0.3% Heparinoid cream | 6264 | |
| 24.08.2001 | 23.05.1993 | M | | 1006 | 1011 | (R) eye injury from a tennis ball | Referred to Ophthalmologist | 6341 | Erythromycin allergy. |
| 29.08.2001 | 01.01.1924 | M | | 1653 | 1658 | Night cramps in the legs | Quinine Sulphate | 6353 | |
| 22.08.2001 | 04.02.1918 | F | URTI | 1708 | 1716 | Sore throat | Amoxycillin | 6559 | |
| 23.08.2001 | 22.07.1920 | F | Rash | 956 | 1006 | Generalised itchy rash | Cetirizine | 6599 | For U/Es, LFTs & FBC. |
| 22.08.2001 | 04.05.1937 | F | | 1725 | 1737 | Advised to discuss with the Rheumatologist about her persistent abnormal LFTs | | 6723 | |

Result of a query that lists all consultations from the 22$^{nd}$ to the end of August 2001 (ConsultationsSeenFrom22ndTillEndOfAug2001)

| SurgeryDate | DateOfBirth | Sex | Diagnosis | TimeIn | TimeOut | Complaints | Treatments | NumbersID | Notes |
|---|---|---|---|---|---|---|---|---|---|
| 23.08.2001 | 20.09.1943 | F | | 1816 | 1821 | Script for Pravastatin given | | 6781 | Penicillin allergy. Patient had been on Cerivastatin. |
| 23.08.2001 | 22.06.1999 | F | | 930 | 938 | Fits of vomiting & not eating well | Referred to Paediatrician | 6837 | |
| 24.08.2001 | 16.10.1979 | M | S/Leave | 939 | 946 | Pain (R) knee - Private | | 6859 | Script for Ibuprofen & Co-dydramol given. |
| 30.08.2001 | 18.08.1962 | M | RTI | 1707 | 1711 | Cough | Amoxycillin | 6868 | |
| 30.08.2001 | 02.11.1977 | F | | 1808 | 1813 | Headaches & recurrent sinus problems | Referred to ENT Surgeon (Basildon hospital) | 6877 | |
| 30.08.2001 | 25.06.1949 | F | URTI | 1717 | 1720 | Sinusitis | Amoxycillin | 6964 | |
| 24.08.2001 | 05.07.1968 | F | | 1747 | 1750 | Urine smells | Cefalexin | 6966 | |
| 29.08.2001 | 24.04.1981 | F | Deafness | 1722 | 1732 | Wax in ears | Waxsol | 6970 | |
| 22.08.2001 | 09.08.1971 | M | Rash | 1808 | 1816 | Itchy rash, ?Scabies | Lyclear Dermal cream | 6978 | Penicillin allergy. |
| 29.08.2001 | 17.03.1968 | F | | 1734 | 1744 | Stressed | To observe | 7008 | 13/40 gestation. |
| 28.08.2001 | 04.12.1926 | M | | 931 | 944 | Advised to contact the hospital regarding the treatment for his eye problem | | 7037 | Penicillin allergy. |
| 22.08.2001 | 22.02.2001 | F | Conjunctivitis | 1040 | 1048 | Sticky (R) eye | Chloramphenicol eye drops | 7049 | |
| 23.08.2001 | 20.09.1959 | F | S/Leave | 1024 | 1029 | Pain lower back & both sides | | 7060 | |

Result of a query that lists all consultations from the 22nd to the end of August 2001 (ConsultationsSeenFrom22ndTillEndOfAug2001)

| SurgeryDate | DateOfBirth | Sex | Diagnosis | TimeIn | TimeOut | Complaints | Treatments | NumbersID | Notes |
|---|---|---|---|---|---|---|---|---|---|
| 23.08.2001 | 29.09.1945 | F | | 1017 | 1024 | Awaiting old records to be given sick certificate | | 7075 | |
| 29.08.2001 | 17.07.2000 | F | Rash | 1018 | 1023 | Rash on arms | Aqueous cream | 7076 | |
| 23.08.2001 | 29.09.1945 | F | S/Leave | 1639 | 1645 | Plantar fasciitis (R) foot & (L) Hip pain | | 7095 | |
| 30.08.2001 | 02.08.1975 | F | Rash | 1025 | 1031 | Moles on breast | Referred to Dermatologist (Basildon hospital) | 7111 | |
| 23.08.2001 | 09.05.2001 | M | | 1040 | 1047 | Oral thrush | Nystatin oral suspension | 7133 | (R) eye is still weepy, Rx. Chloramphenicol eye drops. |
| 22.08.2001 | 18.01.1939 | F | | 1001 | 1010 | Diarrhoea | Electrolade, Ciprofloxacin & Lomotil | 7143 | |
| 24.08.2001 | 08.09.1978 | M | Rash | 1712 | 1724 | Red rash on back | Fucidin-H cream | 7168 | Script for Clotrimazole cream given. |
| 22.08.2001 | 05.11.1980 | M | | 939 | 943 | Headaches & sweating | Amoxycillin & Co-dydramol | 7169 | |
| 23.08.2001 | 11.01.1939 | F | Pain | 1010 | 1017 | Low back pain | For Physiotherapy | 71767 | |
| 23.08.2001 | 02.03.1984 | F | | 1821 | 1825 | Recurrent sore throats | Referred to ENT Surgeon (Basildon hospital) | 730 | |

Result of a query that lists all consultations from the 22nd to the end of August 2001 (ConsultationsSeenFrom22ndTillEndOfAug2001)

| SurgeryDate | DateOfBirth | Sex | Diagnosis | TimeIn | TimeOut | Complaints | Treatments | NumbersID | Notes |
|---|---|---|---|---|---|---|---|---|---|
| 29.08.2001 | 24.01.1960 | M | Pain | 1643 | 1649 | Back Pain | For X-Ray Lumbar Spine | 889 | |
| 28.08.2001 | 29.06.1915 | M | Hypertension | 1905 | 1920 | BP 170/100 | Atenolol & Bendrofluazide | 937 | Dizziness & vomiting, Rx. Betahistine. Script for Aspirin Dispersible given. Home visit. |
| 29.08.2001 | 20.10.1925 | F | Conjunctivitis | 941 | 949 | Sore & red (R) eye | Chloramphenicol eye ointment | 952 | Penicillin & Aspirin allergy. Script for Losartan given. |

Result of a query that lists all consultations from the 22nd to the end of August 2003 (ConsultationsSeenFrom22ndTillEndOfAug2003)

| SurgeryDate | DateOfBirth | Sex | Diagnosis | TimeIn | TimeOut | Complaints | Treatments | NumbersID | Notes |
|---|---|---|---|---|---|---|---|---|---|
| 22.08.2003 | 08.02.1939 | F | | 908 | 913 | Heavy-headed & congested | Erythromycin | 113 | Trimethoprim allergy. |
| 29.08.2003 | 17.09.1986 | F | | 1722 | 1731 | Her hairs are falling off | Referred to Dermatologist | 1173 | |
| 29.08.2003 | 28.02.1959 | M | Pain | 1006 | 1018 | Back Pain | Diclofenac enteric coated & Co-codamol | 1308 | |
| 27.08.2003 | 02.08.1934 | M | Revisit | 939 | 950 | Still has chesty cough | Erythromycin | 1369 | |
| 28.08.2003 | 22.07.1939 | F | | 901 | 907 | For serum Cholesterol | | 1546 | Sulpha allergy. |

Result of a query that lists all consultations from the 22nd to the end of August 2003 (ConsultationsSeenFrom22ndTillEndOfAug2003)

| SurgeryDate | DateOfBirth | Sex | Diagnosis | TimeIn | TimeOut | Complaints | Treatments | NumbersID | Notes |
|---|---|---|---|---|---|---|---|---|---|
| 26.08.2003 | 23.08.1925 | F | | 1706 | 1715 | Script for Co-codamol given | | 1613 | |
| 22.08.2003 | 01.01.1951 | F | | 1631 | 1638 | X-Ray (R) elbow shows evidence of osteo-arthritis | | 1769 | |
| 28.08.2003 | 02.09.1941 | F | | 923 | 927 | To keep Orthopaedic appointment | | 1797 | |
| 27.08.2003 | 29.03.1969 | F | | 1702 | 1712 | Vaginal thrush | Clotrimazole pessary | 1963 | For FBC & Fasting Glucose. |
| 29.08.2003 | 06.06.1969 | M | | 1731 | 1736 | Dizzy spells | Prochlorperazine | 2065 | |
| 26.08.2003 | 18.09.1980 | F | Pain | 1807 | 1811 | Pain (L) shoulder | Diclofenac enteric coated & Co-codamol | 2193 | |
| 29.08.2003 | 13.03.1932 | M | | 909 | 915 | He has Gilberts syndrome | | 2202 | |
| 26.08.2003 | 31.07.1924 | M | | 1230 | 1310 | Bad (R) leg ulcer & necrotic tissue under (R) big toe | To Surgical Dr. on call, SGH | 2275 | Home visit. |
| 27.08.2003 | 28.05.1987 | M | Rash | 1712 | 1716 | Impetigo-like rash on (R) ear lobe & near mouth | Flucloxacillin & Fusidic Acid cream | 2672 | |
| 26.08.2003 | 25.09.1989 | M | URTI | 1640 | 1645 | (L) ear ache | Amoxycillin | 2695 | |
| 27.08.2003 | 05.02.1933 | F | Pain | 1641 | 1649 | (L) wrist is painful | Diclofenac enteric coated & Ranitidine | 276 | For Rheumatoid Factor. |
| 26.08.2003 | 09.02.1956 | M | Revisit | 1656 | 1706 | Still has pain back of (L) thigh | Referred to Orthopaedic Surgeon (BUPA) | 2846 | |

## Result of a query that lists all consultations from the 22nd to the end of August 2003 (ConsultationsSeenFrom22ndTillEndOfAug2003)

| SurgeryDate | DateOfBirth | Sex | Diagnosis | TimeIn | TimeOut | Complaints | Treatments | NumbersID | Notes |
|---|---|---|---|---|---|---|---|---|---|
| 22.08.2003 | 17.02.1958 | M | | 1806 | 1812 | Fungal infection (L) big toe | Terbinafine cream | 3 | Tender cyst (L) chin, Rx. Fusidic Acid cream & Flucloxacillin. |
| 27.08.2003 | 25.02.1986 | F | | 1754 | 1758 | FBC normal | | 3035 | FP1001 (GMS4) form signed. |
| 29.08.2003 | 29.12.1954 | F | Revisit | 901 | 909 | Still gets chest pain & breathless | Referred to Cardiologist | 3128 | Script for GTN spray given. |
| 27.08.2003 | 31.07.1959 | F | | 950 | 1004 | USScan of Pelvis - Fibroids | Referred to Gynaecologist (Basildon Hospital) | 3327 | |
| 22.08.2003 | 14.08.1935 | M | URTI | 1024 | 1030 | Bilateral ear ache | Amoxycillin & Otomize ear spray | 3353 | |
| 29.08.2003 | 12.05.1973 | M | | 1808 | 1813 | For FBC & Fasting Glucose | | 3442 | Penicillin allergy. |
| 26.08.2003 | 28.10.1930 | F | | 1016 | 1020 | To see P/Nurse in 9/12 for repeat FBC | | 359 | |
| 22.08.2003 | 16.08.1927 | F | Rash | 925 | 932 | Scabby mole on (L) side of chest & (R) wrist | Referred to Dermatologist | 3717 | Bilateral pedal oedema, Rx. Frusemide. |
| 27.08.2003 | 12.09.1947 | F | | 1806 | 1813 | Dysuria | Trimethoprim | 3908 | |
| 28.08.2003 | 31.03.1986 | F | | 1005 | 1011 | Script for Microgynon-30 given | | 4001 | |
| 29.08.2003 | 05.05.1960 | M | | 947 | 953 | Hearing is muffled | Sodium bicarbonate ear drops | 4024 | |

Result of a query that lists all consultations from the 22nd to the end of August 2003 (ConsultationsSeenFrom22ndTillEndOfAug2003)

| SurgeryDate | DateOfBirth | Sex | Diagnosis | TimeIn | TimeOut | Complaints | Treatments | NumbersID | Notes |
|---|---|---|---|---|---|---|---|---|---|
| 27.08.2003 | 08.04.1961 | F | S/Leave | 903 | 907 | Laparoscopic Cholecystectomy | | 407 | |
| 27.08.2003 | 29.02.1944 | F | | 921 | 929 | For LFT's & Fasting Cholesterol | | 432 | Canesten & Metronidazole allergy. |
| 26.08.2003 | 09.10.1926 | M | | 1006 | 1016 | Statins don't agree with him | | 4367 | Penicillin allergy. |
| 27.08.2003 | 17.09.1938 | M | | 1758 | 1806 | Epistaxes (R) nostril | Naseptin cream | 4448 | |
| 22.08.2003 | 15.02.1927 | F | | 1654 | 1659 | Script for Co-codamol given | | 4495 | |
| 28.08.2003 | 24.11.1973 | M | Pain | 927 | 931 | Painful (L) shoulder | Diclofenac enteric coated & Co-codamol | 4565 | |
| 22.08.2003 | 24.09.1930 | F | | 932 | 942 | Script for Co-Careldopa 25/100 given | | 4666 | |
| 22.08.2003 | 21.09.1923 | M | | 1020 | 1024 | Black spots in the mouth | Amoxycillin | 4692 | |
| 27.08.2003 | 13.03.1932 | M | | 1632 | 1637 | Injection Zoladex given | | 4699 | |
| 29.08.2003 | 15.04.1921 | M | | 1759 | 1808 | Script for Diazepam given | | 4795 | His friend came to the Surgery. |
| 27.08.2003 | 28.10.1991 | M | Conjunctivitis | 1649 | 1702 | Sore (L) eye | Chloramphenicol eye ointment | 4896 | |
| 27.08.2003 | 26.10.1995 | M | Rash | 919 | 921 | Mole on the back of the neck | Referred to Dermatologist | 5080 | Penicillin allergy. |

Result of a query that lists all consultations from the 22nd to the end of August 2003 (ConsultationsSeenFrom22ndTillEndOfAug2003)

| SurgeryDate | DateOfBirth | Sex | Diagnosis | TimeIn | TimeOut | Complaints | Treatments | NumbersID | Notes |
|---|---|---|---|---|---|---|---|---|---|
| 29.08.2003 | 04.12.1995 | M | Rash | 1740 | 1743 | Impetigo-like rash on the (L) side of chest | Erythromycin & Mupirocin cream | 5091 | Penicillin allergy. |
| 26.08.2003 | 02.05.1985 | F | URTI | 1000 | 1006 | Sore throat | Amoxycillin | 5114 | |
| 27.08.2003 | 26.05.1976 | M | | 1041 | 1119 | Metropolitan Police Service Examination done | | 512 | |
| 26.08.2003 | 07.10.1944 | M | Hypertension | 925 | 940 | BP 161/92 | Atenolol | 5141 | |
| 28.08.2003 | 20.04.1955 | F | | 952 | 1001 | Outbreak of scabies at the Nursing home where she works | Permethrin 5% cream | 5253 | |
| 28.08.2003 | 05.12.1988 | F | Rash | 1011 | 1028 | Facial acne rash | Topicycline lotion | 5347 | Script for Microgynon-30 given. |
| 29.08.2003 | 06.04.1950 | M | URTI | 1813 | 1817 | Bilateral ear ache | Amoxycillin & Otomize ear spray | 535 | |
| 27.08.2003 | 13.11.1996 | F | RTI | 1637 | 1641 | Chesty cough | Amoxycillin | 5440 | |
| 27.08.2003 | 25.06.1921 | M | | 1018 | 1024 | Lesion on the lower lip | 1% Hydrocortisone cream & Co-codamol | 5474 | |
| 26.08.2003 | 19.05.1988 | F | UTI | 1634 | 1640 | Dysuria | Amoxycillin | 5579 | |
| 22.08.2003 | 22.02.1936 | F | Revisit | 913 | 920 | Still coughing | For CXR | 5595 | Penicillin allergy. Script for Ranitidine given. |
| 29.08.2003 | 17.08.1947 | F | RTI | 1716 | 1722 | Hacking cough | Cefpodoxime | 56 | Script for Fluconazole given. |

Result of a query that lists all consultations from the 22nd to the end of August 2003 (ConsultationsSeenFrom22ndTillEndOfAug2003)

| SurgeryDate | DateOfBirth | Sex | Diagnosis | TimeIn | TimeOut | Complaints | Treatments | NumbersID | Notes |
|---|---|---|---|---|---|---|---|---|---|
| 28.08.2003 | 26.10.1962 | F | | 1043 | 1055 | Alcohol problem | Referred to ROCHE unit & to P/Counsellor | 5691 | |
| 22.08.2003 | 19.11.1937 | M | | 944 | 949 | Script for Ranitidine given | | 5776 | |
| 26.08.2003 | 13.08.1997 | M | RTI | 1811 | 1815 | Cough | Amoxycillin | 5785 | |
| 22.08.2003 | 23.03.1926 | M | URTI | 1003 | 1020 | Catarrh in the head & ear ache | Amoxycillin & Otomize ear spray | 5954 | |
| 29.08.2003 | 09.05.1997 | M | | 1702 | 1706 | Script for Methylphenidate given | | 6253 | |
| 22.08.2003 | 27.10.1998 | M | URTI | 1812 | 1818 | Sore throat & viral rash | Amoxycillin, Paracetamol & Calamine lotion | 6289 | |
| 27.08.2003 | 21.06.1942 | M | RTI | 1037 | 1041 | Chesty cough | Amoxycillin | 6335 | |
| 26.08.2003 | 09.11.1941 | F | UTI | 1715 | 1719 | Dysuria | Trimethoprim | 6442 | |
| 26.08.2003 | 21.02.1959 | F | S/Leave | 1756 | 1807 | Stress - Private | | 6621 | |
| 29.08.2003 | 21.02.1959 | F | S/Leave | 940 | 947 | Stress | | 6621 | |
| 26.08.2003 | 14.10.1997 | F | URTI | 1753 | 1756 | Bad throat | Amoxycillin & Paracetamol | 6626 | |
| 22.08.2003 | 13.01.1941 | F | | 1735 | 1806 | Dizzy spell, heavy head nausea | Prochlorperazine & Amoxycillin | 673 | BP 156/92, Rx. Atenolol. For FBC, Fasting Glucose, U/Es, LFTs & Cholesterol. |

804

Result of a query that lists all consultations from the 22nd to the end of August 2003 (ConsultationsSeenFrom22ndTillEndOfAug2003)

| SurgeryDate | DateOfBirth | Sex | Diagnosis | TimeIn | TimeOut | Complaints | Treatments | NumbersID | Notes |
|---|---|---|---|---|---|---|---|---|---|
| 27.08.2003 | 11.01.1951 | F | | 1716 | 1729 | Hot flushes | Prempak C | 6735 | Chest infection & exacerbation of asthma, Rx. Amoxycillin, Formoterol/Budesonide & Prednisolone enteric coated. |
| 29.08.2003 | 11.04.1963 | M | Revisit | 1706 | 1710 | Still coughing | For CXR | 6798 | |
| 27.08.2003 | 27.05.1968 | M | S/Leave | 1729 | 1744 | Injury (L) chest - Private | | 6947 | Bitten on (L) chest by a thief, Rx. Co-Amoxiclav & Co-codamol. |
| 22.08.2003 | 25.06.1949 | F | URTI | 920 | 925 | Sore throat & sore ears | Amoxycillin & Otomize ear spray | 6964 | |
| 26.08.2003 | 31.10.2000 | M | URTI | 1751 | 1753 | Bad throat | Erythromycin | 6986 | |
| 22.08.2003 | 03.07.1974 | F | | 1649 | 1654 | Late Period | For Pregnancy test | 7005 | |
| 22.08.2003 | 09.10.1976 | F | | 1659 | 1704 | Cervical spine X-Ray: No bony abnormality. Apparent loss of the normal Cervical lordosis may be due to spasm | | 7064 | |
| 22.08.2003 | 03.04.1980 | M | URTI | 1641 | 1649 | Pain (R) ear | Erythromycin & Otomize ear spray | 7118 | Sebaceous cysts on the scrotum, referred to Surgeon. Penicillin allergy. |

Result of a query that lists all consultations from the 22nd to the end of August 2003 (ConsultationsSeenFrom22ndTillEndOfAug2003)

| SurgeryDate | DateOfBirth | Sex | Diagnosis | TimeIn | TimeOut | Complaints | Treatments | NumbersID | Notes |
|---|---|---|---|---|---|---|---|---|---|
| 28.08.2003 | 09.05.2001 | M | Rash | 1055 | 1101 | Urticarial-type rash all over | Desloratadine suspension & Calamine lotion | 7133 | |
| 22.08.2003 | 04.09.1970 | M | | 949 | 1003 | To see P/Nurse in 1/12 for BP check | | 7154 | |
| 29.08.2003 | 31.05.1972 | F | URTI | 1710 | 1716 | Dull ache in (R) ear | Flucloxacillin & Otomize ear spray | 7176 | |
| 29.08.2003 | 25.03.1947 | F | | 1030 | 1047 | Her dad died from MRSA | Swabs taken from nostril, throat, axillae & groins, & sent for sensitivity | 7209 | |
| 26.08.2003 | 14.08.1947 | F | | 940 | 944 | To take own Paracetamol for pain in her (L) hand | | 7237 | |
| 28.08.2003 | 29.08.1981 | F | | 1028 | 1033 | Mouth infection | Amoxycillin | 7238 | |
| 27.08.2003 | 02.02.1968 | F | | 1004 | 1018 | Script for Citalopram given | | 7269 | |
| 28.08.2003 | 21.08.1934 | F | | 907 | 913 | To stop Fluoxetine & to continue with Amitriptyline | | 7287 | Penicillin allergy. |
| 29.08.2003 | 17.08.1952 | F | | 915 | 923 | To keep menstrual chart | | 7291 | |
| 28.08.2003 | 13.03.1973 | F | URTI | 1001 | 1005 | Sore throat | Amoxycillin | 7346 | |
| 26.08.2003 | 13.02.2002 | F | URTI | 1747 | 1751 | Infected rhinorrhoea & diarrhoea | Erythromycin, Paracetamol & Dioralyte | 7392 | |

Result of a query that lists all consultations from the 22nd to the end of August 2003 (ConsultationsSeenFrom22ndTillEndOfAug2003)

| SurgeryDate | DateOfBirth | Sex | Diagnosis | TimeIn | TimeOut | Complaints | Treatments | NumbersID | Notes |
|---|---|---|---|---|---|---|---|---|---|
| 29.08.2003 | 17.03.1967 | F | | 1743 | 1752 | Constipated | Bisacodyl | 7409 | Lump on the volar aspect of (L) index finger, referred to Orthopaedic Surgeon (Basildon Hospital) |
| 29.08.2003 | 06.06.1970 | M | | 1752 | 1759 | Options to where he could get vasectomy done explained to him | | 7412 | |
| 29.08.2003 | 03.05.1944 | F | | 1634 | 1650 | Script for Rabeprazole & Amitriptyline given | | 7499 | Lamotrigine allergy. |
| 29.08.2003 | 28.03.1960 | F | S/Leave | 1650 | 1702 | Depression - Private | | 7518 | Script for Rabeprazole given. |
| 26.08.2003 | 14.01.1947 | F | Hypertension | 1033 | 1049 | BP 172/83 | Bendrofluazide | 7519 | Penicillin allergy. |
| 26.08.2003 | 31.08.1971 | M | | 919 | 925 | Script for Amoxycillin & Diclofenac enteric coated given | | 7523 | |
| 26.08.2003 | 24.02.1952 | F | S/Leave | 1631 | 1634 | Abdominal hysterectomy | | 7567 | |
| 29.08.2003 | 27.10.1966 | M | Revisit | 1736 | 1740 | Rash on the hand is weepy | Fusidic Acid 2% + 0.01% Betamethasone cream | 7571 | |
| 27.08.2003 | 18.10.1966 | F | | 1029 | 1037 | Headaches & dizziness | Amoxycillin & Co-codamol | 7634 | For FBC, TFTs & Fasting Glucose. |
| 26.08.2003 | 07.02.1948 | M | URTI | 1729 | 1742 | Sore throat | Amoxycillin | 7684 | Script for Co-codamol given. |

807

Result of a query that lists all consultations from the 22nd to the end of August 2003 (ConsultationsSeenFrom22ndTillEndOfAug2003)

| SurgeryDate | DateOfBirth | Sex | Diagnosis | TimeIn | TimeOut | Complaints | Treatments | NumbersID | Notes |
|---|---|---|---|---|---|---|---|---|---|
| 26.08.2003 | 23.12.1946 | M | RTI | 944 | 1000 | Cough | Amoxycillin | 7761 | Script for Gliclazide, Rabeprazole, Metformin & Multivitamins given. |
| 28.08.2003 | 30.09.1931 | F | | 1033 | 1043 | Script for Fusemide & Fusidic Acid 2% + 1% Hydrocortisone cream | | 7788 | |
| 26.08.2003 | 27.05.2003 | M | URTI | 1742 | 1747 | Infected rhinorrhoea | Amoxycillin | 7802 | |
| 22.08.2003 | 18.01.1937 | M | Revisit | 1704 | 1707 | Rash on face & arms has persisted | Referred to Dermatologist | 7804 | |
| 27.08.2003 | 05.03.1953 | F | | 907 | 919 | She would think about going on HRT | | 7819 | |
| 26.08.2003 | 23.08.1944 | F | S/Leave | 915 | 919 | Fractured (L) Humerus - Med. 5 | | 7841 | Script for Dihydrocodeine given. |
| 26.08.2003 | 25.06.1940 | M | | 1719 | 1724 | Epigastric discomfort | Esomeprazole | 7844 | |
| 22.08.2003 | 19.10.1938 | M | | 903 | 908 | He will observe the blockage in his (L) nostril for now | | 7847 | |
| 27.08.2003 | 08.08.2003 | F | | 1024 | 1029 | Umbilical hernia | To observe | 7871 | |
| 27.08.2003 | 25.10.1966 | M | | 929 | 934 | Script for Sibutramine given | | 800 | |
| 28.08.2003 | 20.10.1925 | F | | 937 | 952 | Script for Simvastatin & Thyroxine given | | 952 | Aspirin allergy. |
| 28.08.2003 | 25.05.1950 | M | | 917 | 923 | For Physiotherapy | | 968 | |

Result of a query that lists all consultations from the 22nd to the end of August 2004 (ConsultationsSeenFrom22ndTillEndOfAug2004)

| SurgeryDate | DateOfBirth | Sex | Diagnosis | TimeIn | TimeOut | Complaints | Treatments | NumbersID | Notes |
|---|---|---|---|---|---|---|---|---|---|
| 27.08.2004 | 06.08.1928 | F | URTI | 1635 | 1639 | (L) ear is painful | Erythromycin & Dexamethasone with neomycin ear spray | 1074 | Penicillin allergy. |
| 23.08.2004 | 08.02.1939 | F | URTI | 931 | 936 | Sore throat | Amoxycillin | 113 | Trimethoprim allergy. |
| 26.08.2004 | 22.05.1931 | F | | 916 | 929 | Script for Co-codamol, Simvastatin & Quinine Sulphate given | | 1183 | |
| 24.08.2004 | 20.02.1930 | M | | 934 | 942 | To get OTC "tonics" which he requested for | | 1254 | Erythromycin & Penicillin allergy. Possible Digger trial involvement. |
| 27.08.2004 | 15.07.1936 | F | | 1803 | 1835 | 1st & 2nd visits of the PAR study | | 1309 | |
| 27.08.2004 | 18.11.1946 | F | | 1715 | 1720 | Keeps losing her balance & legs going numb | Referred to Neurologist | 1367 | |
| 25.08.2004 | 21.09.1924 | F | Hypertension | 1646 | 1657 | BP 170/75 | Atenolol | 1419 | |
| 24.08.2004 | 08.01.1942 | F | | 1735 | 1738 | To contact Lady Mc Caden Breast Unit regarding her aching (L) breast | | 1435 | |
| 23.08.2004 | 09.10.1924 | F | | 1702 | 1712 | Script for Erythromycin & Glandosane given | | 1477 | |

Result of a query that lists all consultations from the 22nd to the end of August 2004 (ConsultationsSeenFrom22ndTillEndOfAug2004)

| SurgeryDate | DateOfBirth | Sex | Diagnosis | TimeIn | TimeOut | Complaints | Treatments | NumbersID | Notes |
|---|---|---|---|---|---|---|---|---|---|
| 25.08.2004 | 06.05.1984 | F | | 1756 | 1800 | To stop the Microgynon to see if the Migraine will improve | | 1697 | |
| 23.08.2004 | 08.11.1981 | M | | 1645 | 1650 | to continue with Co-codamol for his headaches | | 1699 | |
| 26.08.2004 | 28.01.1920 | F | Pain | 1310 | 1325 | Pain in the (L) knee | Referred to Orthopaedic Surgeon (Basildon Hospital) | 1730 | Home visit. Penicillin & Trimethoprim allergy. |
| 25.08.2004 | 03.10.1939 | M | | 1037 | 1043 | Haemoptysis | For CXR | 1849 | |
| 23.08.2004 | 04.01.1962 | F | URTI | 920 | 928 | Sore throat & (L) ear ache | Erythromycin, Dexamethasone ear spray with neomycin & Co-codamol | 1884 | Trimethoprim allergy. |
| 27.08.2004 | 11.04.1986 | F | Revisit | 1639 | 1642 | Still has (L) ear ache | Referred to ENT Surgeon | 1970 | |
| 25.08.2004 | 02.10.1935 | M | | 1043 | 1047 | To take own Piriton for the itchy rash | | 1991 | |
| 24.08.2004 | 06.11.1915 | M | | 1049 | 1055 | For B12, Folate & Ferritin | | 229 | |
| 27.08.2004 | 19.07.1925 | F | | 924 | 932 | Loose motions | Mist Kaolin et Morph | 2290 | Stool for C&S. |
| 25.08.2004 | 26.08.1987 | F | | 1731 | 1736 | She wants her period postponed whilst on holidays | Norethisterone | 2332 | |

810

Result of a query that lists all consultations from the 22nd to the end of August 2004 (ConsultationsSeenFrom22ndTillEndOfAug2004)

| SurgeryDate | DateOfBirth | Sex | Diagnosis | TimeIn | TimeOut | Complaints | Treatments | NumbersID | Notes |
|---|---|---|---|---|---|---|---|---|---|
| 26.08.2004 | 16.03.1927 | F | | 904 | 913 | To persevere with Atenolol | | 2415 | |
| 23.08.2004 | 07.11.1984 | F | | 1635 | 1645 | Pregnancy test positive | | 2438 | |
| 24.08.2004 | 08.06.1984 | M | S/Leave | 1756 | 1803 | Tender cyst (L) upper eye lid - Private | | 2670 | |
| 27.08.2004 | 15.02.1946 | F | Conjunctivitis | 1642 | 1652 | Blood shot (R) eye | Chloramphenicol eye drops | 2729 | |
| 27.08.2004 | 24.03.1973 | M | S/Leave | 907 | 911 | Pain (R) toe - Med. 5 | | 2784 | |
| 25.08.2004 | 27.11.1992 | F | RTI | 1707 | 1715 | Script for Erythromycin & Prochlorperazine given | | 2797 | |
| 25.08.2004 | 27.09.1937 | F | Revisit | 902 | 911 | Wound on the leg hasn't healed adequately | Flucloxacillin & Fusidic Acid cream | 2893 | |
| 24.08.2004 | 21.09.1991 | M | Rash | 1038 | 1049 | Weepy wound behind (L) ear | Flucloxacillin & Fusidic Acid cream | 2917 | Script for Bendrofluazide given. Referred to Dermatologist (Basildon Hospital, urgent). Possible Digger Trial participant. |
| 25.08.2004 | 25.07.1938 | F | Pain | 958 | 1009 | Neck Pain | Co-codamol | 2964 | |
| 26.08.2004 | 27.10.1961 | F | | 955 | 1003 | Script for Omeprazole given | | 2973 | |
| 25.08.2004 | 11.09.1914 | F | Hypertension | 926 | 942 | BP 193/104 | Atenolol | 3004 | |

811

Result of a query that lists all consultations from the 22nd to the end of August 2004 (ConsultationsSeenFrom22ndTillEndOfAug2004)

| SurgeryDate | DateOfBirth | Sex | Diagnosis | TimeIn | TimeOut | Complaints | Treatments | NumbersID | Notes |
|---|---|---|---|---|---|---|---|---|---|
| 24.08.2004 | 10.10.1990 | F | Rash | 928 | 934 | Eczema on fingers is quite bad & weepy | Flucloxacillin & Fusidic Acid 2% + 0.1% Betamethasone cream | 3039 | |
| 23.08.2004 | 15.12.1939 | M | | 1754 | 1812 | Script for Allopurinol given | | 3272 | Visit 3 (final visit) of PAR study. |
| 26.08.2004 | 02.12.1923 | M | Hypertension | 1246 | 1306 | BP 170/95 | Bendrofluazide | 3429 | Dizzy, Rx. Prochlorperazine. Home visit. Possible Digger trial participant. |
| 26.08.2004 | 13.12.1966 | M | | 929 | 937 | Boil on the (R) of the scrotum | Flucloxacillin & Fusidic Acid cream | 3512 | |
| 27.08.2004 | 02.05.1992 | M | | 905 | 907 | Ears are not sore again since being treated whilst on holidays | | 3606 | |
| 25.08.2004 | 05.12.1931 | M | RTI | 942 | 958 | Chesty cough | Amoxycillin | 3646 | Private script for Viagra given. |
| 25.08.2004 | 26.10.1943 | F | Revisit | 911 | 916 | Still has ankle oedema | Frusemide | 365 | |
| 25.08.2004 | 23.05.1927 | M | | 1022 | 1037 | Bleeding wound on the tip of the nose | Fusidic Acid cream | 3716 | Penicillin allergy. |
| 25.08.2004 | 16.08.1927 | F | | 1013 | 1022 | Pancreatic cysts on USScan | Referred to General Surgeon | 3717 | |
| 23.08.2004 | 02.11.1973 | F | | 1712 | 1716 | Late period | For Pregnancy test | 3864 | |
| 24.08.2004 | 06.03.1973 | F | Rash | 1657 | 1700 | Probable Chicken Pox | Acyclovir | 3896 | |

Result of a query that lists all consultations from the 22nd to the end of August 2004 (ConsultationsSeenFrom22ndTillEndOfAug2004)

| SurgeryDate | DateOfBirth | Sex | Diagnosis | TimeIn | TimeOut | Complaints | Treatments | NumbersID | Notes |
|---|---|---|---|---|---|---|---|---|---|
| 25.08.2004 | 01.08.1947 | F | S/Leave | 916 | 921 | Urinary Tract Infection | | 398 | Script for Prochlorperazine given. |
| 24.08.2004 | 18.01.1968 | M | | 1803 | 1811 | Came in to enquire about vasectomy | | 3992 | |
| 23.08.2004 | 19.05.1964 | M | S/Leave | 1655 | 1702 | Unwell | | 3995 | |
| 24.08.2004 | 09.12.1928 | M | | 901 | 912 | Wax in the ears | Sodium bicarbonate ear drops | 4269 | |
| 25.08.2004 | 24.01.1957 | M | Hypertension | 1736 | 1742 | BP 151/105 | Atenolol | 4354 | |
| 26.08.2004 | 16.05.1993 | F | | 1021 | 1032 | Septic burn wound on the (R) leg | Flucloxacillin & Fusidic Acid cream | 4397 | |
| 27.08.2004 | 26.12.1932 | F | UTI | 911 | 924 | Pain (L) loin & frequency of micturition | Amoxycillin | 4437 | Script for Atenolol given. For MSU. |
| 25.08.2004 | 29.06.1946 | F | | 1058 | 1108 | She will like to be referred to Gastro-enterologist privately | | 444 | |
| 26.08.2004 | 29.06.1946 | F | S/Leave | 950 | 955 | Unwell & vomiting | | 444 | |
| 27.08.2004 | 13.03.1932 | M | | 1051 | 1056 | Injection Zoladex given | | 4699 | |
| 25.08.2004 | 04.05.1956 | M | Rash | 1144 | 1150 | Urticarial type itchy rash | Fexofenadine | 4859 | |
| 23.08.2004 | 24.04.1956 | F | | 1720 | 1735 | For HBA1c in 4 weeks | | 4863 | |
| 24.08.2004 | 09.04.1926 | M | | 1012 | 1030 | Script for Atenolol given | | 5248 | |

Result of a query that lists all consultations from the 22nd to the end of August 2004 (ConsultationsSeenFrom22ndTillEndOfAug2004)

| SurgeryDate | DateOfBirth | Sex | Diagnosis | TimeIn | TimeOut | Complaints | Treatments | NumbersID | Notes |
|---|---|---|---|---|---|---|---|---|---|
| 25.08.2004 | 08.06.1996 | M | | 1009 | 1013 | To observe scar on his face | | 5324 | |
| 25.08.2004 | 01.02.1996 | M | | 1742 | 1748 | He is disruptive & will not listen | Referred to Child Psychiatrist | 5336 | Mum came to Surgery. |
| 23.08.2004 | 09.02.1963 | F | S/Leave | 913 | 920 | Depression - Med. 5 | | 5567 | Script for Fluoxetine given. |
| 24.08.2004 | 23.02.1927 | F | Rash | 942 | 954 | Itchy scalp | Clobetasol scalp application 0.05% | 5580 | Script for Bendrofluazide given. |
| 27.08.2004 | 24.04.1935 | F | URTI | 1016 | 1027 | (L) ear discharge | Dexamethasone with neomycin ear spray | 5770 | Script for Lansoprazole orodispersible given. |
| 23.08.2004 | 03.05.1991 | F | | 928 | 931 | Mole on the tip of the (R) nostril | Referred to ENT Surgeon | 5849 | |
| 26.08.2004 | 21.05.1958 | F | Revisit | 937 | 950 | Still has (R) sided lower abdominal pain | For USScan of the lower abdomen & pelvis (urgent) | 6209 | |
| 24.08.2004 | 18.06.1959 | M | Pain | 1738 | 1749 | Back Pain | Co-codamol | 6557 | For MSU. |
| 23.08.2004 | 25.01.1988 | F | | 940 | 948 | Back Pain | For MSU | 6586 | |
| 25.08.2004 | 19.12.1974 | F | RTI | 1657 | 1701 | Cough | Amoxycillin | 6729 | |
| 24.08.2004 | 26.01.1953 | F | | 1700 | 1714 | Her repeat prescriptions were issued for her | | 686 | |
| 27.08.2004 | 25.06.1949 | F | | 1710 | 1715 | Blood test are normal | | 6964 | |

Result of a query that lists all consultations from the 22nd to the end of August 2004 (ConsultationsSeenFrom22ndTillEndOfAug2004)

| SurgeryDate | DateOfBirth | Sex | Diagnosis | TimeIn | TimeOut | Complaints | Treatments | NumbersID | Notes |
|---|---|---|---|---|---|---|---|---|---|
| 27.08.2004 | 28.10.1931 | M | | 932 | 949 | Script for Nifedipine m/r capsules & Sodium bicarbonate ear drops given | | 7031 | Possible Digger trial participant. |
| 26.08.2004 | 07.07.1980 | M | | 913 | 916 | I explained to him that the local psychiatrist is the Tourette syndrome expert | | 7057 | |
| 25.08.2004 | 06.02.1952 | F | Pain | 1701 | 1707 | Pain in the (L) wrist | Referred to Orthopaedic Surgeon (Basildon Hospital) | 7106 | |
| 27.08.2004 | 15.02.1948 | M | | 1733 | 1742 | Stepped on a nail, septic | Phenoxymethylpenicillin & Flucloxacillin | 7251 | |
| 23.08.2004 | 09.09.1944 | M | | 904 | 913 | Script for Bendrofluazide given | | 7324 | Private script for Viagra given. |
| 25.08.2004 | 26.02.1915 | F | Pain | 1640 | 1646 | Pain in the (R) wrist | For X-Ray | 7334 | Penicillin & Erythromycin allergy. |
| 24.08.2004 | 28.12.1921 | M | RTI | 1030 | 1038 | Chesty cough | Amoxycillin | 7407 | Script for Normal Saline nebules given. |
| 23.08.2004 | 01.10.1937 | F | | 1716 | 1720 | Tender glands | Amoxycillin | 7489 | |
| 25.08.2004 | 05.03.1954 | F | S/Leave | 1047 | 1058 | Release of (R) middle trigger finger | | 7492 | |
| 27.08.2004 | 14.12.1944 | F | | 1752 | 1803 | Script for Atenolol given | | 7534 | |

815

Result of a query that lists all consultations from the 22$^{nd}$ to the end of August 2004 (ConsultationsSeenFrom22ndTillEndOFAug2004)

| SurgeryDate | DateOfBirth | Sex | Diagnosis | TimeIn | TimeOut | Complaints | Treatments | NumbersID | Notes |
|---|---|---|---|---|---|---|---|---|---|
| 24.08.2004 | 26.07.1960 | F | | 958 | 1012 | Referred to local GP (BUPA) for acupuncture for her back | | 7591 | |
| 27.08.2004 | 05.12.2002 | M | URTI | 1742 | 1752 | (R) ear ache | Amoxycillin | 7632 | |
| 24.08.2004 | 13.04.1967 | M | | 1753 | 1756 | To observe the black on his arms | | 7688 | |
| 25.08.2004 | 01.06.1947 | F | Rash | 921 | 926 | Itchy & weepy rash under the breasts | Miconazole 2% + 1% Hydrocortisone cream | 7754 | Penicillin allergy. |
| 23.08.2004 | 08.04.1942 | M | | 936 | 940 | Septic insect bite around the (L) eye lid | Flucloxacillin | 7774 | |
| 23.08.2004 | 18.10.1974 | F | | 948 | 1000 | Referred to Neurologist (Basildon Hospital) for a second opinion regarding possible MS | | 784 | |
| 24.08.2004 | 22.11.1978 | F | | 1749 | 1753 | To attend FP Clinic regarding her contraception | | 7901 | |
| 24.08.2004 | 02.08.2003 | F | Rash | 916 | 928 | Nappy rash | Hydrocortisone with nystatin dimeticone & benzalkonium cream | 7917 | |

Result of a query that lists all consultations from the 22nd to the end of August 2004 (ConsultationsSeenFrom22ndTillEndOfAug2004)

| SurgeryDate | DateOfBirth | Sex | Diagnosis | TimeIn | TimeOut | Complaints | Treatments | NumbersID | Notes |
|---|---|---|---|---|---|---|---|---|---|
| 24.08.2004 | 18.08.1963 | M | | 1719 | 1726 | Reception staff to enquire if he can have MRI scan locally following referral by his GP | | 7920 | |
| 25.08.2004 | 21.02.1982 | M | Rash | 1753 | 1756 | Itchy rash in the (R) groin | Miconazole 2% + 1% Hydrocortisone cream | 834 | |
| 24.08.2004 | 28.09.1958 | M | S/Leave | 1726 | 1735 | Pain (L) elbow - Med. 5 | | 905 | |
| 24.08.2004 | 04.12.2002 | F | Rash | 954 | 958 | Possible Chicken Pox | To apply own Calamine lotion | NP (ALM) | |
| 23.08.2004 | 09.01.1987 | F | URTI | 1735 | 1741 | Sore throat & rash | Fexofenadine & Amoxycillin | NP (JW) | |
| 23.08.2004 | 20.04.1945 | F | Pain | 1650 | 1655 | Pain in the (R) knee | For X-Ray | NP (KY) | |
| 24.08.2004 | 12.05.1983 | M | URTI | 1714 | 1719 | Sore throat | Amoxycillin | NP (NDM) | |
| 25.08.2004 | 07.02.1972 | F | Pain | 1748 | 1753 | Pain (L) lower abdomen | For MSU | NP (SR) | For MSU. |
| 24.08.2004 | 13.02.1985 | F | | 912 | 916 | Script for Marvelon given | | Temp | |
| 24.08.2004 | 05.07.1980 | M | URTI | 1055 | 1100 | (L) ear ache | Amoxycillin & Dexamethasone with neomycin ear spray | Temp | |

Result of a query that lists all consultations from the 22nd to the end of August 2005 (ConsultationsSeenFrom22ndTillEndOfAug2005)

| SurgeryDate | DateOfBirth | Sex | Diagnosis | TimeIn | TimeOut | Complaints | Treatments | NumbersID | Notes |
|---|---|---|---|---|---|---|---|---|---|
| 24.08.2005 | 24.02.1942 | M | | 902 | 919 | Script for Acarbose given | | 1031 | |
| 22.08.2005 | 08.02.1939 | F | URTI | 1746 | 1750 | Sore throat | Erythromycin | 113 | Trimethoprim allergy. |
| 26.08.2005 | 14.11.1963 | F | S/Leave | 1715 | 1725 | (L) Breast Cancer | | 1185 | |
| 25.08.2005 | 20.02.1930 | M | | 901 | 914 | To stop Atorvastatin for one month | | 1254 | Penicillin & Erythromycin allergy. |
| 22.08.2005 | 24.10.1929 | F | | 925 | 934 | Script for 1% Hydrocortisone cream & Fexofenadine given | | 1255 | |
| 26.08.2005 | 06.08.1944 | M | Hypertension | 1636 | 1647 | BP 187/98 | Bendrofluazide | 1304 | |
| 23.08.2005 | 21.02.1961 | F | | 1651 | 1658 | Script for Trimethoprim & Omeprazole given | | 131 | |
| 26.08.2005 | 19.01.1967 | M | | 903 | 919 | Script for Citalopram & Diazepam | | 136 | |
| 23.08.2005 | 19.01.1967 | M | S/Leave | 1131 | 1151 | Stress | | 156 | Agitated & paranoid, referred to Mental Health Team. |
| 25.08.2005 | 19.01.1967 | M | | 928 | 936 | To get holiday cancellation form from Insurance Company | | 156 | |
| 24.08.2005 | 05.08.1942 | M | | 949 | 958 | Informed that he has been referred to Orthopaedic Surgeon | | 1573 | |

## Result of a query that lists all consultations from the 22nd to the end of August 2005 (ConsultationsSeenFrom22ndTillEndOfAug2005)

| SurgeryDate | DateOfBirth | Sex | Diagnosis | TimeIn | TimeOut | Complaints | Treatments | NumbersID | Notes |
|---|---|---|---|---|---|---|---|---|---|
| 23.08.2005 | 15.10.1923 | F | RTI | 1722 | 1732 | Chesty cough | Amoxycillin | 1711 | |
| 25.08.2005 | 30.05.1916 | M | | 943 | 948 | Fixed flexion of the dipj of the (R) Ring finger | Referred to Orthopaedic Surgeon (Basildon Hospital) | 1712 | |
| 30.08.2005 | 21.11.1954 | M | URTI | 1737 | 1742 | Sore throat | Amoxycillin | 2018 | |
| 22.08.2005 | 17.10.1953 | F | URTI | 1038 | 1043 | Sore throat | Amoxycillin | 2020 | |
| 25.08.2005 | 16.09.1971 | F | S/Leave | 1722 | 1725 | Non-Hodgkin's Lymphoma | | 2053 | |
| 30.08.2005 | 02.03.0918 | F | | 928 | 943 | Script for Aspirin dispersible given | | 2134 | |
| 22.08.2005 | 02.04.1959 | F | | 934 | 939 | To use OTC Ferrous Sulphate | | 2310 | Erythromycin allergy. |
| 30.08.2005 | 24.02.1944 | F | | 1650 | 1701 | Script for Tolterodine m/r given | | 2330 | |
| 26.08.2005 | 07.11.1984 | F | | 1700 | 1715 | Script for Fluoxetine given | | 2438 | |
| 24.08.2005 | 26.03.1987 | M | S/Leave | 1005 | 1009 | Whiplash injury | | 2439 | |
| 26.08.2005 | 06.01.1955 | M | | 1734 | 1737 | Private script for Viagra given | | 2556 | |
| 22.08.2005 | 09.05.1955 | M | S/Leave | 905 | 910 | Back injury | | 2650 | |
| 30.08.2005 | 09.05.1955 | M | S/Leave | 947 | 952 | Back injury - Med. 5 | | 2650 | |
| 25.08.2005 | 24.03.1973 | M | S/Leave | 936 | 943 | Injury (R) ankle - Private & Med. 5 | | 2784 | |
| 25.08.2005 | 15.02.1946 | F | | 1725 | 1732 | Script for Fosamax given | | 2792 | |
| 30.08.2005 | 28.03.1926 | F | | 1029 | 1035 | Septic insect bite (L) thigh | Flucloxacillin | 2837 | |

819

Result of a query that lists all consultations from the 22nd to the end of August 2005 (ConsultationsSeenFrom22ndTillEndOfAug2005)

| SurgeryDate | DateOfBirth | Sex | Diagnosis | TimeIn | TimeOut | Complaints | Treatments | NumbersID | Notes |
|---|---|---|---|---|---|---|---|---|---|
| 24.08.2005 | 27.09.1937 | F | | 1000 | 1005 | BP 124/79 | | 2893 | |
| 23.08.2005 | 03.11.1971 | F | Pain | 1755 | 1801 | Pain & tingling (L) median nerve distribution | Referred to Orthopaedic Surgeon (Basildon Hospital) | 3015 | |
| 24.08.2005 | 01.03.1934 | F | | 919 | 929 | X-Ray (R) knee - No recent fracture shown | | 3114 | Penicillin allergy. |
| 24.08.2005 | 24.07.1956 | M | | 1635 | 1639 | Script for Omeprazole given | | 3169 | |
| 25.08.2005 | 22.02.1944 | M | UTI | 1022 | 1029 | Dysuria | Amoxycillin | 3203 | For MSU. Trimethoprim allergy. |
| 24.08.2005 | 26.04.1942 | F | | 1639 | 1704 | To take Gliclazide 40mg daily | | 3497 | |
| 30.08.2005 | 08.04.1971 | F | UTI | 1811 | 1818 | Dysuria | Nitrofurantoin | 3633 | For MSU. |
| 23.08.2005 | 24.04.1986 | M | | 1121 | 1131 | Pyrexial & swollen glands | Amoxycillin | 3659 | |
| 26.08.2005 | 24.04.1986 | M | | 1753 | 1800 | Advised to see how he feels on Tuesday before going on holidays | | 3659 | |
| 30.08.2005 | 02.02.1976 | F | | 952 | 1007 | Vaginal thrush | Clotrimazole pessary | 3762 | |
| 23.08.2005 | 02.10.1992 | M | | 1739 | 1750 | Fractured 4th (R) toe | Referred to Fracture Clinic | 3788 | |
| 24.08.2005 | 14.01.1965 | M | URTI | 1733 | 1744 | Throat feels raw & sore | Amoxycillin | 3837 | |
| 24.08.2005 | 02.11.1973 | F | | 929 | 942 | Increased facial hair | Referred to Endocrinologist | 3864 | |

Result of a query that lists all consultations from the 22nd to the end of August 2005 (ConsultationsSeenFrom22ndTillEndOfAug2005)

| SurgeryDate | DateOfBirth | Sex | Diagnosis | TimeIn | TimeOut | Complaints | Treatments | NumbersID | Notes |
|---|---|---|---|---|---|---|---|---|---|
| 30.08.2005 | 01.08.1947 | F | | 1636 | 1644 | For X-Ray of hips & pelvis | | 398 | |
| 30.08.2005 | 29.11.1962 | M | S/Leave | 1022 | 1029 | Flu symptoms - Private | | 4135 | Script for Amoxycillin given. |
| 25.08.2005 | 13.08.1923 | F | | 1633 | 1639 | Script for Gaviscon Advance | | 424 | Penicillin allergy. |
| 22.08.2005 | 10.03.1936 | M | | 947 | 1000 | PSA – 5.5 mcg/L, elevated | Referred to Urologist | 425 | Script for Simvastatin given. |
| 23.08.2005 | 10.03.1936 | M | URTI | 1706 | 1713 | Sore throat | Amoxycillin | 425 | |
| 24.08.2005 | 27.09.1984 | M | | 1031 | 1045 | He will put in a self-certificate for the first week | | 434 | |
| 25.08.2005 | 27.09.1984 | M | S/Leave | 1732 | 1740 | Stressed from looking after dad who has Waldenstrom's Macroglobulinemia - Med. 5 | | 434 | |
| 22.08.2005 | 10.08.1985 | F | | 1712 | 1718 | Script for Clotrimazole pessary & Tetracycline topical solution given | | 4429 | |
| 30.08.2005 | 10.08.1985 | F | | 1731 | 1737 | Unable to contact the GUM clinic | | 4429 | |
| 23.08.2005 | 13.05.1994 | M | | 1750 | 1755 | Septic (R)IGTN | Flucloxacillin | 4432 | |
| 25.08.2005 | 29.09.1932 | F | RTI | 956 | 1008 | Cough & Clammy | Amoxycillin | 4487 | |
| 30.08.2005 | 09.04.1938 | M | Pain | 1701 | 1713 | (R) knee pain | Etodolac capsules & Co-codamol | 4519 | Tetracycline allergy. |

Result of a query that lists all consultations from the 22nd to the end of August 2005 (ConsultationsSeenFrom22ndTillEndOfAug2005)

| SurgeryDate | DateOfBirth | Sex | Diagnosis | TimeIn | TimeOut | Complaints | Treatments | NumbersID | Notes |
|---|---|---|---|---|---|---|---|---|---|
| 23.08.2005 | 19.07.1994 | F | | 1713 | 1722 | Deafness in the (L) ear | Referred to ENT Surgeon | 4535 | |
| 23.08.2005 | 09.10.1926 | M | Pain | 1220 | 1230 | (R) shoulder pain | Dihydrocodeine | 4567 | Penicillin & Statins allergy. |
| 22.08.2005 | 21.02.1976 | F | S/Leave | 939 | 947 | Strress | | 4585 | |
| 26.08.2005 | 29.11.1969 | M | | 1737 | 1741 | Septic (R)IGTN | Flucloxacillin | 4619 | Referred to Podiatrist. |
| 26.08.2005 | 22.04.1975 | F | URTI | 1741 | 1745 | Sore throat | Erythromycin | 4810 | |
| 26.08.2005 | 17.04.1945 | F | | 919 | 930 | Abdominal pain & irregular bowel habits | Referred to Gastro-enterologist | 5207 | Co-dydramol & Penicillin allergy. |
| 24.08.2005 | 25.04.1909 | F | | 1427 | 1440 | Pyrexial & arms ache | Amoxycillin, soluble Paracetamol & Aspirin dispersible | 5257 | Home visit. |
| 24.08.2005 | 17.12.1981 | F | URTI | 1022 | 1031 | Sore & deafness (L) ear | Amoxycillin & Dexamethasone with neomycin ear spray | 5384 | |
| 30.08.2005 | 17.01.1956 | F | S/Leave | 900 | 918 | Back Pain & Acute Renal failure | | 5796 | |
| 23.08.2005 | 31.01.1941 | F | | 905 | 923 | Script for Peppermint oil e/c m/r capsules given | | 5867 | |
| 25.08.2005 | 19.04.1984 | F | | 1639 | 1645 | Pregnancy test positive | | 5884 | |

822

Result of a query that lists all consultations from the 22nd to the end of August 2005 (ConsultationsSeenFrom22ndTillEndOfAug2005)

| SurgeryDate | DateOfBirth | Sex | Diagnosis | TimeIn | TimeOut | Complaints | Treatments | NumbersID | Notes |
|---|---|---|---|---|---|---|---|---|---|
| 26.08.2005 | 23.03.1926 | M | | 1002 | 1025 | Advised to complete & send off the DVL form | | 5954 | |
| 24.08.2005 | 08.03.1961 | M | Pain | 1045 | 1058 | pain (R) elbow | Referred to Orthopaedic Surgeon (Basildon Hospital) | 6198 | |
| 22.08.2005 | 27.08.1948 | F | | 1738 | 1746 | Burning sensation in the upper & lower limbs | Referred to Neurologist | 6538 | |
| 23.08.2005 | 11.12.1968 | F | Pain | 1042 | 1053 | Crampy abdominal pain | Hyoscine butylbromide & Metoclopramide | 6579 | |
| 25.08.2005 | 09.04.1944 | F | | 1008 | 1022 | Script for Amitriptyline & Injection MethylPrednisolone with Lidocaine given | | 6592 | |
| 26.08.2005 | 02.11.1984 | F | | 930 | 938 | Burst condom | Levonorgestrel | 6604 | |
| 22.08.2005 | 27.09.1984 | M | | 1756 | 1808 | Bruises easily & anaemia as a child | For FBC, TFTs, Clotting Screen & TFTs | 6668 | |
| 23.08.2005 | 19.10.1924 | F | | 1630 | 1651 | To reduce dose of Lisinopril | | 677 | Penicillin allergy. |
| 23.08.2005 | 16.01.1998 | F | | 923 | 931 | For FBC | | 6809 | |
| 30.08.2005 | 23.11.1946 | M | S/Leave | 1754 | 1800 | Back Pain - Med. 5 | | 6822 | |
| 30.08.2005 | 07.09.1928 | M | | 1644 | 1650 | Gum infection | Amoxycillin | 6915 | |
| 24.08.2005 | 11.01.1964 | F | URTI | 1744 | 1750 | Sore throat | Amoxycillin | 6976 | |

Result of a query that lists all consultations from the 22nd to the end of August 2005 (ConsultationsSeenFrom22ndTillEndOfAug2005)

| SurgeryDate | DateOfBirth | Sex | Diagnosis | TimeIn | TimeOut | Complaints | Treatments | NumbersID | Notes |
|---|---|---|---|---|---|---|---|---|---|
| 22.08.2005 | 04.01.1932 | F | | 1718 | 1731 | Script for Erythromycin given | | 7247 | Ciproxin allergy. |
| 23.08.2005 | 06.10.1944 | F | | 959 | 1006 | To bring in the result of the lower spine X-Ray she had done privately | | 7262 | |
| 25.08.2005 | 14.02.1952 | M | | 1740 | 1744 | MSU & PSA normal | | 7298 | |
| 22.08.2005 | 24.03.1972 | M | | 1750 | 1756 | Feels low & depressed | Fluoxetine | 7350 | Penicillin allergy. |
| 22.08.2005 | 28.12.1921 | M | | 1637 | 1640 | He will observe the patches of non-itchy brownish rash on his body | | 7407 | |
| 24.08.2005 | 01.10.1937 | F | | 942 | 949 | Tongue burns | Referred to Maxillo-facial Surgeon | 7489 | Cyst on the (L) upper eye lid, referred to Ophthalmologist. Aspirin & Septrin allergy. |
| 30.08.2005 | 11.06.1930 | M | | 1713 | 1722 | For repeat CXR post antibiotics | | 7576 | |
| 30.08.2005 | 28.02.1986 | F | S/Leave | 1007 | 1022 | Diarrhoea & Headaches - Med. 5 | | 7583 | Script for Loperamide & Co-codamol given. |
| 23.08.2005 | 07.02.1940 | F | | 1019 | 1042 | Script for Tolterodine given | | 7600 | The Parking Badge Scheme for Disabled People Medical Practitioner Report completed. |

824

## Result of a query that lists all consultations from the 22nd to the end of August 2005 (ConsultationsSeenFrom22ndTillEndOfAug2005)

| SurgeryDate | DateOfBirth | Sex | Diagnosis | TimeIn | TimeOut | Complaints | Treatments | NumbersID | Notes |
|---|---|---|---|---|---|---|---|---|---|
| 25.08.2005 | 27.08.1952 | F | S/Leave | 914 | 928 | Low back pain - Med. 4 | | 7676 | Script for Omeprazole given. |
| 23.08.2005 | 28.04.1957 | M | S/Leave | 931 | 941 | Chest infection | | 7698 | |
| 26.08.2005 | 28.04.1957 | M | | 1725 | 1729 | Script for Erythromycin given | | 7698 | |
| 25.08.2005 | 07.01.1944 | M | | 1029 | 1037 | To continue with Dihydrocodeine & Diclofenac for the moderate to severe osteoarthritis of his knees | | 7714 | |
| 25.08.2005 | 07.11.1968 | F | Conjunctivitis | 948 | 956 | Swollen, sore & sticky (L) eye | Chloramphenicol eye drops & Amoxycillin | 7739 | |
| 22.08.2005 | 08.04.1942 | M | S/Leave | 1000 | 1025 | Stress - Private | | 7774 | |
| 30.08.2005 | 24.11.1960 | F | | 1800 | 1811 | Burst condom | Levonorgestrel | 7782 | |
| 30.08.2005 | 29.01.1941 | M | UTI | 918 | 928 | Dysuria & frequency of micturition | Amoxycillin | 7839 | For MSU. |
| 25.08.2005 | 03.10.1958 | F | Revisit | 1750 | 1802 | Pain in (R) foot has persisted | Referred to Orthopaedic Surgeon (Basildon Hospital) | 7891 | Penicillin allergy. |
| 22.08.2005 | 29.11.1937 | F | | 1043 | 1105 | Diabetic Clinic | | 7918 | Script for Gliclazide, Quinine Sulphate & Erythromycin given. |

825

Result of a query that lists all consultations from the 22nd to the end of August 2005 (ConsultationsSeenFrom22ndTillEndOfAug2005)

| SurgeryDate | DateOfBirth | Sex | Diagnosis | TimeIn | TimeOut | Complaints | Treatments | NumbersID | Notes |
|---|---|---|---|---|---|---|---|---|---|
| 24.08.2005 | 13.09.1918 | M |  | 1704 | 1733 | Script for Alfuzosin given |  | 841 |  |
| 23.08.2005 | 04.03.1947 | M | Depressed | 1053 | 1110 | Feels low & cries easily | Referred to Practice Counsellor | 88 | Script for Atorvastatin given. |
| 26.08.2005 | 04.12.2002 | F | Rash | 1745 | 1753 | Rash in the perineum | Mebendazole & Hydrocortisone with nystatin & benzalkonium cream | NP (ALM) |  |
| 26.08.2005 | 22.01.1991 | M | Lump | 1652 | 1700 | Lump (R) testicle | For USScan of the testicles (urgent) | NP (BH) |  |
| 26.08.2005 | 08.08.1953 | M | S/Leave | 958 | 1002 | Back Pain |  | NP (BP) |  |
| 25.08.2005 | 15.10.1974 | M |  | 1716 | 1722 | Tender small cyst on face | Flucloxacillin | NP (CP) |  |
| 30.08.2005 | 25.02.1950 | F |  | 1722 | 1731 | Neck pain | Diclofenac e/c & Co-codamol | NP (CS) |  |
| 22.08.2005 | 30.09.1941 | M |  | 911 | 925 | Diarrhoea | Co-phenotrope 2.5mg + 25mcg & oral rehydration salts oral powder | NP (DGC) |  |
| 25.08.2005 | 13.11.2004 | F |  | 1655 | 1700 | To use OTC Calamine lotion for her rash |  | NP (EP) |  |
| 23.08.2005 | 27.07.1979 | F | UTI | 1658 | 1706 | Frequency of micturition | Amoxycillin | NP (ER) | For MSU. |

Result of a query that lists all consultations from the 22nd to the end of August 2005 (ConsultationsSeenFrom22ndTillEndOfAug2005)

| SurgeryDate | DateOfBirth | Sex | Diagnosis | TimeIn | TimeOut | Complaints | Treatments | NumbersID | Notes |
|---|---|---|---|---|---|---|---|---|---|
| 22.08.2005 | 29.05.1937 | M | | 1649 | 1701 | Script for Clopidogrel, Simvastatin & Co-danthrusate given | | NP (FAS) | |
| 23.08.2005 | 01.04.1920 | F | Lump | 941 | 953 | (R) breast lump | Referred to Breast Surgeon (Cancer Referral) | NP (HW) | |
| 22.08.2005 | 24.04.1931 | F | Conjunctivitis | 1701 | 1704 | Sore, red & weepy (R) eye | Chloramphenicol eye ointment | NP (JB) | Aspirin allergy. |
| 22.08.2005 | 29.10.1985 | M | | 1731 | 1738 | T.A.T.T. | For FBC & Fasting Glucose | NP (JB) | |
| 22.08.2005 | 04.06.1958 | F | | 1031 | 1038 | To put in self certificate for the first week | | NP (JC) | |
| 26.08.2005 | 04.06.1958 | F | S/Leave | 938 | 948 | Abdominal pain | | NP (JC) | |
| 24.08.2005 | 01.05.1987 | F | | 1750 | 1801 | Script for Ferrous fumarate with low dose folic acid | | NP (JD) | |
| 22.08.2005 | 27.11.2004 | F | URTI | 1025 | 1031 | Infected rhinorrhoea | Erythromycin | NP (JLR) | |
| 30.08.2005 | 01.12.1933 | F | Hypertension | 1742 | 1754 | BP 185/93 | Bendrofluazide | NP (JM) | Penicillin allergy. |
| 22.08.2005 | 31.01.1938 | F | | 1640 | 1649 | Referred to Chest Physician (urgent) regarding her persistent pleural effusion | | NP (JS) | |
| 26.08.2005 | 10.12.1983 | F | | 948 | 958 | Panic attacks & headaches | Propranolol | NP (KP) | (R)IGTN, referred to Podiatrist. |
| 30.08.2005 | 14.04.1948 | F | S/Leave | 943 | 947 | Arthritis of the knees | | NP (LM) | |

Result of a query that lists all consultations from the 22nd to the end of August 2005 (ConsultationsSeenFrom22ndTillEndOfAug2005)

| SurgeryDate | DateOfBirth | Sex | Diagnosis | TimeIn | TimeOut | Complaints | Treatments | NumbersID | Notes |
|---|---|---|---|---|---|---|---|---|---|
| 26.08.2005 | 18.01.1977 | F | Pain | 1041 | 1058 | (L) ankle pain | Dihydrocodeine & Ibuprofen | NP (MP) | Script for Peppermint oil capsules. For X-Ray. |
| 26.08.2005 | 02.01.1952 | F | URTI | 1729 | 1734 | Pain (L) ear | Amoxycillin & Dexamethasone with neomycin ear spray | NP (PD) | |
| 30.08.2005 | 26.10.1921 | F | Rash | 1340 | 1355 | Itchy rash all over the body | Calamine lotion, Fexofenadine & Permethrin cream 0.5% | NP (RJ) | Home visit. |
| 25.08.2005 | 16.04.1995 | F | URTI | 1711 | 1716 | Sore throat & fever | Amoxycillin & Paracetamol | NP (SG) | |
| 26.08.2005 | 07.02.1972 | F | | 1647 | 1652 | To come in later for Montelukast if necessary | | NP (SR) | |
| 24.08.2005 | 26.05.1936 | M | | 1009 | 1022 | For repeat MSU in one week | | NP (TC) | |
| 23.08.2005 | 14.10.1978 | F | S/Leave | 953 | 959 | Depression | | NP (TI) | |
| 23.08.2005 | 19.09.1978 | F | | 1110 | 1122 | For USScan of the abdomen (urgent) & MSU | | NP (VW) | |
| 23.08.2005 | 21.09.1983 | M | S/Leave | 1006 | 1019 | Whiplash injury - Private | | Temp | |
| 23.08.2005 | 08.06.1976 | M | Pain | 1801 | 1810 | Pain in the legs & back following Motor-bike accident | Dihydrocodeine & Diclofenac e/c | Temp | Script for Diclofenac e/c & Co-codamol given. |

828

Result of a query that lists all consultations from the 22nd to the end of August 2006 (ConsultationsSeenFrom22ndTillEndOFAug2006)

| SurgeryDate | DateOfBirth | Sex | Diagnosis | TimeIn | TimeOut | Complaints | Treatments | Initials | Notes |
|---|---|---|---|---|---|---|---|---|---|
| 22.08.2006 | 20.02.2002 | F | | 952 | 1000 | USScan of the kidneys normal | | SJB | |
| 22.08.2006 | 25.09.1961 | F | | 1000 | 1008 | Script for Norethisterone given | | CAS | |
| 22.08.2006 | 08.03.1946 | F | UTI | 1008 | 1016 | Dysuria | Cefalexin | GRC | For MSU. |
| 22.08.2006 | 08.08.1918 | M | | 1016 | 1032 | For Lumbar Spine X-Ray | | VHS | |
| 22.08.2006 | 03.08.1948 | M | S/Leave | 1032 | 1043 | Infection in the (L) leg | | EAP | |
| 22.08.2006 | 02.07.1924 | M | | 1043 | 1100 | To get the medications for his stay in Australia for 3 months | | TCC | |
| 22.08.2006 | 04.01.1962 | F | | 1100 | 1109 | Script for Lactulose given | | CEC | |
| 22.08.2006 | 01.06.1932 | M | | 1109 | 1119 | Script for Flucloxacillin given | | IGH | |
| 22.08.2006 | 03.04.1980 | M | URTI | 1119 | 1124 | Sore throat | Erythromycin | JK | Penicillin allergy. |
| 22.08.2006 | 04.07.1938 | F | | 1124 | 1142 | Script for Diclofenac suppositories, Erythromycin & Omeprazole given | | BJT | |
| 22.08.2006 | 05.12.1988 | F | | 1142 | 1150 | Script for Flucloxacillin & Fusidic acid cream given | | CLL | |

Result of a query that lists all consultations from the 22nd to the end of August 2006 (ConsultationsSeenFrom22ndTillEndOfAug2006)

| SurgeryDate | DateOfBirth | Sex | Diagnosis | TimeIn | TimeOut | Complaints | Treatments | Initials | Notes |
|---|---|---|---|---|---|---|---|---|---|
| 22.08.2006 | 24.04.1931 | F | | 1150 | 1157 | Script for Co-codamol & Quinine sulphate given | | JWB | |
| 22.08.2006 | 01.10.1920 | M | | 1157 | 1212 | Script for Simvastatin given | | JM | |
| 22.08.2006 | 05.12.1956 | M | | 1649 | 1652 | Script for Amoxycillin & Fusidic eye drops given | | DTB | |
| 22.08.2006 | 21.08.1946 | F | | 1652 | 1705 | Script for Dihydrocodeine given | | JK | |
| 22.08.2006 | 11.08.1980 | F | | 1708 | 1738 | Script for Diazepam & Fluoxetine given | | MD | Referred to Physiotherapist regarding (L) wrist pain. |
| 22.08.2006 | 24.10.1989 | F | | 1738 | 1744 | Script for Amoxycillin & Neomycin Sulphate with Chlorhexidine given | | MC | Mupirocin nasal ointment prescribed as they can't get naseptin cream. |
| 22.08.2006 | 08.03.1961 | M | | 1744 | 1757 | Pain in (R) elbow - Private | | RAB | Script for Co-codamol & Diclofenac e/c given. |
| 22.08.2006 | 24.04.1956 | F | S/Leave | 1757 | 1807 | Depression | | CAP | |
| 22.08.2006 | 31.03.1967 | F | | 1807 | 1814 | For X-Rays of hips & Lumbar spine | | LJS | |
| 22.08.2006 | 13.09.1969 | M | S/Leave | 1814 | 1832 | General discussion about contacts of letters from haematologist | | KDA | |

Result of a query that lists all consultations from the 22$^{nd}$ to the end of August 2006 (ConsultationsSeenFrom22ndTillEndOfAug2006)

| SurgeryDate | DateOfBirth | Sex | Diagnosis | TimeIn | TimeOut | Complaints | Treatments | Initials | Notes |
|---|---|---|---|---|---|---|---|---|---|
| 22.08.2006 | 07.07.1943 | F |  | 1832 | 1840 | Script for Prednisolone e/c given |  | GM |  |
| 23.08.2006 | 05.01.1969 | F |  | 947 | 1000 | Routine ante-natal examination done |  | NS |  |
| 23.08.2006 | 27.04.1939 | F |  | 1000 | 1009 | Script to Ezetimibe given |  | DBS |  |
| 23.08.2006 | 12.05.1936 | M |  | 1011 | 1023 | Script for Macrogol compound npf oral powder & peppermint oil e/c m/r given |  | AM |  |
| 23.08.2006 | 31.10.1940 | F |  | 1023 | 1030 | Script for Cefalexin given |  | CF |  |
| 23.08.2006 | 03.02.1965 | M |  | 1033 | 1044 | Referred to Colo-rectal surgeon regarding his rectal bleeding |  | DF |  |
| 23.08.2006 | 26.01.1959 | F |  | 1044 | 1059 | For LFTs |  | SAM |  |
| 23.08.2006 | 23.05.1932 | M |  | 1059 | 1114 | Script for Ezetimibe & Lisinopril given |  | EB |  |
| 23.08.2006 | 04.07.1959 | F |  | 1114 | 1120 | Script for Sofradex ear drops given |  | SAB |  |
| 23.08.2006 | 18.02.1961 | M |  | 1120 | 1132 | Referred to Physiotherapist regarding his back pain |  | MMA |  |
| 23.08.2006 | 10.08.1952 | F |  | 1132 | 1153 | Script for Ezetimibe, Metformin & Lisinopril given |  | SAG |  |

Result of a query that lists all consultations from the 22nd to the end of August 2006 (ConsultationsSeenFrom22ndTillEndOfAug2006)

| SurgeryDate | DateOfBirth | Sex | Diagnosis | TimeIn | TimeOut | Complaints | Treatments | Initials | Notes |
|---|---|---|---|---|---|---|---|---|---|
| 23.08.2006 | 05.03.1973 | F | | 1153 | 1212 | Routine 6 weeks post-natal check | | HAAF | |
| 23.08.2006 | 23.07.1920 | F | | 1330 | 1355 | Unwell & very dizzy | Referred to Medical Dr. on call, SGH | GR | Home visit. |
| 23.08.2006 | 23.09.1990 | F | | 1645 | 1658 | Script for Amoxycillin & Tetracycline topical solution given | | LET | |
| 23.08.2006 | 06.09.1958 | F | | 1658 | 1709 | Septic blisters on the (R) foot | Flucloxacillin & Fusidic acid cream | SDI | For FBC & Fasting Glucose. |
| 23.08.2006 | 22.02.1968 | M | Rash | 1709 | 1720 | Itchy red rash in groins & in the abdominal fold | Trimovate cream | ADB | For FBC & Fasting Glucose. |
| 23.08.2006 | 03.08.1948 | M | | 1720 | 1730 | He will look well for his misplaced certificate before asking for a duplicate | | EAP | |
| 23.08.2006 | 02.11.1989 | M | Rash | 1730 | 1735 | Multiple warts on arms & hands | Salicylic acid topical solution | CJRR | |
| 23.08.2006 | 18.04.1930 | F | | 1740 | 1805 | Contents of letter of 17.08.06 explained to patient | | IDB | |
| 23.08.2006 | 08.06.1974 | M | URTI | 1805 | 1810 | Sore throat | Amoxycillin | SWM | |
| 23.08.2006 | 21.08.1979 | F | | 1810 | 1821 | Routine ante-natal check done | | NAA | |
| 24.08.2006 | 18.04.1978 | F | | 946 | 1006 | Routine ante-natal check done | | SL | |

Result of a query that lists all consultations from the 22nd to the end of August 2006 (ConsultationsSeenFrom22ndTillEndOfAug2006)

| SurgeryDate | DateOfBirth | Sex | Diagnosis | TimeIn | TimeOut | Complaints | Treatments | Initials | Notes |
|---|---|---|---|---|---|---|---|---|---|
| 24.08.2006 | 07.05.1938 | F | | 1006 | 1015 | Script for Dermol cream given | | ILB | |
| 24.08.2006 | 05.10.1960 | M | | 1015 | 1026 | Script for Prednisolone tablets given | | RCB | |
| 24.08.2006 | 12.11.1950 | M | | 1026 | 1034 | Script for Diclofenac c/c given | | MJP | |
| 24.08.2006 | 30.09.1933 | M | | 1034 | 1050 | Script for Bendrofluazide given | | RBAR | |
| 24.08.2006 | 11.04.2006 | F | | 1050 | 1102 | To try Olive oil for her cradle cap | | BCW | |
| 24.08.2006 | 24.08.1918 | F | | 1136 | 1155 | Script for Flucloxacillin, Fusidic acid with hydrocortisone cream & Lisinopril given | | GPE | |
| 24.08.2006 | 26.05.1936 | M | | 1315 | 1405 | Script for Citalopram, Movicol, Ensure Plus, Enlive & Amoxycillin given | | TC | Home visit. |
| 24.08.2006 | 28.03.1985 | F | | 1648 | 1708 | Routine ante-natal check done | | LEB | Script for Gaviscon Advance given |
| 24.08.2006 | 09.05.1964 | F | | 1708 | 1715 | Script for Amitriptyline given | | CAC | |
| 24.08.2006 | 03.08.1948 | M | S/Leave | 1715 | 1721 | Infection in (L) leg - Med. 5 (Duplicate given) | | EAP | |

Result of a query that lists all consultations from the 22nd to the end of August 2006 (ConsultationsSeenFrom22ndTillEndOfAug2006)

| SurgeryDate | DateOfBirth | Sex | Diagnosis | TimeIn | TimeOut | Complaints | Treatments | Initials | Notes |
|---|---|---|---|---|---|---|---|---|---|
| 24.08.2006 | 30.09.1961 | F | | 1721 | 1745 | Letter to whom it may concern that she suffer from manic attacks | | TJB | |
| 24.08.2006 | 15.04.1953 | M | | 1745 | 1802 | Referred to Urologist (BUPA) regarding pain in his (L) testicle | | KGS | |
| 24.08.2006 | 21.07.1983 | M | | 1810 | 1817 | Script for Lansoprazole given | | Temp (JH) | |
| 24.08.2006 | 31.03.1986 | F | | 1817 | 1838 | Information regarding alleged assault on his face obtained | | NAK | |
| 25.08.2006 | 08.11.1931 | F | | 947 | 1007 | Script for Ferrous Sulphate & Senna given | | JC | |
| 25.08.2006 | 02.03.1918 | F | | 1007 | 1021 | For repeat FBC in one month | | YV | |
| 25.08.2006 | 07.02.1940 | F | | 1021 | 1059 | Script for Doxazosin given | | MEC | |
| 25.08.2006 | 18.03.1983 | F | | 1059 | 1103 | Pregnancy test positive | | HLK | |
| 25.08.2006 | 29.04.1935 | F | | 1103 | 1112 | Script for 1% Hydrocortisone cream given | | CM | |
| 25.08.2006 | 27.03.1940 | F | | 1112 | 1119 | Referred to Orthopaedic Surgeon regarding painful knees & loose body in the (L) knee | | MAD | |

Result of a query that lists all consultations from the 22nd to the end of August 2006 (ConsultationsSeenFrom22ndTillEndOfAug2006)

| SurgeryDate | DateOfBirth | Sex | Diagnosis | TimeIn | TimeOut | Complaints | Treatments | Initials | Notes |
|---|---|---|---|---|---|---|---|---|---|
| 25.08.2006 | 05.03.1954 | F | S/Leave | 1119 | 1140 | Acute coronary syndrome | | PSC | Script for Ramipril given. |
| 25.08.2006 | 31.05.1930 | F | | 1140 | 1153 | For MSU | | JVJ | |
| 25.08.2006 | 08.03.1959 | F | | 1153 | 1212 | She will try to change her gynaecology appointment to Basildon hospital on line | | DM | |
| 25.08.2006 | 27.07.2006 | F | | 1212 | 1220 | Script for E45 cream given | | ML | |
| 25.08.2006 | 22.02.1936 | F | | 1641 | 1700 | Yearly Diabetic Monitoring check done | | RPM | |
| 25.08.2006 | 02.02.1928 | M | | 1700 | 1708 | Script for Acyclovir tablets given | | DH | |
| 25.08.2006 | 04.06.1958 | F | | 1708 | 1718 | Script for Prednisolone with Cinchocaine ointment & suppositories given | | JDC | |
| 25.08.2006 | 03.04.1920 | F | | 1734 | 1748 | Script for Atenolol given | | JA | |
| 25.08.2006 | 26.03.1958 | F | | 1748 | 1853 | She may need sick leave in view of her painful (L) ankle | | JLA | |
| 25.08.2006 | 09.03.1966 | M | | 1753 | 1803 | For FBC, Fasting Glucose, ESR & Fasting Cholesterol | | MS | |
| 25.08.2006 | 06.02.1968 | F | | 1803 | 1812 | Script for Citalopram given | | TW | |

Result of a query that lists all consultations from the 22nd to the end of August 2006 (ConsultationsSeenFrom22ndTillEndOfAug2006)

| SurgeryDate | DateOfBirth | Sex | Diagnosis | TimeIn | TimeOut | Complaints | Treatments | Initials | Notes |
|---|---|---|---|---|---|---|---|---|---|
| 25.08.2006 | 22.10.1976 | F | | 1812 | 1821 | For USScan of the upper abdomen | | HJE | |
| 29.08.2006 | 04.09.1958 | F | S/Leave | 941 | 948 | (R) foot operation | | LKW | Script for Dihydrocodeine given. |
| 29.08.2006 | 08.10.1938 | M | | 948 | 957 | Script for Ezetimibe given | | TAC | |
| 29.08.2006 | 01.10.1963 | M | | 957 | 1005 | Script for Miconazole with hydrocortisone & Amoxycillin given | | PDD | |
| 29.08.2006 | 01.09.1958 | F | S/Leave | 1005 | 1015 | Fractured (R) lower ribs | Otomize ear spray | RM | |
| 29.08.2006 | 13.09.1918 | M | | 1015 | 1030 | Script for Simvastatin given | | EJG | |
| 29.08.2006 | 25.05.1939 | F | RTI | 1030 | 1045 | Chesty cough & sticky eyes | Amoxycillin & Chloramphenicol eye drops | DET | |
| 29.08.2006 | 04.04.1953 | M | | 1045 | 1058 | Script for Ciprofloxacin, Co-phenotrope, Hyoscine butylbromide & Oral rehydration salts oral powder given | | GC | |
| 29.08.2006 | 06.11.1981 | F | | 1058 | 1104 | Burst condom | Levonorgestrel | CF | |
| 29.08.2006 | 25.09.1989 | M | | 1107 | 1115 | Script for Co-codamol & Ibuprofen given | | BDG | |

Result of a query that lists all consultations from the 22nd to the end of August 2006 (ConsultationsSeenFrom22ndTillEndOfAug2006)

| SurgeryDate | DateOfBirth | Sex | Diagnosis | TimeIn | TimeOut | Complaints | Treatments | Initials | Notes |
|---|---|---|---|---|---|---|---|---|---|
| 29.08.2006 | 25.06.2001 | M | | 1115 | 1128 | Mum to contact the child psychiatrist regarding ADHD problem | | JJP | |
| 29.08.2006 | 25.07.1942 | F | | 1128 | 1135 | Script for Dexamethasone given | | ICM | |
| 29.08.2006 | 16.11.1984 | F | | 1135 | 1148 | Routine ante-natal clinic check done | | ILH | Hypertensive, discussed with Gynae. Dr. on call, to Ward MB1, SGH. |
| 29.08.2006 | 14.12.1944 | F | | 1645 | 1654 | Script for Lisinopril given | | PEG | |
| 29.08.2006 | 30.05.1988 | M | S/Leave | 1654 | 1705 | (R) ankle injury - Med. 5 | | RLA | |
| 29.08.2006 | 24.11.1954 | F | | 1705 | 1710 | For repeat MSU | | HD | |
| 29.08.2006 | 22.07.1939 | F | | 1710 | 1717 | For X-Rays of the upper lip to exclude foreign body | | AP | |
| 29.08.2006 | 20.11.1988 | M | S/Leave | 1717 | 1726 | Stab wound to (L) thigh - Med. 5 | | CSB | |
| 29.08.2006 | 21.05.1953 | F | | 1726 | 1733 | Script for Erythromycin & Hyoscine butylbromide given | | CB | |
| 29.08.2006 | 13.12.1986 | F | | 1742 | 1749 | (L) ear ache | Amoxycillin | SAP | |

837

Result of a query that lists all consultations from the 22nd to the end of August 2006 (ConsultationsSeenFrom22ndTillEndOfAug2006)

| SurgeryDate | DateOfBirth | Sex | Diagnosis | TimeIn | TimeOut | Complaints | Treatments | Initials | Notes |
|---|---|---|---|---|---|---|---|---|---|
| 29.08.2006 | 30.09.1941 | M | | 1749 | 1758 | Script for Flucloxacillin & Co-codamol given | | DGC | |
| 29.08.2006 | 07.08.1972 | F | | 1802 | 1810 | Referred to ENT Surgeon regarding feeling of sound muffling in the ears | | SCB | |
| 29.08.2006 | 17.10.1998 | M | | 1810 | 1819 | Script for Amoxycillin given | | KRC | |
| 29.08.2006 | 25.04.1984 | F | | 1819 | 1827 | Script for Co-codamol given | | WDB | |
| 30.08.2006 | 05.01.1969 | F | | 946 | 958 | Routine ante-natal clinic check done | | NS | |
| 30.08.2006 | 18.09.1954 | F | | 958 | 1007 | For blood tests regarding her tiredness & bruising | | CAC | |
| 30.08.2006 | 05.04.1952 | M | S/Leave | 1007 | 1010 | Back Pain | | LFC | |
| 30.08.2006 | 15.04.1973 | F | | 1010 | 1019 | Script for Dianette, Flucloxacillin & Fusidic acid with hydrocortisone cream given | | LJB | |
| 30.08.2006 | 17.10.1933 | M | | 1019 | 1024 | Script for Olanzapine given | | FDF | |
| 30.08.2006 | 23.03.1926 | M | | 1033 | 1044 | To use own Quinine Sulphate for his leg cramp | | JWH | |
| 30.08.2006 | 17.03.1940 | F | | 1044 | 1050 | Script for Mebeverine given | | MER | |

Result of a query that lists all consultations from the 22nd to the end of August 2006 (ConsultationsSeenFrom22ndTillEndOfAug2006)

| SurgeryDate | DateOfBirth | Sex | Diagnosis | TimeIn | TimeOut | Complaints | Treatments | Initials | Notes |
|---|---|---|---|---|---|---|---|---|---|
| 30.08.2006 | 26.01.1959 | F | | 1055 | 1105 | Script for Dihydrocodeine given | | SAM | |
| 30.08.2006 | 13.11.1952 | F | | 1105 | 1111 | The injection to the coccyx | | LH | |
| 30.08.2006 | 15.01.1935 | F | | 1113 | 1127 | Script for Loratadine given | | JRS | |
| 30.08.2006 | 05.12.1956 | M | | 1650 | 1655 | Script for Ciprofloxacin given | | DTB | |
| 30.08.2006 | 08.12.1930 | M | | 1655 | 1705 | Script for Ciprofloxacin given | | FSR | |
| 30.08.2006 | 15.05.1937 | M | | 1705 | 1720 | Referred to Physiotherapy regarding his back pain | | JHR | |
| 30.08.2006 | 20.02.1937 | F | | 1720 | 1728 | Sinusitis | Amoxycillin | RFP | |
| 30.08.2006 | 08.12.1962 | F | | 1728 | 1741 | Script for Ciprofloxacin, Co-phenotrope & Hyoscine butylbromide given | | BJM | Stool for C&S. |
| 30.08.2006 | 28.02.1986 | F | S/Leave | 1741 | 1747 | Depression & Stressed | | JEM | Referred to Dermatologist regarding recurrent wounds on the neck. |
| 30.08.2006 | 24.11.1943 | M | | 1747 | 1757 | Script for Flucloxacillin & Fusidic acid cream given | | JTP | |

### Result of a query that lists all consultations from the 22nd to the end of August 2006 (ConsultationsSeenFrom22ndTillEndOfAug2006)

| SurgeryDate | DateOfBirth | Sex | Diagnosis | TimeIn | TimeOut | Complaints | Treatments | Initials | Notes |
|---|---|---|---|---|---|---|---|---|---|
| 30.08.2006 | 23.07.1919 | F | | 1757 | 1814 | Script for Enlive Plus, Ensure Plus & Vitamin bpc given | | KF | |
| 30.08.2006 | 16.07.1967 | F | | 1814 | 1825 | Script for Diclofenac e/c given | | MJN | Referred to Practice Counsellor. |
| 30.08.2006 | 26.04.1943 | M | RTI | 1825 | 1830 | Chesty cough | Erythromycin | WWH | Penicillin allergy. |
| 30.08.2006 | 22.04.1975 | F | | 1830 | 1838 | Script for Amoxycillin given | | SAG | |
| 30.08.2006 | 04.05.1937 | F | | 1838 | 1848 | Wound on the (R) leg | Flucloxacillin | DMB | |
| 30.08.2006 | 29.12.1930 | F | | 1848 | 1856 | Referred to Medical Dr. on call, SGH regarding possible (L) DVT | | AK | |

### Result of a query that lists all consultations from the 22nd to the end of August 2007 (ConsultationsSeenFrom22ndTillEndOfAug2007)

| SurgeryDate | DateOfBirth | Sex | Diagnosis | TimeIn | TimeOut | Complaints | Treatments | Initials | Notes |
|---|---|---|---|---|---|---|---|---|---|
| 22.08.2007 | 05.10.1960 | M | | 950 | 959 | Script for Acyclovir tablets given | | RCB | |
| 22.08.2007 | 08.05.1990 | F | | 1002 | 1019 | For MSU & for Pregnancy test | | SPK | |
| 22.08.2007 | 17.05.1935 | F | | 1019 | 1025 | Script for Chloramphenicol eye drops given | | CSS | |
| 22.08.2007 | 22.01.1932 | M | | 1025 | 1033 | Script for Quinine sulphate given | | RM | For CXR. |

Result of a query that lists all consultations from the 22nd to the end of August 2007 (ConsultationsSeenFrom22ndTillEndOfAug2007)

| SurgeryDate | DateOfBirth | Sex | Diagnosis | TimeIn | TimeOut | Complaints | Treatments | Initials | Notes |
|---|---|---|---|---|---|---|---|---|---|
| 22.08.2007 | 29.04.1935 | F | | 1033 | 1050 | For B12, FBC, Folate & Ferritin by the end of November | | CM | |
| 22.08.2007 | 11.12.1943 | F | | 1050 | 1112 | Script for Amoxycillin given | | PAH | |
| 22.08.2007 | 05.02.1946 | F | | 1112 | 1122 | Script for Flucloxacillin given | | ML | For FBC. |
| 22.08.2007 | 01.06.1947 | F | | 1122 | 1131 | Script for Diclofenac e/c, Dihydrocodeine & Omeprazole given | | VP | |
| 22.08.2007 | 16.07.1938 | F | | 1131 | 1142 | To take own Paracetamol for the pain in her (L) leg which is improving | | EG | |
| 22.08.2007 | 24.02.1981 | M | | 1142 | 1149 | Script for Flucloxacillin given | | PRB | |
| 22.08.2007 | 21.08.1934 | F | | 1643 | 1655 | Script for Trimethoprim given | | IEW | |
| 22.08.2007 | 11.12.1944 | F | | 1655 | 1703 | Script for Topiramate given | | GNW | |
| 22.08.2007 | 09.01.1949 | M | | 1703 | 1727 | Referred to Nephrologist regarding abnormal Creatinine levels | | DFH | |
| 22.08.2007 | 23.09.1951 | F | | 1727 | 1739 | For B12, Folate & Ferritin | | DJS | |

Result of a query that lists all consultations from the 22nd to the end of August 2007 (ConsultationsSeenFrom22ndTillEndOfAug2007)

| SurgeryDate | DateOfBirth | Sex | Diagnosis | TimeIn | TimeOut | Complaints | Treatments | Initials | Notes |
|---|---|---|---|---|---|---|---|---|---|
| 22.08.2007 | 15.02.1929 | F | | 1739 | 1751 | Referred to General Surgeon regarding sebaccous cyst on the back of her head | | NLA | For X-Ray of the (L) hip & Lumbar Spine. For MSU. |
| 22.08.2007 | 03.08.2005 | F | | 1751 | 1801 | Script for Loratadine & Calamine lotion given | | MEM | Referred to Dermatologist regarding worsening rash all over. |
| 22.08.2007 | 02.10.1943 | M | | 1801 | 1806 | Script for Flucloxacillin given | | SHS | |
| 22.08.2007 | 24.07.1952 | F | | 1806 | 1818 | Okay for her to have cryotherapy to skin tag on her neck | | JMM | |
| 22.08.2007 | 13.03.1944 | F | | 1818 | 1830 | Script for Simvastatin given | | BCO | |
| 22.08.2007 | 17.07.1956 | M | | 1830 | 1842 | Script for Amoxycillin, Prednisolone with Cinchocaine ointment & Prednisolone with Cinchocaine suppository given | | BR | |
| 23.08.2007 | 12.02.1959 | F | | 945 | 951 | Script for Diclofenac c/c given | | JEG | |
| 23.08.2007 | 23.05.1932 | M | | 951 | 1001 | For FBC, TFTs, U/Es & Fasting Glucose | | EB | |

Result of a query that lists all consultations from the 22nd to the end of August 2007 (ConsultationsSeenFrom22ndTillEndOfAug2007)

| SurgeryDate | DateOfBirth | Sex | Diagnosis | TimeIn | TimeOut | Complaints | Treatments | Initials | Notes |
|---|---|---|---|---|---|---|---|---|---|
| 23.08.2007 | 11.11.1934 | M | | 1005 | 1015 | Referred to Haematologist regarding elevated Lymphocyte count | | VRB | |
| 23.08.2007 | 07.05.1938 | F | | 1015 | 1025 | Script for Amoxycillin, Beclomethasone inhaler & Fusidic acid with hydrocortisone cream | | ILB | For CXR. |
| 23.08.2007 | 15.04.1927 | M | URTI | 1025 | 103 | (R) ear ache & discharge | Amoxycillin | JB | |
| 23.08.2007 | 28.10.1930 | F | | 1043 | 1053 | Script for Lisinopril given | | KBC | |
| 23.08.2007 | 20.12.1922 | F | | 1053 | 1101 | Script for Macrogol compound npf oral powder 13.8g given | | DEA | |
| 23.08.2007 | 27.03.1931 | F | | 1101 | 1108 | Script for Trimethoprim given | | MMA | For MSU. |
| 23.08.2007 | 27.03.1943 | F | | 1108 | 1117 | Script for Chloramphenicol eye drops given | | CFW | Referred to Dermatologist regarding mole on side of face. |
| 23.08.2007 | 07.11.1984 | F | | 1117 | 1123 | For Urine Pregnancy test | | LMW | |
| 23.08.2007 | 25.12.1942 | M | | 1123 | 1143 | Injection Depo-Medrone with Lidocaine given to the (L) heel | | RFL | |

Result of a query that lists all consultations from the 22nd to the end of August 2007 (ConsultationsSeenFrom22ndTillEndOfAug2007)

| SurgeryDate | DateOfBirth | Sex | Diagnosis | TimeIn | TimeOut | Complaints | Treatments | Initials | Notes |
|---|---|---|---|---|---|---|---|---|---|
| 23.08.2007 | 30.03.1923 | M | | 1405 | 1425 | Script for Fluoxetine given | | PH | Home visit. |
| 23.08.2007 | 14.01.1994 | F | | 1647 | 1659 | Script for Amoxycillin given | | GJG | |
| 23.08.2007 | 20.01.1941 | F | | 1653 | 1705 | Script for Co-codamol given | | BDD | |
| 23.08.2007 | 06.09.1961 | F | | 1705 | 1716 | For X-Rays of the (L) elbow | | TMF | |
| 23.08.2007 | 27.04.1925 | M | | 1716 | 1728 | For MSU | | RWF | |
| 23.08.2007 | 09.04.1975 | F | | 1731 | 1745 | Script for Prochlorperazine given | | SAE | |
| 23.08.2007 | 03.02.1968 | M | | 1745 | 1751 | Script for Sodium bicarbonate ear drops given | | MP | |
| 23.08.2007 | 13.05.1992 | F | | 1751 | 1758 | Referred to Dr. Gen regarding her painful knees | | ZLB | |
| 23.08.2007 | 13.01.1966 | M | | 1758 | 1806 | To see the nurse for monthly BP checks | | PJB | |
| 23.08.2007 | 14.01.1987 | F | | 1806 | 1812 | Script for Norethisterone given | | ECC | |
| 23.08.2007 | 19.12.1949 | M | | 1812 | 1823 | Script for Omeprazole given | | DJB | |
| 23.08.2007 | 13.07.1957 | M | | 1823 | 1831 | Script for Omeprazole & Diclofenac e/c given | | ARM | |

Result of a query that lists all consultations from the 22nd to the end of August 2007 (ConsultationsSeenFrom22ndTillEndOfAug2007)

| SurgeryDate | DateOfBirth | Sex | Diagnosis | TimeIn | TimeOut | Complaints | Treatments | Initials | Notes |
|---|---|---|---|---|---|---|---|---|---|
| 24.08.2007 | 26.09.1973 | F | | 929 | 936 | Referred to Dermatologist regarding rash all over the body except on the face | | SJS | |
| 24.08.2007 | 19.05.1981 | F | | 943 | 951 | Referred to Dermatologist regarding moles on her (R) upper arm | | LAC | Penicillin allergy. |
| 24.08.2007 | 28.03.1945 | M | | 951 | 959 | Script for Dihydrocodeine given | | APD | |
| 24.08.2007 | 14.04.2007 | M | | 1005 | 1015 | Referred to Rapid Access clinic, SGH regarding swollen (R) side of scrotum | | JJH | |
| 24.08.2007 | 01.04.1994 | F | RTI | 1015 | 1019 | Cough | Amoxycillin | KLB | |
| 24.08.2007 | 11.10.1992 | F | RTI | 1019 | 1023 | Cough | Amoxycillin | LRB | |
| 24.08.2007 | 02.11.1937 | F | | 1051 | 1104 | Script for Acyclovir, Co-codamol & Simvastatin given | | JMC | |
| 24.08.2007 | 20.04.1921 | F | | 1104 | 1113 | Referred to Dermatologist regarding lesion on her (L) temple | | ELH | |
| 24.08.2007 | 07.01.2007 | M | | 1118 | 1134 | Script for Clotrimazole with hydrocortisone cream given | | CHS | For USScan of the testicles/scrotum. |

Result of a query that lists all consultations from the 22nd to the end of August 2007 (ConsultationsSeenFrom22ndTillEndOfAug2007)

| SurgeryDate | DateOfBirth | Sex | Diagnosis | TimeIn | TimeOut | Complaints | Treatments | Initials | Notes |
|---|---|---|---|---|---|---|---|---|---|
| 24.08.2007 | 18.12.1968 | F | | 1134 | 1152 | For repeat MSU for fastidious organisms, FBC, U//Es, TFTs & Fasting Glucose | | DH | |
| 24.08.2007 | 28.11.2006 | F | | 1152 | 1157 | Cough | Amoxycillin | BC | |
| 28.08.2007 | 10.07.1962 | F | | 948 | 954 | She can stop the Norethisterone now that she has Mirena IUCD in situ | | PL | |
| 28.08.2007 | 24.12.1975 | M | | 954 | 957 | USScan of the testes showed a 4mm cyst, otherwise normal testes noted | | DWDS | |
| 28.08.2007 | 30.05.1955 | F | | 957 | 1003 | Script for Amoxycillin & Eflornithine cream given | | 42795 | |
| 28.08.2007 | 30.03.1962 | F | | 1006 | 1016 | Script for GTN spray given | | CW | |
| 28.08.2007 | 27.12.1959 | F | S/Leave | 1026 | 1048 | Hypertension | | KDI | Script for Lisinopril given. |
| 28.08.2007 | 13.12.1966 | M | | 1043 | 1051 | Script for Flucloxacillin given | | AL | |
| 28.08.2007 | 16.06.1915 | M | | 1051 | 1100 | Script for Flucloxacillin given | | LB | |
| 28.08.2007 | 24.03.1959 | M | S/Leave | 1103 | 1109 | Excess Alcohol Intake | | KMH | |
| 28.08.2007 | 07.11.1984 | F | | 1109 | 1115 | Urine Pregnancy test positive | | LMW | |

Result of a query that lists all consultations from the 22nd to the end of August 2007 (ConsultationsSeenFrom22ndTillEndOfAug2007)

| SurgeryDate | DateOfBirth | Sex | Diagnosis | TimeIn | TimeOut | Complaints | Treatments | Initials | Notes |
|---|---|---|---|---|---|---|---|---|---|
| 28.08.2007 | 04.05.1937 | F | | 1125 | 1139 | Referred to Dermatologist regarding redness & pain on her (R) leg | | DMB | |
| 28.08.2007 | 20.10.1983 | F | URTI | 1139 | 1147 | Sore throat | Amoxycillin | ARS | |
| 28.08.2007 | 28.07.1961 | F | | 1152 | 1205 | Script for Co-codamol given | | KTN | |
| 28.08.2007 | 16.10.1921 | F | | 1425 | 1440 | Script for Trimethoprim given | | EF | Home visit. |
| 28.08.2007 | 19.02.1975 | F | | 1645 | 1654 | To try OTC hypnotics in the first instance for her insomnia | | JIM | |
| 28.08.2007 | 21.09.1924 | F | | 1654 | 1704 | Her daughter stopped the anti-depressant as it was adversely affecting her | | GPM | Her daughter came to Surgery. |
| 28.08.2007 | 27.10.1966 | M | S/Leave | 1704 | 1711 | Flu symptoms & diarrhoea - Private | | DJW | |
| 28.08.2007 | 05.03.1994 | M | URTI | 1711 | 1717 | (L) ear ache | Erythromycin | JMW | |
| 28.08.2007 | 23.08.2001 | M | | 1717 | 1723 | Script for Hydrocortisone cream 0.05% given | | GAB | |
| 28.08.2007 | 02.05.1987 | F | | 1723 | 1733 | Referred to General Surgeon regarding possible removal of metal on her upper lip | | JT | |

847

Result of a query that lists all consultations from the 22$^{nd}$ to the end of August 2007 (ConsultationsSeenFrom22ndTillEndOfAug2007)

| SurgeryDate | DateOfBirth | Sex | Diagnosis | TimeIn | TimeOut | Complaints | Treatments | Initials | Notes |
|---|---|---|---|---|---|---|---|---|---|
| 28.08.2007 | 11.03.1968 | F | | 1741 | 1753 | To see nurse in 3 months for repeat TFTs & LFTs | | EJA | |
| 28.08.2007 | 29.01.1956 | M | S/Leave | 1753 | 1758 | Injury to the back - Med. 5 | | AJH | |
| 28.08.2007 | 04.02.1963 | F | S/Leave | 1813 | 1822 | Shingles - Med. 5 | | SAL | Script for Flucloxacillin given. |
| 29.08.2007 | 06.04.1924 | F | | 943 | 954 | For Urinalysis monthly for proteinuria with the nurse | | EAS | |
| 29.08.2007 | 05.06.1953 | F | | 954 | 1013 | BP 143/100 | | CAE | |
| 29.08.2007 | 11.03.1930 | F | | 1013 | 1026 | For Urinalysis monthly for proteinuria with the nurse | | DLP | Daughter came to Surgery. |
| 29.08.2007 | 26.01.1991 | M | | 1026 | 1046 | Repeat X-Rays form for Chest X-Rays & X-Rays of the (L) elbow given to the patient as he has mislaid the original form | | LTM | |
| 29.08.2007 | 09.04.1926 | M | | 1046 | 1056 | Script for Glandosane saliva oral spray given | | TS | |
| 29.08.2007 | 20.12.1931 | M | | 1056 | 1103 | For HbA1c | | FWR | |

Result of a query that lists all consultations from the 22nd to the end of August 2007 (ConsultationsSeenFrom22ndTillEndOfAug2007)

| SurgeryDate | DateOfBirth | Sex | Diagnosis | TimeIn | TimeOut | Complaints | Treatments | Initials | Notes |
|---|---|---|---|---|---|---|---|---|---|
| 29.08.2007 | 18.01.1939 | F | | 1103 | 1116 | Script for Levothyroxine & Simvastatin given | | FAB | |
| 29.08.2007 | 07.04.1921 | F | | 1116 | 1139 | BP 181/93 | | EDW | |
| 29.08.2007 | 24.06.1969 | M | | 1139 | 1201 | For HbA1c, cholesterol & LFTs | | DPM | |
| 29.08.2007 | 21.07.1919 | M | | 1201 | 1217 | His wife doesn't feel he needs Citalopram | | SEB | His wife came to the Surgery. |
| 29.08.2007 | 22.06.1921 | F | | 1217 | 1230 | For FBC, serum Ferritin, Folate & B12 | | FCH | |
| 29.08.2007 | 08.08.1918 | M | | 1230 | 1241 | For FBC, U/Es, TFTs, LFTs, BNP, Fasting Glucose, Fasting Cholesterol & CXR | | VHS | |
| 29.08.2007 | 03.12.1994 | F | | 1241 | 1302 | Script for Metoclopramide, oral rehydration salts oral powder & Paracetamol given | | NTN | |
| 29.08.2007 | 28.06.1956 | M | | 1645 | 1657 | Referred to ENT Surgeon regarding funny throat & voice change | | BGM | |
| 29.08.2007 | 08.12.1930 | M | | 1657 | 1707 | Script for Ciprofloxacin given | | FSR | |
| 29.08.2007 | 27.10.1931 | F | | 1707 | 1719 | She has gone back onto the Co-Amilofruse | | JEID | |

## Result of a query that lists all consultations from the 22nd to the end of August 2007 (ConsultationsSeenFrom22ndTillEndOfAug2007)

| SurgeryDate | DateOfBirth | Sex | Diagnosis | TimeIn | TimeOut | Complaints | Treatments | Initials | Notes |
|---|---|---|---|---|---|---|---|---|---|
| 29.08.2007 | 25.04.1935 | M | | 1719 | 1725 | He is due back in the Memory clinic in December | | KGB | |
| 29.08.2007 | 28.06.1959 | M | | 1725 | 1736 | BP 140/86 | | SCU | |
| 29.08.2007 | 24.03.1969 | M | | 1736 | 1749 | I explained to him that there is no reason why he cannot have steroid injection to his injured wrist area | | PO | |
| 29.08.2007 | 18.05.1952 | F | | 1749 | 1801 | Script for Evorel 50 patch given | | CAE | |
| 29.08.2007 | 15.11.1940 | F | URTI | 1801 | 1805 | Sore throat | Amoxycillin | | |
| 29.08.2007 | 25.08.1961 | F | | 1805 | 1813 | Script for Prochlorperazine & Trimethoprim given | | MFD | |
| 29.08.2007 | 18.12.2005 | M | | 1813 | 1818 | Mouth ulcers | Erythromycin | FM | |
| 29.08.2007 | 06.07.1936 | F | | 1818 | 1833 | Script for Coracten XL, Lisinopril & Prochlorperazine given | | MLW | |
| 29.08.2007 | 08.03.1964 | M | | 1833 | 1839 | Script for Flucloxacillin & Penicillin V given | | DDM | |
| 29.08.2007 | 21.04.1990 | M | URTI | 1839 | 1842 | (R) sore ear | Amoxycillin | BFC | |
| 30.08.2007 | 11.05.1962 | F | | 945 | 956 | Script for Lisinopril given | | JAB | For CXR. |
| 30.08.2007 | 30.12.1952 | F | | 956 | 1003 | For X-Rays of the (L) knee | | PBS | |

Result of a query that lists all consultations from the 22nd to the end of August 2007 (ConsultationsSeenFrom22ndTillEndOfAug2007)

| SurgeryDate | DateOfBirth | Sex | Diagnosis | TimeIn | TimeOut | Complaints | Treatments | Initials | Notes |
|---|---|---|---|---|---|---|---|---|---|
| 30.08.2007 | 16.07.1936 | F | | 1003 | 1009 | Phlebitis (L) leg | Flucloxacillin | EG | |
| 30.08.2007 | 06.10.1933 | M | | 1009 | 1021 | Script for Simvastatin given | | RJK | |
| 30.08.2007 | 16.07.1952 | F | | 1035 | 1044 | Script for Amitriptyline given | | KAM | Referred to Pain Management Consultant. |
| 30.08.2007 | 23.10.1941 | M | | 1044 | 1048 | He has abnormal BNP & enlarged heart on CXR for which he has appointment to be seen at the Heart & Chest clinic, SGH | | RJH | |
| 30.08.2007 | 21.06.1959 | M | | 1048 | 1054 | Script for Diclofenac e/c given | | SJW | |
| 30.08.2007 | 22.06.1983 | F | | 1054 | 1108 | Referred to Gynaecologist regarding PCO & dysfunctional uterine bleeding | | DIW | |
| 30.08.2007 | 19.06.1930 | F | | 1108 | 1115 | Script for Dihydrocodeine given | | RTA | |
| 30.08.2007 | 05.10.1969 | F | | 1118 | 1128 | Referred to Dermatologist regarding rash on arms & abdomen | | NJS | For blood test for antibodies to Herpes Zooster virus. |
| 30.08.2007 | 05.04.1964 | F | | 1128 | 1135 | Script for Fluoxetine given | | JL | |

## Result of a query that lists all consultations from the 22nd to the end of August 2007 (ConsultationsSeenFrom22ndTillEndOfAug2007)

| SurgeryDate | DateOfBirth | Sex | Diagnosis | TimeIn | TimeOut | Complaints | Treatments | Initials | Notes |
|---|---|---|---|---|---|---|---|---|---|
| 30.08.2007 | 11.05.1959 | F | | 1135 | 1141 | BP 111/76 | | LJE | |
| 30.08.2007 | 15.04.1927 | M | | 1141 | 1147 | Script for Sofradex ear drops given | | JB | |
| 30.08.2007 | 29.08.2007 | M | | 1405 | 1415 | Script for Co-Amoxiclav given | | VRH | Home visit. |
| 30.08.2007 | 03.10.1915 | F | | 1420 | 1432 | May need referral to Gastro-enterologist regarding her rectal bleeding if her children agree, which they did | | MG | Home visit. |
| 30.08.2007 | 13.12.1925 | M | | 1643 | 1650 | For Urinalysis monthly for proteinuria with the nurse | | GWF | |
| 30.08.2007 | 09.05.1937 | F | | 1650 | 1701 | She will contact the Neurologist's secretary to find out when she would next be seen | | KMN | |
| 30.08.2007 | 07.07.1992 | M | | 1701 | 1709 | Referred to Physiotherapist regarding his (L) painful & clicking shoulder | | MJP | |
| 30.08.2007 | 31.07.1945 | M | | 1709 | 1713 | Script for Erythromycin given | | TJS | Penicillin allergy. |
| 30.08.2007 | 24.07.1956 | M | | 1713 | 1727 | Script for Bendroflumethiazide & Lisinopril given | | SS | |

Result of a query that lists all consultations from the 22nd to the end of August 2007 (ConsultationsSeenFrom22ndTillEndOfAug2007)

| SurgeryDate | DateOfBirth | Sex | Diagnosis | TimeIn | TimeOut | Complaints | Treatments | Initials | Notes |
|---|---|---|---|---|---|---|---|---|---|
| 30.08.2007 | 27.04.1939 | F | | 1727 | 1733 | For LFTs | | DBS | |
| 30.08.2007 | 23.02.1940 | M | | 1738 | 1746 | Script for Omeprazole given | | BWH | |
| 30.08.2007 | 17.07.1956 | M | | 1751 | 1800 | BP 126/83 | | BR | |
| 30.08.2007 | 01.09.1983 | F | | 1800 | 1807 | Script for Amoxycillin given | | KLM | For MSU & FBC. Co-trimoxazole allergy. |
| 30.08.2007 | 06.11.1961 | F | | 1807 | 1812 | For FSH | | BSM | |
| 30.08.2007 | 01.09.1983 | M | | 1812 | 1818 | Private script for Viagra given | | LPCE | |

Result of a query that lists all consultations from the 22nd to the end of August 2008 (ConsultationsSeenFrom22ndTillEndOfAug2008)

| SurgeryDate | DateOfBirth | Sex | Diagnosis | TimeIn | TimeOut | Complaints | Treatments | Initials | Notes |
|---|---|---|---|---|---|---|---|---|---|
| 22.08.2008 | 21.05.1949 | M | | 924 | 929 | For LFTs | | JJH | |
| 22.08.2008 | 16.08.1927 | F | | 929 | 942 | Script for Simvastatin given | | EFM | |
| 22.08.2008 | 26.04.1944 | F | | 942 | 952 | For X-Rays of the (R) foot | | AW | |
| 22.08.2008 | 11.06.1950 | F | | 952 | 1000 | Referred to Orthopaedic Surgeon regarding marked osteo arthritic (L) knee | | ADB | |

853

Result of a query that lists all consultations from the 22nd to the end of August 2008 (ConsultationsSeenFrom22ndTillEndOfAug2008)

| SurgeryDate | DateOfBirth | Sex | Diagnosis | TimeIn | TimeOut | Complaints | Treatments | Initials | Notes |
|---|---|---|---|---|---|---|---|---|---|
| 22.08.2008 | 03.08.1935 | M | | 1000 | 1007 | Script for Injection Hydroxocobalamin given | | RH | For Pernicious anaemia screen. |
| 22.08.2008 | 20.04.1921 | F | | 1007 | 1020 | Medication Review Done | | ELH | |
| 22.08.2008 | 11.08.1962 | F | UTI | 1024 | 1030 | Dysuria | Trimethoprim | KRD | For MSU. |
| 22.08.2008 | 17.10.1928 | M | | 1036 | 1050 | Script for Ropinirole & Cetirizine given | | CDW | |
| 22.08.2008 | 26.01.1959 | F | | 1058 | 1108 | Script for Lisinopril given | | SAM | |
| 22.08.2008 | 30.12.1925 | M | | 1427 | 1442 | Script for Amoxycillin & Co-codamol given | | WHF | Home visit. |
| 26.08.2008 | 23.04.1923 | F | | 946 | 957 | Script for Otomize ear spray given | | JD | |
| 26.08.2008 | 15.08.1959 | M | S/Leave | 957 | 1005 | Back & Neck Pain | | SGS | |
| 26.08.2008 | 20.12.1943 | F | | 1007 | 1014 | Medication Review Done | | BAR | |
| 26.08.2008 | 08.04.1948 | M | | 1014 | 1029 | Referred to Urologist regarding persistent haematuria & (L) loin pain | | WRT | |
| 26.08.2008 | 31.10.1943 | M | | 1029 | 1040 | Referred to ENT Surgeon regarding bilateral deafness | | NFH | |
| 26.08.2008 | 06.04.1930 | M | | 1040 | 1047 | Medication Review Done | | JHS | |
| 26.08.2008 | 02.03.1969 | M | RTI | 1047 | 1053 | Chesty cough | Erythromycin | DAH | Penicillin allergy. |
| 26.08.2008 | 18.02.1968 | F | S/Leave | 1053 | 1058 | Chesty Infection | | PAC | |

854

## Result of a query that lists all consultations from the 22nd to the end of August 2008 (ConsultationsSeenFrom22ndTillEndOfAug2008)

| SurgeryDate | DateOfBirth | Sex | Diagnosis | TimeIn | TimeOut | Complaints | Treatments | Initials | Notes |
|---|---|---|---|---|---|---|---|---|---|
| 26.08.2008 | 20.10.1935 | F | | 1058 | 1105 | Script for Primidone given | | MM | |
| 26.08.2008 | 04.09.1963 | F | | 1103 | 1117 | Script for Ferrous Sulphate given | | AR | |
| 26.08.2008 | 19.06.1930 | F | | 1327 | 1353 | Referred to Neurologist regarding recurrent dysarthria & dysphonia | | RTA | Script for Lisinopril given. Home visit. |
| 26.08.2008 | 18.09.1989 | M | | 1649 | 1654 | Referred to Podiatrist regarding (R) in growing toe nail | | CH | |
| 26.08.2008 | 23.09.1951 | M | | 1654 | 1715 | He will come back later for his sickness certificate | | JWH | |
| 26.08.2008 | 13.04.1944 | M | UTI | 1715 | 1720 | Urine smells strong & cloudy | Ciprofloxacin | RAP | |
| 26.08.2008 | 16.06.1967 | M | | 1720 | 1726 | Script for Amoxycillin & Co-codamol | | PBK | |
| 26.08.2008 | 27.09.1987 | F | | 1726 | 1731 | For X-Rays of the (R) foot | | JTR | |
| 26.08.2008 | 21.09.1943 | M | | 1731 | 1735 | Script for Amoxycillin given | | TAG | |
| 26.08.2008 | 20.04.1945 | F | | 1735 | 1752 | Script for Prochlorperazine & Sibutramine given | | KCY | For letter to whom it may concern regarding getting bigger leg room in plane. For X-Rays of both knees. |

## Result of a query that lists all consultations from the 22nd to the end of August 2008 (ConsultationsSeenFrom22ndTillEndOfAug2008)

| SurgeryDate | DateOfBirth | Sex | Diagnosis | TimeIn | TimeOut | Complaints | Treatments | Initials | Notes |
|---|---|---|---|---|---|---|---|---|---|
| 26.08.2008 | 01.06.2007 | M | Rash | 1752 | 1757 | Impetigo rash on arm & behind the (L) ear | Flucloxacillin & Fusidic acid cream | AJH | |
| 26.08.2008 | 08.06.1974 | M | RTI | 1757 | 1802 | Chesty cough | Amoxycillin | SWM | |
| 26.08.2008 | 13.01.2001 | F | RTI | 1802 | 1805 | Chesty cough | Amoxycillin | RJM | |
| 27.08.2008 | 25.08.1961 | M | | 947 | 951 | She will come back later for the extension of her sick leave certificate | | MFD | |
| 27.08.2008 | 22.09.1967 | F | S/Leave | 951 | 1000 | Neck Pain - Med. 5 | | SG | |
| 27.08.2008 | 03.02.1970 | M | | 1000 | 1013 | Script for Olanzapine given | | DM | |
| 27.08.2008 | 22.07.1961 | M | | 1013 | 1019 | Script for Prochlorperazine given | | PWL | For FBC, Fasting Cholesterol & Fasting Glucose. |
| 27.08.2008 | 24.01.1958 | F | | 1025 | 1040 | Script for Fusidic acid with hydrocortisone cream given | | JDB | Referred to ENT Surgeon regarding lesion in the (L) ear lobe concha. |
| 27.08.2008 | 15.10.1937 | F | | 1040 | 1045 | Script for Salbutamol nebulising solution given | | GS | |
| 27.08.2008 | 09.10.1974 | F | | 1045 | 1055 | For MSU | | MJF | |
| 27.08.2008 | 07.05.1974 | M | | 1055 | 1102 | He will come back later for his sick leave | | SBK | |
| 27.08.2008 | 09.10.1924 | F | | 1102 | 1109 | Script for Amoxycillin & Co-codamol given | | VOM | |

Result of a query that lists all consultations from the 22nd to the end of August 2008 (ConsultationsSeenFrom22ndTillEndOfAug2008)

| SurgeryDate | DateOfBirth | Sex | Diagnosis | TimeIn | TimeOut | Complaints | Treatments | Initials | Notes |
|---|---|---|---|---|---|---|---|---|---|
| 27.08.2008 | 23.09.1951 | M | S/Leave | 1109 | 1136 | Irritable Bowel Syndrome - Med. 5 | | JWH | |
| 27.08.2008 | 07.02.1940 | F | | 1136 | 1155 | To use OTC Cryogesic to nail when she attends the Chiropodist | | MED | |
| 27.08.2008 | 16.04.1951 | F | Pain | 1159 | 1207 | (L) heel pain | Diclofenac e/c & Omeprazole | MM | |
| 27.08.2008 | 20.11.1923 | M | | 1645 | 1654 | To see the nurse twice monthly for urinalysis check for protein & for repeat U/Es in 6 weeks | | WEG | |
| 27.08.2008 | 23.09.1990 | F | | 1654 | 1701 | Referred to Dermatologist regarding her bead facial acne | | LET | |
| 27.08.2008 | 08.10.1981 | F | RTI | 1701 | 1708 | Chesty cough | Amoxycillin | SG | |
| 27.08.2008 | 28.06.1959 | M | | 1708 | 1716 | For repeat FBC & serum Ferritin by August 2009 | | SCU | |
| 27.08.2008 | 07.03.1955 | F | | 1721 | 1729 | Script for Lisinopril given | | DN | |
| 27.08.2008 | 18.06.1951 | M | | 1733 | 1741 | Script for Clonidine given | | AL | |
| 27.08.2008 | 27.10.1988 | F | | 1741 | 1749 | For Pregnancy test | | RC | |
| 27.08.2008 | 04.09.1958 | F | URTI | 1749 | 1754 | Sore throat | Amoxycillin | LKW | |

## Result of a query that lists all consultations from the 22nd to the end of August 2008 (ConsultationsSeenFrom22ndTillEndOfAug2008)

| SurgeryDate | DateOfBirth | Sex | Diagnosis | TimeIn | TimeOut | Complaints | Treatments | Initials | Notes |
|---|---|---|---|---|---|---|---|---|---|
| 27.08.2008 | 19.05.1969 | F | | 1754 | 1807 | Referred to Vascular Surgeon regarding her painful legs varicose veins | | LH | |
| 27.08.2008 | 28.02.1960 | F | | 1807 | 1824 | Referred to Breast Surgeon regarding bilateral breast pain | | JS | |
| 28.08.2008 | 02.06.1942 | M | | 944 | 954 | Script for Doxazosin given | | DBW | |
| 28.08.2008 | 13.08.1985 | M | | 954 | 1010 | Script for Fusidic acid cream given | | KJH | Referred to Practice Counsellor regarding being stressed. |
| 28.08.2008 | 23.05.1927 | M | | 1010 | 1018 | Paronychia (R) big toe | Erythromycin | JHM | Penicillin allergy. |
| 28.08.2008 | 16.03.1956 | F | | 1018 | 1024 | Advised to bathe her breast wounds with Savlon solution | | SPD | |
| 28.08.2008 | 12.11.1950 | M | | 1024 | 1030 | Referred to Dermatologist regarding his toe nails falling off | | MJP | |
| 28.08.2008 | 15.04.1956 | M | | 1030 | 1037 | Cellulitis (R) leg | Flucloxacillin | MAO | |
| 28.08.2008 | 21.07.1959 | F | | 1037 | 1044 | For X-Rays of the feet | | LMO | |
| 28.08.2008 | 06.07.1948 | M | | 1050 | 1056 | Referred to Dermatologist regarding spots on his (R) arm & (R) leg which are changing colour | | PAM | |

Result of a query that lists all consultations from the 22$^{nd}$ to the end of August 2008 (ConsultationsSeenFrom22ndTillEndOfAug2008)

| SurgeryDate | DateOfBirth | Sex | Diagnosis | TimeIn | TimeOut | Complaints | Treatments | Initials | Notes |
|---|---|---|---|---|---|---|---|---|---|
| 28.08.2008 | 09.10.1949 | M | | 1056 | 1104 | Referred to Audiology clinic regarding her bilateral deafness | | DS | |
| 28.08.2008 | 09.02.1969 | F | | 1111 | 1118 | Referred to ENT Surgeon regarding re-occurring feeling of something stuck in her throat for the past year | | OLB | |
| 28.08.2008 | 05.10.1988 | F | | 1648 | 1654 | For repeat Pregnancy test in 3 weeks | | SLR | |
| 28.08.2008 | 15.10.2007 | M | | 1654 | 1700 | Script for Calamine lotion & Paracetamol given | | BADR | |
| 28.08.2008 | 13.07.1946 | F | | 1700 | 1709 | To see the Dermatologist as arranged regarding her leg wound | | JFRH | |
| 28.08.2008 | 23.03.1926 | M | | 1709 | 1717 | Medication Review Done | | JWH | |
| 28.08.2008 | 29.11.1986 | M | | 1717 | 1724 | Script for Simvastatin given | | ALF | |
| 28.08.2008 | 21.08.1979 | F | | 1724 | 1730 | She is already taking folic acid as she is trying for a baby | | NAA | |
| 28.08.2008 | 14.10.1969 | F | | 1730 | 1739 | Referred to Practice Counsellor regarding feeling weepy & depressed | | LB | |

859

Result of a query that lists all consultations from the 22nd to the end of August 2008 (ConsultationsSeenFrom22ndTillEndOfAug2008)

| SurgeryDate | DateOfBirth | Sex | Diagnosis | TimeIn | TimeOut | Complaints | Treatments | Initials | Notes |
|---|---|---|---|---|---|---|---|---|---|
| 28.08.2008 | 25.11.1949 | M | | 1739 | 1749 | Script for Diclofenac e/c, Dihydrocodeine & Omeprazole given | | PVD | |
| 28.08.2008 | 04.10.1947 | F | | 1749 | 1755 | Script for Trimethoprim given | | CAG | For MSU. |
| 28.08.2008 | 11.02.1960 | F | | 1758 | 1804 | Referred to Dermatologist regarding spots on the back of her hand | | CAG | |
| 28.08.2008 | 30.04.1988 | F | | 1813 | 1829 | Referred to Gynaecologist regarding dyspareunia & secondary infertility | | ECJ | |
| 28.08.2008 | 18.10.1920 | F | | 1920 | 1930 | Script for Cefalexin given | | QK | Home visit. |
| 29.08.2008 | 03.08.1957 | F | | 934 | 947 | Script for Erythromycin given | | CK | For Chest X-Rays. |
| 29.08.2008 | 27.04.1928 | M | | 947 | 952 | For repeat U/Es | | RFV | |
| 29.08.2008 | 08.11.1941 | F | | 952 | 1010 | Script for Ezetimibe given | | PET | |
| 29.08.2008 | 25.02.1943 | F | Rash | 1010 | 1020 | Impetigo | Flucloxacillin & Fusidic acid cream | CB | |
| 29.08.2008 | 15.05.1937 | M | | 1020 | 1032 | The Parking Badge Scheme for Disabled People Medical Practitioner Report form completed with the patient | | JHR | |

Result of a query that lists all consultations from the 22nd to the end of August 2008 (ConsultationsSeenFrom22ndTillEndOfAug2008)

| SurgeryDate | DateOfBirth | Sex | Diagnosis | TimeIn | TimeOut | Complaints | Treatments | Initials | Notes |
|---|---|---|---|---|---|---|---|---|---|
| 29.08.2008 | 12.12.1959 | M | | 1032 | 1044 | Script for Co-codamol, Diclofenac e/c, Erythromycin & Omeprazole given | | RJW | Penicillin allergy. |
| 29.08.2008 | 16.08.1927 | F | | 1044 | 1052 | Referred to Rheumatologist regarding multiple joints pains | | EFM | Script for Quinine Sulphate & Cinchocaine with Hydrocortisone ointment given. |
| 29.08.2008 | 05.06.1935 | F | | 1052 | 1101 | Referred to Physiotherapist regarding upper back pain | | PCB | Script for Diclofenac e/c & Omeprazole given. |
| 29.08.2008 | 20.04.1929 | F | | 1101 | 1109 | Referred to DVT Clinic regarding possible (L) leg DVT | | JMG | |
| 29.08.2008 | 05.02.1960 | F | | 1109 | 1120 | Script for Amoxycillin, Dihydrocodeine & Erythromycin given | | SJW | |
| 29.08.2008 | 31.05.1997 | F | | 1120 | 1128 | Referred to Dermatologist regarding itchy dry lesion on her (R) arm | | SC | |
| 29.08.2008 | 17.05.1943 | M | | 1128 | 1138 | Constipation | Movicol | PJC | |
| 29.08.2008 | 26.02.1973 | M | | 1138 | 1153 | Referred to Practice Counsellor regarding being unable to cope | | ADC | Script for Citalopram given. |

## Result of a query that lists all consultations from the 22nd to the end of August 2008 (ConsultationsSeenFrom22ndTillEndOfAug2008)

| SurgeryDate | DateOfBirth | Sex | Diagnosis | TimeIn | TimeOut | Complaints | Treatments | Initials | Notes |
|---|---|---|---|---|---|---|---|---|---|
| 29.08.2008 | 20.04.1921 | F | | 1153 | 1203 | Referred to ENT Surgeon regarding gruff voice with weight loss | | ELH | Script for Ensure Plus given. |
| 29.08.2008 | 23.09.1951 | F | | 1256 | 1301 | Infected insect bite on the (L) hand | Flucloxacillin | DJS | |
| 29.08.2008 | 11.01.1964 | F | | 1441 | 1453 | Script for Amitriptyline & Diclofenac given | | TJR | |

## Result of a query that lists all consultations from the 22nd to the end of August 2009 (ConsultationsSeenFrom22ndTillEndOfAug2009)

| SurgeryDate | DateOfBirth | Sex | Diagnosis | TimeIn | TimeOut | Complaints | Treatments | Initials | Notes |
|---|---|---|---|---|---|---|---|---|---|
| 24.08.2009 | 22.03.1933 | F | | 944 | 1000 | Script for Bendroflumethiazide given | | LLW | |
| 24.08.2009 | 20.03.1945 | M | | 1000 | 1007 | Referred to Dermatologist regarding a possible BCC on the (L) temple region | | MPC | |
| 24.08.2009 | 20.01.1941 | F | | 1007 | 1015 | Referred to Orthopaedic Surgeon regarding possible (R) carpal tunnel syndrome | | BDD | Script for Erythromycin given. |

Result of a query that lists all consultations from the 22nd to the end of August 2009 (ConsultationsSeenFrom22ndTillEndOfAug2009)

| SurgeryDate | DateOfBirth | Sex | Diagnosis | TimeIn | TimeOut | Complaints | Treatments | Initials | Notes |
|---|---|---|---|---|---|---|---|---|---|
| 24.08.2009 | 02.12.1995 | F | URTI | 1015 | 1022 | (L) ear ache | Amoxycillin | JAM | Script for Clobetasol scalp solution given. |
| 24.08.2009 | 10.08.1985 | F | | 1022 | 1031 | Urine Pregnancy test positive | | HNN | |
| 24.08.2009 | 25.01.1939 | F | | 1031 | 1044 | The Captopril was recently stopped by the Cardiologist | | PMC | |
| 24.08.2009 | 12.11.1944 | F | | 1048 | 1057 | Infected insect bit on both thighs | Flucloxacillin | PM | For FBC, U/Es, LFTs & Fasting cholesterol. |
| 24.08.2009 | 21.08.1934 | F | | 1057 | 1106 | Nausea & Epigastric pain | Metoclopramide & Omeprazole | IEW | |
| 24.08.2009 | 06.10.1952 | M | | 1106 | 1119 | Script for Co-codamol & Nafridrofuryl given | | CJG | |
| 24.08.2009 | 07.04.1966 | M | | 1119 | 1134 | Script for Amoxycillin given | | SG | |
| 24.08.2009 | 20.02.1932 | M | | 1134 | 1141 | Script for Co-codamol given | | KDC | For X-Rays of the (L) knee. |
| 24.08.2009 | 11.09.1947 | M | | 1642 | 1700 | Referred to Orthopaedic Surgeon (BUPA) regarding his back pain | | TSN | Script for Tramadol capsules given. |
| 24.08.2009 | 20.10.1953 | M | | 1700 | 1710 | Referred to Dermatologist regarding the darkish mole on his (R) lower back | | PJH | Referred to General Surgeon regarding the cyst on his head. |

Result of a query that lists all consultations from the 22nd to the end of August 2009 (ConsultationsSeenFrom22ndTillEndOfAug2009)

| SurgeryDate | DateOfBirth | Sex | Diagnosis | TimeIn | TimeOut | Complaints | Treatments | Initials | Notes |
|---|---|---|---|---|---|---|---|---|---|
| 24.08.2009 | 30.05.1964 | M | | 1710 | 1724 | | | ED | Referred to General Surgeon regarding possible lipoma in the epigastric region. Script for Omeprazole given. |
| 24.08.2009 | 19.04.1996 | M | | 1724 | 1737 | Referred to Counsellor regarding difficulty coping with his wife and children | | SAM | |
| 24.08.2009 | 20.08.1939 | F | | 1737 | 1745 | Referred to Paediatrician regarding possible autism or ADHD development | | SLT | |
| 24.08.2009 | 28.08.1946 | F | | 1745 | 1757 | Script for Bendroflumethiazide & Prochlorperazine given | | MPB | |
| 24.08.2009 | 09.02.1969 | F | | 1757 | 1804 | Script for Fusidic acid cream & Miconazole/ Hydrocortisone cream given | | OLB | |
| 24.08.2009 | 03.03.1984 | M | | 1804 | 1809 | Script for Ferrous Sulphate given | | PWK | |
| 25.08.2009 | 16.08.1981 | M | S/Leave | 945 | 957 | Script for Omeprazole given | | REH | |
| 25.08.2009 | 23.02.1940 | M | | 957 | 1013 | Operation on the (R) shoulder | | BWH | |
| 25.08.2009 | 08.10.1950 | F | | 1013 | 1022 | Referred to DVT clinic regarding swollen (R) calf | | CAH | |
| | | | | | | Script for Diazepam given | | | |

864

Result of a query that lists all consultations from the 22nd to the end of August 2009 (ConsultationsSeenFrom22ndTillEndOfAug2009)

| SurgeryDate | DateOfBirth | Sex | Diagnosis | TimeIn | TimeOut | Complaints | Treatments | Initials | Notes |
|---|---|---|---|---|---|---|---|---|---|
| 25.08.2009 | 02.06.1936 | M | URTI | 1022 | 1029 | Feels congested | Amoxycillin | AJG | |
| 25.08.2009 | 25.04.1951 | F | S/Leave | 1032 | 1048 | Headaches & Diarrhoea - Med. 5 | | SM | |
| 25.08.2009 | 04.09.1952 | M | | 1048 | 1106 | For PSA | | DJB | |
| 25.08.2009 | 25.09.1968 | F | | 1106 | 1124 | Script for Lisinopril give | | JAF | |
| 25.08.2009 | 03.05.1996 | F | | 1124 | 1130 | Referred to Dermatologist (urgent) regarding darkish mole on (R) buttock area | | EMH | |
| 25.08.2009 | 17.06.1960 | F | | 1130 | 1143 | Holiday cancellation form partially completed, to be fully completed | | RT | |
| 25.08.2009 | 18.01.1958 | F | | 1143 | 1149 | Script for Amoxycillin given | | LRG | |
| 25.08.2009 | 12.01.1992 | F | | 1644 | 1652 | Script for Omeprazole given | | SAL | |
| 25.08.2009 | 20.02.1930 | M | | 1652 | 1702 | For B12, Folate, Ferritin & Fasting Glucose | | AL | |
| 25.08.2009 | 03.08.1935 | M | | 1706 | 1712 | For Folate & serum Ferritin | | RH | |
| 25.08.2009 | 06.01.1941 | F | | 1712 | 1724 | For X-Rays of the (R) wrist | | JRM | |

865

Result of a query that lists all consultations from the 22nd to the end of August 2009 (ConsultationsSeenFrom22ndTillEndOfAug2009)

| SurgeryDate | DateOfBirth | Sex | Diagnosis | TimeIn | TimeOut | Complaints | Treatments | Initials | Notes |
|---|---|---|---|---|---|---|---|---|---|
| 25.08.2009 | 09.12.1945 | F | | 1724 | 1732 | Referred to Dermatologist regarding mole on the (L) cheek | | AML | |
| 25.08.2009 | 06.11.1990 | M | | 1740 | 1748 | Script for Hyoscine transdermal patch given | | MJEL | |
| 25.08.2009 | 07.07.1961 | F | RTI | 1759 | 1809 | Chesty cough | Erythromycin | SSA | Penicillin allergy. |
| 25.08.2009 | 27.05.1978 | M | URTI | 1824 | 1830 | Sore throat | Amoxycillin | TRS | |
| 26.08.2009 | 15.07.1955 | F | | 946 | 957 | Script for Irbesartan given | | JDU | |
| 26.08.2009 | 30.09.1925 | M | | 957 | 1004 | Script for Macrogol compound half-strength oral powder given | | JCA | Penicillin allergy. |
| 26.08.2009 | 05.12.1973 | F | | 1011 | 1020 | To do a repeat home pregnancy test in 3 to 4 weeks | | VNB | |
| 26.08.2009 | 27.08.1952 | F | | 1020 | 1049 | Medical Review Done | | KLB | |
| 26.08.2009 | 28.08.1994 | F | | 1049 | 1058 | For X-Rays of the (L) knee (urgent) | | GJH | |
| 26.08.2009 | 02.10.1992 | M | | 1058 | 1109 | Medical Review Done | | LF | |
| 26.08.2009 | 15.01.1942 | M | | 1109 | 1112 | Private script for Cialis 20mg given | | SJF | |
| 26.08.2009 | 18.05.1952 | F | | 1645 | 1702 | Script for Dixarit given | | CAE | For DEXA Scan. |
| 26.08.2009 | 08.04.1948 | M | | 1702 | 1716 | Medical Review Done | | WRT | |
| 26.08.2009 | 26.08.1982 | M | | 1716 | 1730 | BP 135/85 | | BLS | |
| 26.08.2009 | 28.06.1991 | F | URTI | 1730 | 1737 | Sore throat | Amoxycillin | LC | |

Result of a query that lists all consultations from the 22nd to the end of August 2009 (ConsultationsSeenFrom22ndTillEndOfAug2009)

| SurgeryDate | DateOfBirth | Sex | Diagnosis | TimeIn | TimeOut | Complaints | Treatments | Initials | Notes |
|---|---|---|---|---|---|---|---|---|---|
| 26.08.2009 | 15.01.1980 | M | | 1747 | 1808 | Referred to Cardiologist regarding regular ECGs as he is a carrier for Myotonic dystrophy | | NJCL | For Chest X-Rays. |
| 27.08.2009 | 06.07.1948 | M | | 947 | 1000 | Referred to Psychiatrist regarding being very tormented with stress | | PAM | |
| 27.08.2009 | 06.06.1947 | F | | 1000 | 1007 | Referred to Orthopaedic Surgeon regarding pain in the (R) Achilles tendon & pain in the (L) knee | | MM | |
| 27.08.2009 | 30.09.1961 | F | | 1007 | 1020 | Referred to Podiatrist regarding pain in her outer (R) 3 toes | | TJB | Script for Dihydrocodeine given |
| 27.08.2009 | 23.05.1932 | M | | 1022 | 1044 | Referred to Physiotherapist regarding back pain | | EB | Script for Tramadol m/r given |
| 27.08.2009 | 23.07.1943 | F | | 1044 | 1056 | Medication Review Done | | JFA | |
| 27.08.2009 | 02.08.1931 | M | | 1056 | 1107 | Inj. Zoladex 10.8mg implant given sc | | PEW | |
| 27.08.2009 | 30.03.1923 | M | | 1107 | 1116 | Inj. Zoladex 10.8mg implant given sc | | PGH | |
| 27.08.2009 | 07.10.1933 | M | | 1116 | 1130 | For serum Ferritin, Folate & B12 | | FDF | |

## Result of a query that lists all consultations from the 22nd to the end of August 2009 (ConsultationsSeenFrom22ndTillEndOfAug2009)

| SurgeryDate | DateOfBirth | Sex | Diagnosis | TimeIn | TimeOut | Complaints | Treatments | Initials | Notes |
|---|---|---|---|---|---|---|---|---|---|
| 27.08.2009 | 28.03.1985 | F | | 1235 | 1245 | Routine post-natal check done | | LEB | |
| 27.08.2009 | 25.11.1943 | M | | 1646 | 1702 | For Modified GTT | | AES | |
| 27.08.2009 | 05.06.1960 | M | | 1702 | 1711 | Referred to Cardiologist regarding pain that goes down his (L) arm & up into his jaw | | GWP | |
| 27.08.2009 | 15.07.1936 | F | | 1711 | 1726 | Referred to Orthopaedic Surgeon regarding her upper back pain | | TRL | |
| 27.08.2009 | 03.07.1950 | F | | 1726 | 1732 | Referred to Orthopaedic Surgeon regarding lump on her (R) thigh | | YC | |
| 27.08.2009 | 21.10.1982 | M | Rash | 1732 | 1736 | Pityriasis versicolor | Ketoconazole cream | JLW | |
| 27.08.2009 | 21.09.1947 | M | | 1736 | 1750 | Script for Macrogol compound half-strength oral powder sachets given | | DL | |
| 27.08.2009 | 13.09.1918 | M | | 1750 | 1804 | Script for Furosemide given | | EJG | |
| 27.08.2009 | 02.08.1956 | M | | 1804 | 1810 | For repeat U/Es & serum cholesterol in 3 to 6 months with the nurse | | KRC | |

Result of a query that lists all consultations from the 22nd to the end of August 2009 (ConsultationsSeenFrom22ndTillEndOfAug2009)

| SurgeryDate | DateOfBirth | Sex | Diagnosis | TimeIn | TimeOut | Complaints | Treatments | Initials | Notes |
|---|---|---|---|---|---|---|---|---|---|
| 27.08.2009 | 24.04.1950 | M | | 1810 | 1820 | He will speak to the cancer specialist nurse about having genetics test | | IGH | |
| 28.08.2009 | 04.07.1961 | F | S/Leave | 931 | 939 | Depression | | JB | |
| 28.08.2009 | 18.07.1956 | F | S/Leave | 939 | 947 | Fractured (R) Humerus | | MTC | |
| 28.08.2009 | 22.04.1951 | M | S/Leave | 949 | 956 | Injury to the (R) knee | | PJT | |
| 28.08.2009 | 20.10.1983 | F | S/Leave | 958 | 1007 | Generalised itching | | ARS | |
| 28.08.2009 | 01.06.1947 | F | | 1007 | 1019 | Script for Atorvastatin & Conjugated Oestrogens vaginal cream given | | VP | |
| 28.08.2009 | 05.07.1931 | F | | 1019 | 1028 | Script for Omeprazole given | | AVD | |
| 28.08.2009 | 19.01.1940 | F | | 1028 | 1039 | Script for Fusidic acid with Hydrocortisone cream given | | VS | |
| 28.08.2009 | 28.07.1939 | F | | 1040 | 1100 | Restless legs | Ropinirole | RMM | Script for Lactulose given. Referred to Podiatrist regarding blister on (R) foot & redness on the toes. |
| 28.08.2009 | 08.02.1939 | F | URTI | 1100 | 1110 | Sore throat | Amoxycillin | IB | Referred to Physiotherapist regarding her back pain. |

Result of a query that lists all consultations from the 22nd to the end of August 2009 (ConsultationsSeenFrom22ndTillEndOfAug2009)

| SurgeryDate | DateOfBirth | Sex | Diagnosis | TimeIn | TimeOut | Complaints | Treatments | Initials | Notes |
|---|---|---|---|---|---|---|---|---|---|
| 28.08.2009 | 09.10.1926 | M | | 1110 | 1123 | Script for Trimethoprim given | | RAC | For USScan of the testicles. |
| 28.08.2009 | 09.05.1955 | M | URTI | 1123 | 1127 | Sore throat | Amoxycillin | SL | |
| 28.08.2009 | 05.11.1926 | F | | 1127 | 1135 | Septic insect bite on (L) leg | Flucloxacillin | JJ | |
| 28.08.2009 | 21.07.1923 | M | RTI | 1319 | 1348 | Chesty cough | Cefalexin | RU | |

Result of a query that lists all consultations from the 22nd to the end of August 2010 (ConsultationsSeenFrom22ndTillEndOfAug2010)

| SurgeryDate | DateOfBirth | Sex | Diagnosis | TimeIn | TimeOut | Complaints | Treatments | Initials | Notes |
|---|---|---|---|---|---|---|---|---|---|
| 23.08.2010 | 18.02.1968 | F | S/Leave | 945 | 954 | Med. 3 04/10 given for Abdominal Wound Infection from 22.08.10 until 23.08.10 | | PAC | |
| 23.08.2010 | 10.04.1971 | F | | 954 | 959 | to come back for medications recommended by Neurologist for her migraine if required | | KS | |
| 23.08.2010 | 27.05.1941 | F | | 1000 | 1007 | Script for Clobetasol ointment & Dihydrocodeine given | | MDR | |
| 23.08.2010 | 24.10.1946 | F | | 1007 | 1018 | Medication Review Done | | MW | |

Result of a query that lists all consultations from the 22nd to the end of August 2010 (ConsultationsSeenFrom22ndTillEndOfAug2010)

| SurgeryDate | DateOfBirth | Sex | Diagnosis | TimeIn | TimeOut | Complaints | Treatments | Initials | Notes |
|---|---|---|---|---|---|---|---|---|---|
| 23.08.2010 | 03.04.1944 | M | | 1018 | 1024 | Referred to ENT Surgeon regarding recurrent smelly discharge from the (L) ear | | DJW | |
| 23.08.2010 | 31.01.2006 | M | | 1024 | 1034 | Referred to Paediatrician regarding being very hyperactive & not sleeping at night | | HEWD | |
| 23.08.2010 | 12.12.1934 | F | | 1034 | 1040 | Referred to Breast Surgeon (One Stop Breast Clinic) regarding noticing that the (L) breast is bigger that the right one | | SDH | |
| 23.08.2010 | 01.07.1966 | M | | 1058 | 1110 | Referred to Physiotherapist regarding tingling with pins & needles across his lower back | | KFA | |
| 23.08.2010 | 21.04.1949 | M | | 1110 | 1118 | Referred for Colonoscopy regarding recurrent diarrhoea & rectal bleeding | | RL | |

871

Result of a query that lists all consultations from the 22nd to the end of August 2010 (ConsultationsSeenFrom22ndTillEndOFAug2010)

| SurgeryDate | DateOfBirth | Sex | Diagnosis | TimeIn | TimeOut | Complaints | Treatments | Initials | Notes |
|---|---|---|---|---|---|---|---|---|---|
| 23.08.2010 | 10.08.1950 | M | | 1648 | 1656 | Referred to Vascular Surgeon regarding varicose veins, ache & swelling in the (L) leg | | JD | |
| 23.08.2010 | 07.10.1933 | M | | 1656 | 1700 | Script for Ferrous Sulphate given | | FDF | |
| 23.08.2010 | 06.10.1952 | M | | 1700 | 1710 | Script for Hydrocortisone with Fusidic acid cream given | | CJG | |
| 23.08.2010 | 19.02.1942 | F | | 1710 | 1725 | Referred to Haematologist regarding her elevated Paraproteinemia | | EF | Script for Ferrous Sulphate given. |
| 23.08.2010 | 28.06.1956 | M | | 1725 | 1733 | Referred for Gastroscopy regarding his abdominal pain & indigestion | | BGM | |
| 23.08.2010 | 27.02.1945 | M | | 1733 | 1745 | For MSU, FBC, U/Es, Fasting Glucose & PSA | | GFS | |
| 23.08.2010 | 09.02.1956 | M | | 1745 | 1756 | Script for Co-Amoxiclav given | | TH | |
| 23.08.2010 | 20.10.1983 | F | | 1756 | 1802 | Script for Amoxycillin & Prednisolone e/c given | | ARS | |

Result of a query that lists all consultations from the 22nd to the end of August 2010 (ConsultationsSeenFrom22ndTillEndOfAug2010)

| SurgeryDate | DateOfBirth | Sex | Diagnosis | TimeIn | TimeOut | Complaints | Treatments | Initials | Notes |
|---|---|---|---|---|---|---|---|---|---|
| 23.08.2010 | 04.07.1986 | F | S/Leave | 1807 | 1814 | Med. 3 04/10 given for Diarrhoea & Vomiting from 23.08.10 until 25.08.10 | | CA | |
| 24.08.2010 | 08.04.1945 | M | | 945 | 954 | Medication Review Done | | GTW | |
| 24.08.2010 | 10.04.1937 | F | | 954 | 1019 | Medication Review Done | | MC | |
| 24.08.2010 | 31.05.1930 | F | | 1019 | 1028 | Script for Co-codamol & Erythromycin given | | SAW | For Cervical Spine X-Rays. Penicillin allergy. |
| 24.08.2010 | 23.08.1925 | F | | 1028 | 1051 | Referred to Chest Physician as suggested by Cardiologist in view of her worsening breathlessness | | REP | The Blue Badge Parking Scheme of Parking Concessions for Disabled and Blind Medical Practitioner Report form ECC1190 (ESS208B) completed with the patient in the Surgery. |
| 24.08.2010 | 13.07.2008 | M | Conjunctivitis | 1051 | 1054 | Bilateral sticky eyes | Chloramphenicol eye drops | MJD | |
| 24.08.2010 | 28.10.1930 | F | | 1054 | 1059 | Referred to Ophthalmologist regarding cyst in her (L) upper eye lid | | KBC | |

## Result of a query that lists all consultations from the 22nd to the end of August 2010 (ConsultationsSeenFrom22ndTillEndOfAug2010)

| SurgeryDate | DateOfBirth | Sex | Diagnosis | TimeIn | TimeOut | Complaints | Treatments | Initials | Notes |
|---|---|---|---|---|---|---|---|---|---|
| 24.08.2010 | 02.07.1926 | M | | 1059 | 1107 | For MSU | | BLB | |
| 24.08.2010 | 01.09.1946 | M | | 1107 | 1115 | Referred for Sigmoidoscopy regarding his persistent soft stools which is unusual for him | | PAH | |
| 24.08.2010 | 23.10.1929 | F | | 1115 | 1127 | Referred to Audiology Clinic regarding her worsening deafness | | MOL | |
| 24.08.2010 | 03.04.1918 | F | | 1318 | 1342 | Script for Amoxycillin & Oramorph given | | JMR | Home visit. |
| 24.08.2010 | 21.09.1919 | M | | 1650 | 1700 | Script for Ferrous Sulphate & Gaviscon Advance given | | VB | His Daughter in law came in to the Surgery. |
| 24.08.2010 | 09.10.1926 | M | | 1700 | 1714 | Script for Metformin given | | RAC | |
| 24.08.2010 | 17.04.1940 | F | | 1714 | 1724 | Script for Simvastatin given | | JAB | |
| 24.08.2010 | 26.03.1935 | F | | 1724 | 1736 | Script for Flucloxacillin given | | JJ | For U/Es. |
| 24.08.2010 | 27.09.1931 | M | | 1736 | 1745 | Script for Flucloxacillin given | | TJN | For X-Rays of the knees. |
| 24.08.2010 | 02.12.1992 | M | | 1745 | 1750 | Referred to Dermatologist regarding his worsening facial acne | | TJN | |
| 24.08.2010 | 11.03.1944 | M | Pain | 1750 | 1756 | Pain in the (L) leg | Diclofenac e/c & Dihydrocodeine | KRW | |

Result of a query that lists all consultations from the 22nd to the end of August 2010 (ConsultationsSeenFrom22ndTillEndOfAug2010)

| SurgeryDate | DateOfBirth | Sex | Diagnosis | TimeIn | TimeOut | Complaints | Treatments | Initials | Notes |
|---|---|---|---|---|---|---|---|---|---|
| 24.08.2010 | 26.02.1960 | F | | 1801 | 1813 | Script for Erythromycin, Otomize ear spray, Prochlorperazine & Dixarit given | | JS | |
| 24.08.2010 | 14.11.1963 | F | S/Leave | 1823 | 1837 | Med. 3 04/10 given for Voice Hoarseness & Dysphagia for 3 months from 24.08.10 | | SJK | |
| 24.08.2010 | 29.07.1947 | F | | 1318 | 1342 | Medication Review Done | | KM | |
| 25.08.2010 | 22.04.1951 | M | S/Leave | 946 | 955 | Med. 3 04/10 given for Injury to the (R) knee from 25.08.10 for 3 months | | PJT | |
| 25.08.2010 | 08.10.1969 | F | | 957 | 1021 | Script for Citalopram given | | DMDM | |
| 25.08.2010 | 09.03.1947 | F | | 1021 | 1030 | Referred to ENT Surgeon (BUPA) regarding mole on the (R) ear lobe | | PAN | |
| 25.08.2010 | 27.03.1940 | F | | 1030 | 1035 | For X-Rays of the hips & of the Cervical spine | | MAN | |
| 25.08.2010 | 14.06.1945 | M | | 1035 | 1040 | Script for Ferrous sulphate given | | BL | |
| 25.08.2010 | 16.03.1978 | M | | 1045 | 1056 | Referred for Vasectomy | | JWPS | |

Result of a query that lists all consultations from the 22nd to the end of August 2010 (ConsultationsSeenFrom22ndTillEndOfAug2010)

| SurgeryDate | DateOfBirth | Sex | Diagnosis | TimeIn | TimeOut | Complaints | Treatments | Initials | Notes |
|---|---|---|---|---|---|---|---|---|---|
| 25.08.2010 | 05.01.1984 | M | | 1056 | 1116 | Script for Fucidin 2% ointment given | | AGTN | |
| 25.08.2010 | 20.11.1991 | F | S/Leave | 1116 | 1126 | Med. 3 04/10 given for Sore Throat from 25.08.10 until 26.08.10 | | BS | |
| 25.08.2010 | 23.07.1953 | M | | 1126 | 1136 | Referred to Physiotherapist regarding neck pain | | THM | |
| 25.08.2010 | 01.03.1934 | F | | 1335 | 1345 | Script for Erythromycin given | | BLR | Penicillin allergy. Home visit. |
| 25.08.2010 | 06.08.1921 | F | | 1646 | 1657 | Script for Salbutamol inhaler given | | EE | |
| 25.08.2010 | 04.03.1982 | F | | 1705 | 1715 | Script for Flucloxacillin given | | GV | |
| 25.08.2010 | 13.04.1944 | M | | 1715 | 1723 | Medication Review Done | | RAP | |
| 25.08.2010 | 27.05.1978 | M | | 1728 | 1735 | Script for Flucloxacillin given | | TRS | For FBC, U/Es & Fasting Glucose. |
| 25.08.2010 | 29.04.1984 | M | | 1735 | 1738 | Advised to still keep the Urologist appointment even though the penile cyst has busted | | PAB | |
| 25.08.2010 | 21.01.1960 | F | | 1741 | 1751 | Referred to Chest Physician regarding her breathlessness on exertion | | SBW | For serum Ferritin, B12 & Folate. |

876

Result of a query that lists all consultations from the 22nd to the end of August 2010 (ConsultationsSeenFrom22ndTillEndOfAug2010)

| SurgeryDate | DateOfBirth | Sex | Diagnosis | TimeIn | TimeOut | Complaints | Treatments | Initials | Notes |
|---|---|---|---|---|---|---|---|---|---|
| 25.08.2010 | 22.01.1937 | M | | 1751 | 1758 | Script for Macrogol compound half-strength oral powder sachets NPF given | | AM | |
| 26.08.2010 | 22.07.1939 | F | | 945 | 952 | Medication Review Done | | AP | |
| 26.08.2010 | 01.02.1931 | M | | 952 | 957 | Medication Review Done | | MDS | |
| 26.08.2010 | 17.06.1965 | F | | 957 | 1003 | Referred to Orthopaedic Surgeon regarding her back pain | | JLP | |
| 26.08.2010 | 15.06.1940 | M | | 1003 | 1014 | Script for Hydrocortisone with Miconazole cream given | | RAB | |
| 26.08.2010 | 19.06.1927 | F | | 1014 | 1025 | Referred to Heart & Chest Clinic for ECG | | GEG | |
| 26.08.2010 | 03.08.1933 | F | | 1045 | 1100 | The Blue Badge Parking Scheme of Parking Concessions for Disabled & Blind Medical Practitioner Report form ECC1190 (ESS208B) completed with the patient in the Surgery | | BB | |

877

Result of a query that lists all consultations from the 22nd to the end of August 2010 (ConsultationsSeenFrom22ndTillEndOfAug2010)

| SurgeryDate | DateOfBirth | Sex | Diagnosis | TimeIn | TimeOut | Complaints | Treatments | Initials | Notes |
|---|---|---|---|---|---|---|---|---|---|
| 26.08.2010 | 02.09.1977 | F | | 1100 | 1108 | Referred to Physiotherapist regarding her back pain | | RMS | Script for Co-codamol given. |
| 26.08.2010 | 13.07.1957 | M | | 1108 | 1124 | Script for Venlafaxine given | | ARM | For MSU & PSA. |
| 26.08.2010 | 31.10.1951 | F | | 1124 | 1133 | Insomnia | Amitriptyline | BAL | |
| 26.08.2010 | 25.02.1934 | M | | 1645 | 1654 | Script for Ensure Plus, Hyoscine butylbromide, Loperamide & oral rehydration salts oral powder | | BAC | |
| 26.08.2010 | 25.01.1944 | F | | 1654 | 1703 | Referred to Orthopaedic Surgeon regarding pain in the (L) knee | | HPS | |
| 26.08.2010 | 13.06.1994 | F | | 1703 | 1721 | Script for Amoxycillin & Desogestrel | | TAB | |
| 26.08.2010 | 08.05.1939 | F | | 1721 | 1725 | For repeat MSU for fastidious organisms | | JCH | |
| 26.08.2010 | 03.07.1950 | F | | 1725 | 1734 | Referred to Dermatologist regarding red itchy rash on the feet | | YC | Referred to Physiotherapist regarding her painful index finger. |
| 26.08.2010 | 13.09.1992 | F | | 1734 | 1739 | Urine Pregnancy test positive | | MRW | |

Result of a query that lists all consultations from the 22nd to the end of August 2010 (ConsultationsSeenFrom22ndTillEndOfAug2010)

| SurgeryDate | DateOfBirth | Sex | Diagnosis | TimeIn | TimeOut | Complaints | Treatments | Initials | Notes |
|---|---|---|---|---|---|---|---|---|---|
| 26.08.2010 | 25.03.1972 | M | | 1745 | 1754 | Script for Nicotine 25mg/16hrs patch given | | SAM | |
| 26.08.2010 | 12.12.1961 | F | | 1754 | 1804 | Script for Trimethoprim given | | KSO | |
| 26.08.2010 | 08.05.1962 | M | | 1804 | 1810 | Script for Amoxycillin & Gliclazide given | | JJO | |
| 26.08.2010 | 05.07.1955 | F | | 1817 | 1824 | Script for Co-codamol & Flucloxacillin given | | SPER | |
| 27.08.2010 | 07.03.1955 | F | | 935 | 942 | Medication Review Done | | DN | |
| 27.08.2010 | 01.08.1947 | F | | 942 | 958 | Patient informed that she has got Diabetes Mellitus | | JLC | |
| 27.08.2010 | 09.11.1941 | F | | 958 | 1009 | Script for Co-codamol & Metoclopramide given | | LMD | |
| 27.08.2010 | 21.09.1947 | M | | 1009 | 1014 | Referred to ENT Surgeon regarding fluid in the (R) ear | | DL | |
| 27.08.2010 | 06.01.1943 | F | | 1014 | 1021 | Script for Gliclazide given | | PC | |
| 27.08.2010 | 11.03.1968 | F | | 1021 | 1041 | Patient advised not to go back to work in Iceland until we sort out from hospital regarding her Shigella boydii infection | | EJA | |

879

## Result of a query that lists all consultations from the 22ⁿᵈ to the end of August 2010 (ConsultationsSeenFrom22ndTillEndOfAug2010)

| SurgeryDate | DateOfBirth | Sex | Diagnosis | TimeIn | TimeOut | Complaints | Treatments | Initials | Notes |
|---|---|---|---|---|---|---|---|---|---|
| 27.08.2010 | 10.08.1931 | M | Pain | 1041 | 1050 | Back Pain | Ibuprofen & Dihydrocodeine | REW | |
| 27.08.2010 | 09.08.1971 | M | | 1050 | 1059 | Script for Simvastatin given | | JCW | |
| 27.08.2010 | 28.02.1971 | F | | 1059 | 1102 | Infected wound lower end of the chest scar | Flucloxacillin | SJW | |
| 27.08.2010 | 06.06.2004 | M | | 1108 | 1118 | Epistaxis from the (L) nostril | Naseptin cream | JMT | |
| 27.08.2010 | 01.03.1947 | M | | 1118 | 1128 | Script for Loperamide & oral rehydration salts oral powder given | | JRW | |

## Result of a query that lists all consultations from the 22ⁿᵈ to the end of August 2011 (ConsultationsSeenFrom22ndTillEndOfAug2011)

| SurgeryDate | DateOfBirth | Sex | Diagnosis | TimeIn | TimeOut | Complaints | Treatments | Initials | Notes |
|---|---|---|---|---|---|---|---|---|---|
| 22.08.2011 | 01.05.1949 | F | Rash | 952 | 1006 | (R) C2 shingles rash | Acyclovir tablets | LPR | |
| 22.08.2011 | 28.06.1959 | F | | 1006 | 1017 | Medication Review Done | | PIS | |
| 22.08.2011 | 04.11.1991 | F | | 1017 | 1029 | BP 102/74 | | SSOOS | |
| 22.08.2011 | 31.10.1951 | F | | 1029 | 1034 | Fungal nail infection of the (L) Great toe | Amorolfine paint | BAL | |
| 22.08.2011 | 19.07.1925 | F | Rash | 1034 | 1040 | Rash on arms | Fusidic acid with hydrocortisone cream | RMW | |
| 22.08.2011 | 05.06.1930 | F | | 1047 | 1100 | Script for Propranolol given | | JMF | |

Result of a query that lists all consultations from the 22nd to the end of August 2011 (ConsultationsSeenFrom22ndTillEndOfAug2011)

| SurgeryDate | DateOfBirth | Sex | Diagnosis | TimeIn | TimeOut | Complaints | Treatments | Initials | Notes |
|---|---|---|---|---|---|---|---|---|---|
| 22.08.2011 | 03.05.1990 | F | RTI | 1106 | 1114 | Chesty cough | Amoxycillin | HLW | For Pregnancy test. |
| 22.08.2011 | 25.03.2011 | M | | 1248 | 1257 | Fever | Amoxycillin | JAB | |
| 22.08.2011 | 06.12.1946 | F | | 1647 | 1656 | Script for Amitriptyline given | | KMT | |
| 22.08.2011 | 28.07.1939 | F | | 1656 | 1705 | Script for Omeprazole given | | RMM | |
| 22.08.2011 | 21.02.1961 | F | | 1705 | 1721 | Script for Citalopram given | | CHO | |
| 22.08.2011 | 09.07.1964 | F | URTI | 1721 | 1727 | Sore throat | Amoxycillin | JJ | |
| 22.08.2011 | 07.04.1950 | M | Conjunctivitis | 1730 | 1735 | Sticky (L) eye | Chloromycetin Redidrops | DML | |
| 22.08.2011 | 07.02.1948 | M | | 1735 | 1750 | Script for Codeine & Trimethoprim given | | GRC | For MSU & TFTs. |
| 22.08.2011 | 14.01.1994 | F | | 1750 | 1808 | BP 112/77 | | GJG | |
| 22.08.2011 | 23.12.1974 | M | | 1808 | 1822 | Script for Amoxycillin given | | SB | Referred to ENT Surgeon (urgent) regarding enlarged (R) sub-mandibular gland. |
| 23.08.2011 | 21.11.1954 | M | | 948 | 955 | Script for Fusidic acid with Hydrocortisone cream given | | GLS | |
| 23.08.2011 | 17.10.1953 | F | RTI | 955 | 1002 | Chesty cough | Amoxycillin | MS | |
| 23.08.2011 | 24.03.1935 | M | | 1002 | 1015 | Script for Amitriptyline & Lansoprazole given | | PW | Referred to Physiotherapist regarding low back pain. |

Result of a query that lists all consultations from the 22nd to the end of August 2011 (ConsultationsSeenFrom22ndTillEndOfAug2011)

| SurgeryDate | DateOfBirth | Sex | Diagnosis | TimeIn | TimeOut | Complaints | Treatments | Initials | Notes |
|---|---|---|---|---|---|---|---|---|---|
| 23.08.2011 | 13.03.1934 | M | | 1015 | 1034 | Script for Diltiazem & Naftidrofuryl given | | KRF | |
| 23.08.2011 | 16.09.1936 | M | | 1037 | 1041 | Private script for Viagra given | | LPCE | |
| 23.08.2011 | 12.08.1936 | F | | 1041 | 1051 | To see the nurse for ear syringing | | RHP | |
| 23.08.2011 | 15.10.1923 | F | | 1059 | 1113 | Script for Flucloxacillin & Heparinoid cream given | | DWR | |
| 23.08.2011 | 14.01.1974 | F | | 1132 | 1140 | Script for Erythromycin given | | LBA | |
| 23.08.2011 | 30.08.1979 | F | | 1648 | 1708 | Script for Citalopram & Senna given | | JJG | |
| 23.08.2011 | 04.10.1947 | F | | 1658 | 1708 | Cryotherapy treatment applied to verrucae on the soles of the feet | | PVD | |
| 23.08.2011 | 18.06.2010 | M | | 1708 | 1718 | For USScan of the testicles (urgent) | | CPM | |
| 23.08.2011 | 06.02.1944 | M | | 1718 | 1726 | For Rheumatoid factor | | AMC | Script for Co-codamol given. |
| 23.08.2011 | 20.09.1988 | M | | 1726 | 1736 | For FBC, MSU, U/Es & Fasting Glucose | | SJG | |
| 23.08.2011 | 03.05.1990 | F | | 1736 | 1741 | Script for Paracetamol given | | HLW | |
| 23.08.2011 | 31.05.1967 | M | | 1741 | 1749 | Script for Fusidic acid cream given | | GKP | |
| 23.08.2011 | 16.09.1980 | F | URTI | 1749 | 1753 | Sore throat | Erythromycin | LCY | Penicillin allergy. |

Result of a query that lists all consultations from the 22nd to the end of August 2011 (ConsultationsSeenFrom22ndTillEndOfAug2011)

| SurgeryDate | DateOfBirth | Sex | Diagnosis | TimeIn | TimeOut | Complaints | Treatments | Initials | Notes |
|---|---|---|---|---|---|---|---|---|---|
| 23.08.2011 | 26.01.1966 | F | | 1803 | 1822 | Script for Citalopram given | | MI | Referred to Physiotherapist regarding her whiplash injuries after RTA. For X-Rays of the (R) knee. |
| 24.08.2011 | 02.11.1978 | M | | 948 | 956 | Referred to Ophthalmologist regarding his keratoconus & blurred vision in the (L) eye | | SCC | |
| 24.08.2011 | 26.10.1943 | F | | 957 | 1010 | Script for Furosemide given | | APM | |
| 24.08.2011 | 06.12.1940 | F | | 1010 | 1017 | Script for Amoxycillin & Lidocaine/ Hydrocortisone ointment given | | MC | |
| 24.08.2011 | 04.12.1957 | F | | 1017 | 1028 | Script for Clobetasol 0.05% cream given | | TA | |
| 24.08.2011 | 15.03.1984 | F | | 1103 | 1117 | Routine post-natal check done | | SLL | |
| 24.08.2011 | 05.01.1984 | M | | 1122 | 1137 | Referred to Counsellor regarding stress | | AGTN | For FBC, U/Es, TFTs & Fasting Glucose. |
| 24.08.2011 | 24.02.1932 | F | | 1330 | 1345 | Script for Citalopram given | | EM | Home visit. |

Result of a query that lists all consultations from the 22$^{nd}$ to the end of August 2011 (ConsultationsSeenFrom22ndTillEndOfAug2011)

| SurgeryDate | DateOfBirth | Sex | Diagnosis | TimeIn | TimeOut | Complaints | Treatments | Initials | Notes |
|---|---|---|---|---|---|---|---|---|---|
| 24.08.2011 | 08.04.1971 | F | | 1648 | 1700 | Referred to Gynaecologist regarding her heavy period | | JRB | Referred to Gastroenterologist regarding her B12 deficiency. |
| 24.08.2011 | 02.04.1959 | F | | 1700 | 1713 | Referred to Vascular Surgeon regarding her prominent varicose vein on her (L) leg causing aching of the leg | | JW | |
| 24.08.2011 | 12.06.1943 | M | | 1713 | 1721 | Script for Zomorph capsules given | | PB | |
| 24.08.2011 | 17.05.1939 | M | | 1721 | 1734 | Script for Trimethoprim given | | JTN | For USScan of the testicles. |
| 24.08.2011 | 19.04.1996 | M | | 1734 | 1741 | To be referred to Lighthouse Centre as requested by his Social Worker according to his dad | | SAM | His dad came to the Surgery. |
| 24.08.2011 | 26.08.1982 | M | | 1741 | 1752 | Advised to get the Social Services to write me directly for any query they require | | BLS | |
| 24.08.2011 | 30.04.1988 | F | | 1809 | 1815 | Infected insect bite on arm | Cefalexin | ECJ | |
| 25.08.2011 | 02.09.1941 | F | | 944 | 954 | Script for Calcipotriol/ Betamethasone ointment & Pizotifen given | | MS | |

884

Result of a query that lists all consultations from the 22nd to the end of August 2011 (ConsultationsSeenFrom22ndTillEndOfAug2011)

| SurgeryDate | DateOfBirth | Sex | Diagnosis | TimeIn | TimeOut | Complaints | Treatments | Initials | Notes |
|---|---|---|---|---|---|---|---|---|---|
| 25.08.2011 | 27.04.1925 | M | URTI | 1050 | 1105 | Sore throat | Amoxycillin | RWF | Script for Gaviscon given. Referred to rapid access chest pain clinic regarding his recurrent chest pains. |
| 25.08.2011 | 14.07.1991 | F | S/Leave | 1645 | 1702 | Med. 03 04/10 given for Migraine for one week from 23.08.11 | | BG | Script for Paracetamol with Metoclopramide. |
| 25.08.2011 | 24.12.1972 | F | | 1702 | 1712 | Script for Oramorph given | | CC | |
| 25.08.2011 | 08.03.1994 | F | | 1712 | 1720 | Script for Levonorgestrel given | | RHB | |
| 25.08.2011 | 10.11.1962 | F | S/Leave | 1724 | 1730 | Med. 03 04/10 given for (L) Carpal tunnel decompression from 25.08.11 until 26.08.11 | | PL | |
| 25.08.2011 | 17.05.1955 | M | | 1730 | 1735 | For X-Rays of the (R) shoulder | | SJL | |
| 25.08.2011 | 23.11.1960 | M | | 1747 | 1752 | To get his health Insurance Company to put in writing what type of medical examination they require | | DNT | |

885

Result of a query that lists all consultations from the 22nd to the end of August 2011 (ConsultationsSeenFrom22ndTillEndOfAug2011)

| SurgeryDate | DateOfBirth | Sex | Diagnosis | TimeIn | TimeOut | Complaints | Treatments | Initials | Notes |
|---|---|---|---|---|---|---|---|---|---|
| 25.08.2011 | 05.03.1972 | M | S/Leave | 1752 | 1758 | Med. 03 04/10 given for Abdominal Pain & Depression from 20.08.11 for 3 months | | EDJGW | |
| 25.08.2011 | 18.11.1979 | M | | 1758 | 1806 | Script for Flucloxacillin given | | JAS | |
| 26.08.2011 | 22.04.1951 | M | S/Leave | 933 | 939 | Med. 03 04/10 given for Injury to the (R) knee from 26.08.11 for 6 months | | PTJ | |
| 26.08.2011 | 28.02.1975 | F | Rash | 939 | 947 | Intertrigo rash in the lower abdomen area | Daktacort cream | SN | |
| 26.08.2011 | 03.03.1946 | M | | 950 | 1004 | To increase the Omeprazole from 20mg to 40mg daily | | SP | |
| 26.08.2011 | 10.04.1937 | F | | 1004 | 1015 | Referred to Orthopaedic Surgeon regarding pain & locking of the (L) knee | | MC | |
| 26.08.2011 | 09.06.1934 | M | | 1015 | 1022 | He wanted the diagnosis on the last letter from the Rheumatologist explained to him, which I did | | MKC | |
| 26.08.2011 | 27.09.1931 | M | | 1033 | 1044 | Script for Amoxycillin given | | JJ | |

886

Result of a query that lists all consultations from the 22nd to the end of August 2011 (ConsultationsSeenFrom22ndTillEndOfAug2011)

| SurgeryDate | DateOfBirth | Sex | Diagnosis | TimeIn | TimeOut | Complaints | Treatments | Initials | Notes |
|---|---|---|---|---|---|---|---|---|---|
| 26.08.2011 | 04.10.1968 | F | | 1044 | 1053 | Script for Ferrous Gluconate given | | AW | |
| 26.08.2011 | 06.08.1921 | F | | 1053 | 1107 | Script for Ensure Plus & Ropinirole given | | EE | |
| 30.08.2011 | 17.03.1958 | M | | 947 | 956 | Script for Candesartan given | | KEW | |
| 30.08.2011 | 09.01.1962 | F | | 956 | 1003 | She may come back later with view to be referred to Physiotherapist regarding pain in her (L) leg | | VVB | |
| 30.08.2011 | 06.06.1945 | M | | 1003 | 1011 | Script for Omeprazole given | | LJB | |
| 30.08.2011 | 26.05.1936 | M | | 1011 | 1019 | Script for Gliclazide given | | TC | |
| 30.08.2011 | 15.03.1984 | F | | 1019 | 1024 | She will come back if the mole on her head gets bigger | | SLL | |
| 30.08.2011 | 23.08.1925 | F | | 1024 | 1040 | Script for Rosuvastatin given | | REP | |
| 30.08.2011 | 26.09.2003 | F | | 1040 | 1052 | Script for Dicycloverine given | | ENF | |
| 30.08.2011 | 19.05.1964 | M | S/Leave | 1052 | 1058 | Med. 03 04/10 given for Operation on the (R) ankle for one week from 30.08.11 | | VPH | |

Result of a query that lists all consultations from the 22nd to the end of August 2011 (ConsultationsSeenFrom22ndTillEndOfAug2011)

| SurgeryDate | DateOfBirth | Sex | Diagnosis | TimeIn | TimeOut | Complaints | Treatments | Initials | Notes |
|---|---|---|---|---|---|---|---|---|---|
| 30.08.2011 | 30.04.1946 | F | | 1058 | 1105 | Referred to General Surgeon regarding the pedunculated lipoma/fibroma on her anterior chest wall | | LMM | |
| 30.08.2011 | 25.07.1964 | M | | 1648 | 1654 | Script for Compression hosiery class 2 below knee stocking given | | SJP | |
| 30.08.2011 | 03.02.1966 | F | | 1654 | 1700 | Script for Amoxycillin given | | LJR | |
| 30.08.2011 | 01.01.1951 | F | | 1700 | 1707 | Script for Lisinopril given | | CR | |
| 30.08.2011 | 22.04.1975 | F | | 1707 | 1716 | For Chest X-Rays | | SAG | |
| 30.08.2011 | 06.12.1940 | F | | 1716 | 1738 | Script for Ensure Plus, Paracetamol & Temazepam given | | MC | Referred to Counsellor regarding her panic attacks. |
| 30.08.2011 | 25.06.1940 | M | | 1738 | 1748 | Script for Transvasin Heat Rub cream given | | RAB | For X-Rays of the Lumbar Spine & hips. |
| 30.08.2011 | 26.10.1995 | M | | 1748 | 1754 | Script for Clenil Modulite inhaler given | | JWW | |
| 30.08.2011 | 17.04.1945 | F | | 1754 | 1800 | Script for Dixarit given | | MC | |
| 30.08.2011 | 01.07.1961 | M | | 1802 | 1808 | USScan of the abdomen normal | | CJG | |

Result of a query that lists all consultations from the 22nd to the end of August 2012 (ConsultationsSeenFrom22ndTillEndOfAug2012)

| SurgeryDate | DateOfBirth | Sex | Diagnosis | TimeIn | TimeOut | Complaints | Treatments | Initials | Notes |
|---|---|---|---|---|---|---|---|---|---|
| 22.08.2012 | 09.08.1946 | F | | 940 | 956 | Referred to Pain Management specialist regarding her back & (L) hip pain | | JMW | Referred to Orthopaedic Surgeon regarding her back pain. |
| 22.08.2012 | 13.05.1992 | F | | 956 | 1002 | Awaiting appointment to see the Rheumatologist | | AVB | |
| 22.08.2012 | 23.05.1927 | M | | 1002 | 1014 | To continue with the Pregabalin for his pain | | JM | |
| 22.08.2012 | 23.01.1926 | F | | 1014 | 1024 | For urinary Bence Jones protein | | FGN | |
| 22.08.2012 | 17.02.1957 | F | | 1024 | 1029 | Medication Review Done | | VMC | |
| 22.08.2012 | 24.10.2000 | F | | 1029 | 1034 | To add her creams from Dermatologist to her repeat medications | | NMC | |
| 22.08.2012 | 19.08.1939 | F | | 1044 | 1054 | To see nurse for serum Calcium in 3 months | | JEN | |
| 22.08.2012 | 15.03.1984 | F | S/Leave | 1701 | 1707 | Med. 3 04/10 given for Crohn's Disease & Psoriasis from 22.08.12 for 3 months | | SLL | |
| 22.08.2012 | 03.12.1960 | M | | 1710 | 1720 | Script for Lisinopril given | | GTR | |
| 22.08.2012 | 11.01.1964 | F | | 1720 | 1724 | Script for Sumatriptan & Amitripyline given | | TJR | |

Result of a query that lists all consultations from the 22nd to the end of August 2012 (ConsultationsSeenFrom22ndTillEndOfAug2012)

| SurgeryDate | DateOfBirth | Sex | Diagnosis | TimeIn | TimeOut | Complaints | Treatments | Initials | Notes |
|---|---|---|---|---|---|---|---|---|---|
| 22.08.2012 | 19.09.1962 | M | | 1729 | 1739 | He will come back if his (R) knee pain gets worse | | KPW | |
| 22.08.2012 | 04.10.1968 | F | | 1744 | 1751 | For USScan of the Thyroid gland | | AW | |
| 22.08.2012 | 12.03.1954 | M | | 1751 | 1801 | Script for Rosuvastatin given | | JFL | For FBC, U/Es, HbA1c, serum cholesterol & LFTs. |
| 23.08.2012 | 17.03.1958 | M | | 941 | 951 | Script for Mesren m/r given | | KEW | |
| 23.08.2012 | 10.09.1981 | F | | 951 | 1003 | Script for Ferrous Fumarate given | | HAS | |
| 23.08.2012 | 16.01.1986 | M | S/Leave | 1003 | 1011 | Med. 3 04/10 given for Back Pain from 23.08.12 for 2 weeks | | ANI | |
| 23.08.2012 | 30.09.1967 | F | | 1015 | 1024 | Script for Amoxycillin given | | SEF | |
| 23.08.2012 | 15.09.1939 | F | | 1024 | 1030 | To see the nurse regarding cholesterol lowering dietary advice | | EH | |
| 23.08.2012 | 17.11.1937 | F | | 1030 | 1038 | Script for Amitriptyline given | | JIC | |
| 23.08.2012 | 19.12.1949 | M | | 1038 | 1045 | Referred to Podiatrist regarding cramps in the soles of both feet | | DJB | |

Result of a query that lists all consultations from the 22ⁿᵈ to the end of August 2012 (ConsultationsSeenFrom22ndTillEndOfAug2012)

| SurgeryDate | DateOfBirth | Sex | Diagnosis | TimeIn | TimeOut | Complaints | Treatments | Initials | Notes |
|---|---|---|---|---|---|---|---|---|---|
| 23.08.2012 | 02.12.1973 | F | | 1045 | 1049 | To see the nurse regarding dietary advice for weight loss | | MC | |
| 23.08.2012 | 18.05.1952 | F | | 1049 | 1057 | Script for Amoxycillin given | | CAE | Referred to ENT Surgeon regarding her snoring & sleep apnoea. |
| 23.08.2012 | 18.09.1946 | F | | 1058 | 1102 | Script for Trimethoprim given | | SL | |
| 23.08.2012 | 24.08.2010 | F | | 1102 | 1112 | Referred to Paediatric Dr. on call, SGH, regarding the blisters on his hand, foot & knee | | JIS | |
| 23.08.2012 | 22.02.2012 | M | RTI | 1112 | 1117 | Chesty cough | Amoxycillin | RNEL | |
| 23.08.2012 | 20.09.1984 | M | | 1640 | 1649 | Cryotherapy blasts x2 applied to seborrheic keratitis on the anterior abdominal wall | | PD | |
| 23.08.2012 | 15.07.1956 | M | | 1652 | 1702 | Script for Driclor Solution given | | DHC | For FBC, U/Es, LFTs & serum cholesterol. |
| 23.08.2012 | 29.06.1947 | F | | 1702 | 1709 | Script for Cetraben cream given | | SLS | |
| 23.08.2012 | 18.11.1946 | F | | 1709 | 1718 | Referred to Orthopaedic Surgeon regarding her (R) knee pain | | JML | Referred for Gastroscopy regarding her dysphagia. |

Result of a query that lists all consultations from the 22nd to the end of August 2012 (ConsultationsSeenFrom22ndTillEndOfAug2012)

| SurgeryDate | DateOfBirth | Sex | Diagnosis | TimeIn | TimeOut | Complaints | Treatments | Initials | Notes |
|---|---|---|---|---|---|---|---|---|---|
| 23.08.2012 | 13.10.1955 | F | | 1721 | 1729 | BP 125/78 | | TK | |
| 23.08.2012 | 13.10.1955 | M | | 1729 | 1735 | Referred to Counsellor regarding his anger problems | | KB | |
| 23.08.2012 | 01.04.1940 | M | | 1735 | 1744 | Script for Codeine tablets given | | MCW | |
| 23.08.2012 | 10.04.1984 | M | | 1805 | 1814 | Cryotherapy blasts x2 applied to wart on the sole of the (R) foot | | BM | |
| 24.08.2012 | 24.10.1959 | M | S/Leave | 944 | 1017 | Med. 3 04/10 given for Laparoscopic Cholecystectomy from 24.08.12 for 4 weeks | | BRH | Script for Levothyroxine given. For B12, Folate & Ferritin. |
| 24.08.2012 | 16.05.1964 | M | | 1017 | 1025 | Referred to Orthopaedic Surgeon with view to having MRI scan as suggested by the Chiropractor for his back pain | | GDC | |
| 24.08.2012 | 08.06.1959 | F | | 1025 | 1035 | Script for Simvastatin given | | TAE | |
| 24.08.2012 | 06.01.1969 | F | S/Leave | 1035 | 1040 | Med. 3 04/10 given for (R) knee arthroscopy from 24.08.12 for 2 weeks | | KEL | |
| 24.08.2012 | 22.03.1931 | F | | 1040 | 1052 | For FBC, U/Es, LFT's & Ferritin | | HH | |

Result of a query that lists all consultations from the 22$^{nd}$ to the end of August 2012 (ConsultationsSeenFrom22ndTillEndOfAug2012)

| SurgeryDate | DateOfBirth | Sex | Diagnosis | TimeIn | TimeOut | Complaints | Treatments | Initials | Notes |
|---|---|---|---|---|---|---|---|---|---|
| 24.08.2012 | 28.07.1939 | F | | 1052 | 1118 | Script for Amoxicillin, Optive eye drops & Pregabalin given | | RMM | |
| 24.08.2012 | 02.06.1970 | M | | 1118 | 1123 | Script for Co-codamol given | | DLM | |
| 24.08.2012 | 29.08.1939 | M | | 1123 | 1136 | Script for Lansoprazole given | | JFP | |
| 24.08.2012 | 11.03.1972 | M | | 1136 | 1142 | Medication Review Done | | NRB | |
| 24.08.2012 | 26.06.1955 | F | | 1142 | 1147 | Script for Naproxen given | | JAP | |
| 24.08.2012 | 17.03.1961 | M | | 1147 | 1158 | Script for Codeine given | | LDM | Referred to Neurologist regarding first episode of epileptic fit. |
| 24.08.2012 | 04.07.1929 | M | | 1158 | 1202 | For X-Rays of the (L) knee | | RMC | |
| 24.08.2012 | 31.01.1933 | M | | 1202 | 1210 | For FBC, U/Es, TFTs & Fasting Glucose | | MPB | |
| 28.08.2012 | 05.04.1952 | M | S/Leave | 944 | 954 | Med. 3 04/10 given for Myocardial Infarction from 28.08.12 to 29.08.12 (phased return) | | LFC | Script for Bisoprolol given. |
| 28.08.2012 | 08.10.1976 | M | | 954 | 1000 | Script for Co-codamol & Naproxen given | | LG | |

Result of a query that lists all consultations from the 22nd to the end of August 2012 (ConsultationsSeenFrom22ndTillEndOfAug2012)

| SurgeryDate | DateOfBirth | Sex | Diagnosis | TimeIn | TimeOut | Complaints | Treatments | Initials | Notes |
|---|---|---|---|---|---|---|---|---|---|
| 28.08.2012 | 18.10.1949 | M | | 1021 | 1037 | Script for Enoxaparin injection given | | BJG | |
| 28.08.2012 | 04.12.1957 | F | | 1037 | 1046 | Script for Erythromycin, Prednisolone tablets, Salbutamol inhaler & Seretide 500 Accuhaler given | | TA | |
| 28.08.2012 | 20.10.1983 | F | | 1046 | 1054 | To see the nurse regarding dieting | | ARS | |
| 28.08.2012 | 27.03.1940 | F | | 1054 | 1102 | Referred to Orthopaedic Surgeon regarding painful (L) knee | | MAD | |
| 28.08.2012 | 27.03.1931 | F | | 1102 | 1110 | Script for Erythromycin, Prednisolone, Qvar 50 inhaler & Salbutamol inhaler given | | MMA | |
| 28.08.2012 | 04.04.1953 | M | S/Leave | 1110 | 1127 | Med. 3 04/10 given for (L) ankle arthroscopy from 28.08.12 for 2 weeks | | GC | |
| 28.08.2012 | 03.04.1987 | F | | 1644 | 1657 | For FBC, U/Es, TFTs, Fasting Glucose, Fasting Lipids, LFTs & HbA1c | | LJP | |

Result of a query that lists all consultations from the 22nd to the end of August 2012 (ConsultationsSeenFrom22ndTillEndOfAug2012)

| SurgeryDate | DateOfBirth | Sex | Diagnosis | TimeIn | TimeOut | Complaints | Treatments | Initials | Notes |
|---|---|---|---|---|---|---|---|---|---|
| 28.08.2012 | 27.10.1960 | F | S/Leave | 1657 | 1704 | Med. 3 04/10 given for Back Pain from 22.08.12 for 3 months | | DLK | Script for Cetraben cream, Co-dydramol & Oramorph given. |
| 28.08.2012 | 14.01.1974 | F | | 1704 | 1714 | Script for Norethisterone given | | LBA | For MSU. |
| 28.08.2012 | 03.02.1957 | M | S/Leave | 1714 | 1735 | Med. 3 04/10 given for Diabetic ulcer on (R) foot from 22.05.12 for 5 months | | ER | Script for Candesartan given. |
| 28.08.2012 | 16.06.1915 | M | | 1735 | 1749 | For Chest X-Rays | | LB | |
| 28.08.2012 | 25.01.1958 | M | | 1749 | 1754 | Medication Review Done | | TSE | |
| 28.08.2012 | 08.04.1995 | F | | 1754 | 1800 | Script for Amoxycillin given | | SB | |
| 28.08.2012 | 22.07.1961 | M | | 1800 | 1805 | Script for Calamine lotion given | | PWL | |
| 28.08.2012 | 12.12.1961 | F | | 1845 | 1850 | Script for Flucloxacillin given | | KSO | |
| 28.08.2012 | 08.05.1962 | M | | 1850 | 1800 | Script for Amoxycillin & Omeprazole given | | JJO | For Chest X-Rays. |
| 29.08.2012 | 28.07.1946 | M | | 948 | 958 | BP 119/83 | | PWD | |
| 29.08.2012 | 07.02.1948 | M | | 958 | 1015 | Script for Trimethoprim & Movicol-Half oral powder given | | GRC | For MSU. |

895

Result of a query that lists all consultations from the 22nd to the end of August 2012 (ConsultationsSeenFrom22ndTillEndOfAug2012)

| SurgeryDate | DateOfBirth | Sex | Diagnosis | TimeIn | TimeOut | Complaints | Treatments | Initials | Notes |
|---|---|---|---|---|---|---|---|---|---|
| 29.08.2012 | 04.11.1966 | F | | 1015 | 1023 | Referred for Coloscopy in view of her iron deficiency anaemia & family history of bowel cancer | | SJOB | |
| 29.08.2012 | 16.11.1944 | F | | 1023 | 1037 | Script for Amoxycillin, Bendroflumethiazide & Lansoprazole given | | JH | |
| 29.08.2012 | 08.10.1938 | M | | 1037 | 1048 | Referred to Dermatologist regarding the non-healing wound on his fore-head | | TAC | |
| 29.08.2012 | 28.12.1962 | M | S/Leave | 1048 | 1057 | Med. 3 04/10 given for Back & (L) hip pain due to leg prosthesis from 29.08.12 for 6 months | | KF | |
| 29.08.2012 | 17.04.1930 | M | | 1057 | 1106 | Script for Amoxycillin given | | FL | Referred for Colonoscopy in view of his iron deficiency anaemia. For Chest X-Rays. |
| 29.08.2012 | 05.03.1965 | F | | 1106 | 1112 | BP 134/76 | | ALC | |
| 29.08.2012 | 24.04.1966 | M | | 1112 | 1123 | Script for Amoxycillin given | | BSE | For Chest X-Rays. |

Result of a query that lists all consultations from the 22nd to the end of August 2012 (ConsultationsSeenFrom22ndTillEndOfAug2012)

| SurgeryDate | DateOfBirth | Sex | Diagnosis | TimeIn | TimeOut | Complaints | Treatments | Initials | Notes |
|---|---|---|---|---|---|---|---|---|---|
| 29.08.2012 | 27.09.1931 | M | | 1646 | 1656 | Script for Erythromycin & Prednisolone tablets given | | JJ | |
| 29.08.2012 | 04.02.1963 | F | S/Leave | 1656 | 1716 | Med. 3 04/10 given for Fainted from 21.08.12 for 3 weeks | | SAL | Referred to Counsellor regarding crying easily. For FBC, Fasting Glucose, TFT, LFTs, Fasting Lipids, U/Es & FSH. |
| 29.08.2012 | 09.09.1993 | M | | 1716 | 1721 | To continue with the Salbutamol inhaler | | MPC | |
| 29.08.2012 | 22.06.1979 | M | S/Leave | 1721 | 1728 | Med. 3 04/10 given for Depression from 29.08.12 for 6 months | | DC | |
| 29.08.2012 | 17.06.1965 | F | | 1728 | 1737 | Script for Scheriproct suppositories & Scheriproct ointment given | | JLP | |
| 29.08.2012 | 10.11.2000 | M | | 1737 | 1741 | Script for Clenil Modulite inhaler given | | CJM | |
| 29.08.2012 | 16.09.1989 | F | | 1741 | 1746 | Script for Prochlorperazine given | | SLW | |

Result of a query that lists all consultations from the 22nd to the end of August 2012 (ConsultationsSeenFrom22ndTillEndOfAug2012)

| SurgeryDate | DateOfBirth | Sex | Diagnosis | TimeIn | TimeOut | Complaints | Treatments | Initials | Notes |
|---|---|---|---|---|---|---|---|---|---|
| 29.08.2012 | 10.12.1986 | F | | 1757 | 1807 | For Pregnancy test | | HEB | Referred for Termination of Pregnancy. |
| 30.08.2012 | 05.07.1931 | F | | 944 | 959 | Script for Gliclazide & Naftidrofuryl given | | AVD | |
| 30.08.2012 | 23.01.1926 | F | | 959 | 1006 | For X-Rays of the hips/pelvis | | FGN | |
| 30.08.2012 | 07.11.1957 | F | | 1006 | 1013 | For Rheumatoid factor & CRP | | DJE | |
| 30.08.2012 | 24.01.1957 | M | S/Leave | 1016 | 1027 | Med. 3 04/10 given for Back Pain from 27.08.12 for 2 weeks | | PGI | |
| 30.08.2012 | 20.08.1939 | F | | 1027 | 1038 | Script for Canesten HC cream given | | SLT | For Pelvic/Lower abdominal USScan. |
| 30.08.2012 | 03.03.1937 | M | | 1038 | 1052 | Script for MST continus & Oramorph given | | EJC | |
| 30.08.2012 | 01.12.1934 | F | | 1052 | 1104 | For Clotting screen & FBC in 2 months | | LFM | |
| 30.08.2012 | 16.08.1927 | F | | 1104 | 1112 | Script for Oramorph & Paracetamol given | | EFM | |
| 30.08.2012 | 01.12.1989 | F | | 1112 | 1121 | Script for Amoxycillin given | | PB | |
| 30.08.2012 | 09.04.1938 | M | | 1644 | 1651 | Script for Hyoscine butylbromide given | | NWH | |
| 30.08.2012 | 17.05.1943 | M | | 1651 | 1658 | Script for Tranvasin cream given | | PJC | |

Result of a query that lists all consultations from the 22nd to the end of August 2012 (ConsultationsSeenFrom22ndTillEndOfAug2012)

| SurgeryDate | DateOfBirth | Sex | Diagnosis | TimeIn | TimeOut | Complaints | Treatments | Initials | Notes |
|---|---|---|---|---|---|---|---|---|---|
| 30.08.2012 | 11.08.1935 | F |  | 1701 | 1707 | Script for Tranvasin cream & Paracetamol given |  | CH |  |
| 30.08.2012 | 08.04.1971 | F | S/Leave | 1707 | 1712 | Med. 3 04/10 given for Back Pain from 27.08.12 for 1 week |  | JRB |  |
| 30.08.2012 | 19.09.1962 | M |  | 1716 | 1728 | Referred to Physiotherapist regarding pain down the (R) arm |  | KPW | Referred to Orthopaedic Surgeon regarding pain in the (R) knee. |
| 30.08.2012 | 14.01.1994 | F |  | 1733 | 1742 | To try OTC anti-histamine to see if it will help with prickly heat when she goes on holidays |  | GJG |  |
| 30.08.2012 | 19.12.1972 | F |  | 1745 | 1752 | Script for Erythromycin given |  | AJH | Penicillin allergy. |

Result of a query that lists all consultations from the 22nd to the end of August 2012 (ConsultationsSeenFrom22ndTillEndOfAug2012)

| SurgeryDate | DateOfBirth | Sex | Diagnosis | TimeIn | TimeOut | Complaints | Treatments | Initials | Notes |
|---|---|---|---|---|---|---|---|---|---|
| 22.08.2012 | 09.08.1946 | F | | 940 | 956 | Referred to Pain Management specialist regarding her back & (L) hip pain | | JMW | Referred to Orthopaedic Surgeon regarding her back pain. |
| 22.08.2012 | 13.05.1992 | F | | 956 | 1002 | Awaiting appointment to see the Rheumatologist | | AVB | |
| 22.08.2012 | 23.05.1927 | M | | 1002 | 1014 | To continue with the Pregabalin for his pain | | JM | |
| 22.08.2012 | 23.01.1926 | F | | 1014 | 1024 | For urinary Bence Jones protein | | FGN | |
| 22.08.2012 | 17.02.1957 | F | | 1024 | 1029 | Medication Review Done | | VMC | |
| 22.08.2012 | 24.10.2000 | F | | 1029 | 1034 | To add her creams from Dermatologist to her repeat medications | | NMC | |
| 22.08.2012 | 19.08.1939 | F | | 1044 | 1054 | To see nurse for serum Calcium in 3 months | | JEN | |
| 22.08.2012 | 15.03.1984 | F | S/Leave | 1701 | 1707 | Med. 3 04/10 given for Crohn's Disease & Psoriasis from 22.08.12 for 3 months | | SLL | |
| 22.08.2012 | 03.12.1960 | M | | 1710 | 1720 | Script for Lisinopril given | | GTR | |
| 22.08.2012 | 11.01.1964 | F | | 1720 | 1724 | Script for Sumatriptan & Amitriptyline given | | TJR | |

Result of a query that lists all consultations from the 22nd to the end of August 2012 (ConsultationsSeenFrom22ndTillEndOfAug2012)

| SurgeryDate | DateOfBirth | Sex | Diagnosis | TimeIn | TimeOut | Complaints | Treatments | Initials | Notes |
|---|---|---|---|---|---|---|---|---|---|
| 22.08.2012 | 19.09.1962 | M | | 1729 | 1739 | He will come back if his (R) knee pain gets worse | | KPW | |
| 22.08.2012 | 04.10.1968 | F | | 1744 | 1751 | For USScan of the Thyroid gland | | AW | |
| 22.08.2012 | 12.03.1954 | M | | 1751 | 1801 | Script for Rosuvastatin given | | JFL | For FBC, U/Es, HbA1c, serum cholesterol & LFTs. |
| 23.08.2012 | 17.03.1958 | M | | 941 | 951 | Script for Mesren m/r given | | KEW | |
| 23.08.2012 | 10.09.1981 | F | | 951 | 1003 | Script for Ferrous Fumarate given | | HAS | |
| 23.08.2012 | 16.01.1986 | M | S/Leave | 1003 | 1011 | Med. 3 04/10 given for Back Pain from 23.08.12 for 2 weeks | | ANI | |
| 23.08.2012 | 30.09.1967 | F | | 1015 | 1024 | Script for Amoxycillin given | | SEF | |
| 23.08.2012 | 15.09.1939 | F | | 1024 | 1030 | To see the nurse regarding cholesterol lowering dietary advice | | EH | |
| 23.08.2012 | 17.11.1937 | F | | 1030 | 1038 | Script for Amitriptyline given | | JIC | |
| 23.08.2012 | 19.12.1949 | M | | 1038 | 1045 | Referred to Podiatrist regarding cramps in the soles of both feet | | DJB | |

901

Result of a query that lists all consultations from the 22nd to the end of August 2012 (ConsultationsSeenFrom22ndTillEndOfAug2012)

| SurgeryDate | DateOfBirth | Sex | Diagnosis | TimeIn | TimeOut | Complaints | Treatments | Initials | Notes |
|---|---|---|---|---|---|---|---|---|---|
| 23.08.2012 | 02.12.1973 | F | | 1045 | 1049 | To see the nurse regarding dietary advice for weight loss | | MC | |
| 23.08.2012 | 18.05.1952 | F | | 1049 | 1057 | Script for Amoxycillin given | | CAE | Referred to ENT Surgeon regarding her snoring & sleep apnoea. |
| 23.08.2012 | 18.09.1946 | F | | 1058 | 1102 | Script for Trimethoprim given | | SL | |
| 23.08.2012 | 24.08.2010 | F | | 1102 | 1112 | Referred to Paediatric Dr. on call, SGH, regarding the blisters on his hand, foot & knee | | JIS | |
| 23.08.2012 | 22.02.2012 | M | RTI | 1112 | 1117 | Chesty cough | Amoxycillin | RNEL | |
| 23.08.2012 | 20.09.1984 | M | | 1640 | 1649 | Cryotherapy blasts x2 applied to seborrheic keratitis on the anterior abdominal wall | | PD | |
| 23.08.2012 | 15.07.1956 | M | | 1652 | 1702 | Script for Driclor Solution given | | DHC | For FBC, U/Es, LFTs & serum cholesterol. |
| 23.08.2012 | 29.06.1947 | F | | 1702 | 1709 | Script for Cetraben cream given | | SLS | |
| 23.08.2012 | 18.11.1946 | F | | 1709 | 1718 | Referred to Orthopaedic Surgeon regarding her (R) knee pain | | JML | Referred for Gastroscopy regarding her dysphagia. |

Result of a query that lists all consultations from the 22nd to the end of August 2012 (ConsultationsSeenFrom22ndTillEndOfAug2012)

| SurgeryDate | DateOfBirth | Sex | Diagnosis | TimeIn | TimeOut | Complaints | Treatments | Initials | Notes |
|---|---|---|---|---|---|---|---|---|---|
| 23.08.2012 | 13.10.1955 | F | | 1721 | 1729 | BP 125/78 | | TK | |
| 23.08.2012 | 13.10.1955 | M | | 1729 | 1735 | Referred to Counsellor regarding his anger problems | | KB | |
| 23.08.2012 | 01.04.1940 | M | | 1735 | 1744 | Script for Codeine tablets given | | MCW | |
| 23.08.2012 | 10.04.1984 | M | | 1805 | 1814 | Cryotherapy blasts x2 applied to wart on the sole of the (R) foot | | BM | |
| 24.08.2012 | 24.10.1959 | M | S/Leave | 944 | 1017 | Med. 3 04/10 given for Laparoscopic Cholecystectomy from 24.08.12 for 4 weeks | | BRH | Script for Levothyroxine given. For B12, Folate & Ferritin. |
| 24.08.2012 | 16.05.1964 | M | | 1017 | 1025 | Referred to Orthopaedic Surgeon with view to having MRI scan as suggested by the Chiropractor for his back pain | | GDC | |
| 24.08.2012 | 08.06.1959 | F | | 1025 | 1035 | Script for Simvastatin given | | TAE | |
| 24.08.2012 | 06.01.1969 | F | S/Leave | 1035 | 1040 | Med. 3 04/10 given for (R) knee arthroscopy from 24.08.12 for 2 weeks | | KEL | |
| 24.08.2012 | 22.03.1931 | F | | 1040 | 1052 | For FBC, U/Es, LFTs & Ferritin | | HH | |

Result of a query that lists all consultations from the 22nd to the end of August 2012 (ConsultationsSeenFrom22ndTillEndOfAug2012)

| SurgeryDate | DateOfBirth | Sex | Diagnosis | TimeIn | TimeOut | Complaints | Treatments | Initials | Notes |
|---|---|---|---|---|---|---|---|---|---|
| 24.08.2012 | 28.07.1939 | F | | 1052 | 1118 | Script for Amoxycillin, Optive eye drops & Pregabalin given | | RMM | |
| 24.08.2012 | 02.06.1970 | M | | 1118 | 1123 | Script for Co-codamol given | | DLM | |
| 24.08.2012 | 29.08.1939 | M | | 1123 | 1136 | Script for Lansoprazole given | | JFP | |
| 24.08.2012 | 11.03.1972 | M | | 1136 | 1142 | Medication Review Done | | NRB | |
| 24.08.2012 | 26.06.1955 | F | | 1142 | 1147 | Script for Naproxen given | | JAP | |
| 24.08.2012 | 17.03.1961 | M | | 1147 | 1158 | Script for Codeine given | | LDM | Referred to Neurologist regarding first episode of epileptic fit. |
| 24.08.2012 | 04.07.1929 | M | | 1158 | 1202 | For X-Rays of the (L) knee | | RMC | |
| 24.08.2012 | 31.01.1933 | M | | 1202 | 1210 | For FBC, U/Es, TFTs & Fasting Glucose | | MPB | |
| 28.08.2012 | 05.04.1952 | M | S/Leave | 944 | 954 | Med. 3 04/10 given for Myocardial Infarction from 28.08.12 to 29.08.12 (phased return) | | LFC | Script for Bisoprolol given. |
| 28.08.2012 | 08.10.1976 | M | | 954 | 1000 | Script for Co-codamol & Naproxen given | | LG | |

Result of a query that lists all consultations from the 22nd to the end of August 2012 (ConsultationsSeenFrom22ndTillEndOfAug2012)

| SurgeryDate | DateOfBirth | Sex | Diagnosis | TimeIn | TimeOut | Complaints | Treatments | Initials | Notes |
|---|---|---|---|---|---|---|---|---|---|
| 28.08.2012 | 18.10.1949 | M | | 1021 | 1037 | Script for Enoxaparin injection given | | BJG | |
| 28.08.2012 | 04.12.1957 | F | | 1037 | 1046 | Script for Erythromycin, Prednisolone tablets, Salbutamol inhaler & Seretide 500 Accuhaler given | | TA | |
| 28.08.2012 | 20.10.1983 | F | | 1046 | 1054 | To see the nurse regarding dieting | | ARS | |
| 28.08.2012 | 27.03.1940 | F | | 1054 | 1102 | Referred to Orthopaedic Surgeon regarding painful (L) knee | | MAD | |
| 28.08.2012 | 27.03.1931 | F | | 1102 | 1110 | Script for Erythromycin, Prednisolone, Qvar 50 inhaler & Salbutamol inhaler given | | MMA | |
| 28.08.2012 | 04.04.1953 | M | S/Leave | 1110 | 1127 | Med. 3 04/10 given for (L) ankle arthroscopy from 28.08.12 for 2 weeks | | GC | |
| 28.08.2012 | 03.04.1987 | F | | 1644 | 1657 | For FBC, U/Es, TFTs, Fasting Glucose, Fasting Lipids, LFTs & HbAlc | | LJP | |

Result of a query that lists all consultations from the 22nd to the end of August 2012 (ConsultationsSeenFrom22ndTillEndOfAug2012)

| SurgeryDate | DateOfBirth | Sex | Diagnosis | TimeIn | TimeOut | Complaints | Treatments | Initials | Notes |
|---|---|---|---|---|---|---|---|---|---|
| 28.08.2012 | 27.10.1960 | F | S/Leave | 1657 | 1704 | Med. 3 04/10 given for Back Pain from 22.08.12 for 3 months | | DLK | Script for Cetraben cream, Co-dydramol & Oramorph given. |
| 28.08.2012 | 14.01.1974 | F | | 1704 | 1714 | Script for Norethisterone given | | LBA | For MSU. |
| 28.08.2012 | 03.02.1957 | M | S/Leave | 1714 | 1735 | Med. 3 04/10 given for Diabetic ulcer on (R) foot from 22.05.12 for 5 months | | ER | Script for Candesartan given. |
| 28.08.2012 | 16.06.1915 | M | | 1735 | 1749 | For Chest X-Rays | | LB | |
| 28.08.2012 | 25.01.1958 | M | | 1749 | 1754 | Medication Review Done | | TSE | |
| 28.08.2012 | 08.04.1995 | F | | 1754 | 1800 | Script for Amoxycillin given | | SB | |
| 28.08.2012 | 22.07.1961 | M | | 1800 | 1805 | Script for Calamine lotion given | | PWL | |
| 28.08.2012 | 12.12.1961 | F | | 1845 | 1850 | Script for Flucloxacillin given | | KSO | |
| 28.08.2012 | 08.05.1962 | M | | 1850 | 1800 | Script for Amoxycillin & Omeprazole given | | JJO | For Chest X-Rays. |
| 29.08.2012 | 28.07.1946 | M | | 948 | 958 | BP 119/83 | | PWD | |
| 29.08.2012 | 07.02.1948 | M | | 958 | 1015 | Script for Trimethoprim & Movicol-Half oral powder given | | GRC | For MSU. |

906

Result of a query that lists all consultations from the 22nd to the end of August 2012 (ConsultationsSeenFrom22ndTillEndOfAug2012)

| SurgeryDate | DateOfBirth | Sex | Diagnosis | TimeIn | TimeOut | Complaints | Treatments | Initials | Notes |
|---|---|---|---|---|---|---|---|---|---|
| 29.08.2012 | 04.11.1966 | F | | 1015 | 1023 | Referred for Coloscopy in view of her iron deficiency anaemia & family history of bowel cancer | | SJOB | |
| 29.08.2012 | 16.11.1944 | F | | 1023 | 1037 | Script for Amoxycillin, Bendroflumethiazide & Lansoprazole given | | JH | |
| 29.08.2012 | 08.10.1938 | M | | 1037 | 1048 | Referred to Dermatologist regarding the non-healing wound on his fore-head | | TAC | |
| 29.08.2012 | 28.12.1962 | M | S/Leave | 1048 | 1057 | Med. 3 04/10 given for Back & (L) hip pain due to leg prosthesis from 29.08.12 for 6 months | | KF | |
| 29.08.2012 | 17.04.1930 | M | | 1057 | 1106 | Script for Amoxycillin given | | FL | Referred for Colonoscopy in view of his iron deficiency anaemia. For Chest X-Rays. |
| 29.08.2012 | 05.03.1965 | F | | 1106 | 1112 | BP 134/76 | | ALC | |
| 29.08.2012 | 24.04.1966 | M | | 1112 | 1123 | Script for Amoxycillin given | | BSE | For Chest X-Rays. |

Result of a query that lists all consultations from the 22nd to the end of August 2012 (ConsultationsSeenFrom22ndTillEndOfAug2012)

| SurgeryDate | DateOfBirth | Sex | Diagnosis | TimeIn | TimeOut | Complaints | Treatments | Initials | Notes |
|---|---|---|---|---|---|---|---|---|---|
| 29.08.2012 | 27.09.1931 | M | | 1646 | 1656 | Script for Erythromycin & Prednisolone tablets given | | JJ | |
| 29.08.2012 | 04.02.1963 | F | S/Leave | 1656 | 1716 | Med. 3 04/10 given for Fainted from 21.08.12 for 3 weeks | | SAL | Referred to Counsellor regarding crying easily. For FBC, Fasting Glucose, TFT, LFTs, Fasting Lipids, U/Es & FSH. |
| 29.08.2012 | 09.09.1993 | M | | 1716 | 1721 | To continue with the Salbutamol inhaler | | MPC | |
| 29.08.2012 | 22.06.1979 | M | S/Leave | 1721 | 1728 | Med. 3 04/10 given for Depression from 29.08.12 for 6 months | | DC | |
| 29.08.2012 | 17.06.1965 | F | | 1728 | 1737 | Script for Scheriproct suppositories & Scheriproct ointment given | | JLP | |
| 29.08.2012 | 10.11.2000 | M | | 1737 | 1741 | Script for Clenil Modulite inhaler given | | CJM | |
| 29.08.2012 | 16.09.1989 | F | | 1741 | 1746 | Script for Prochlorperazine given | | SLW | |
| 29.08.2012 | 10.12.1986 | F | | 1757 | 1807 | For Pregnancy test | | HEB | Referred for Termination of Pregnancy. |

Result of a query that lists all consultations from the 22nd to the end of August 2012 (ConsultationsSeenFrom22ndTillEndOfAug2012)

| SurgeryDate | DateOfBirth | Sex | Diagnosis | TimeIn | TimeOut | Complaints | Treatments | Initials | Notes |
|---|---|---|---|---|---|---|---|---|---|
| 30.08.2012 | 05.07.1931 | F | | 944 | 959 | Script for Gliclazide & Naftidrofuryl given | | AVD | |
| 30.08.2012 | 23.01.1926 | F | | 959 | 1006 | For X-Rays of the hips/pelvis | | FGN | |
| 30.08.2012 | 07.11.1957 | F | | 1006 | 1013 | For Rheumatoid factor & CRP | | DJE | |
| 30.08.2012 | 24.01.1957 | M | S/Leave | 1016 | 1027 | Med. 3 04/10 given for Back Pain from 27.08.12 for 2 weeks | | PGI | |
| 30.08.2012 | 20.08.1939 | F | | 1027 | 1038 | Script for Canesten HC cream given | | SLT | For Pelvic/Lower abdominal USScan. |
| 30.08.2012 | 03.03.1937 | M | | 1038 | 1052 | Script for MST continus & Oramorph given | | EJC | |
| 30.08.2012 | 01.12.1934 | F | | 1052 | 1104 | For Clotting screen & FBC in 2 months | | LFM | |
| 30.08.2012 | 16.08.1927 | F | | 1104 | 1112 | Script for Oramorph & Paracetamol given | | EFM | |
| 30.08.2012 | 01.12.1989 | F | | 1112 | 1121 | Script for Amoxycillin given | | PB | |
| 30.08.2012 | 09.04.1938 | M | | 1644 | 1651 | Script for Hyoscine butylbromide given | | NWH | |
| 30.08.2012 | 17.05.1943 | M | | 1651 | 1658 | Script for Tranvasin cream given | | PJC | |
| 30.08.2012 | 11.08.1935 | F | | 1701 | 1707 | Script for Tranvasin cream & Paracetamol given | | CH | |

Result of a query that lists all consultations from the 22nd to the end of August 2012 (ConsultationsSeenFrom22ndTillEndOfAug2012)

| SurgeryDate | DateOfBirth | Sex | Diagnosis | TimeIn | TimeOut | Complaints | Treatments | Initials | Notes |
|---|---|---|---|---|---|---|---|---|---|
| 30.08.2012 | 08.04.1971 | F | S/Leave | 1707 | 1712 | Med. 3 04/10 given for Back Pain from 27.08.12 for 1 week | | JRB | |
| 30.08.2012 | 19.09.1962 | M | | 1716 | 1728 | Referred to Physiotherapist regarding pain down the (R) arm | | KPW | Referred to Orthopaedic Surgeon regarding pain in the (R) knee. |
| 30.08.2012 | 14.01.1994 | F | | 1733 | 1742 | To try OTC anti-histamine to see if it will help with prickly heat when she goes on holidays | | GJG | |
| 30.08.2012 | 19.12.1972 | F | | 1745 | 1752 | Script for Erythromycin given | | AJH | Penicillin allergy. |

Result of a query that lists all consultations from the 22nd to the end of August 2013 (ConsultationsSeenFrom22ndTillEndOfAug2013)

| SurgeryDate | DateOfBirth | Sex | Diagnosis | TimeIn | TimeOut | Complaints | Treatments | Initials | Notes |
|---|---|---|---|---|---|---|---|---|---|
| 22.08.2013 | 06.11.1961 | F | S/Leave | 945 | 1002 | Med. 3 04/10 given for Hypothyroidism for 1 week from 19.08.13 | | BSM | |
| 22.08.2013 | 08.04.1995 | F | | 1002 | 1012 | Script for Trimethoprim given | | SB | For MSU. |
| 22.08.2013 | 19.02.1942 | F | | 1012 | 1034 | For B12, Folate & Ferritin | | EF | |

**Result of a query that lists all consultations from the 22nd to the end of August 2013 (ConsultationsSeenFrom22ndTillEndOfAug2013)**

| SurgeryDate | DateOfBirth | Sex | Diagnosis | TimeIn | TimeOut | Complaints | Treatments | Initials | Notes |
|---|---|---|---|---|---|---|---|---|---|
| 22.08.2013 | 27.03.1935 | M | | 1034 | 1041 | Script for Flucloxacillin given | | RH | |
| 22.08.2013 | 19.08.1917 | F | | 1056 | 1120 | Script for Aymes shake sample pack given | | VL | |
| 22.08.2013 | 27.09.1931 | M | | 1648 | 1655 | Cryotherapy blasts x 2 applied to wart on his (L) wrist area | | JJ | |
| 22.08.2013 | 29.12.1975 | F | | 1701 | 1707 | To see the nurse in 3 to 6 months for repeat FBC | | JC | |
| 22.08.2013 | 15.04.1953 | M | | 1707 | 1714 | Referred to ENT Surgeon regarding the feeling of something getting stuck on the (L) side of the throat | | KGS | |
| 22.08.2013 | 02.12.1992 | M | | 1720 | 1726 | Reassured about the benign-looking dimple on his (R) lower leg | | TJN | |
| 22.08.2013 | 19.08.1939 | F | | 1726 | 1734 | Patient informed that the chest X-Rays result has not changed from the previous one | | JEN | |
| 22.08.2013 | 23.11.1960 | M | | 1746 | 1754 | For X-Rays of the Thoracic Spine | | DNT | |

Result of a query that lists all consultations from the 22nd to the end of August 2013 (ConsultationsSeenFrom22ndTillEndOfAug2013)

| SurgeryDate | DateOfBirth | Sex | Diagnosis | TimeIn | TimeOut | Complaints | Treatments | Initials | Notes |
|---|---|---|---|---|---|---|---|---|---|
| 22.08.2013 | 19.05.1992 | F | | 1759 | 1804 | Script for Clobetasol 0.05% ointment given | | FLM | |
| 22.08.2013 | 31.01.1969 | M | | 1804 | 1814 | Referred to Neurologist regarding his ongoing migraine as he missed his last hospital appointment | | DRA | |
| 23.08.2013 | 17.03.1961 | M | | 949 | 955 | Script for Sertraline & Sumatriptan given | | LDM | |
| 23.08.2013 | 26.09.1937 | M | | 955 | 1010 | Script for Calamine lotion | | DJD | |
| 23.08.2013 | 16.08.1968 | M | | 1010 | 1016 | For X-Rays of the (R) hand | | WB | |
| 23.08.2013 | 28.03.1945 | M | | 1016 | 1025 | Script for Chloramphenicol eye drops & Tears Naturale eye drops given | | APD | |
| 23.08.2013 | 09.05.1933 | M | | 1025 | 1034 | To see the nurse in 3 months for repeat serum Ferritin | | JS | |
| 23.08.2013 | 25.01.1955 | F | | 1053 | 1110 | Script for Levothyroxine given | | CYR | |
| 27.08.2013 | 14.03.1934 | M | | 941 | 1005 | Advised to go to A/E when next he gets his funny turns | | KRF | |
| 27.08.2013 | 04.10.1968 | F | | 1005 | 1013 | Script for Codeine tablets given | | AW | |

912

Result of a query that lists all consultations from the 22nd to the end of August 2013 (ConsultationsSeenFrom22ndTillEndOfAug2013)

| SurgeryDate | DateOfBirth | Sex | Diagnosis | TimeIn | TimeOut | Complaints | Treatments | Initials | Notes |
|---|---|---|---|---|---|---|---|---|---|
| 27.08.2013 | 10.03.1936 | M | | 1013 | 1022 | Medications Review Done | | TCC | |
| 27.08.2013 | 26.04.1943 | M | | 1022 | 1038 | Medications Review Done | | WWH | |
| 27.08.2013 | 07.11.1957 | F | | 1038 | 1043 | She says the pain on the (L) side of her face has got much better | | DJE | |
| 27.08.2013 | 16.04.1995 | F | | 1043 | 1050 | Advised to inform the hospital about the status of his grandfather's MEN1 status | | SMG | |
| 27.08.2013 | 28.03.1945 | M | | 1050 | 1054 | Script for Azelaic acid 15% gel given | | APD | |
| 27.08.2013 | 18.02.1968 | F | | 1054 | 1108 | Referred to Dietician regarding her obesity | | PAC | For Fasting Glucose, TFTs, B12, Folate & Ferritin. |
| 27.08.2013 | 20.05.1949 | M | | 1106 | 1116 | Medications Review Done | | RJP | |
| 27.08.2013 | 03.04.1987 | F | | 1127 | 1143 | Routine 6 weeks post-natal check done | | LJP | |
| 27.08.2013 | 27.11.1930 | F | | 1400 | 1415 | Script for Stemetil given | | VRG | Home visit. Penicillin allergy. |
| 27.08.2013 | 20.12.1928 | M | | 1645 | 1657 | Script for Flucloxacillin given | | RM | For BNP & U/Es. |
| 27.08.2013 | 15.05.1948 | M | | 1657 | 1704 | Script for Salbutamol inhaler & Omeprazole given | | NRL | |

Result of a query that lists all consultations from the 22nd to the end of August 2013 (ConsultationsSeenFrom22ndTillEndOfAug2013)

| SurgeryDate | DateOfBirth | Sex | Diagnosis | TimeIn | TimeOut | Complaints | Treatments | Initials | Notes |
|---|---|---|---|---|---|---|---|---|---|
| 27.08.2013 | 27.10.1960 | F | S/Leave | 1704 | 1716 | Med. 3 04/10 given for Back Pain for 3 months from 22.08.13 | | DLK | Script for Oramorph, Cetraben cream, Co-dydramol & Laxido Orange given. |
| 27.08.2013 | 17.04.1942 | F | | 1716 | 1729 | Referred to DVT Clinic regarding swelling of the (L) leg | | MRH | |
| 27.08.2013 | 29.11.1946 | F | | 1729 | 1737 | Referred to Vascular Surgeon regarding the painful varicose veins on the (L) lower leg | | PW | |
| 27.08.2013 | 22.03.1986 | F | | 1746 | 1850 | Fostering Medical Examination Done | | KAS | |
| 27.08.2013 | 21.07.1996 | F | | 1850 | 1900 | Script for Amoxycillin & Otosporin ear drops given | | LAPB | |
| 28.08.2013 | 06.09.1974 | M | | 948 | 1001 | Script for Lisinopril given | | DGH | |
| 28.08.2013 | 04.05.1963 | M | | 1001 | 1014 | For USScan of the testicles & for PSA | | DPF | |
| 28.08.2013 | 28.09.1959 | F | | 1014 | 1023 | Script for Amoxycillin & Amitriptyline given | | CAW | Referred to ENT Surgeon regarding her recurrent (L) ear ache. |
| 28.08.2013 | 04.03.1982 | F | | 1023 | 1032 | Script for Amoxycillin given | | GV | |

914

Result of a query that lists all consultations from the 22nd to the end of August 2013 (ConsultationsSeenFrom22ndTillEndOfAug2013)

| SurgeryDate | DateOfBirth | Sex | Diagnosis | TimeIn | TimeOut | Complaints | Treatments | Initials | Notes |
|---|---|---|---|---|---|---|---|---|---|
| 28.08.2013 | 25.04.1935 | M |  | 1032 | 1043 | To go on permanent Vit. B12 in view of his pernicious anaemia diagnosis |  | KGB |  |
| 28.08.2013 | 18.03.1979 | F |  | 1049 | 1059 | For Urine Pregnancy test & TOP |  | MJH |  |
| 28.08.2013 | 20.11.1944 | M |  | 1059 | 1106 | Referred to Audiology clinic regarding worsening deafness in his (L) ear |  | JE |  |
| 28.08.2013 | 17.04.1945 | F |  | 1106 | 1115 | DEXA scan results explained to the patient |  | MC | Penicillin allergy. |
| 28.08.2013 | 11.07.1962 | M |  | 1645 | 1655 | Referred to Cardiologist regarding his recurrent chest pains |  | JEG | Script for Nitrolingual spray given. |
| 28.08.2013 | 03.05.1946 | F |  | 1655 | 1700 | For X-Rays of the hips & pelvis |  | JP |  |
| 28.08.2013 | 09.03.1947 | F |  | 1700 | 1708 | BP 128/78 |  | PAN |  |
| 28.08.2013 | 10.07.1962 | F |  | 1708 | 1715 | Her FSH is 88.3 which makes her post-menopausal |  | PL |  |
| 28.08.2013 | 15.12.1935 | F |  | 1715 | 1727 | Script for Trimethoprim given |  | DL | For MSU. |
| 28.08.2013 | 17.03.1985 | F |  | 1734 | 1740 | Script for Buscopan, Co-codamol & Naproxen given |  | KAB |  |

Result of a query that lists all consultations from the 22nd to the end of August 2013 (ConsultationsSeenFrom22ndTillEndOfAug2013)

| SurgeryDate | DateOfBirth | Sex | Diagnosis | TimeIn | TimeOut | Complaints | Treatments | Initials | Notes |
|---|---|---|---|---|---|---|---|---|---|
| 28.08.2013 | 11.11.1961 | M | | 1740 | 1752 | Script for Glycerol suppositories & Laxido Orange oral powder sachets given | | AMP | |
| 28.08.2013 | 05.04.1964 | F | | 1752 | 1800 | Script for Fluoxetine & Ramipril given | | JL | |
| 28.08.2013 | 25.04.1951 | F | | 1804 | 1820 | Script for Forxiga & Lisinopril given | | SM | Referred to Physiotherapist regarding pains in her knees & feet. |
| 29.08.2013 | 02.10.1943 | M | | 941 | 947 | Script for Flucloxacillin given | | SS | |
| 29.08.2013 | 08.10.1940 | F | | 947 | 951 | The red spot on her chest has improved with the antibiotics | | MRH | |
| 29.08.2013 | 04.07.1929 | M | | 951 | 1003 | Script for Erythromycin given | | RMC | Penicillin allergy. |
| 29.08.2013 | 23.01.1926 | F | | 1003 | 1014 | Script for Transvasin Heat Rub cream given | | FGN | |
| 29.08.2013 | 14.08.1935 | M | | 1014 | 1035 | Results of his recent blood test result was explained to him | | RAT | |
| 29.08.2013 | 17.04.1936 | M | | 1043 | 1101 | Script for Nicorandil, Seebri Breezhaler & Symbicort given | | RB | |
| 29.08.2013 | 24.02.1981 | F | | 1101 | 1105 | BP 111/78 | | KLM | |
| 29.08.2013 | 18.12.1925 | F | | 1105 | 1122 | Script for Codeine tablets, Laxido Orange & Phenobarbital was given | | AL | |
| 29.08.2013 | 19.08.1917 | F | | 1122 | 1139 | BP 133/67 | | VL | |

Result of a query that lists all consultations from the 22nd to the end of August 2013 (ConsultationsSeenFrom22ndTillEndOfAug2013)

| SurgeryDate | DateOfBirth | Sex | Diagnosis | TimeIn | TimeOut | Complaints | Treatments | Initials | Notes |
|---|---|---|---|---|---|---|---|---|---|
| 29.08.2013 | 07.02.1952 | M | | 1305 | 1315 | Advised to go to A/E for X-Rays regarding his injured (R) wrist | | GAH | Home visit. |
| 29.08.2013 | 05.08.1936 | F | | 1635 | 1648 | Script for Codeine tablets given | | SAMN | |
| 29.08.2013 | 13.05.1992 | F | | 1648 | 1655 | Script for Fucidin H cream given | | ZLB | |
| 29.08.2013 | 10.11.1969 | F | | 1655 | 1702 | Script for Codeine tablets given | | PS | |
| 29.08.2013 | 19.08.1939 | F | | 1702 | 1709 | Script for Citalopram given | | JEN | |
| 29.08.2013 | 04.04.1953 | M | | 1727 | 1739 | Script for Fucidin H cream & Erythromycin given | | GC | Penicillin allergy. |
| 29.08.2013 | 03.05.1990 | F | | 1739 | 1744 | Script for Co-Phenotrope given | | HLW | |
| 29.08.2013 | 02.01.1952 | F | | 1744 | 1750 | Script for Amoxycillin, Prednisolone & Salbutamol inhaler given | | PAD | For Chest X-Rays. |
| 29.08.2013 | 18.01.1958 | F | | 1756 | 1812 | BP 129/79 | | LRG | |
| 30.08.2013 | 06.01.1943 | F | | 945 | 1004 | Script for Lisinopril given | | PC | For U/Es, B12, Folate, Ferritin & FBC. |
| 30.08.2013 | 26.10.1944 | M | | 1004 | 1012 | BP 117/66 | | DJW | |
| 30.08.2013 | 01.07.1997 | F | URTI | 1012 | 1016 | (R) ear ache | Amoxycillin | MJB | |

Result of a query that lists all consultations from the 22nd to the end of August 2013 (ConsultationsSeenFrom22ndTillEndOfAug2013)

| SurgeryDate | DateOfBirth | Sex | Diagnosis | TimeIn | TimeOut | Complaints | Treatments | Initials | Notes |
|---|---|---|---|---|---|---|---|---|---|
| 30.08.2013 | 18.06.1959 | M | | 1016 | 1026 | Script for Amoxycillin, Prednisolone & Salbutamol inhaler given | | SRF | |
| 30.08.2013 | 09.10.2009 | F | | 1026 | 1032 | Referred to Paediatrician regarding her recurrent constipation | | LP | |
| 30.08.2013 | 18.05.1935 | M | | 1036 | 1046 | For PSA | | AFB | |
| 30.08.2013 | 13.12.1934 | F | | 1046 | 1056 | For X-Rays of the (R) Humerus (urgent) | | SDH | |
| 30.08.2013 | 06.05.1971 | M | | 1056 | 1106 | Script for Dermovate scalp application given | | RHG | |
| 30.08.2013 | 27.03.1931 | F | | 1106 | 1113 | Script for Ferrous Fumarate given | | MMA | |
| 30.08.2013 | 23.02.1991 | M | | 1113 | 1119 | Script for Flucloxacillin given | | MSK | |
| 30.08.2013 | 14.06.1945 | M | | 1119 | 1122 | Script for Trimethoprim given | | BL | |
| 30.08.2013 | 07.03.1958 | M | | 1122 | 1137 | Script for Co-Amoxiclav given | | JDP | Referred to Orthopaedic Surgeon regarding his persistent (R) shoulder pain. |
| 30.08.2013 | 14.04.1946 | F | | 1137 | 1147 | Script for Trimethoprim given | | VBB | |

Result of a query that lists all consultations from the 22nd to the end of August 2014 (ConsultationsSeenFrom22ndTillEndOfAug2014)

| SurgeryDate | DateOfBirth | Sex | Diagnosis | TimeIn | TimeOut | Complaints | Treatments | Initials | Notes |
|---|---|---|---|---|---|---|---|---|---|
| 22.08.2014 | 21.02.1952 | M | | 949 | 956 | He may come back later to have his sick leave extended | | JPB | |
| 22.08.2014 | 10.04.1958 | F | | 956 | 1005 | Script for Ibuprofen given | | DAB | |
| 22.08.2014 | 20.02.1990 | M | | 1021 | 1035 | Referred back to Orthopaedic Surgeon (Mr. Greer) regarding his painful (R) knee as he missed his follow-up appointment following MRI scan | | JLG | |
| 22.08.2014 | 18.11.1982 | F | URTI | 1035 | 1041 | (L) ear ache | Doxycycline | VAB | Penicillin allergy. |
| 22.08.2014 | 08.05.1942 | M | | 1041 | 1047 | His (L) hernia repair wound is healing well | | GJHC | |
| 22.08.2014 | 14.07.1929 | M | | 1047 | 1056 | Eprex 2000iu/0.5ml given in (L) Deltoid | | RMC | |
| 22.08.2014 | 31.01.1941 | F | | 1127 | 1140 | Script for Doxycycline, Loratadine & Terbinafine 1% cream given | | JAE | |
| 26.08.2014 | 20.05.1987 | F | | 943 | 959 | Awaiting appointment to see the counsellor | | DADS | |

919

Result of a query that lists all consultations from the 22nd to the end of August 2014 (ConsultationsSeenFrom22ndTillEndOfAug2014)

| SurgeryDate | DateOfBirth | Sex | Diagnosis | TimeIn | TimeOut | Complaints | Treatments | Initials | Notes |
|---|---|---|---|---|---|---|---|---|---|
| 26.08.2014 | 17.08.1912 | F | | 959 | 1024 | For Chest X-Rays in 2 months, form given to the patient | | IAA | Referred to Dermatologist (urgent) regarding pigmented lesion on the (R) sided of her cheek. |
| 26.08.2014 | 11.07.1962 | M | | 1024 | 1038 | Script for Candesartan given | | JEG | Referred to Neurologist regarding his frequent & recurrent blackouts. |
| 26.08.2014 | 14.03.1984 | F | | 1038 | 1044 | Advised to take no more than 2 litres in any 24 hour period | | MJW | |
| 26.08.2014 | 07.12.1998 | F | | 1044 | 1054 | Referred to Gynaecologist regarding her late menarche | | JNF | For USScan of the abdomen. |
| 26.08.2014 | 25.03.1944 | M | | 1054 | 1101 | Referred to Orthopaedic Surgeon regarding the severe pain in the (L) knee | | RFB | |
| 26.08.2014 | 16.04.1995 | F | | 1125 | 1200 | Referred to ENT Surgeon regarding the lumpy feeling on the (R) side of her throat | | SMG | |
| 26.08.2014 | 01.07.2014 | M | | 1200 | 1210 | Referred to Paediatrician regarding the dimple at the lower end of the sacral region | | KRMF | |

Result of a query that lists all consultations from the 22nd to the end of August 2014 (ConsultationsSeenFrom22ndTillEndOfAug2014)

| SurgeryDate | DateOfBirth | Sex | Diagnosis | TimeIn | TimeOut | Complaints | Treatments | Initials | Notes |
|---|---|---|---|---|---|---|---|---|---|
| 26.08.2014 | 04.10.1947 | F | S/Leave | 1710 | 1720 | Med. 3 04/10 given for (R) Sciatica for 2 weeks from 21.08.14 | | PVD | |
| 26.08.2014 | 24.08.2012 | M | | 1720 | 1726 | Referred to Paediatrician regarding the peeling rash on both soles of the feet & involving the toes | | FSDPH | |
| 26.08.2014 | 04.04.1938 | M | | 1726 | 1741 | Script for Piroxicam 0.5% gel given | | DB | |
| 26.08.2014 | 16.09.1997 | F | | 1741 | 1750 | To use alarm, to wake her up, in the first instance for her bed wetting problems | | GJJ | |
| 26.08.2014 | 18.11.1999 | M | | 1750 | 1756 | He is due to see the Paediatrician for his widespread rash on 15.10.14 | | KOF | |
| 26.08.2014 | 24.04.1951 | M | | 1758 | 1806 | Script for Co-Amoxiclav & Fexofenadine given | | CJL | |
| 26.08.2014 | 05.12.2007 | F | | 1806 | 1828 | Script for Co-Amoxiclav given | | ABH | Referred to Paediatrician (urgent) regarding her recurrent UTIs. For USScan of the kidneys (urgent). |
| 27.08.2014 | 16.05.1944 | M | | 945 | 954 | For FBC | | CEJY | |

Result of a query that lists all consultations from the 22nd to the end of August 2014 (ConsultationsSeenFrom22ndTillEndOfAug2014)

| SurgeryDate | DateOfBirth | Sex | Diagnosis | TimeIn | TimeOut | Complaints | Treatments | Initials | Notes |
|---|---|---|---|---|---|---|---|---|---|
| 27.08.2014 | 14.09.1947 | F | | 954 | 1014 | Script for Gliclazide given | | JRL | |
| 27.08.2014 | 13.03.1938 | F | | 1014 | 1026 | Script for Indapamide m/r given | | DGP | |
| 27.08.2014 | 15.12.1939 | M | | 1026 | 1032 | Script for Fucidin H cream given | | ERC | |
| 27.08.2014 | 28.02.1941 | F | | 1032 | 1047 | Referred to Haematologist (urgent) regarding her tiredness & hypogammaglobulinemia | | SJW | For FBC, U/Es, Bone profile, LFTs & urine Bence Jones Protein. |
| 27.08.2014 | 22.03.1933 | F | | 1047 | 1055 | Script for Fenbid 5% gel given | | LLW | For X-Rays of the (R) knee. |
| 27.08.2014 | 04.11.1924 | F | | 1055 | 1118 | Script for Indapamide tablets given | | OJR | |
| 27.08.2014 | 04.07.1929 | M | | 1118 | 1128 | Eprex 2000iu/0.5ml given in (L) Deltoid | | RMC | |
| 27.08.2014 | 06.09.1924 | M | | 1330 | 1345 | To refer him to Incontinent services | | FE | Home visit. |
| 27.08.2014 | 21.02.1952 | M | S/Leave | 1642 | 1649 | Med. 3 04/10 given for Pain in both hands for 6 months from 26.08.14 | | JPB | |
| 27.08.2014 | 31.05.1967 | F | | 1649 | 1704 | Script for Oxybutynin & Ventolin Evohaler given | | GKP | For MSU & PSA. |
| 27.08.2014 | 16.07.1968 | F | S/Leave | 1704 | 1715 | Med. 3 04/10 given for Breathlessness for 1 month from 26.08.14 | | JLF | Script for Qvar inhaler & Ventolin Evohaler given. |

Result of a query that lists all consultations from the 22nd to the end of August 2014 (ConsultationsSeenFrom22ndTillEndOfAug2014)

| SurgeryDate | DateOfBirth | Sex | Diagnosis | TimeIn | TimeOut | Complaints | Treatments | Initials | Notes |
|---|---|---|---|---|---|---|---|---|---|
| 27.08.2014 | 16.08.1983 | F | | 1717 | 1727 | Script for Amoxycillin & Otomize ear spray given | | RJN | |
| 27.08.2014 | 01.12.1934 | F | | 1727 | 1739 | Script for Gaviscon & Paracetamol given | | LFM | |
| 27.08.2014 | 08.09.1957 | M | | 1739 | 1749 | He is at present being investigated for his visual problems at Harlow hospital | | TJG | |
| 27.08.2014 | 05.08.1984 | M | S/Leave | 1749 | 1755 | Med. 3 04/10 given for Chest Infection for 2 weeks from 16.08.14 | | RML | |
| 27.08.2014 | 11.09.1947 | M | | 1800 | 1809 | Script for 1% Hydrocortisone cream given | | TSN | Referred to Dermatologist (Community) regarding his lichen planus on his feet. |
| 28.08.2014 | 01.12.1942 | M | | 944 | 952 | Medications Review Done | | CLH | |
| 28.08.2014 | 22.09.1967 | M | RTI | 952 | 959 | Chesty cough | Doxycycline | SRB | For Chest X-Rays. |
| 28.08.2014 | 06.09.1963 | F | | 959 | 1010 | Script for Ferrous Fumarate given | | JYH | |
| 28.08.2014 | 10.10.1964 | F | | 1010 | 1020 | Script for Adcal-D3 & Alendronic acid given | | KF | |
| 28.08.2014 | 31.05.1930 | F | | 1020 | 1032 | Referred to Neurologist (BUPA) regarding her tremor to rule out early Parkinson's disease development | | SAW | |

Result of a query that lists all consultations from the 22nd to the end of August 2014 (ConsultationsSeenFrom22ndTillEndOfAug2014)

| SurgeryDate | DateOfBirth | Sex | Diagnosis | TimeIn | TimeOut | Complaints | Treatments | Initials | Notes |
|---|---|---|---|---|---|---|---|---|---|
| 28.08.2014 | 03.12.1924 | F | | 1032 | 1040 | For repeat urine microalbumin in one month, form given to the patient | | AH | |
| 28.08.2014 | 14.06.1945 | M | | 1042 | 1049 | Medications Review Done | | BL | |
| 28.08.2014 | 14.10.1968 | F | | 1049 | 1056 | Referred to Endocrinologist regarding feeling as if she is hypothyroid despite being on the therapeutic dose of Levothyroxine and normal TFTs | | AW | |
| 28.08.2014 | 02.01.1955 | M | S/Leave | 1049 | 1056 | Med. 3 04/10 given for Stress for 1 week from 28.08.14 | | TRE | |
| 28.08.2014 | 28.11.1925 | F | | 1303 | 1315 | Script for Flucloxacillin given | | JJF | Home visit. |
| 28.08.2014 | 21.11.1948 | M | S/Leave | 1645 | 1658 | Med. 3 04/10 given for Pain in the (R) knee for 3 days from 25.08.14 | | PCB | |
| 28.08.2014 | 23.09.1948 | M | | 1658 | 1708 | Script for Amoxycillin given | | KWK | Referred to Neurologist regarding the burning sensation he has on the (L) side of his body. |

Result of a query that lists all consultations from the 22nd to the end of August 2014 (ConsultationsSeenFrom22ndTillEndOfAug2014)

| SurgeryDate | DateOfBirth | Sex | Diagnosis | TimeIn | TimeOut | Complaints | Treatments | Initials | Notes |
|---|---|---|---|---|---|---|---|---|---|
| 28.08.2014 | 13.05.1992 | F | | 1708 | 1714 | Referred to Dermatologist (Community) regarding mole on her (L) breast | | AVB | |
| 28.08.2014 | 16.06.1965 | M | | 1714 | 1727 | Script for Lisinopril & Loperamide given | | MJH | Stool for C&S. |
| 28.08.2014 | 26.03.1974 | M | S/Leave | 1727 | 1740 | Med. 3 04/10 given for Wound on the (R) leg from 24.08.14 to 28.08.14 | | PMF | |
| 28.08.2014 | 11.12.2008 | M | | 1740 | 1745 | Script for Occlusal 26% solution given | | MBB | |
| 28.08.2014 | 23.06.1941 | M | | 1745 | 1755 | Script for Amoxycillin given | | RWS | For FBC, U/Es, Fasting Glucose, TFTs, LFTs, Cholesterol & MSU. |
| 28.08.2014 | 02.10.1943 | M | | 1755 | 1805 | Script for Codeine tablets & Canesten HC cream given | | SHS | |
| 29.08.2014 | 16.12.1970 | F | | 943 | 954 | Referred to Neurologist (Dr. Gall) regarding her persistent headaches | | KMB | |
| 29.08.2014 | 14.08.1935 | M | | 954 | 1011 | Script for Ferrous Fumarate & Doxycycline given | | RAT | |

925

Result of a query that lists all consultations from the 22nd to the end of August 2014 (ConsultationsSeenFrom22ndTillEndOfAug2014)

| SurgeryDate | DateOfBirth | Sex | Diagnosis | TimeIn | TimeOut | Complaints | Treatments | Initials | Notes |
|---|---|---|---|---|---|---|---|---|---|
| 29.08.2014 | 11.10.1942 | M | | 1011 | 1019 | For serum Ferritin, Folate & B12 | | RWA | |
| 29.08.2014 | 17.04.1945 | F | | 1019 | 1029 | For FBC & serum Ferritin | | MC | |
| 29.08.2014 | 28.02.1941 | F | | 1029 | 1049 | Referred to Medical Dr. on call SGH regarding her tiredness, listlessness, very low Hb & platelets | | SJW | |
| 29.08.2014 | 20.09.1934 | M | | 1049 | 1109 | Script for Amoxycillin & Paracetamol given | | EWM | Referred to Counsellor regarding his low mood & depression. |
| 29.08.2014 | 04.07.1929 | M | | 1107 | 1116 | Eprex 2000iu/0.5ml given in (L) Deltoid | | RMC | |

CPSIA information can be obtained
at www.ICGtesting.com
Printed in the USA
LVHW020657160622
721416LV00001B/1